# HUMAN NUTRITION

# HUMAN NUTRITION

Its Physiological, Medical and Social Aspects

## A Series of Eighty-Two Essays

*By*

**JEAN MAYER**
Ph.D., D.Sc., A.M. (hon.), M.D. (hon.)

*Professor of Nutrition*
*Harvard University*
*Boston, Massachusetts*

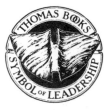

CHARLES C THOMAS • PUBLISHER
*Springfield • Illinois • U.S.A.*

*Published and Distributed Throughout the World by*

CHARLES C THOMAS • PUBLISHER

Bannerstone House

301-327 East Lawrence Avenue, Springfield, Illinois, U.S.A

©*1972, by* CHARLES C THOMAS • PUBLISHER

ISBN 0-398-02359-X

Library of Congress Catalog Card Number: 72-175081

*Printed in the United States of America*
*RN-1*

*This book is dedicated to the memory of*
André Mayer (1875-1956)
*Physiologist, Physician and Social Reformer*

# PREFACE

THE first essay in this volume is one on nutrition written in 1959. As I look at it twelve years later, it seems to me that there are four aspects that have become clearer. First, it is becoming evident that nutrition cannot continue to be considered a purely environmental science. The realization that inborn intestinal saccharidase deficiencies are more common than once thought, the finding that there are different types of hyperlipidemic reactions to diet, the demonstration that only certain types appear to be susceptible to obesity are reestablishing the balance between constitutional and external factors in our understanding of disease. Work relating nutritional problems to heredity and to body type is still scanty, but awareness of the importance of that area is growing.

Secondly, it is clearer to us, after the great civil rights movement of the sixties — translated in the health field into the hunger movement and culminating in the McGovern Committee hearings and the White House Conference and its aftereffects — that malnutrition due to poverty subsists even in a country as rich as the United States and must be dealt with not only by overall social action, but within the context of the health care delivery system as well. Massive federal programs — food stamps, school lunch, meals for the aged, etc., supported by appropriations approaching four billion dollars — are beginning to lift up the burden of malnutrition due to poverty from the shoulders of our underprivileged fellow citizens; however, our hospitals and other health institutions have yet to fully understand that insuring that poor patients be properly nourished is an integral part of the practice of good medicine from prenatal care to geriatrics.

The third aspect is related to the foods we eat: in the past decade it has become obvious that our food supply is undergoing an extremely rapid change, from primary foods to highly processed convenience foods. Our ability to manipulate the composition of these foods to improve the health of the consumers — by decreasing their sugar, their saturated fat or their salt content — has hardly been used. Instead, there took place, at least until the alarm was sounded at the White House Conference, a steady erosion of the nutritional content of our food supply which has been only in part arrested by fortification of flour-based foods with a few vitamins and iron. Furthermore, advertising, by constantly pressing for an increased consumption of the least valuable foods (snacks, candy, soft drinks) is threatening to destroy sound familial eating habits. The media, instead of being used for a massive nutrition education effort, are often perverters of sound nutrition. It must be noted that an increasing number of persons, professionals, consumers and even industrialists, are concerned over these developments; we can hope that the next decade will see a reversal of the present trends.

Fourth and finally, if we now consider the world at large, it is becoming more evident that as the introduction of "miracle" cereals and the improvement in methods of production, processing and distribution of food push back the specter of a worldwide famine, the interrelationship of nutrition and of other social developments becomes more evident: if food is not the only or the main "limiting" factor in the growth of the world population, what other factors threaten our survival as the earth becomes more and more crowded?

I do not flatter myself that this book answers all the questions I just raised. Most of the essays it contains are articles I wrote for my readers in *Postgraduate Medicine,* a monthly journal primarily addressed to general practitioners. They contain didactic material with a heavy clinical orientation. I trust, however, that they reflect many of the new preoccupations of the period. Some of the articles, particularly in Parts IX and X are derived from other sources. Because I was so intimately involved in the "hunger movement" from the mid-sixties on, I have included a number of documents such as my testimony (the opening professional statement) at the McGovern hearings as well as key statements before, at, and following the White House Conference. I have also included one general analysis of the role of nutrition in economic development (my example was West Africa) as well as statements reflecting my anxieties over the ethical aspects of several major nutritional issues. My 1966 letter on "Crop Destruction in Vietnam" to *Science,* which was at the time reproduced in many newspapers and magazines, was, I believe, the first article calling attention to this outrageous program. It took five years of additional articles by many others as well as by myself to eventually lead the President to officially forbid the continuation of chemical destruction of crops. My article on Biafra is an account of the only professional U.S. mission to have looked into this disaster while the war was still going on. Many of the observations are applicable to other famines (and other war situations). Biafra, too, incidentally, was an example of famine and malnutrition being used as an instrument of genocide and of terror by one side and as an instrument of propaganda by the other. My letter to *The New York Times* on the outlawing of famine as a weapon of war and on the creation of an international disaster relief organization seems to have triggered action by international legal societies, by the United Nations and by private foundations to try to reach both objectives. It is included, therefore, as a note of hope in what is otherwise a grim part of the book.

JEAN MAYER

# CONTENTS

## PART V

## Inborn Errors of Metabolism and Nutrition

## PART VI

## Nutrition and Disease

## PART VII

### The Safety of Foods

## PART VIII

### Dietetics

## PART IX

### The White House Conference, Hunger and Nutrition Policy

**PART X**

**Nutrition and the World**

# HUMAN NUTRITION

# NUTRITION

IT has become a truism in medical education that the physician must learn to treat the whole patient and not just the disease. This is never any truer than where diet is concerned. If it is to succeed, any nutritional program or dietary regimen must take into account the patient's financial status, his level of education, in some instances his religious practices, the familial background of food preparation, and, of course, the local availability of foodstuffs. The casual advice, "Better cut down on calories," or "Cut down on fats," or "Keep the proteins up" may be unintelligible to the patient or may entail such difficulties that he is unable to heed it without help. Even the technic of assessing the nutritional intake of a cooperative patient is fraught with difficulties involving economics, food analysis, cooking practices, etc. Yet, as the immediate threat of infectious diseases recedes as one of the main causes of death and as Americans are increasingly felled by degenerative diseases, cardiovascular, renal and hepatic syndromes, diabetes, all conditions often aggravated in frequency and in severity by obesity, the metabolic and nutritional factors loom larger in the thinking of practicing physicians.

## EARLY HISTORY

In nutrition, as in other fields, the present is the child of the past. It may be useful at the outset of this series to remind the reader of the general lines of the evolution which has made the science of nutrition what it is today. Very broadly this evolution can be divided into four periods: (1) the prescientific period, extending from the dim beginnings of the Stone Age to the second

Reprinted from *Postgraduate Medicine, 25* (No. 1), January, 1959.

half of the the eighteenth century, following Lavoisier's introduction of the calorimetric concepts and measurements; (2) the age of
study of caloric and nitrogen balance, the nineteenth century; (3)
the era of the discovery of trace elements, vitamins and essential
amino acids and the era of deficiency diseases, extending from
Hopkins to the 1940s; and (4) since the end of World War II, the
development of the study of the role of nutrition in degenerative
diseases and the recognition of the fact that what is in the diet can
be almost as important as what is missing from the diet.

An instinctive knowledge of food is necessary for survival. In a
long series of trials and errors — sometimes mortal errors — the
number of animals and plants which can provide food has been
extended. The idea that food does more than assuage hunger is
very old. Certain beliefs, such as the idea that consumption of the
heart or flesh of brave or strong animals would confer the same
virtues to the warriors of the tribe, appeared with the dawn of
human history. Food taboos also appeared during the Stone Age.
While some of these taboos may well have had something to do
with the wholesomeness of certain foods (e.g. the Biblical
prohibition of pork may have been based on the recognition of
frequent infestation of swine with *Trichinella)* most of these edicts
seem to have had no basis in fact. Examples of such practices were
the Egyptian prohibition of beef or chicken for kings and the
Biblical edict against hare.

Closely allied with the problem of taboos and superstitious
beliefs was the search for foodstuffs which also would be
remedies. Many herbs and parts of plants or animals were
prescribed because of their shape, their color or some other
property unrelated to any demonstrable pharmacologic effect. But
the recommendations of the "Ebers Papyrus" (1600 B.C.), of
Hippocrates (fifth century B.C.), of medieval writers who advocated liver for eye diseases and night blindness, and of Cartier's
Indians, who used evergreen needle infusions for scurvy are early
examples of prescriptions for deficiency diseases. Incidentally,
Hippocrates, the founder of scientific medicine, paid considerable
attention to nutrition in his writings. Many of his opinions are
difficult to justify, for example, his belief that beef is more
difficult to digest than pork, or that fish should be roasted rather

than boiled for feverish patients. But this abhorrence both of extreme abstemiousness and diet restriction and of excessive intake without corresponding physical labor is still good nutritional advice.

## LAVOISIER'S INVESTIGATIONS

Probably the greatest turning point in the history of biology and of medicine was the investigation of combustion conducted by Lavoisier (1743 to 1794). In addition to introducing measurements in biologic and chemical studies, Lavoisier in these experiments laid the basis for our understanding of caloric expenditures and requirements. The summary of the experiments conducted on his collaborator Seguin in 1785 illustrates well the modern outlook of this great innovator: of every 100 parts oxygen Seguin absorbed in respiration, only 81 parts reappeared as carbonic acid gas, the remaining 19 parts being combined with hydrogen to form water. He absorbed the lowest amount of oxygen when in a state of rest at a comfortable temperature after an overnight fast (now called basal metabolism). When fasting, Seguin absorbed a greater amount of oxygen at a temperature of 12° C than at 26° C (effect of cold on stimulating oxidations). When he took food but remained at rest, he absorbed more oxygen than when he had had no food (specific dynamic action). The greatest increase in oxygen absorption (up to 200% or 300%) came from doing mechanical work. Nevertheless, even 170 years after Lavoisier's experiments, the increase in caloric expenditure due to exercise is still too often belittled when reducing regimens are prescribed.

## NINETEENTH-CENTURY DEVELOPMENTS

The results of Lavoisier's work were extended by the work of the nineteenth-century physiologists and chemists. Vauquelin, Magendie, Prout, Mulder and, especially, Von Liebig (1803 to 1873) developed concepts and methods of analyses permitting the establishment of food composition tables. These are still the essential tool of the nutritionist, since any reassessment of the value of a diet and any dietary recommendations eventually must be translated in terms of foods in order to be of practical use.

Boussingault (1802 to 1887) studied absorption and digestion of foodstuffs. The proportion of carbohydrate, protein and fat and their contribution to the caloric content of foodstuffs became the basis of nutrition, with only scant attention being given to the minerals and almost none to the other nutritional factors.

Atwater, who returned to this country in 1892 following a period of European study, tried to put all of practical nutrition on the basis of cost of calories and protein. In effect, he advocated deriving the diet from cereals, peas and beans, and omitting fruits and garden vegetables. Both Von Voit and Atwater recommended large amounts of protein for adults (approximately 150 gm per day), in spite of Chittenden's experiments showing that men could live and work with less than one-third this amount of protein intake.

## ESSENTIAL NUTRIENTS

Another great turning point came at the beginning of this century when the concepts of essential nutrients came into existence. This was tantamount to recognizing that while the organism is a good chemist, it is not perfect; while it can synthesize thousands of complicated molecules, there are a number of structures – vitamins and essential amino and fatty acids – which it cannot synthesize. Hopkins showed that tryptophan was such an indispensable nutrient. Osborn and Mendel showed that the addition of tryptophan and lysine considerably improved the biologic value of corn proteins; the chief corn protein zein is particularly low in these amino acids. Systematically using semisynthetic experimental diets, McCollum and Davis showed that the minimum adequate diet for the rat must provide, in addition to the long-known nutrients, two unidentified factors which they called "fat-soluble A" and "water-soluble B."

It is remarkable that while clinicians – Linde, Trousseau and Eijkman – first implicated nutrition in diseases such as scurvy, rickets and beriberi, it is to chemists – Hopkins, Mendel,

McCollum and others — that we owe the concept of deficiency diseases as clinical entities. It seems almost incredible that barely a century ago Charles Caldwell, one of the most prominent clinicians of his time, was writing a 95-page pamphlet to denounce Von Liebig and proclaim that chemistry had nothing to contribute to medical science!

## LATER ADVANCES

It is unnecessary to point out the extreme speed at which our understanding of the deficiency diseases, the characterization and synthesis of vitamins, and the translation of experimental nutrition into clinical advancement have progressed between World War I and World War II. The pasteurian revolution is the only comparable explosion of knowledge in the history of medicine.

Rickets, once the most prevalent disease condition in Western cities, was almost wiped out in 10 years by the widespread use of fish-liver oils and by the fortification of milk with vitamin D. Goiter was eliminated from entire populations by the addition of iodine to salt. Flour enrichment and diet improvement have so effectively dealt with pellagra that it has been impossible for several years to locate a pellagrous patient in the whole state of Georgia to demonstrate the once-common signs of the disease to the students of the Medical College of Georgia.

At the same time that our experimental and clinical knowledge improved, our sense of social responsibility increased. It was believed that educated nations could not tolerate the fact that diseases which could be easily prevented should continue to kill and disable millions of human beings. In his famous book, *Diet, Health and Income,* John Boyd Orr showed that in Scotland poor growth and morbidity were much more prevalent among the poor classes than among the wealthy. Hazel Stiebeling in this country and André Mayer in France conducted nutritional surveys which demonstrated that many children and adults, particularly in the poorer classes, were undernourished or malnourished.

In the 1930's the League of Nations called together a committee of physiologists which promulgated the first set of recommended dietary allowances as well as a practical handbook on the assessment of the nutritional status of populations. This impetus was further accelerated by the preoccupation with food problems during World War II. Scientific advisory bodies, such as the United States National Research Council Food and Nutrition Board, came into existence on several continents. More important, over 60 nations combined their efforts to improve nutrition all over the world. The Food and Agriculture Organization of the United Nations, the Nutrition Section of the World Health Organization and the United Nations International Children's Emergency Fund were some of the offspring of this great movement. In many regions the emergency measures taken by some of the "crisis committees" created by FAO averted the widespread starvation which otherwise would have followed the end of the war. UNICEF has started and encouraged child feeding programs covering millions of children in Asia, Africa and Latin America. FAO and WHO have initiated, supported and publicized epidemiologic and clinical studies of kwashiorkor, the most widespread deficiency syndrome found in poor areas, which apparently is due to lack of good-quality proteins in the diet during early childhood following weaning.

## DIET AND DEGENERATIVE DISEASES

The renewed interest in undernutrition during World War II resulted directly in an interest in overnutrition. Observers were struck by the drastic decrease in the number of patients hospitalized with cardiovascular conditions during the famine accompanying the siege of Leningrad. When the siege was broken and the famine relieved, the "refeeding" period was accompanied by an upsurge in cardiovascular conditions. Statistics accumulated by life insurance companies emphasized the positive correlation of excess weight and mortality not only from cardiovascular diseases but also from liver conditions, diabetes, increased operative risk, etc. This in turn stimulated interest in the etiology and pathogenesis of obesity and in its associative and causative links to disease.

Considerable interest also was generated by Keys' suggestion that the presence of a high proportion of fat in the diet was associated with hypercholesteremia, atherosclerosis and coronary disease. A lively and constructive experimental controversy still rages as to the relative influence on cholesterol levels of the proportion of animal and vegetable fats, degree of saturation of the fat, concentration of polyunsaturated (essential) fatty acids, presence of plant sterols, etc.

## LONG-TERM STUDIES

Another recent development has been the recognition that the time factor should be accorded more attention in nutrition. For example, Best showed in experimental animals that choline deficiency during growth may result in renal hypertension in old age; many investigators have produced congenital malformations by feeding to pregnant animals deficient diets at certain crucial periods during pregnancy. The links between diet and degenerative diseases also point to the need for longer-term studies.

This introduction of longer duration in nutritional problems reemphasized the fact, known by experienced physicians since Hippocrates, that to understand how a given disease affects a given patient one must consider not only the disease agent but also the patient's individual constitution. Recent trends emphasize the importance of studying the interaction of constitutional and nutritional factors. For example, it is becoming clear that there are strong genetic determinants in the ability of an organism to switch from high carbohydrate to a high fat diet without accumulating excessive adiposity. It is also apparent that there are constitutional differences in the ability to regulate food intake at low exercise levels; in other words, the appetite of certain individuals is reduced proportionately when their activity is reduced to low levels; others are constitutionally prone to overeat if their activity is too low.

## RECOGNITION OF OTHER NUTRITIONAL PROBLEMS

There are many other nutritional problems which are receiving renewed attention, such as the relationship of diet to aging, to physical and intellectual performance, and to reproduction and the special nutritional problems of adolescence, arising in part from the recognition of the widespread character of iron deficiency anemia in this age group. Parenteral nutrition, especially when prolonged, urgently raises the whole problem of nutritional requirements. Advances in general nutrition have led to a critical reexamination of many of the classic special diets. Is the high-fat ulcer diet dangerous from the viewpoint of atherosclerosis? Is the rice diet deficient in protein? What of electrolyte balance in the low-salt diet? The problem of food additives, of contamination with insecticides, is one which should raise more serious toxicologic consideration than it has in the past.

Study of the mode of action of antimetabolites (a general class of substances which comprise many of the antibiotics) has focused attention on the problem of "differential" nutrition, balancing the requirements of the host (patient) against those of the parasites. There are indications that the understanding of the mode of action of viruses and of malignant cells may involve similar problems.

The development of cultural anthropology also has placed renewed emphasis on what may be called the non-nutritional aspects of foods. Certain food practices and certain dishes may have a symbolic significance which rejoins through conscious and subconscious associations the taboos of an earlier age as well as buried childhood memories. Realization of these overtones may be of considerable importance to the psychiatrist or to the general practitioner trying to reeducate his patient to better nutrition.

The relationship of alcoholism to nutritional factors is also of great importance in our society. The addiction of many patients to fad diets, "nature foods," etc. causes an unnecessary drain on their budgets, often results in an unbalanced diet, and may be a symptom of more serious psychologic difficulties which can be understood only in terms of their general emotional background.

## SUMMARY

It can be seen that, far from coming to a dead end with the solving of the classic deficiencies, the scope of the science of nutrition has expanded considerably in the past few years. The nutritional aspect should be considered in the treatment of any patient, not just the pediatric, obstetric or postoperative patient. In many ways nutrition is the single most important aspect of the environment of a patient.

# PART I
## Calories and Needs for Energy

*Chapter 1*

# CALORIES

$A$T a time when so much of the physician's and dietitian's attention is devoted to weight reduction, it probably would be helpful to recall that primary nutritional requirement is the need for calories. Caloric undernutrition, if sufficiently prolonged, is such an overriding factor that no diet can be considered adequate unless the energy balance is considered – a fact which should be drilled into the consciousness of many patients, particularly teen-age girls desiring to be excessively slim and nursing mothers determined to recover their figure as soon as possible.

I can think of few words as commonly used with as little understanding of meaning as the word "Calorie."* Readers will remember that the Calorie, or kilocalorie, is the amount of heat energy which is required to raise the temperature of 1 kg of water 1° C, from 14.5° to 15.5° C, and that the caloric equivalent of mechanical energy may be calculated by multiplying the units of mechanical energy (joules) by the factor 4.18. It is probably important to pause at this point, however, and reflect on the fact that many patients have never thought of the first law of thermodynamics or about the equivalence of chemical potential energy in foods, mechanical energy in physical exercise, and chemical energy used in synthesis of tissues, milk or body fat. Thus, it is essential that this concept be made clear to them before any further dietary instruction can be given profitably. The idea that five slices of white bread, an hour of walking at moderated

---

*Properly speaking, Calorie, the unit used in nutrition, should always be spelled with a capital "C" when a measure of intake or output is given. The word "calorie" with a small "c" refers to the gram-calorie, a thousandth of the Calorie. The word "calorie" can be used when speaking of calories in general. In fact, the distinction is often not made, and calorie with a small "c" is often used improperly in lieu of Calorie.
Reprinted from *Postgraduate Medicine, 25* (No. 2), February, 1959.

speed, and an ounce of body fat are roughly equivalent from an energy standpoint is not as readily understood by patients as busy practitioners would like to believe.

## FOOD COMPOSITION

The main sources of calories for man are carbohydrate, fat and protein. Again, from the viewpoint of energy, the three foodstuffs are interchangeable in accordance with their caloric equivalent. This was first shown by Rubner and further elaborated in this country by Atwater and his collaborators at the beginning of this century. These workers determined not only the composition of all common American foodstuffs but also their digestibility; thus, they could determine with great precision their energy content. They found that the proteins, fats and carbohydrates contained in the various foods were not strictly equivalent gram for gram from the viewpoint of energy; for example, a gram of starch contains a little more energy than a gram of glucose, and a gram of steak protein has a little more energy than a gram of protein from bread. However, consider such differences as small, so that when we consider the usual mixed diets, such as those consumed in this country, an excellent approximation of the total energy content can be obtained by using the caloric equivalents four, nine and four for carbohydrate, fat and protein, respectively. Further, these "net caloric factors" consider digestibility and can be applied as such to the composition of the whole diet.

Food composition tables are still prepared along the same principles. In the United States, the tables usually seen by practicing physicians are reproductions, summaries and adaptations of the food composition tables prepared by the United States Department of Agriculture. The famous blue* booklet (1) issued by this department gives the caloric value of 751 foods in terms of pounds "as purchased," "common household units" (slices, cupfuls, portions, etc.), and in 100 gm edible portions. For anyone interested in diet analysis, this handbook is a constant reference.

It must be realized that the availability of date concerning a given foodstuff is not sufficient to assess the caloric content of a

---

*The latest edition is red, does not include all types of units.

dish based on this foodstuff. Actual samples may differ widely in composition from the average value published in the food composition table. For example, the composition of a certain variety of pears consumed in August is unlikely to coincide with the median values for fifty varieties of pears consumed during a large part of the year all over the United States. The weight of the latter is calculated on the basis of survey data on varieties consumed in larger quantities over longer periods. The variability in caloric content is likely to be even much greater in cuts of meat than in fruits. Variations in fat content which appear small in terms of dry weight from animal to animal and from cut to cut will be translated into large differences in caloric equivalents. In addition, individual cooking practices vary: Some cooks will add butter when cooking steak; others will not. The drippings may or may not be eliminated from the dish as served.

Finally, individual attitudes toward table fats are difficult to ascertain. Some patients will cut the fat from ham; others will eat the whole slice. Some patients eschew gravy; others eat liberal quantities, using bread to avoid wasting any. Such differences in practice may entail 100 per cent differences in the actual caloric content of two consumed portions of what appeared to be, a priori, the same dish.

Children present a particularly difficult problem because of the greater variability of their attitudes and appetites. Unless these causes of variations are investigated and the results quantified, the appraisal of a diet is worthless from the viewpoint of caloric intake, even though a more cursory evaluation can still be valuable from the viewpoint of less variable nutrients.

## COMPONENTS OF ENERGY EXPENDITURE

The appraisal of caloric balance is rendered even more difficult by the fact that energy output depends on a number of factors other than intake, some of which may vary from day to day. Classically, the components of energy expenditure are (1) basal metabolism, (2) specific dynamic action, (3) extra heat production for maintenance of body temperature in a cold environment, (4) physical activity, and (5) growth, tissue repairs, pregnancy and lactation.

## Basal Metabolism

Basal metabolism represents the energy expenditure of the fasting resting subject as thermal neutrality — about 25° C. The familiar clinical determination is conducted on the person who is awake and lying at rest at a comfortable temperature at least 14 hours after ingesting food. Other things being equal, larger persons show a greater basal metabolic rate (B.M.R.) than smaller persons, the difference being roughly proportional to the difference in body surface.

A number of theoretical and empirical formulas have been proposed to express this "surface law." the empirical equation of DuBois and DuBois is most often used in the United States. The index obtained by dividing the basal metabolism by the body surface is the well-known basal metabolic rate, a parameter found to be characteristic for healthy individuals of the same age and sex. Basal Metabolic rate values for women are about 10 per cent smaller than those for men of the same size, a fact which has been ascribed to the finding that kilogram for kilogram the active body mass of women is smaller than that of men; i.e., women's bodies are normally higher in fat and lower in protein than are men's bodies. Basal metabolic rates decrease slowly with age. For example, the rate for a 35-year-old man is usually about 40 calories per square meter per hour. (The body surface of the 155-lb. man is slightly under 2 sq m) The same person at age 65 will usually show a B.M.R. of about 35 calories per square meter per hour. Again this decline is ascribed to the fact that even if there is no weight change in the intervening 30 years, a shift of body composition occurs, so that the body of the 65-year-old man contains less protein and more fat than it did at age 35.

The basal metabolic rate is often expressed in terms of percentage above or below the normal B.M.R. standards. A rate of +10 corresponds to a basal heat production of 10 per cent above the standard; a rate of −15 corresponds to a basal heat production of 15 per cent below the standard. In using these standards, it is well to remember the following facts:

1. The current standards are based mostly on averages of first tests and give values 5 to 10 per cent too high when compared

with values obtained with trained subjects. This has been confirmed in particular by E. F. DuBois.

2. The empirical formula used as a basis for the standards was based on data obtained for persons of various weights (including overweight persons) considered clinically to be free from disease, particularly thyroid diseases, and devised in such a way that the formula would give a good representation of their basal metabolism. To reverse the situation, as has occasionally been done, and say, "Most obese persons have a B.M.R. which fits the basal metabolism formula, and therefore, their metabolism is normal," is not a legitimate proposition for two reasons. The formula was established so that the persons examined who were free from thyroid disease would fit it, and the word "metabolism" is being used with two very different meanings. The basal metabolism of most diabetic persons is normal, yet their metabolism is not.

3. Small variations — particularly, downward variations — from the standards have no diagnostic significance per se and should not be used to justify thyroid therapy without additional supporting evidence (e.g. protein-bound iodine, thyroid iodine uptake, clinical signs and symptoms). This is especially important in considering children and adolescents, for whom B.M.R. standards and interpretations are particularly uncertain, and obese individuals, in whom not only weight and surface (taken into account in the standards) but also body composition (proportion of active body mass) may be very abnormal.

In a recent survey conducted in the Adolescent Clinic of the Children's Hospital in Boston, it was found that many obese adolescents who had been "put on thyroid" by their physician did not exhibit any hypothyroidism when subjected to thorough clinical and metabolic appraisal. Thyroid or thyroxin therapy without convincing prior diagnosis of hypothyroidism is a highly questionable practice.

It has often been stated that, in addition to its influence on the component of energy expenditure concerned with maintaining body temperature in the cold, basal metabolism is depressed by prolonged exposure to a warm climate and elevated by exposure to a cold climate. The evidence is poor and contradictory. It appears that if the B.M.R. is measured, as it should be, in a thermoneutral environment, climate has no significant effect on basal metabolism. Claims of racial differences in the B.M.R. have never been substantiated.

## Specific Dynamic Action

The simple experimental concept of specific dynamic action (S.D.A.) is usually taught in such a way as to give the medical student a confused impression which opens his mind, when he becomes a practitioner, either to beliefs of exaggerated variability of this parameter (particularly in relation to high protein diets) or, possibly by reaction, to the curious conviction that the existence of the S.D.A. has been "disproved." Actually, all that is involved is that the recent ingestion of food by a resting individual in a comfortable environment brings about an increase in heat production and heat loss, which is called the specific dynamic action of the foodstuffs ingested.

It is true that when single nutrients are ingested under laboratory conditions there are differences between the S.D.A. of proteins (ingesting 100 calories of protein raises the heat production by 30 calories, leaving 70 net calories available – a 30% S.D.A.), that of carbohydrates (8% to 10%), and that of fat (4% to 6%). However, the S.D.A. of mixed meals – the only ones of practical dietary significance – varies between relatively narrow limits (about 10% to 15%). In other words, the S.D.A. of a meal is not the sum of the specific dynamic action of the carbohydrates, fats and proteins contained in the meal. High protein meals may be preferable to low protein meals in certain circumstances, particularly in reducing diets. But, it is not because the S.D.A. of the two types of diet represents an appreciable caloric fraction.

## Heat Production and Heat Loss

One of the most fundamental facts about man is that he is homothermal, i.e. an organism which regulates its body temperature within a very narrow range. Deviations from the normal have a diagnostic significance; if they are excessive in either direction, they may be fatal. The nature and function of the thermostat through which a constant temperature of $37 \pm 0.5°$ C is achieved in man is still largely unknown. My investigations in collaboration with T. R. A. Davis showed that two types of control of heat production seemed to be involved: a nonmuscular (chemical) thermogenesis, apparently regulated by the variations of internal temperature, and a muscular (physical) thermogenesis, expressly from shivering and apparently regulated by differences between internal and skin temperatures.

The mechanism of heat loss, the other factor in the balance, is better known. Heat loss from a resting man occurs through radiation and convection, through the latent heat of evaporation of water through skin and lungs (the so-called insensible perspiration already demonstrated by Sanctorius at the end of the sixteenth century), and through the warming of inspired air and of ingested food and water. This heat loss is a function of many factors other than the environmental temperature. Clothing, wind, humidity, time spent indoors, etc. combine to define the individual "microenvironment" and the "effective temperature" at which a given subject lives.

In trying to evaluate the quantitative effect of temperature on human energy needs, the first and second committees on Calorie requirements called by the Food and Agriculture Organization of the United Nations and the World Health Organization had available the results of a study of United States and Canadian soldiers stationed in various parts of the world in which geographical situations ranged from arctic to dry and tropical environments. The study showed a linear relationship between decreasing environmental temperature and increasing caloric intake. This principle of linearity was retained by the first Calorie committee for calculations on civilian populations. Deviations from this relationship were observed in practice. The second Calorie committee estimated that for the general population the caloric requirement increases by 3 per cent for each 10° C below an average mean annual temperature of 10° C (typified by Minneapolis), and it decreases by 5 per cent for each 10° C above this average. The difference results from the fact that man protects himself better against cold than against heat. The recommendations of these committees were essentially adopted by the Food and Nutrition Board of the United States Research Council.

When trying to estimate the caloric requirements of an individual patient, the physician can use such figures only as a very general guide and should estimate the amount of actual exposure to outside temperatures. Thus even in a cold environment, for example, Chicago in the winter, the amount of actual exposure to cold for an individual commuting in a heated car from home to office may be negligible.

## Physical Activity

Physical activity is the most variable component of the total energy expenditure. It can be subdivided into two types: that related to body size (walking, moving the arms and hands, etc.) and that unrelated to body size (lifting and pushing objects). The first component is roughly proportional to body weight; the second is influenced only very little by body weight.

An enormous amount of experimental work, started in the nineteenth century and pursued throughout this century, has made available the energy cost of all the usual occupations, games, household chores, etc. Knowing the schedule of a given individual, it is true that skill and training will modify the expenditure required by a given task or exercise; it is also true that the "microschedule," the number and duration of pauses during a given task or exercise, also should be considered in such estimates. Still the available data make it possible for an experienced physician or nutritionist to arrive at a moderately good idea of how many calories a given individual expends every day, an operation which is essential in prescribing a reducing diet in which after all, the magnitude of the caloric deficit is only estimated. As is well known, the considerable differences in cost of activities, ranging from 10 calories (writing) to 700 calories (sawing) or more per hour, lead to differences in allowances which range from 2400 calories per day for a sedentary man to a 4500 calories for a very active man, with a rare maximum of 6000 or more for the most strenuous athletic or other extremely ardous occupations. Tables giving the expenditure corresponding to various occupations have been published by Passmore and Durnin (2).

It is essential that the physician or dietitian who is trying to determine the energy expenditure of a patient pay particular attention to time spent on each major occupation as well as to cost. If the time spent at rest in bed, sitting, standing, walking, occupations requiring physical effort, and sports is accurately recorded, other incidental energy expenditures are secondary. The mere designation "farmer" or "miner" gives very little information on the energy expenditure of the patient. A farmer may have a wide range of physical activities, depending on his job on the farm, the type of farming, and the extent of mechanization. Similarly, a miner is anyone who works in a mine. He may use a pick and shovel, carry and handle a pneumatic drill, or sit at a desk keeping track of coal cars coming out of a gallery.

Christensen has classified physical work in five categories: very light work (office work), less than 2.5 calories per minute; light work (leisurely walking, painting), 2.5 to 4.9 calories per minute; moderate work (brisk walking, light plumbing work, laying bricks), 5.0 to 7.4 calories per minute; heavy work (blacksmithing, bicycling, skating), 7.5 to 9.9 calories per minute; and very heavy work (swimming, climbing, shoveling), more than 10 calories per minute. These classifications can be used to establish an approximate picture of a man's daily expenditure (Table 1-1).

### Growth

Growth in its broadest sense (body growth, repairs, pregnancy, lactation) is accompanied by an increase in energy requirements. The caloric requirements of children are given in Table 1-2. It must be noted that these are extremely approximate in that the variability of activity in children is such that the standard deviation is probably about one-fourth the expenditure. In other words, many children will require 25 per cent more calories than the average, and a substantial proportion of children will require more than 50 per cent more than the average, because of their activity.

Pregnancy has been calculated to correspond to an increased

*Human Nutrition*

## TABLE 1-1

### CALORIES USED IN DAILY ENERGY EXPENDITURES

Case 1—A 25-year-old, 154-lb. house painter living in a suburb of Minneapolis, which has a mean annual temperature of 10° C.

|  |  |
|---|---:|
| Working activity (10 hours) | |
|     8 hours standing and painting (3 calories per minute) | 1,450 |
|     2 hours gardening or sports (5 calories per minute) | 600 |
| Nonoccupational activity (6 hours) | |
|     1 hour washing, dressing, etc. (2.5 calories per minute) | 150 |
|     4 hours driving, sitting, etc. (1.7 calories per minute) | 400 |
|     1 hour domestic work (3.5 calories per minute) | 200 |
| Rest in bed at B.M.R. (8 hours) | 500 |
| Total | 3300 |

Case 2—A 50-year-old, 170-lb. office worker living in Minneapolis.

|  |  |
|---|---:|
| Working activity (8 hours) | |
|     Office work, sitting (1.6 calories per minute) | 760 |
| Nonoccupational activity (8 hours) | |
|     1 hour washing, dressing, etc. (3 calories per minute) | 180 |
|     6 hours driving, sitting (1.8 calories per minute) | 640 |
|     1 hour domestic work, standing (2.5 calories per minute) | 150 |
| Rest in bed at B.M.R. (8 hours) | 500 |
| Total | 2200 |

Case 3—A 21-year-old, 121-lb. housewife, lactating, living in California, which has a mean annual temperature of 20° C.

|  |  |
|---|---:|
| Working activity (10 hours) | |
|     Domestic work, care of baby, etc. (2 calories per minute) | 1200 |
| Nonoccupational activity (6 hours) | |
|     1 hour washing, dressing, etc. (2 calories per minute) | 120 |
|     1 hour walking at 3 mph and shopping (3.2 calories per minute) | 200 |
|     2 hours playing golf or gardening (3.0 calories per minute) | 360 |
|     2 hours sitting (1.2 calories per minute) | 140 |
| Rest in bed at B.M.R. (8 hours) | 400 |
| Lactation allowance (600 to 700 cc milk) | 800 |
| Total | 3200 |

Case 4—A 35-year-old, 132-lb housewife living in Minneapolis.

|  |  |
|---|---:|
| Working activity (8 hours) | |
|     Domestic work (1.9 calories per minute) | 910 |
| Nonoccupational activity (8 hours) | |
|     1 hour washing, dressing, etc. (2 calories per minute) | 120 |
|     1 hour shopping and driving (1.8 calories per minute) | 100 |
|     6 hours sitting (1.3 calories per minute) | 470 |
| Rest in bed at B.M.R. (8 hours) | 400 |
| Total | 2000 |

requirement of about 80,000 calories for the over-all nine-month period. The extra calorie needs imposed by pregnancy can however, be covered in two ways: either by increased food intake or, in part at least, by reduced physical activity. The balance between the two is determined by the personal habits, conditions of employment, presence of older children to be cared for, etc. A few women will thus require the full amount of extra calories as food. This would correspond to an average of 300 calories per day or, more generally, no increase during the first trimester and an increase of 400 to 500 calories during the next two trimesters. However, most women will achieve the desired weight of approximately 20 lb for the entire pregnancy with a much smaller increase in food intake. In fact, in our society many women will achieve this increase solely on the basis of decreased physical

TABLE 1-2

DAILY DIETARY ALLOWANCES FOR CALORIES*

| Subjects | Age (years) | Weight (kg) | (lb) | Height (cm) | (in) | Calories |
|---|---|---|---|---|---|---|
| Men | 25 | 70 | 154 | 175 | 69 | 3200 |
| | 45 | 70 | 154 | 175 | 69 | 3000 |
| | 65 | 70 | 154 | 175 | 69 | 2550 |
| Women† | 25 | 58 | 128 | 163 | 64 | 2330 |
| | 45 | 58 | 128 | 163 | 64 | 2200 |
| | 65 | 58 | 128 | 163 | 64 | 1800 |
| Infants | 0 to 1/12 | | | | | |
| | 2/12 to 6/12 | 6 | 13 | 60 | 24 | kg x 120 |
| | 7/12 to 12/12 | 9 | 20 | 70 | 28 | kg x 100 |
| Children | 1 to 3 | 12 | 27 | 87 | 34 | 1300 |
| | 4 to 6 | 18 | 40 | 109 | 43 | 1700 |
| | 7 to 9 | 27 | 60 | 129 | 51 | 2100 |
| | 10 to 12 | 36 | 79 | 144 | 57 | 2500 |
| Boys | 13 to 15 | 49 | 108 | 163 | 64 | 3100 |
| | 16 to 19 | 63 | 139 | 175 | 69 | 3600 |
| Girls | 13 to 15 | 49 | 108 | 160 | 63 | 2600 |
| | 16 to 19 | 54 | 120 | 162 | 64 | 2400 |

*Allowances for normally active persons in a temperate climate, according to 1958 revised recommendations of the Food and Nutrition Board, National Research Council.
†A woman in the second half of pregnancy should have +300 calories daily. A woman with a daily lactation of 850 ml should have +1000 calories.

activity. This has important consequences for the practicing obstetrician: If an extracaloric intake corresponds to excessive weight gain during pregnancy for such women, the obvious way to improve their diet is not simply by prescribing additional milk, eggs, etc., but by eliminating some of the "empty" calories and replacing them with foodstuffs of higher nutritional values.

The problem of lactation is one which is particularly important and often neglected. Obstetricians have a strong tendency to stress the importance of a good diet during pregnancy and to neglect to check the diet during lactation. Yet the daily accretion of tissue during pregnancy represents a much smaller nutritional stress than the secretion of large quantities of milk (850 ml milk corresponds to about 1000 calories). The lactation period also usually represents a time of return to normal activity; in fact, very often it is a time of increased physical activity. In addition to previous commitments, the mother must take care of a small baby, so that caloric compensations by inactivity no longer occur. The pregnant woman could not ignore her physiologic state, especially during the last trimester of pregnancy, and "took care of herself" for fear of harming her unborn baby; however, the lactating mother has a tendency not to worry any more about her nutrition, even though she has to provide more protein, more calcium, etc. Too often she wants to get back "as fast as possible" to her prepregnancy figure. The physician must remember that the caloric requirement during lactation is dominated by the amount of milk output. For satisfactory lactation the increment over the normal intake should be not less than 800 calories per day.

## REFERENCES

1. Watt, B. K. and Merrill, A. L.: Composition of Foods — Raw, Processed, Prepared. Handbook No. 8. Washington, D. C., United States Department of Agriculture, 1950.
2. Passmore, R. and Durnin, J. V. G. A.: Human energy expenditure. Physiol. Rev., 37:801-840, 1955.

## Chapter 2

# EXERCISE AND WEIGHT CONTROL

In the past one or two decades, especially on this side of the Atlantic, the role of exercise in weight control has been minimized, if not ridiculed, by a number of lay health educators and sometimes (let us recognize it) by professional workers as well. The basis of this repeated denial has not been experimental work or clinical observations. Nor has it been the weight of the accumulated experience of the centuries, which has always contrasted the lean, hard, active soldier or hunter with the fat, sedentary merchant or clerk. Disparagement of the role of exercise in weight control has been based on two plausible misconceptions. These erroneous beliefs are usually expressed in the two following statements: (1) Exercise requires relatively little caloric expenditure and, therefore, increased physical activity hardly changes the caloric balance; and (2) an increase in physical activity is always automatically followed by an increase in appetite and food intake and may, therefore, actually impair the success of a weight reduction program. Let us examine these two propositions in detail.

## CALORIC EXPENDITURE IN EXERCISE

The first misconception, minimizing the caloric expenditure due to physical activity, should be avoided by anyone who has ever looked at a table of energy expenditure. Such tables illustrate the fact that the cost of expenditure can be high. Similarly, the National Research Council table of recommemded dietary allowances for men gives a range of 2400 to 4500 calories per day, depending on the level of activity. The figure of 4500 calories per day does not represent an upper limit: Laborers, soldiers in the

Reprinted from *Postgraduate Medicine, 25* (No. 3), March, 1959.

field, and athletes may require more than 6000 calories per day.

One frequently hears or reads such contrasting statements as the following: The caloric equivalent of 1 lb fat can be matched only by walking for 36 hours, splitting wood for 7 hours, or playing volleyball for 11 hours. These unattainable extremes of physical activity are used to demonstrate that it is impossible to lose weight by exercise. The implicit postulate is that the cost of exercise depends completely on its being done at one stretch. Actually, of course, the cost of splitting wood for 7 hours is equivalent to 1 lb fat, even though the seven hours may not be consecutive. Although splitting wood for seven consecutive hours would be difficult for anyone other than a Paul Bunyan, splitting wood for one-half hour every day is by no means an impossible task for a healthy man, and this would add up to seven hours in a fortnight. If it represented a regular practice, it would, by the very reasoning of the detractors of exercise, be the caloric equivalent of 26 lb body fat in a year. A half-hour of handball or squash a day would be equivalent to 16 lb a year.

It seems more useful, however, simply to recall the measured costs of different types of physical exercise. Table 2-1, modified and summarized from the work of Orr and Leitch (1) and from Passmore and Durnin (2), gives approximate requirements per hour of exercise over basal rate, established for young men of average size (145 to 170 lb).

It will be seen from Table 2-1 that for the average man examples of energy expenditure over the cost of sitting (which is about 15 calories an hour over lying at rest) are: walking, about 250 calories per hour; swimming, up to 900 calories; cycling, up to 700 calories. These hourly rates of energy expenditure above the sitting level do not include the admittedly short-duration peaks of activity reached in competition, which may be as high as 1500 calories per hour. (A Scandinavian journal recently published a study showing that athletes expend between 4000 and 5000 calories during three hours of cross-country skiing!) An expenditure of 500 to 600 calories per hour above the resting level represents a rate of physical activity which the average middle-aged adult not in training can endure for a period of 30 minutes without undue discomfort. A healthy young adult, even if untrained, can, of course, tolerate such rates of expenditure for much longer periods. A few years ago, in an experiment conducted in the nutrition department at Harvard, undergraduates were made to double their food intake, already in the vicinity of 3000 calories, without increasing their weight. These boys had to work hard to achieve this result, expecially since classes limited the time

TABLE 2-1

CALORIE REQUIREMENTS FOR VARIOUS ACTIVITIES*

| Activities | Calories per Hour | Activities | Calories per Hour |
|---|---|---|---|
| Domestic occupations | | Running | 800-1000 |
| Sewing | 10-30 | Cycling | |
| Writing | 20 | 5 mph | 250 |
| Sitting at rest | 15 | 10 mph | 450 |
| Standing relaxed | 20 | 14 mph | 700 |
| Dressing and undressing | 30-40 | Horseback riding | |
| Ironing (with 5-lb. iron) | 60 | Walking | 150 |
| Dishwashing | 60 | Trotting | 500 |
| Sweeping or dusting | 80-130 | Galloping | 600 |
| Polishing | 150-200 | Dancing | 200-400 |
| | | | |
| Industrial occupations | | Gymnastics | 200-500 |
| Tailoring | 50-100 | Golfing | 300 |
| Shoemaking | 80-100 | Playing tennis | 400-500 |
| Bookbinding | 75-100 | Playing soccer | 550 |
| Locksmithing | 150-200 | Canoeing | |
| House painting | 150-200 | 2.5 mph | 180 |
| Carpentering | 150-200 | 4.0 mph | 420 |
| Joinering | 200 | Sculling | |
| Cartwrighting | 200 | 50 strokes per minute | 420 |
| Smithing (light work) | 250-300 | 97 strokes per minute | 670 |
| Smithing (heavy work) | 300-400 | Rowing (peak effort) | 1200 |
| Riveting | 300 | Swimming | |
| Coal mining (avg. for shift) | 200-400 | Breast and back stroke | 300-650 |
| Stone masoning | 300-400 | Crawl | 700-900 |
| Sawing wood | 400-600 | Playing squash | 600-700 |
| | | | |
| Physical exercise | | | |
| Walking | | Climbing | 700-900 |
| 2 mph | 200 | Skiing | 600-700 |
| 3 mph | 270 | Skating (fast) | 300-700 |
| 4 mph | 350 | Wrestling | 900-1000 |

Figures obtained for 150-lb. subject. To be added to B.M.R. plus 10 per cent for specific dynamic action.
*Modified from Orr and Leitch[1] and from Passmore and Durnin.[2]

during which they could exercise, but they did manage to "lose" an extra 3000 calories per day.

The only heavy object moved in most types of exercise is the entire body or parts of it. Therefore, the energy cost of exercise is proportional to body weight. If excess body weight is so great that it impairs body movement, this relationship will no longer strictly apply, and the cost of exercise will actually increase faster than will body weight.

If the energy cost of exercise is approximately proportional to body weight, it follows that the overweight person will require more energy and hence burn more body reserves for the same amount of exercise than will a slimmer person. If a person is 20 per cent overweight, it will increase the cost of walking, tennis playing, golfing and such by 20 per cent. This represents a much greater proportional increase than that introduced by the increase in basal metabolism due to excess weight, which is proportional only to a fractional power of the body weight.

Thus, any increase of the caloric intake above balance level in a physically active person will cause only a modest increase in weight because of the energy cost of moving the extra poundage. On the other hand, a sedentary person will expend less energy in moving the extra weight; hence, weight gain will be more rapid and more pronounced. Therefore, a sedentary person will be exposed to the danger of overweight to a much greater extent than will a person who makes a practice of daily or, at least, frequent physical exercise.

Data from studies of experimental obesity support these concepts. In the hereditary obese-hyperglycemic syndrome of mice, a recessive form of obesity extensively studied in my laboratory, more than half the extra calories available for fat synthesis comes from inactivity rather from hypergphagia. Measurement of the spontaneous activity of nonfasted animals in activity cages shows that obese animals are 50 to 100 times less active than nonobese animals. This inactivity is not the result of extreme obesity but, in fact, precedes it, as is shown by comparing the activity rates of mature nonobese animals with those of young obese animals of the same weight. It can thus be considered as one of the etiologic factors in the syndrome determined by the obese-hyperglycemic gene. Nonobese animals maintained at a constant weight consume about 20 calories per day, of which 10 cover basal expenditure and two cover specific dynamic action, leaving eight for the cost of activity. Obese littermates consume about 25 calories per day and may gain up to 1 gm (nine calories) daily. Their basal is, again, about 10 calories per day, with specific dynamic action two and one-half calories per day. When the eight calories expended daily on activity by the nonobese mouse are ascribed to fat synthesis in the obese mouse, the rapid development of extreme adiposity is no longer a thermodynamic impossibility.

The weight gain of genetically obese mice can be drastically reduced by treadmill exercise. The obese members of the strain who carry the "waltzing" gene and are in constant rotary movement in their cages show a weight gain only about 30 per cent greater than that of the nonobese mice, instead of the 200 or 300 per cent shown by sedentary obese mice.

There are many forms of experimental obesities. (These various conditions may be models for a similar variety of human obesities.) The obese-hyperglycemic syndrome is a metabolic (endocrine form) obesity probably due to primary hypertrophy of the islands of Langerhans, with resulting hypersecretion of insulin and of the pancreatic hyperglycemic-glycogenolytic factor (glucagon).

Among the six or seven other forms of mouse obesity which have been described in my laboratory is hypothalamic obesity. This can be achieved by specifically destroying the ventromedial area of the hypothalamus by surgical eletrocoagulation or, more conveniently, by the single injection of the chemical gold thioglucose. Mice in which hypothalamic obesity is produced by gold thioglucose differ from those with the hereditary obese-hyperglycemic syndrome in that they are normally active and use all the extra calories which they consume (up to 50% above normal). Yet these animals will still lose weight if exercised on the treadmill or if given the opportunity to exercise in a squirrel-type rotary cage.

Such findings emphasize both the diversity of obesities in regard to spontaneous activities and the importance of exercise as a weight control factor.

## INCREASED FOOD INTAKE IN EXERCISE

A second frequent misconception concerning the value of exercise in weight control is that an increase in physical activity always causes an increase in appetite and food intake which equals or is greater in energy value than that of the energy cost of the exercise.

It is true that in a normal, reasonably exercised animal or person an increase in food intake follows an increase in activity. This explains why the weight of most adult animals and men is relatively constant. Proper adjustments of appetite prevent the body from indefinitely burning away reserves if the person is called on to perform at higher levels of exertion than previously customary. However, experimental results show that this is true only within a certain range, which I call "normal activity range." When the activity of rabbits is restricted by confinement in a small cage, they will consume more calories than they require and thus accumulate fat. The excess food consumed is characteristic of the strain; hence, a hereditary factor is involved. The same phenomenon is illustrated by the fact that rats become obese if they are totally immobilized.

The dependence of food intake and body weight on physical activity has been systematically explored in experimental animals in my laboratory. When mature rats, accustomed to a sedentary (caged) existence, were exercised on a treadmill for increasing daily periods, moderated exercise of short duration (20 minutes to one hour) did not result in a corresponding increase in food intake. Actually, food intake decreased slightly but significantly. Body weight also decreased (sedentary range in Figure 2-1). For longer periods of exercise, (one to five or six hours), food intake increased linearly and weight was maintained (range of proportional response, a normal activity range in Figure 2-1). As a result of very long periods of exercise, the animals lost weight, their food intake decreased and their appearance deteriorated (exhaustion range in Figure 2-1). Both the sedentary and the exhaustion ranges can thus be considered "nonresponsive" with respect to food intake, because in these ranges an increase in activity is not accompanied by a corresponding increase in food intake.

Obviously, the sedentary nonresponsive zone is of particular interest to the problem of obesity. It demonstrates that under abnormal environmental conditions which force partial immobilization or, at least, a sedentary life on the subject the limits below which food intake no longer decreases because of a decrease in activity are overtaken. Adiposity is the unavoidable result. This, of course, has been known empirically to farmers for centuries and explains the practice of cooping or penning cattle, hogs and geese for fattening. Passmore confirmed these findings in a recent systematic study.

Similar observations are available concerning man. Greene

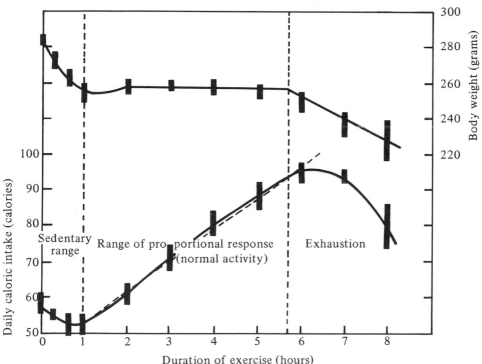

Voluntary caloric intake and body weight
as functions of exercise in normal rats

Figure 2-1. A summary of laboratory experiments, this graph shows that food intake does not necessarily increase with exercise in experimental animals. Although rats exercised for three or four hours daily eat more than those exercised for one hour, they maintain their body weight because of their activity. However, rats exercised for less than one hour daily or not at all eat significantly more, and weight accumulates because of the increased food intake and low activity level.

studied more than 200 overweight adult patients in whom the beginning of obesity could be traced directly to a sudden decrease in activity. In the summer of 1954 I had an opportunity to conduct a study on an industrial population of West Bengal (India), which has a particularly wide range of physical activity, from bazaar tailors and clerks to coolies carrying twice their body weight on their heads for nine hours a day. Figure 2-2 illustrates the findings of that study.

The determination of food intake was facilitated by the fact that most of the persons surveyed did not live in a family situation, but bought their food and cooked for themselves. The lack of storage facilities forced them to shop frequently. The diet was extraordinarily uniform for each person and showed little variety within groups and from group to group. Individual one-day dietary recalls, checked by buying records, and studies on amounts spent per week on food gave results generally identical with exhaustive dietary histories and appeared more representative of long-range intakes than did corresponding data obtained in a Western society.

Activity was determined by detailed schedules, industrial ratings of physical effort, and some Douglas bag determinations. Clerks were further subdivided into four classes, according to the mileage walked daily to and from work. Those in class 1 were the most inactive, actually living within the factory grounds. The various occupations or subgroups were each represented by at least 10 persons and were grouped according to a broad classification of activity. One extreme included the merchants, supervisors and "nonwalking" clerks. At the other extreme were the selectors and pilers, carriers, who carried up to 190 lb jute each, coalmen and ashmen, who carried equally heavy bags of coal and ashes and unloaded them in an awkward manner, and cutters, who spent their whole day swinging heavy cutting knives with practically no pause. Individual weights varied from 67 to 198 lb for men of the same height (5 ft 2 in to 5 ft 4 in).

Economic differences and cultural, religious and ethnic factors could be accounted for and ruled out in analyzing the results. It is readily seen from Figure 2-2 that the curves obtained for food intake and body weight as functions of physical activity are

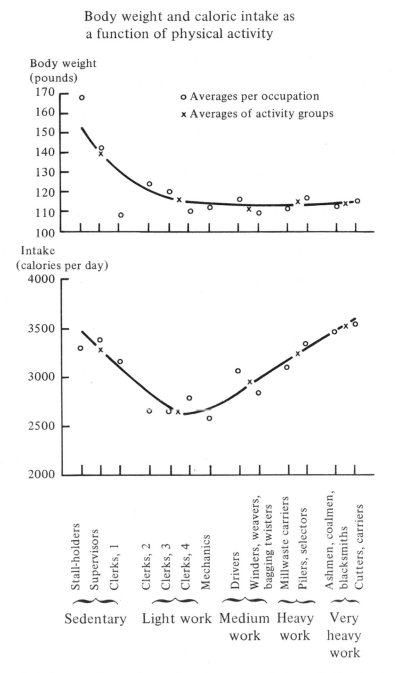

Figure 2-2. Results of a study conducted on a population in India, showing the relation of a wide range of activities to food intake and adiposity. Clerks are grouped according to the daily time spent in walking. As in experimental animals, persons who exercised regularly had the lowest daily food intake. Those who did heavy work ate more to maintain their weight. Inactive persons also ate more and became obese.

strikingly similar to those of Figure 2-1, which were obtained on rats. Again, there is a sedentary range which corresponds to no further decrease in food intake (instead, to an increase) and in which increasing degrees of overweight follow decreasing exercise. Incidentally, the meaning of the actual increase in food intake under extremely sedentary conditions is not clear. It may indicate decreased ready availability of reserves, possibly resulting from circulatory sluggishness due to inactivity.

The work of Taylor and colleagues at the department of physiological hygiene, University of Minnesota, also showed that an increase in exercise above the very sedentary level was not accompanied by an increase in food intake in adult men.

The problem of the relation of weight to activity in children also has been investigated. Bruch found that inactivity was characteristic of the majority of the 160 obese children whom she studied. Only 18 per cent of the boys and 22 per cent of the girls were normally active. 76 per cent of the boys and 88 per cent of the girls were physically inactive. Rony suggested that laziness or a decreased desire to engage in muscular activity is a primary characteristic of the obese subject; it is demonstrated in childhood by avoidance of all unnecessary activity, outdoor play and athletics. Bronstein found that most of the 35 obese children whom he and his associates observed spent most of their leisure time in sedentary activities. Graham reported like observations. Danish workers, particularly Tolstrup and Juel-Nielsen, attempted a semiobjective grading of groups of obese children and found that the lack of activity was characteristic of these subjects. Peckos, studying a large group of Boston children, found that differences in body build and, more specifically, in fat content and distribution were not correlated with caloric intake. Fry determined that obese children with large fat pads did not have higher average caloric intakes than did control children of the same height and age. In her tabulation of "rough psychologic evaluation" a much higher proportion of obese children than of nonobese children are labeled as only moderately active or inactive. This difference was particularly marked in boys; however, no data were given to support this estimate.

In a recent study we attempted to compare systematically both caloric intake and activity in carefully paired groups of obese and normal-weight high school girls. Exhaustive research was conducted on dietary histories and activity schedules covering the year preceding the study. We correlated as accurately as possible the food intake of these teen-agers, with due regard for the difficulties encountered when applied to children and to obese subjects. Checks and counterchecks were conducted until we believed that reliable figures had been obtained. The picture of physical activity was determined by a system of successive examinations. A list of usual activities was established and the subjects were asked how much time they devoted to each on a daily or weekly basis, depending on the type of activity considered. The subjects were then asked to complete the list of activities and schedules, covering the year by seasons. Total hours per week were checked, and in another interview the activities were rechecked again on the same general basis. If the total time per week had been grossly overestimated or underestimated, special efforts were devoted to locating the cause of the error. The activities were rated on the basis of activity tables such as Table 2-1.

We found that suburban high school girls were generally not very active; even the schedule of the nonobese group showed little time devoted to household chores, little participation in active sports, and, at least during the school term, a minimal amount of time devoted to walking or to other physical activity. Even so, there was a marked difference between the obese and nonobese groups. The obese group was much more inactive than the nonobese. Generally speaking, the time spent by the obese group in sports or any sort of exercise (including ballroom dancing) was less than half that spent by the thin girls, the difference being absorbed by "sitting" activities. (It may be worthwhile to mention that many of the obese girls and boys in the school system in which this study was conducted were all too often excused from the sports program by the educational authorities on the basis of a letter from the family physician recommending that they not be required to exercise!) By contrast, caloric intakes were generally larger in the nonobese group. When possible, factors leading to positive energy balance were analyzed. It appeared that for this particular group, even when probable sources of error were recognized as inherent in the dietary interview method and in the type of activity analysis selected, inactivity was of greater importance than was overeating in the development of obesity. These high school girls, both obese and nonobese, attended summer camp each year; almost without exception the enforced strenuous activity caused loss of weight despite simultaneously increased food intake.

In another study a group of obese boys systematically exercised, and the evolution of their total body fat, measured by the determination of skinfold thickness, was followed. (Half the body fat is right under the skin and thus can be measured through the use of special calipers.) These boys did lose fat, and they presented a vastly improved appearance and mental outlook.

## COMMENT

I am convinced that inactivity is the most important factor explaining the frequency of "creeping" overweight in modern Western societies. Natural selection, operating for hundreds of thousands of years, made men physically active and resourceful, well-prepared to become hunters, fishermen or agriculturalists. The regulation of food intake was not designed to adapt to the highly mechanized sedentary conditions of modern life, just as animals were not created to be caged. Adapting to these conditions without developing obesity means either that the individual will have to step up his activity or that he will be mildly or acutely hungry all his life. The first solution is difficult, expecially as present conditions in the United States — particularly in cities — offer little inducement to walking and often have poorly organized facilities for adult exercise. Even among the young, highly competitive sports for the few are emphasized at the expense of individual sports which all could learn and continue to enjoy after the high school and college years are over. But if stepping up activity is difficult, it is well to remember that the alternative (lifetime hunger) is so much more difficult that relying on it for weight control programs will only continue to lead to fiascoes of the past. Strenuous exercise on an irregular basis is obviously not advocated for untrained obese persons. However, a reorganization of one's life to include regular exercise adapted to one's physical potentialities is a justified return to the wisdom of the ages.

If the responsibility of the family physician is not only to treat diseases but also to see that his patients achieve and maintain positive health and full realization of their physical possibilities, it becomes part of his task to see to it that this regular exercise, as well as proper food habits and sufficient rest, becomes an integral part of their daily schedule.

## REFERENCES

1. Orr, J. B. and Leitch, I.: The determinations of the caloric requirements in man. Nutrition Abstr. & Rev., 7:509, 1938.
2. Passmore, R. and Durnin, J. V. G. A.: Human energy expenditure. Physiol. Rev., 35:801, 1955.

*Chapter 3*

# FOOD COMPOSITION TABLES:
# BASIS, USES AND LIMITATIONS

BEFORE the diet of a patient or a group is changed, the reasons for this change must be clear. The analysis of the calorie and nutrient content of the diet, obtained by translating amounts of foodstuffs consumed into amounts of calories and nutrients presumably absorbed, is the first necessary step. The dietitian's essential tool in this procedure is the food composition table. Because these tables thus play a central role in any individual or collective nutrition program, their basis, uses and limitations are of interest to the practitioner.

## CARBOHYDRATES, PROTEINS,
## TOTAL FATS AND CALORIES

### The Atwater System

Interestingly, the unparalleled development of nutrition research in the United States had its start in the establishment of a food composition table: Atwater, a student of Voit, returned to America in 1873 to embark on a comprehensive study of the fuel value of all important food in American dietaries. As this work is still the basis of the values for the caloric content of foods in present-day food composition tables, it may be useful to recall briefly the salient points of Atwater's method as he developed it in his comprehensive report published in 1899 (1). For a comprehensive review of the Atwater system, the reader is invited to turn to the excellent study of Maynard (2).

Atwater began his work by summarizing 185 dietary studies of various groups of people in different areas in the United States.

Reprinted from *Postgraduate Medicine, 28* (No. 3), September, 1960.

The foods concerned were classified in groups (meats, milk, cereals, sugar, vegetables, fruits, and so on). The percentage of protein, fat and carbohydrate contributed by each food group was calculated on the basis of chemical determinations (to be discussed in greater detail later) and results were averaged. The distribution of nutrients corresponding to the "average diet" could thus be established. While Atwater measured the water, fat, protein and ash content of foods directly, the carbohydrate content was determined by difference — the difference between initial weight and the sum of water, fat, protein and ash. Protein was obtained by multiplying the nitrogen content by the factor 6.25, corresponding to a proportion of 16 per cent of the proteins represented by nitrogen.

Atwater next determined the heats of combustion of certain proteins, fats and carbohydrates representative of each food group. He then calculated the average heat of combustion due to protein, fats and carbohydrates in general for each dietary group (e.g. meat, fruits, etc.). The figures for protein were decreased by 1.25 calories per gram — the heat of combustion of the urea formed from 1 gm protein. (This figure had been obtained as an average of 46 determinations on the urine of men consuming mixed diets.) The heats of combustion (minus 1.25 calories per gram for proteins of each group) were then multiplied by the digestibility coefficient determined for this group. Thus, one could ascribe to each food group "specific" fuel values for its fat, protein and carbohydrate. For example, the fuel values of the proteins of eggs, meats, cereals, legumes, fruits and vegetables were 4.35, 4.25, 3.70, 3.20, 3.15, and 2.90 calories per gram respectively. The range of variation was somewhat less for fat (9.00 to 8.35 calories per gram for meat and vegetable fats respectively) and for carbohydrates (4.10 to 3.60 calories per gram for cereals and fruits).

Atwater found that when the fuel values of protein, fat and carbohydrate were averaged for a "normal" U. S. distribution of food groups, the averages for the whole diet were 4.00, 8.90 and 4.00 calories per gram respectively or, according to the well-known approximation, 4, 9, 4. Few coefficients have been so universally used — and, not infrequently, abused.

## Available Carbohydrates

The application of the 4, 9, 4, figures to individual foodstuffs is of necessity, inaccurate. In some cases the errors thus entailed can be significant. Furthermore, even when the correct Atwater figures are employed, certain foodstuffs may fall outside of the list of those he had studied. In that case, it would appear necessary to go through the long and costly processes of calorimetric determinations and digestibility experiments to get the "specific" fuel values to be applied.

While the situation regarding the highly digestible proteins and fats (the indigestible fraction, like the proteins of teguments, is usually removed from food at the "retail" level) is fairly clear-cut, carbohydrates have proved a special problem. The carbohydrates obtained "by difference" include the whole range of digestibility, from the almost totally digestible starches to the almost totally indigestible fibers, and the whole range of physiologic availability, from the totally available hexoses and citric acid to the totally unavailable tartaric acid. Attempting to deal with these complexities, certain British workers, in particular McCance and Widdowson (3), undertook to base their calculations on what they called "available carbohydrates" rather than on "carbohydrates by difference." They determined starch, sugars and dextrins directly, expressed all of these carbohydrates as glucose, and multiplied the total by 3.75, the heat of combustion of this sugar, to obtain calories. This procedure was later modified by the British Medical Research Council which expressed available carbohydrates in terms of their starch equivalent (dividing by 1.055 for disaccharides and by 1.11 for hexoses) before applying the factor 4. This procedure automatically introduces a difference of about 5 per cent from the results obtained by the Atwater system.

## Postwar Developments

The confusion introduced by the multiplicity of existing methods for computing the caloric values of foods became patent in the international planning of food policy during and immediately after World War II. At that time interest in calories, which had receded before the justifiable enthusiasm aroused by the advances in protein metabolism and the discovery of vitamins, was revived by several factors. First and foremost was the prevalence of caloric undernourishment throughout the world; secondly, there was the increased attention given to the role of overeating in the etiology of degenerative diseases and, finally, the realization of the importance of proper caloric intake in therapeutic treatment and growth. In particular, the wartime need for allocating and rationing calories brought into sharp focus the differences introduced in computations by different methods. A difference, say, of 5 per cent in the energy content of a staple food could mean a difference of thousands of tons in terms of national or international food allocations.

The Second Session of the Conference of the Food and Agriculture Organization (4), meeting in 1946, recommended that "FAO should arrange for joint consultation of experts in nutrition and food statistics from various countries who should develop the principles on which average food composition figures used by individual countries should be based and explore the means whereby comparability of data for international use can be obtained including if necessary, the revision of tables now used for this purpose." Similarly, a 1946 resolution of the Food and Nutrition Board of the National Research Council (4) asked that "the FAO be requested to promote, at the earliest possible time, international agreement regarding a common basis for the calculation of the nutritional value of important foodstuffs, giving first consideration to the question of calories.

In accordance with these recommendations, the Nutrition Division of FAO called a meeting of a Committee on Calorie Conversion Factors and Food Composition Tables in Washington in 1947. The Committee concerned itself with four main points: (1) the method of computing energy values, dealing in particular with estimation of carbohydrate calories; (2) the more accurate estimate of protein content from nitrogen value; (3) the problem of the fuel value of alcohol; (4) the fuel value of organic acids (4).

## The FAO Committee Report

The committee, on which, among others, Professor L. A. Maynard of Cornell was particularly active, considered carefully the data available during the period spanned by Atwater's work, the studies of the old Bureau of Home Economics of the United States Department of Agriculture, the data of McCance and Widdowson, as well as analyses and results of digestibility studies from a number of areas. It concluded that "The Committee can find no evidence that Atwater's data, properly used, are not reliable. It must be stressed, however, that Atwater's condensation and averaging of digestion coefficients and energy values to give 4, 9, 4, for protein, fat and carbohydrate, designed to facilitate the estimation of the physiological energy of average United States diets, are erroneously used when applied to diets of different types and to individual foods" (4). Table 3-1 was given to illustrate the misuse of these coefficients. From it, one can immediately see that the use of the 4, 9, 4 coefficients completely masks the 10 per cent difference in availability introduced by substituting whole

TABLE 3-1

GROSS AND PHYSIOLOGIC ENERGY VALUES OF 100 GM OF
WHEAT CALCULATED AT 15 PER CENT MOISTURE [4]

| | | Physiologic Values | | |
|---|---|---|---|---|
| Percentage Extraction | Gross Value Heat of Combustion | Atwater general factors 4, 9, 4 | Individual factors (Atwater method) | McCance et al. 1945[*] |
| 97 to 100 | 380 | 343 | 322 | – |
| 100 | 377 | – | – | 314 |
| 70 to 74 | 379 | 344 | 350 | – |
| 75 | 372 | – | – | 342 |

*McCance, R. A., Widdowson, E. M., Moran, T., Pringle, W. J. S. and Macrae, T. F.: The chemical composition of wheat and rye and of flours derived therefrom. Biochem. J., 39:213-222, 1945.

wheat flour for the 70 per cent extraction flour, a fact that may present considerable economic and physiologic importance in situations where the bulk of the calories comes from bread. The continued use of carbohydrate by difference was thus recommended, with emphatic cautioning against attempts to refine this estimate, for instance, by deduction of fiber. This would lead only to further error since neither the digestion of the residual fraction nor the heat of combustion of the digested portion has been studied, and the coefficient of digestion of carbohydrate by difference could certainly not apply to any such new fraction.

As to protein content, it was emphasized that the usual method of estimation, which consists of determining total nitrogen of a food and multiplying it by 6.25, rests on two assumptions: The first is that all the nitrogen in a food is in the form of protein. All foods, however, contain some nonprotein nitrogen and in some foods, such as tubers, roots and leafy vegetables, the amount of nonprotein nitrogen may be considerable. The other assumption is that all proteins contain 16 percent nitrogen, which again is not true of all foods. New factors were suggested for a variety of foods by the Committee: 6.38 for milk, 5.55 for gelatin, factors varying from 5.18 to 5.71 for enumerated oilseeds and nuts, and specific factors for wheat (5.70 for refined flour and 5.83 for whole wheat, rye, barley, oats and rice).

The special problem of alcohol was circumvented by the Committee, which advised that alcohol should not be included in the computation of dietary energy, but that wherever the amount of alcohol consumed per head is reliably known, it should be indicated as such. (The 1957 International [FAO–WHO] Committee on Calorie Requirements recommended that the value 7.1 calories per gram be applied to alcohol, at least wherever the alcohol consumption does not exceed a certain value, say, 700 calories.) Finally, a special study dealt with the specific fuel values of organic acids, a problem of interest in such cases as the estimate of the energy value of citrus fruits. In the case of lemon juice, 62.5 per cent of the caloric value comes from organic acids which the available carbohydrate method of computation would have omitted.

## Agriculture Handbook No. 8

Two important food composition tables have been issued which applied the Committee's recommendations: in 1949, the FAO Food Composition Tables for International Use, by Chatfield (5), which are suitable for preparing "food balance sheets" (6) and facilitate interregional comparisons; and, more important for the U. S. physician and nutritionist, Agriculture Handbook No. 8 of the United States Department of Agriculture, "Composition of Foods — Raw, Processed, Prepared" (7). In both of these documents, the considerations previously summarized concerning calories, carbohydrates by difference, estimation of protein, and so on, were carefully followed. Agriculture Handbook No. 8 represents the source of reference whenever precise data are required on calories, as well as on nutrients. It is the authorative document used in this country as far as American foods are concerned. All of the "practical," "summarized," etc. "food tables" are based on it, directly or indirectly. Caloric values of individual foods, as well as precise calculations of caloric contents of diets, particularly therapeutic and other diets which do not conform to the "normal" American pattern, should be based on its values. An important example would be the "high-bulk, low-calorie"diets in which the use of the 4, 9, 4 coefficients would produce a considerable overvaluation.*

## Errors in Individual Assessment of Dietary Energy

It would be unfortunate if this discussion led to the idea that the choice of food composition tables and their use are always the limiting factors in assessing caloric intake of individuals when surveys, questionnaires, "recalls," and generally all methods except those resting on weighing and analysis of duplicate samples are used (9). It may be useful to review briefly the possible sources of

---

*The use of "short methods" of computation imply an approximation of the same order and often of even much greater magnitude. They can, therefore, be condoned where precision is not required, but not where accuracy is necessary. The same applies to "share" methods, unless they are based on Agriculture Handbook No. 8. That of Babcock (8) is such a method.

errors and to see where those specifically pertaining to food composition tables fit.

First, too many investigators do not appreciate the variability in time of caloric intake. Unlike intake of other nutrients, caloric requirements are conditioned by activity and environmental temperature. This consideration may help to interpret the findings of Yudkin (10). In a well-controlled study of weekly intakes, he found a difference of up to 68 per cent between the highest and the lowest weekly intakes in one individual, of only 2 per cent between the extremes for another one. Where calories are concerned, the length of a study is often less important than control of environmental conditions.

A second source of error is concerned with the technics of individual surveys and dietary histories. Leitch and Aitken (11) have presented a good critique of the validity and the accuracy of the current methods. It may be useful to add to their comments the point that individual survey methods seem weakest where calories are concerned. Such factors as the frequent partaking of small carbohydrate snacks, the number and size of spoonfuls of sugar in hot beverages, and individual attitude toward fat (see below) may easily account for variations of several hundred calories, yet escape undetected by cross checks usually designed to verify the intake of proteins, minerals and vitamins. For example, as already mentioned, there are wide differences in attitude toward fat among various individuals. Some individuals butter bread, potatoes, etc., others do not. Some like fat gravies, others eschew it. Some persons remove every part of the visible fat of meat, others eat it with relish. Incidentally, even if this is elucidated by especially careful questioning, the degree of fattening of the meat consumed still remains an important source of error. Agriculture Handboook No. 8 gives all figures for "lamb, cooked" in terms of meat of "medium fatness," yet the values for "lamb, carcass or side, raw" vary from 206 to 414 calories per 100 gm, or a ratio of 1 to 2. If one adds to this variability the additional variability of the amount of fat used in cooking, this range can reach 1 to 3. Yet the subject under questioning is not usually asked to (and probably could not) give information on the fat content of the meat he consumes. Similar situations develop in regard to fat content of milk, fried foods, and so on. In all these cases, the fat content (and therefore the caloric content) is the chief variable; proteins, vitamins and minerals are affected to a much lesser degree, Similarly, the use of household measures entails errors bearing in particular on flour, sugar and fat, all foodstuffs essentially of caloric significance.

Different investigators deal with these factors in different ways, making comparisons between figures obtained in the different surveys difficult. In addition, there are some systematic slants. For example, obese individuals, in comparison with normal subjects, will tend to underestimate total caloric intake and, in particular, the intake of fat.

## Assessment of Caloric Intakes of Children

The difficulties and source of errors just mentioned become particularly acute in the case of children. Yet the importance of proper assessment of caloric intake is relatively greater than for adults. First, children have correspondingly larger energy requirements due to their proportionally larger body surface. Second, their growth brings about special additional requirements. The work of Macy (12) clearly demonstrates that, in many cases, inadequate caloric intake may be the limiting factor in growth. Furthermore, as has been shown by others, among them Keys (13), many of the symptoms of protein deficiency are similar to and secondary to caloric deficiency. Reports such as that of Lynch and Snively (14) on "hypoproteinosis of childhood" can only be accepted at their face value if the possibility of caloric deficiency is eliminated. It may be added that in a slow-growing species like man, where the efficiency of growth is poor, the fraction of calories actually stored as body tissue is very small in proportion to those used for maintenance and activity. To detect by dietary history whether this relatively small requirement is provided for would require very precise methods. It may be useful to review briefly these possible causes of inaccuracy in assessing caloric intakes of children.

The first source of difficulties is the variability of requirements and the resultant variability of intakes, even in the case of individuals with good weight control. The principal factors in this variation are irregularities in activity and in exposure to cold. In the case of children, these factors are obviously magnified. Even casual observation of the habits of children reveals enormous differences in physical activity and outdoor exposure from one day to the next. The practice of violent games and sports, emotional factors, and relatively more frequent "small" indispositons make these differences even more acute. When one considers the variability in weekly intake in adults uncovered by Yudkin's (10) study, it is obvious that the variability of intake in children from one week to the next can easily be of the order of 30 to 50 per cent.

The second source of difficulty concerns irregularity in food habits. Here again children present an obviously difficult case. It is often impossible to appraise how much of the portions served are actually consumed; conversely, small caloric snacks and the consumption of candy and sweet beverages are relatively more important and also more variable that for adults and will often escape detection. The proportionately larger surface of children means, of course, a proportionately greater water loss through this surface. Exercise will, therefore, bring about a greater fluid requirement which may be covered alternately by water, fruit juice, sweet beverages, milk and so on, with variable results as far as caloric intake is concerned. To consider estimates of caloric intake by dietary history as accurate in the face of these handicaps is to exhibit considerable optimism.

Finally, it must be recognized that the theoretical basis of food composition tables and the application of their caloric values are insecure in the case of children. All the data on digestibility on which the calculations of Atwater and his successors have been based rested on the results of digestibility trials in adult individuals. The proportion of nutrients actually available to children, and particularly to small children, may be quite different. Similarly, composition of the "average" American diets, on which the Atwater percentage coefficients were based, may not apply to children. Certainly it does not apply to very small children whose diet is made up of relatively few items. The foods themselves may be different. In particular, there is no equivalent

in adult diets of the highly processed "baby foods" where a great
deal, if not all "indigestible" material has been removed. Extra-
polating the values obtained in the digestibility of normal foods by
adults to the digestibility of baby foods by small children seems at
best an approximate procedure.

The only logical conclusion is that whenever metabolic considerations in children are concerned, only complete balance studies,
with analysis of duplicate food samples and determination of the
"fuel value" of the excreta, will do. There is a great need of such
studies and, in particular, of food digestibility experiments on
children. For the time being, it is well to remember that when
dietary histories are used as an investigative or clinical tool, the
range of variation and the possible range of errors for calories
considerably exceed the proportion of calories consumed, which
represents the difference between successful growth and failure of
development.

## NUTRIENTS

### Weighing of Data for Each Foodstuff

The objective of national tables, in particular of the U. S. tables
(8), is to present values representative of foods as they are used
throughout the year in the country as a whole. Generally speaking,
the same sample of food is not analyzed for all the nutrients listed
in these tables. The tables are usually compilations of some
investigations dealing with protein, fat and carbohydrate (and
hence energy content), or investigations dealing with minerals, and
of investigations dealing with one or more vitamins. Some foods
are studied much more frequently with respect to one nutrient
than another; as a result there are great inequalities in the volume
of data available for various nutrients as well as in the volume of
data available for various foods. For example, in the case of
tomatoes, averages in the U. S. Department of Agriculture tables
were based on 956 analyses for ascorbic acid, 73 for thiamine, and
46 for vitamin A.

In order to get at "average" values for each foodstuff, one must
reckon not only with natural variability of foods as affected by

variety, methods of culture and maturity but, in the case of vitamins, with the effects of handling foods after harvesting. In addition, the amount of foods of a given variety and composition may vary from area to area so that an economic weighting as well as taxonomic, seasonal and analytic weighting have to be taken into account so as to obtain representative values.

Production figures are helpful in determining the weight to be given to each variety and to the values corresponding to various seasons. Other elements of judgment enter into the establishment of the tables. For example, it may seem best to exclude experimental strains of fruits or vegetables not in common production, especially if their inclusion might greatly alter the average. Again, it might be argued that ascorbic acid determinations made within two or three hours after harvesting a fruit or vegetable should be excluded on the grounds that store-bought products are never as fresh as this. In many cases, the information needed for this type of decision is not available. Finally, the opinion the compiler has of the relative reliability of various methods and various laboratories may enter into the final conclusions.

## Individual Nutrients

The older food composition tables gave analyses in terms of carbohydrates, proteins and fats, fiber ash and total energy. Present-day tables and in particular the Agriculture Handbook No. 8 (7) (the basis of all U. S. tables used by dietitians) now also give data on calcium, phosphorus, iron, vitamin A value, thiamine, riboflavin, niacin and ascorbic acid (Table 3-2).

The following comments are made in the preamble of these tables and are essential for understanding their use.

As represented in the Handbook, data for calcium, phosphorus and iron show total amounts of these elements present unless otherwise noted. The question of how to treat the calcium content of foods containing relatively large amounts of oxalic acid remains debatable. Total calcium content is given, but it is noted that the possibility exists that all of it may not be available because of the presence of oxalic acid. Likewise, deductions are not made for

TABLE 3-2

COMPOSITION OF FOODS, 100 GM, EDIBLE PORTION*

| Food and Description | Water (Per cent) | Food Energy (Calories) | Protein (Gm) | Fat (Gm) | Carbohydrate (Gm) Total | Carbohydrate (Gm) Fiber | Ash (Gm) | Calcium (Mg) | Phosphorus (Mg) | Iron (Mg) | Vitamin A Value (I.U.) | Thiamine (Mg) | Riboflavin (Mg) | Niacin (Mg) | Ascorbic Acid (Mg) |
|---|---|---|---|---|---|---|---|---|---|---|---|---|---|---|---|
| 1. Almonds, dried, unblanched | 4.7 | 597 | 18.6 | 54.1 | 19.6 | 2.7 | 3.0 | 254 | 475 | 4.4 | 0 | 0.25 | 0.67 | 4.6 | Trace |
| Apples: | | | | | | | | | | | | | | | |
| 2. Raw | 84.1 | 58 | 0.3 | 0.4 | 14.9 | 1.0 | 0.3 | 6 | 10 | 0.3 | 90 | 0.04 | 0.03 | 0.2 | 5 |
| Canned (see applesauce) | | | | | | | | | | | | | | | |
| 3. Dehydrated (small pieces) | 3.0 | 354 | 1.8 | 2.4 | 91.0 | 4.9 | 1.8 | 24 | 61 | 1.8 | (0) | 0.07 | 0.10 | 1.2 | 12 |
| Dried: | | | | | | | | | | | | | | | |
| 4. Uncooked | 23.0 | 277 | 1.4 | 1.0 | 73.2 | 3.9 | 1.4 | 19 | 48 | 1.4 | (0) | 0.10 | 0.10 | 1.0 | 12 |
| Cooked: | | | | | | | | | | | | | | | |
| 5. Unsweetened | 78.1 | 79 | 0.4 | 0.3 | 20.8 | 1.1 | 0.4 | 5 | 14 | 0.4 | (0) | 0.02 | 0.03 | 0.3 | 2 |
| 6. Sweetened | 71.4 | 105 | 0.4 | 0.3 | 27.5 | 1.0 | 0.4 | 5 | 12 | 0.4 | (0) | 0.02 | 0.02 | 0.2 | 2 |
| 7. Apples and apricots canned, strained (infant food) | 82.3 | 63 | 0.4 | 0.3 | 16.5 | 0.5 | 0.5 | 11 | 16 | 1.0 | 1,070 | 0.02 | 0.02 | 0.2 | 2 |

*Reproduced from Agriculture Handbook No. 8.7

phytin present in food. Vitamin values for any one vitamin have been determined by a number of methods. In some cases, the early exploratory procedures have been replaced by methods now thought to be highly reliable, but the more reliable methods have not yet been applied to all foods. The application of better methods will necessitate a revision in some of the figures presented in the Handbook. Vitamin A values are expressed in international units. They are based in part on biologic assay and in part on the physical or chemical determinations of vitamin A itself or of one of its precursors.

The physiologic equivalence of vitamin A and of the carotenes having vitamin A activity has posed difficult questions. Scientists around the globe are not entirely in agreement as to how much carotene is equivalent to an international unit of vitamin A. Values expressed international units of vitamin A on the basis that $0.6\mu g$ of beta carotene and $1.2\mu g$ of other carotenes having vitamin A activity were equivalent to 1 international unit of vitamin A. The problem of deriving suitable values for practical use in evaluating human diets is still further complicated by differences in availability of carotene from different sources. Experimental work with laboratory animals and human subjects has shown that the carotene in some foods is nearly all available and in others only one-third or less is available. Future revisions of vitamin tables will no doubt require considerable change in vitamin A figures appearing in this Handbook.

## B Vitamins

Methods of extraction and assay for the three B vitamins (thiamine, riboflavin, niacin) included in the Agriculture Handbook are still in the process of development. Modifications of the prefered methods are resulting in greater sensitivity and precision and, consequently, in better agreement among methods. Results of applying the improved procedures have not as yet been reported for a great many foods; consequently many of the values in the tables are based on older methods. There is still considerable doubt concerning the adequacy of the present methods for the release of the bound forms of riboflavin; anomalous values are occasionally reported for the retention of this vitamin in foods that have been subjected to heat. All niacin values are derived from data in the literature measuring nicotinamide and related active compounds. Ascorbic acid values reported are based for the most part on determinations of reduced ascorbic acid, because this was the form reported by most workers and is the form in which nearly all of this vitamin occurs in fresh products. Foods that have undergone storage or processing, however, have been found to contain significant quantities of the oxidized form (dehydro-ascorbic acid). Data on total ascorbic acid are used when authors report on both the reduced and the dehydro forms. Since data for estimating total ascorbic acid have been far less often reported, there may be some underestimation of the vitamin C value of the foods. On the other Hand, recent developments in methods for measuring the vitamin C value of products show that some foods contain interfering substances which react chemically like the vitamin but do not have the same physiologic activity. These interfering substances are found especially in foods having a high carbohydrate content that have been subjected to heat or unfavorable storage conditions. Continued research on methods and application of the improved procedures are needed to show what extent present data need revision.

## AMINO ACIDS AND FATTY ACIDS

Recently, additional refinements have been brought into food composition tables. These have been largely the result, on the one hand, of sharpened interest in protein deficiency in under-developed countries and, on the other hand, of increasing realization of the possible importance of certain fatty acids in cholesterol metabolism and hence in heart disease. The U. S. Department of Agriculture has prepared a very useful booklet entitled "Amino Acid Content of Foods" and published as the Home Economics Research Report No. 4 (15). Most of the values used in the tables of this report were based on microbiologic analysis of chemical hydrolysates. In the relatively few instances in which split samples have been hydrolyzed, one portion chemically and the other by enzymes, the results based on analysis of the chemical hydrolysate were usually selected. Sometimes there was good agreement between results. Differences were not consistent in size or direction. If only enzyme hydrolysates had been analyzed by an investigator, the results were not necessarily excluded. To have done so might have meant eliminating data showing the effect of some important variables, even omitting an item entirely.

The methods used for analyzing the hydrolysates may have varied widely in degree of accuracy. Many of the amino acid values on which the United States Department of Agriculture values are based are from studies in which a large number of foods were analyzed by routine procedures. These procedures may not have been equally well adapted to the different types of food being analyzed. Greater accuracy of results from different studies can be expected with the continued discovery of the more important factors that affect results at various steps in analysis.

Many problems in method are recognized, among which are those relating to measurement of sensitivity of specific organiams, suitability of media, optimum pH, time and temperature of incubation, formation of humin, interference of carbohydrates, conditions under which hydrolysates were stored, and purity of standards. Many improvements in amino acid procedures are anticipated as an outgrowth of the renewed interest and study of these problems.

The organization of the summary tables presented a problem for which there was no obvious best solution. The order finally adopted has met with fewer objections than any of the many others considered (Table 3-3). Of the 18 amino acids included in the tables, those of most importance in human nutrition are placed in the positions most readily accessible. The essential amino acids of greatest interest appear in the columns closest to the descriptions of the food items. Cystine and tyrosine, the semi-dispensable amino acids, are adjacent to methionine and phenyl-alanine, respectively, the amino acids for which they are known to have sparing action.

Deficiency of methionine in foods and diets is often reported; therefore, special consideration must be given to the sparing action of the cystine in the foods. Cystine cannot completely replace

TABLE 3-3

AMINO ACID CONTENT OF FOODS, 100 GM, EDIBLE PORTION*

| Item, Protein Content, and Nitrogen Conversion Factor | Trypto-phan (Gm) | Threo-nine (Gm) | Iso-leucinine (Gm) | Leucine (Gm) | Lysine (Gm) | Sulfur Containing | | |
|---|---|---|---|---|---|---|---|---|
| | | | | | | Methionine (gm) | Cystine (gm) | Total (gm) |
| Meat; Poultry; Fish and Shellfish; Their Products | | | | | | | | |
| Meat (protein, N x 6.25) | | | | | | | | |
| 40. Rib roast (17.4% protein) | 0.203 | 0.768 | 0.910 | 1.425 | 1.520 | 0.432 | 0.220 | 0.652 |
| 41. Round (19.5% protein) | 0.228 | 0.861 | 1.020 | 1.597 | 1.704 | 0.484 | 0.246 | 0.730 |
| 42. Rump (16.2% protein) | 0.189 | 0.715 | 0.848 | 1.327 | 1.415 | 0.402 | 0.205 | 0.607 |
| 43. Sirloin (17.3% protein) | 0.202 | 0.764 | 0.905 | 1.417 | 1.511 | 0.429 | 0.219 | 0.648 |
| 44. Beef, canned (25.0% protein) | 0.292 | 1.104 | 1.308 | 2.048 | 2.184 | 0.620 | 0.316 | 0.936 |
| 45. Beef, dried or chipped (34.3% protein) | 0.401 | 1.515 | 1.795 | 2.810 | 2.996 | 0.851 | 0.434 | 1.285 |
| Lamb carcass or side: | | | | | | | | |
| 46. Thin (17.1% protein) | 0.222 | 0.782 | 0.886 | 1.324 | 1.384 | 0.410 | 0.224 | 0.634 |
| 47. Medium fat (15.7% protein) | 0.203 | 0.718 | 0.814 | 1.216 | 1.271 | 0.377 | 0.206 | 0.583 |
| 48. Fat (13.0% protein) | 0.168 | 0.595 | 0.674 | 1.007 | 1.052 | 0.312 | 0.171 | 0.483 |
| Lamb cuts, medium fat: | | | | | | | | |
| 49. Leg (18.0% protein) | 0.233 | 0.824 | 0.933 | 1.394 | 1.457 | 0.432 | 0.236 | 0.668 |
| 50. Rib (14.9% protein) | 0.193 | 0.682 | 0.772 | 1.154 | 1.206 | 0.358 | 0.195 | 0.553 |

*Reproduced from Home Economics Research Report No. 4. 15

TABLE 3-3 (Continued)

AMINO ACID CONTENT OF FOODS, 100 GM, EDIBLE PORTION

| Phenyl-alanine (Gm) | Tyrosine (Gm) | Valine (Gm) | Arginine (Gm) | Histidine (Gm) | Alanine (Gm) | Aspartic Acid (Gm) | Glutamic Acid (Gm) | Glycine (Gm) | Proline (Gm) | Serine (Gm) | Item No. |
|---|---|---|---|---|---|---|---|---|---|---|---|
| 0.715 | 0.590 | 0.966 | 1.122 | 0.604 | 1.005 | 1.623 | 2.634 | 1.077 | 0.857 | 0.729 | 40 |
| 0.802 | 0.661 | 1.083 | 1.257 | 0.677 | 1.126 | 1.819 | 2.952 | 1.207 | 0.961 | 0.817 | 41 |
| 0.666 | 0.550 | 0.899 | 1.045 | 0.562 | 0.936 | 1.511 | 2.452 | 1.003 | 0.798 | 0.679 | 42 |
| 0.711 | 0.587 | 0.960 | 1.116 | 0.601 | 0.999 | 1.614 | 2.619 | 1.071 | 0.853 | 0.725 | 43 |
| 1.028 | 0.848 | 1.388 | 1.612 | 0.868 | 1.444 | 2.332 | 3.784 | 1.548 | 1.232 | 1.048 | 44 |
| 1.410 | 1.163 | 1.904 | 2.212 | 1.191 | 1.981 | 3.200 | 5.192 | 2.124 | 1.690 | 1.438 | 45 |
| 0.695 | 0.594 | 0.843 | 1.114 | 0.476 | 0.955 | 1.576 | 2.594 | 0.999 | 0.791 | 0.684 | 46 |
| 0.638 | 0.545 | 0.774 | 1.022 | 0.437 | 0.877 | 1.447 | 2.381 | 0.917 | 0.726 | 0.628 | 47 |
| 0.528 | 0.451 | 0.641 | 0.847 | 0.362 | 0.726 | 1.198 | 1.972 | 0.759 | 0.601 | 0.520 | 48 |
| 0.732 | 0.625 | 0.887 | 1.172 | 0.501 | 1.005 | 1.659 | 2.730 | 1.051 | 0.832 | 0.720 | 49 |
| 0.606 | 0.517 | 0.734 | 0.970 | 0.415 | 0.832 | 1.373 | 2.260 | 0.870 | 0.689 | 0.596 | 50 |

methionine, but at present information is inadequate for calculating the effective methionine value. On the basis of sulfur content of the molecule, 1.0 gm of cystine would be equivalent to 1.24 gm of methionine. In initial experiments with three young men, cystine replaced from 80 to 89 per cent of the minimum need for methionine. Other replacement factors may be found under different experimental conditions.

The Home Economics Report No. 4 tables include a column showing the total quantity of the sulfur-containing amino acids. The values are the straight sums of the averages for methionine and cystine contents. Considerable change is anticipated in this column when future revisions of the report are published.

The table columns for arginine and histidine follow those for the amino acids known to be essential for the human adult; histidine may be essential for the growing child. Both have been determined in a number of foods. For the remaining amino acids, for which foods were infrequently assayed, an alphabetical order is employed.

The Home Economics Research Report No. 7 (16), also put out by the U. S. Department of Agriculture and which gives the fatty acids in food fats, is designed for practical use by "dietitians, nutritionists, home economists, and others planning and appraising diets." The table comprising this report has been developed from a review and compilation of analytic data available from the literature of 1920 to 1955, showing fatty acids as per cent of total fatty acids (Table 3-4). Although the figures in this table represent the best available, the present pace of research in this field may necessitate early revisions. Few data are available on fruits and vegetables, and many of the other values are based on a limited number of analyses.

Figures for fatty acids per 100 gm of ether extract (crude fat), reported by the Department of Agriculture, have been computed from data on fatty acids as per cent of total fatty acids by correcting for glycerol in the fat and for the content of unsaponifiable matter reported in the ether extract of each food fat. Glycerol values are not included. To calculate fatty acids in foods, it is necessary to only multiply the amount (grams) of fat in a food portion by the value of each fatty acid.

## TABLE 3-4

### FATTY ACID CONTENT OF FOOD FATS, UNSAPONIFIABLE MATTER AND IODINE VALUE GRAMS PER 100 GM ETHER EXTRACT OR CRUDE FAT*

| Food Fat or Oil | Saturated Fatty Acids | | | Unsaturated Fatty Acids | | | | | Unsaponifiable Matter | Iodine Value |
|---|---|---|---|---|---|---|---|---|---|---|
| | Total | Palmitic $C_{16}$ | Stearic $C_{18}$ | Total | Oleic $C_{18}$ (−2H) | Linoleic $C_{18}$ (−4H) | Linolenic $C_{18}$ (−6H) | Other | | |
| **Animal Products** | | | | | | | | | | |
| Meats: | | | | | | | | | | |
| 1. Beef | 48 | 28 | 19 | 47 | 44 | 2 | Trace | 1 | – | 47 |
| 2. Buffalo | 66 | 34 | 28 | 30 | 24 | 1 | – | 5 | Trace | 31 |
| 3. Deer | 63 | 24 | 34 | 32 | 24 | 3 | 2 | 3 | Trace | 36 |
| 4. Goat | 57 | 26 | 24 | 37 | 33 | 2 | – | 2 | 2 | 33 |
| 5. Horse | 30 | 24 | 5 | 60 | 30 | 6 | 13 | 11 | 6 | 75 |
| 6. Lamb | 56 | 29 | 25 | 40 | 36 | 3 | 1 | Trace | – | 40 |
| 7. Luncheon meats | 36 | 24 | 11 | 59 | 45 | 7 | Trace | 7 | – | 61 |
| 8. Pork | | | | | | | | | | |
| a. Back, outer layer | 38 | 26 | 12 | 58 | 46 | 6 | – | 6 | – | 64 |

*Reproduced from Home Economics Research Report No. 7.16

## PRACTICAL CONCLUSIONS

A number of important practical conclusions can be derived from these considerations:

1. Nutrition is a matter of kind and amounts of nutrients. Any dietary prescription entails, therefore, the analysis of the present diet in terms of calories and nutrients, the determinations of changes to be effected, and a prescription retranslating the nutritional changes in terms of altered pattern or altered amounts of foods to be consumed by the patient. It is not sufficient to tell the patient to "cut down on fat" or to "eat more protein," etc.; it is absolutely essential also to tell him how much less or how much more of these nutrients he should eat and what particular foods are rich in these nutrients.

2. The analysis of a diet through the use of food composition tables is not a mechanical translation. The significance and limitations of the method (and of the tables) ought to be clearly understood by the person doing the analysis. When great precision is required, as in metabolic studies, only a chemical analysis of an aliquot of the foodstuffs actually consumed will give sufficient accuracy.

3. Many of the methods in current use (use of the 4, 9, 4 coefficients, use of "short" tables, application of digestibility values obtained in adults to children) may entail a fair degree of error. In the majority of circumstances where extreme accuracy is not sought, this is probably not too important; again, however the physician interested in metabolic balances should keep these limitations in mind.

4. The job of analyzing diets and of making precise dietary prescriptions in terms of foods selected, cooked and consumed by the patient not only is a specialized job, but it is also a time-consuming practice. Most physicians have neither the time nor perhaps the training to do this well. It is, therefore, important that a good dietitian or the dietary outpatient department of the local hospital be brought in as often as is necessary to supplement medical advice concerning nutrition. As a medical auxiliary the dietitian is all too often under-utilized by the physician.

5. Finally, it must be remembered that instruction in food

composition tables may be an essential part of the *treatment* of a nutritional disease. For example, understanding and knowledge of the caloric content of various foods are vital to the success of a weight-reduction program. Here again, effective instruction is likely to take more time than the physician can afford to give, and again the help of a dietitian, this time in her capacity as a health educator, must be sought.

## REFERENCES

1. Atwater, W. O.: Discussions of the Terms Digestibility, Availability, and Fuel Value. Twelfth Annual Report, Storrs Agricultural Experiment Station 69, 1899.
2. Maynard, L. A.: The Atwater system of calculating the caloric value of diets. J. Nutrition, 28:443, 1944.
3. McCance, R. A. and Widdowson, E. M.: The Chemical Composition of Foods. Impression 3. London, H. M. Stationery Office, 1942.
4. Committee on Caloric Conversion Factors and Food Composition Tables: Energy-Yielding Components of Food Computation of Caloric Values. Washington, D. C., Nutrition Division, Food and Agriculture Organization, 1947.
5. Chatfield, C.: Food Composition Tables for International Use. Study No. 3. Washington, D. C., Nutrition Division, Food and Agriculture Organization, 1949.
6. Mayer, J. and Scott, M. L.: Nutrition on the international plane. 2. Some scientific problems. Nutrition Rev., 7:324, 1949.
7. Watt, B. K. and Merrill, A. L.: Composition of Foods – Raw, Processed, Prepared. Agriculture Handbook No. 8. Washington, D. C., U. S. Department of Agriculture, 1950.
8. Babcock, M. J.: Simplification of the "Long Method" for Calculating the Nutritional value of Diets. New Jersey Agric. Exper. Sta. Bull. No. 751, June 1950.
9. Hunscher, H. A. and Macy, I. G.: Dietary study methods. 1. Uses and abuses for dietary study methods. J. Am. Dietet. A., 27:558, 1951.
10. Yudkin, J.: Dietary surveys: Variation in the weekly intake of nutrients. Brit. J. Nutrition, 5:177, 1951.
11. Leitch, I. and Aitken, F. C.: Technique and interpretation of dietary surveys. Nutrition Abstr. & Rev., 19:507, 1950.
12. Macy, I. G.: Nutrition and Chemical Growth in Childhood. Vol. 1. Evaluation. Springfield, Illinois, Charles C Thomas, 1942.
13. Keys, A.: Nitrogen Metabolism After Severe Undernutrition. Seventh Annual Protein Conference, Bureau of Biological Research, Rutgers University, New Brunswick, N. J., 1951.

14. Lynch, H. D. and Snively, W. D., Jr.: Hypoproteinosis of childhood. J.A.M.A., 147:115-119 (September), 1951.
15. Orr, M. L. and Watt, B. K.: Amino Acid Content of Foods. Home Economics Research Report No. 4. Washington, D. C., U. S. Department of Agriculture, 1957.
16. Goddard, V. and Goodall, L.: Fatty Acids in Food Fats. Home Economics Research Report No. 7. Washington, D. C., U. S. Department of Agriculture, 1959.

*Chapter 4*

# ALCOHOL AS CALORIES

FROM the beginning of recorded ages, man has been phenomenally imaginative in recognizing sources of fermentable carbohydrates and producing ethanol for internal consumption. Yeasts have been used in this endeavor even in civilizations that did not pursue other nutritionally more advantageous agricultural practices. The nature of the carbohydrate fermented influences the nature of products other than ethanol that are found in the beverage. The higher alcohols (fusel oils) found in many fermented liquors may cause part or all of the hangover syndrome. Over the centuries, ways have been found to eliminate some of the toxic products of alcoholic fermentation.

## BEERS, ALES AND STOUTS

Beers, ales and stouts are made from malted (germinated) barley. The enzyme diastase is killed by heating after some of the starch has been split. The temperature used determines the color of the brews; dark beers and stout contain caramel. The dried malt is ground with water (mash). Hops are added to the water extract (wort), which is then boiled, cooled, and inoculated with yeast. Because most of the yeast in light ales and lagers is at the bottom of the fermenting vat, these beverages have a high carbon dioxide content. Filtering stops the process of fermentation.

The alcoholic content of these brews is 3 to 7 per cent. The caloric equivalent of alcohol is seven calories per gram. Because these products contain residual carbohydrate after fermentation, the caloric content is higher than is indicated by the alcoholic content alone, ranging from 30 calories per 100 ml in mild draught ale or beer to more than 60 calories in strong beer or stout. The

Reprinted from *Postgraduate Medicine, 47* (No. 5), May 1970. ©McGraw-Hill, Inc.

only vitamins present in significant amounts in beer are nicotinic acid and riboflavin.

## NATIVE BEERS AND CIDERS

In various parts of the world, the alcoholic content of beers made from cereals other than barley and from other sources varies from 1 to 7 per cent, and some beer contains significant amounts of water-soluble vitamins. Fermented ciders, commonly consumed in Britain and Normandy, contain 4 to 10 per cent alcohol and about 40 to 100 calories per 100 ml.

## WINES

The enormous diversity of wines in terms of variety of grapes, soils, exposure to sunshine fermenting schedule, aging, etc., has been given a great deal of empirical consideration, but only recently have more analytic methods been used to correlate kinds of wine and physiologic (or pathologic) effects. The alcoholic content of French wines varies from 8.5 to 10 per cent. Most European wines contain 65 to 75 calories per 100 ml; American wines may contain up to 85 or 90 calories.

The fortified wines such as sherry and port have alcohol and sugar added, which may raise the alcoholic content to 20 per cent. The caloric concentration ranges from 110 calories per 100 ml for a dry sherry (15% alcohol) to about 200 calories for a sweet wine such as sherry or port (20% alcohol).

## SPIRITS

Scotch whisky is usually a mixture of malt whisky (the pure malt product) and grain whisky, which is distilled by being heated directly or through superheated steamed, fractionated, and aged in casks. Casks that have contained sherry are preferred. In Great Britain, whisky is almost uniformly 70 proof, which is equivalent to a 30 per cent alcoholic content. Irish whisky is similar; Irish rye is a mixture of rye and malt. Bourbon is made chiefly of corn, with some barley or wheat added. The color was originally obtained from aging in casks that had held molasses. The alcoholic content is often higher in bourbon than in Scotch.

Brandy is distilled from fermented champagne grapes, and rum from fermented molasses. Gin is almost a pure solution of ethanol, prepared from a diversity of sources and flavored after distillation, traditionally with juniper. Vodka, another neutral spirit (pure alcoholic solution), is prepared from fermented potatoes or rye and is unflavored. Calvados is prepared by distilling hard cider, and applejack by separating the water by freezing. All these beverages at 70 proof have a caloric content of about 225 calories per 100 ml. Sweet liqueurs, which are high in sugar as well as in alcoholic content, have higher caloric equivalents.

## UTILIZATION OF ALCOHOL

Alcohol is a source of calories, and often a major source in alcoholics. For social drinkers who have a tendency to gain weight, the one or two daily cocktails may make the difference between success and failure of a weight-control program.

Ethanol, when combusted in a calorimetric bomb, yields 7.1 calories per gram. The caloric equivalent is the same for a man, provided the alcohol is actually oxidized. The rate of oxidation in

CALORIC CONTENT OF ALCOHOLIC BEVERAGES

| Beverage | Quantity (Oz) | Calories |
| --- | --- | --- |
| Beer | 12 | 150 |
| Rum | 1.5 | 150 |
| Whisky | 1.5 | 110 |
| Grasshopper | 2 | 200 |
| Manhattan | 2 | 160 |
| Martini | 2 | 160 |
| Old-fashioned | 2 | 170 |
| Whisky sour | 2 | 140 |
| Liqueur | 1 | 100 |
| Wine, dry (20%)* | 4 | 160 |
| Wine, light dry (12%)* | 4 | 100 |
| Wine, sweet (20%)* | 4 | 180 |

*Alcoholic content.

the human body is about 100 mg per kilogram per hour (8 gm or 56 calories for a 175 lb man), but varies from 60 to 200 mg per kilogram per hour. The kidney cannot concentrate alcohol, and losses through the lungs and kidneys depend on the alcoholic concentration in the blood. When the concentration is 100 mg per 100 ml (a level at which symptoms of intoxication are usually seen), no more than 5 per cent of alcohol is eliminated in the breath and urine.

## CALORIES FROM ALCOHOL

Atwater and Benedict were the first to show, in 1902, that alcohol can substitute as a source of calories for carbohydrate or fat and can provide up to 65 per cent of the basal calories. This amount cannot be increased by exposure to cold or exercise. The alcohol oxidation rate of 8 gm per hour in a 175-lb man is the equivalent of 1,350 calories in 24 hours. This is equivalent to 2.4 liters of wine, 8.5 pts of beer, or 20 oz of spirits. This variation in range means that some persons cannot oxidize more than 1 liter of wine daily. Although Trémolières, the French nutritionist, reported in 1960 that preoxidase activity in the blood of some chronic alcoholics enables them to eliminate a greater amount of alcohol, it is reasonable to assume that for persons who are not long-term alcoholics, seven calories per gram of alcohol is applicable.

From a nutritional viewpoint, it is worth remembering that with the exception of small amounts of B vitamins and traces of minerals in wine and beer, alcoholic beverages contain an appreciable number of calories and no nutrients. Thus these beverages are the prototype of "empty calories" and are best avoided by those on reducing diets. The idea that calories in alcohol are not fattening has no basis in theory or fact.

*Chapter 5*

# FAMINE

$D$URING our lifetime, millions of men, women and children have died of starvation in great famines in Asia, Europe, Africa and Latin America. Yet so little is ordinarily taught of the physiologic, psychologic and social problems of mass starvation and of their solutions that each new group of physicians and administrators called on to deal with a catastophic situation tends to repeat some of the classic errors of omission and commission. Since more and more of our young physicians are going into the Peace Corps and other technical assistance activities and hundreds more in the Armed Forces are being sent to Vietnam and other trouble spots, a review of what famine is and of what should be done about it seems particularly timely.

## CAUSES

Most recorded famines have been caused by widespread failure of crops due to lack of water (droughts often·followed by dust storms and loss of seeds); various types of diseases (such as fungous blights) or pests (such as locusts); disruption of farming operations due to wars and civil disturbances; or large-scale natural disturbances affecting both crops and farmers (such as floods and earthquakes).

A melancholy testimonial to the frequency of famines recorded up to 1950 appeared in Keys, Brozek and associates' famous book on starvation (1). Since 1950 famines have occurred in India (floods, droughts), in the Middle East (locusts, earthquake), and in Africa (droughts, Congolese civil war).

The four primary causes of famine are still operative and, unfortunately, it is reasonable to expect more famines. For

Reprinted from *Postgraduate Medicine, 38* (No. 5):A-117 t0 A-122, November, 1965.

example, if we examine the first and most frequent cause of crop failure, drought, we may note that there are areas of many square miles in Africa, South America, India and China (and even in North America and Australia) where rains fail periodically. At such times, rainfall may be 80 per cent less than the secular average. By contrast, in Western Europe and usually in New England, a dry year differs from a wet year by less that 20 per cent. Often years of drought alternate with years of flood in which gigantic continental rivers, swollen by excessive rains in the mountains where they originate, burst their banks and destroy all crops.

In many areas of periodic failure of precipitation, erosion has made the situation worse. The Middle East and North Africa are good examples. During the centuries from the dawn of civilization to the end of the Roman Empire, thousands of small and medium-sized dams were built in that vast area which, together with Sicily, was the granary of Rome. With the decay of the Empire, in the course of the great Arab invasion and finally through the ravages of Tamerlane, the dams were destroyed and the irrigation canals abandoned, and the desert now covers what once were some of the great cities of the world. Cyrene and Darius are now but mounds of sand, and the second largest theater in the Roman Empire stands in the Libyan desert as a reminder of how drought, erosion and famine can destroy seemingly permanent civilization.

Whatever the primary natural cause of famine, it is made worse by lack of communication and by social inequality. Certain areas like that bordering the Sahara to the south or the Altiplane of Bolivia are particularly vulnerable to the former. All poor countries are examples of the latter. It may be useful to point out that in as rich a country as England in 1935, with an average daily intake of 3000 calories, at least 10 per cent of the population received insufficient calories, and the diet of 40 per cent of the population was demonstrably too low in certain vitamins. Obviously in a poor country like Egypt, where biblical farming methods can be seen in operation five miles from the modern capital of Cairo, social inequalities are even more acute.

Finally, it is obvious that a country like Vietnam, where farmers are conscripted by both sides into military or labor organizations, where casualties among such farmers are very high, and where villagers are evacuated as a result of terrorism, scorched-earth policies, or for strategic reasons, famine is a constant risk in many areas in spite of the wealth of the land. Poor communications, insecurity of transportation, administrative chaos and profiteering may rapidly make a bad situation much worse.

## PHYSIOLOGIC AND PSYCHOLOGIC EFFECTS

The first and most obvious effect of starvation is the wasting of fat deposits; both the subcutaneous adipose tissue and the deeper fat pads are affected. (A skin-fold caliper is a useful instrument in a famine situation to gauge the extent of the depletion of adipose tissue.) Abdominal and thoracic viscera are affected next; even the size of the liver is drastically diminished. The intestinal mucosa is thin and smooth; it loses some of its absorptive capacity and diarrhea results. Achlorhydria is generally present, and the heart shows a "brown atrophy" characteristic of starvation. Blood pressure falls; in some cases the systolic pressure becomes difficult to estimate and the diastolic pressure may be as low as 75 mm Hg. The pulse rate may fall below 40 per minute.

"Famine edema" generally occurs since the amount of extra-cellular water does not decrease correspondingly as body weight decreases. Causes of famine edema are not yet clearly understood. They may include a disruption of osmotic tension in blood (plasma albumin is generally, although not invariably, decreased); a fall in tissue and interstitial tension, due in turn perhaps to lack of elasticity of the skin, which becomes too big for its content; renal disturbances such as nocturnal polyuria; and endocrine disorders (failure of hormone production and, conversely, deficient inactivation by the liver of estrogens and antidiuretic hormone).

Early effects of starvation are amenorrhea in women and impotence and loss of libido in men. Gynecomastia occurs in young males. Hair is dull and staring and, in children, abnormal lanugo hair grows on the forewarms and the back. The skin acquires the consistency of paper; it is dull, gray and inelastic and not infrequently shows the irreversible dusty brown splotches which are permanent stigmata of starvation. In extreme cases, cancrumoris destroys the lips and parts of the cheeks.

The psychologic state deteriorates rapidly. The individual becomes obsessed with food, mentally restless, physically apathetic, and self-centered to varying degrees. Extremes of behavior are murder and cannibalism.

Decreased calorie requirements due to a decrease in body weight, basal metabolic rate and activity may eventually cause a plateauing of body weight. A precarious equilibrium may thus be created which can endure for several weeks or even months. The terminal events include intractable diarrhea, generally infectious in origin but caused by the intestine's becoming essentially nonfunctional. Cardiovascular collapse can also occur, and infections take their toll of weakened organisms. In infants progressive starvation is essentially similar to marasmus (2).

## SOCIAL EFFECTS

Obviously the main and most immediate effect of a famine is, by definition, widespread deaths from starvation. The number of people dying from starvation is a good index of the severity of the famine. Conversely, the drop in such a number is an index of the effectiveness of the measures employed in combating the famine. It has been repeatedly observed that in famines old persons and young children die first and that women and adolescents tend to survive better than men, although adolescents exposed to prolonged undernutrition are particularly susceptible to tuberculosis.

A second dangerous consequence of famine is the state of social disruption — including large-scale panic — which often accompanies it. People who are starving at home tend to leave if they can and march toward the area where it is rumored that food is available. This increases the prevailing chaos; families are separated and children are lost. Adolescents, finding themselves on their own, band together in foraging gangs which create additional disruption. The prolonged and successful practice of banditry makes it difficult to rehabilitate members of these gangs.

These social disruptions complicate institution of any relief measure. Contrary to a prevalent belief, famines and, for that matter, prolonged severe undernutrition are rarely accompanied by revolution. Severely underfed individuals usually are too feeble and too preoccupied with problems of immediate survival to display the energy, single-mindedness and organization necessary to mount a revolution. Disruption accompanying famine is more likely to entail a large number of unconnected antisocial acts or, at most, regional jacqueries. In turn, revolutions are more likely to take place when food has again been available for some time, but while the memory of actual or supposed governmental corruption or incompetence in dealing with the famine is still fresh.

Finally, a third common catastrophic result of famine is the spead of epidemics. The combination of physiologically weakened human organisms and a disrupted social organism, with the attendant crowding and breakdown of public health installations, lends itself to the explosive spread of infectious diseases. Traditionally, louse-borne typhus has been the great postfamine disease in Europe, and cholera and smallpox the postfamine diseases in Asia, although many other diseases, e.g. plague, influenza, tuberculosis, relapsing fever, etc., have also followed famine. When famine is due to drought, malaria is not usually rampant at the same time, but it is often deadly on a particularly large scale when the rains finally come.

## FAMINE RELIEF

An administrator's most immediate problem in a famine is to gain a clear picture of the situation. With much of society's structure broken down, with rumors flying – and antigovernment sources exaggerating the extent of the catastrophe – it is often difficult to know where the most pressing needs are and the scale of the need. Certification of causes of death may be incomplete and late. The most enfeebled persons – children and old people – may be staying indoors so that the casual observer seeing only ambulatory adolescents and young adults may not realize the scope of the disaster.

All administrative, medical and social agencies must be used to gather and check statistical information. Hospitals and other health agencies must be asked to report causes of death as fast as possible so that any increase in the number of deaths due to starvation and any deaths from epidemic infections can be detected early.

The basis of relief is to obtain and make available sufficient food to stop the developing famine, maintain the population in balance, and eventually rehabilitate it. Table 5-1, adapted from an excellent essay on famine by Passmore and Davidson (3) to which I acknowledge my indebtedness for a number of ideas expressed in this paper, gives reasonable suggestions for the caloric rations permitting emergency subsistence, temporary maintenance, and the generally agreed order of magnitude for the ideal allowances.

Food must not only be purchased – or otherwise acquired on a goverment level – but also be transported, kept safe and distributed. Despite efforts by some of the leaders of the Food and Agricultural Organization such as John Boyd Orr and André

TABLE 5-1

CALORIC ALLOWANCES IN FAMINE AREA

| Age, Sex and Occupation | Emergency Subsistence* (Calories) | Temporary Maintenance† (Calories) |
|---|---|---|
| 0 to 2 Years | 1000 | 1000 |
| 3 to 5 Years | 1250 | 1500 |
| 6 to 9 Years | 1500 | 1750 |
| 10 to 17 Years | 2000 | 2500 |
| Pregnant and nursing women | 2000 | 2500 |
| Normal consumers (sedentary) | | |
| Male | 1900 | 2200 |
| Female | 1600 | 1800 |
| Moderate labor | 2000 | 2500 |
| Heavy labor | 2500 | 3000 |
| Very heavy labor | 3000 | 3500 |

*This allowance would arrest the downward progress of undernutrition leading to social disintegration and mass deaths.
†This allowance would not permit rapid recovery but would maintain the population in a reasonable state of health and permit slow recovery.

Mayer in the late 1940's, a world food bank or regional food banks for emergency situations have not yet come into existence. While there is thus no universal and automatic pathway for famine relief, the continued availability of large surpluses of cereals in the United States, Canada, France and other countries makes relief possible. Yet, in spite of the creation of such national organizations as Food For Peace in the United States, the actual process of relief is often slow and cumbersome.

In the past, available foods have been distributed through various methods. In the nineteenth century and the first half of this one, attempts were made to improve a situation indirectly by supplying money to the starving populace through public health works projects. Food was conveyed to the merchants through the normal channels of trade. This policy, consistent with Adam Smith's laissez-faire philosophy, has had a moderate degree of success in local foreseen shortages, but it has failed miserably in large-scale disasters such as the potato famine in Ireland and the Bengal famine during World War II. Such a plan helps least those groups who are most vulnerable — the very young and the very old. It increases the energy expenditure of men involved in the public works not only through the caloric cost of manual labor but also because such works — usually road building — are at some distance from a worker's domicile. The work is rarely useful; the roads lead "from nowhere in particular to nowhere in general," since important public roads and other projects require careful planning and can rarely be devised and executed properly on the spur of the moment.

In practice, public kitchens and distribution of commodities have proved most valuable, particularly if care is taken to allow food to be doled out under supervised conditions to persons too enfeebled to leave home.

Price control is essential in any famine situation. It must be vigorously enforced. Otherwise, high prices discriminate against the persons most in need. Furthermore, price inflation may tempt traders to withhold food that could end a famine in the hope of perpetuating high prices.

The creation of small famine hospitals in large numbers, even though they may be staffed only with auxiliary personnel and medical students, has proved to be invaluable in checking panic, vaccinating, delousing, disinfecting, distributing insecticides, informing the administration, and taking care of the greater number of starving sick persons. The existence of a large but distant hospital is an invitation to migration and makes relief more difficult. The utmost attention must be given to prevent and check epidemics.

Finally, law and order must be maintained to prevent looting and other abuses. This often means that the police units must be given preferential treatment in regard to food distribution.

## TREATMENT OF STARVATION

Any available, acceptable food is suitable in the treatment of starvation in cases in which diarrhea has not yet begun, although bland foods and skim milk, preferably in small amounts, should be given during the first few days. If these foods are taken well, the patient can progressively be allowed to eat as much as he wants. Intakes above 5000 calories per day with gains of more than 4 lb a week with no apparent ill effects have often been recorded.

If the patient is very enfeebled and particularly if diarrhea is present, bland foods are essential. Skim milk is an ideal element of such a diet. Administering frequent small feedings of 100 ml at a time is a safe and effective way to use skim milk. Skim milk powders are usually reconstituted to a 10 to 15 per cent strength.

Premature use of such foods as canned meat and baked beans was responsible for the death of many World War II concentration camp inmates at their liberation. Fruit juices and glucose should be avoided since they often cause intense discomfort. Slightly sour foods such as yogurt and other curdled milks are usually well accepted and form a good intermediary between reconstituted skim milk and semisolid foods. If edema becomes worse with refeeding, salt should be restricted as much as possible with foods at hand.

If appetite remains poor in spite of the availability of food, and particularly if low blood pressure and diarrhea persist, the prognosis is not good. Intragastric or intravenous feeding must then be administered. Although success does occur and may be spectacular, it is not frequent. It is important to remember also that many treatments and drugs such as anthelmintic agents, which are relatively harmless in normal patients, may be "the straw that breaks the camel's back" in a starving individual.

## REFERENCES

1. Keys, A., Brozek, J., Henschel, A., Michelsen, O. and Taylor, H. L.: The Biology of Human Starvation. Minneapolis, University of Minnesota Press, 1950.
2. Mayer, J.: Kwashiorkor. Postgrad. Med., 26:24, 1959.
3. Passmore R. and Davidson, S.: Human Nutrition and Dietetics. Baltimore, The Williams & Wilkins Company, 1963, p. 757.

# PART II

## Protein, Vitamins, Minerals: Needs for Nutrients

## Chapter 6

# AMINO ACID REQUIREMENTS OF MAN

THE physician practicing in the United States is rarely confronted with a case of protein deficiency (1). In fact, most American adults are subsisting on diets providing two to five times the minimal requirements for protein. In growing children, the margin of safety is by no means as great. There is little evidence, however, that even in children protein shortage is common in America, as is claimed by some authors (2). Probably the only large groups in danger of being deficient in protein, as well as in calories and various nutrients, are young women and adolescent girls who place themselves on faddish reducing diets and attempt to lose weight without much justification and at an excessive rate.

Yet, at the same time, the problem of amino acid requirements is of relevance to the practicing physician. This is due to the fact that an increasing number of foods are fortified with amino acids or are sold to the public on the basis of their "high protein" value. In addition, administration of certain amino acids, such as methionine and glutamic acid, has been advocated in certain pathologic conditions. Actually, requirements for amino acids are quite different from requirements for vitamins and minerals. Essentially, minimal amounts of the latter must be provided to avoid disease or to insure optimum performance, no matter what the rest of the diet may include. Granted, there is some relationship between these minimums and the composition of the diet. For example, a high carbohydrate diet increases the requirement for thiamine. A high protein diet decreases the requirement for nicotinic acid; the availability of a large amount of antioxidants (e.g. vitamin E) in the diet spares vitamin A, etc. Nevertheless, minimal requirements for such nutrients can be

Reprinted from *Postgraduate Medicine, 26* (No. 2), August, 1959.

stated in tables of recommended dietary allowances (3) in terms of so many milligrams or grams per day without detailed reference to dietary composition.

The situation is quite different in regard to amino acids. While early work (4) stated daily amino acid requirements in terms of a minimum (in milligrams per day, sometimes multiplied by two to provide for a margin of safety and to yield an optimum daily requirement), it has come to be realized (5) that such an approach was erroneous. When no less than the minimum or the optimum of a given amino acid has been administered, it is still possible to throw the subject into negative nitrogen balance by administering relative excesses of other essential amino acids. In other words, we are dealing with the need for a "pattern" of essential amino acids. (For that matter, the pattern of nonessential amino acids also may exert some influence.) There is thus no contradiction between the statement that the protein intake of most Americans is much higher than is required and the statement that the problem of amino acid requirements may be of clinical importance even in the United States.

## THE CONCEPT OF ESSENTIAL AMINO ACIDS

The concept of essentiality of amino acids, i.e. the fact that there are amino acids which the body cannot synthesize and which therefore must be provided by the diet, dates back to the demonstration by Willcock and Hopkins in 1906 that rats cannot grow on a diet devoid of tryptophan. Two other pioneers, Osborn and Mendel, working at Yale, demonstrated that the amino acid composition of proteins determines their biologic value, i.e. their value as a source of protein for growth of experimental animals. It is, however, to Rose (4) that we are indebted for a clear and detailed knowledge of indispensable amino acids. He perfected a technic of substituting purified amino acids for protein in the diets of experimental animals and testing, by omitting one amino acid at a time, whether growth stopped and maintenance became impossible, the amino acid was indispensable for maintaining the adult state as well. The work was held up for a number of years by the finding that no known mixture of synthetic amino acids could replace a casein hydrolysate for the growth of rats. Finally, in 1934, this baffling situation was cleared up by the isolation in pure form of a missing amino acid, threonine (6). Considerable work over the years led to the demonstration that certain amino acids could be classified as essential and nonessential for the rat (Table 6-1) (7).

## ESSENTIAL AMINO ACIDS IN MAN

Rose and associates (4, 8, 9) attacked the problem of amino acid requirements in adult man by using mixtures of pure acids as the source of nitrogen in diets. As in the animal studies conducted by Rose, one or more of the amino acids were omitted. The maintenance of nitrogen balance was used as the criterion of essentiality of amino acids. It was thus shown that valine, methionine, threonine, leucine, isoleucine, phenylalanine, tryptophan and lysine are essential. The removal of histidine and

TABLE 6-1

CLASSIFICATION OF THE AMINO ACIDS WITH RESPECT
TO GROWTH EFFECT IN THE RAT

| Essential | Nonessential |
|---|---|
| Lysine | Glycine |
| Tryptophan | Alanine |
| Histidine | Serine |
| Phenylalanine | Cystine† |
| Leucine | Tyrosine‡ |
| Isoleucine | Aspartic acid |
| Threonine | Glutamic acid |
| Methionine | Proline |
| Valine | Hydroxyproline |
| Arginine* | Citrulline |

*Arginine can be synthesized by the rat but not at a rate sufficient to fulfill the requirements for maximal growth. It is thus really in an intermediary status and can be classified either as essential or as nonessential, depending on definition.
†Cystine can replace about one-sixth of the methionine. It has no growth effect in the absence of methionine.
‡Tyrosine can replace about one-half the phenylalanine. It has no growth effect in the absence of phenylalanine.

of arginine did not lead to negative nitrogen balance. It thus appears that these two amino acids are not essential in adult man. The problem of elucidating the nature and the daily need of essential amino acids in infants was undertaken by Holt and Snyderman (10). Many groups of investigators (11-14) have studied this problem in women. In spite of the existence of a considerable body of information thus available, the following limitations to our knowledge must be recognized.

1. The number of subjects used in each experiment, whether adult men or women or infants, was necessarily small. We have thus only limited knowledge of the extent of individual variability in amino acid requirements in man. Data on amino acid excretion suggest that this variability may be appreciable.

2. We have no experimental data on requirements between infancy and adulthood. In particular, we do not know whether the prepuberty growth spurt is accompanied by any qualiative changes in amino acid requirements, an unlikely but by no means impossible eventuality.

3. No explanation is available for the fact that when essential amino acids were fed as pure substances in experiments to determine the amounts required in the diet, it was necessary to provide calories far in excess of normal requirements to obtain nitrogen balance. This was particularly true in Rose's experiments in adult men.

4. The interrelationship among amino acids is such that requirements for one are influenced by intakes of others. The minimal values obtained when one amino acid is dropped from the mixture fed the subject and its intake gradually built up until nitrogen balance is reached are of necessity a function of the intake of the other essential amino acids. For example, while it has been generally thought that imbalance among amino acids was unlikely to occur when only natural foods were ingested, it has been recently shown (15) that the amount of leucine in corn may be large enough to increase the requirements for isoleucine.

5. The human requirements for amino acids are obviously influenced by a number of additional factors, such as the caloric value of the diet, the sparing of protein by carbohydrate and fat, and the timing of the intake of foods containing proteins.

6. The experiments mentioned were carried out under experimental conditions designed to spare the essential amino acids from the need to contribute to the synthesis of the nonessential amino acids. Unless the latter are in ample supply, the need for essential amino acids will be increased. For example, under experimental conditions in which low levels of protein intake are obtained from milk, certain nonessential forms of nitrogen are limiting, and the need to synthesize these creates a demand beyond the minimal requirements (10). Generally speaking, in man as in experimental animals, the pattern as well as the amount of nonessential amino acids may be of importance.

7. Finally, in man as well as in experimental animals, the ability of the nonessential amino acids cystine and tyrosine to spare, respectively, much of the required methionine and phenylalanine is of revelance in determining requirements for these two essential amino acids.

## THE FAO PROVISIONAL PATTERN OF HUMAN AMINO ACID REQUIREMENTS

The international committee which met in 1955 in Rome under the auspices of the Food and Agriculture Organization of the United Nations to draw practical recommendations concerning protein requirements was struck by the fact that while the amounts of essential amino acids found by various investigators to be needed by men, women and infants varied considerably (Table 6-2) the pattern of requirements for each amino acid in relation to the others was much more constant. In particular, we noted that if the amount of tryptophan, for example, found to be required in the experiments cited was taken as a unit and the proportion of other amino acids given in Table 6-2 was recalculated to give the pattern shown in Table 6-3, the variability was not simply an artifact of presentation. This is confirmed by the repeated demonstrations of the interrelationship between requirements for the various amino acids. Another indication of the value of this approach is the remarkable similarity between patterns of human requirements and the patterns of essential amino acids in the proteins of high biologic value (eggs, meat, milk, etc.), i.e. those

TABLE 6-2

AVERAGE MINIMAL REQUIREMENTS FOR ESSENTIAL AMINO ACIDS[5]

Average Minimal Needs
(Milligrams per kilogram of body weight)

| Subjects | Isoleucine | Leucine | Lysine | Phenyl-alanine | Sulfur-containing acids | | | Threonine | Tryptophan | Valine |
|---|---|---|---|---|---|---|---|---|---|---|
| | | | | | Methionine | Cystine | Total | | | |
| Men | 10.4 | 9.9 | 8.8 | 4.3* | 1.5 | 11.6 | 13.1 | 6.5 | 2.9 | 8.8 |
| | | | | 13.3† | 13.2 | 0 | 13.2 | | | |
| Women | 5.2 | 7.1 | 3.3 | 3.1‡ | 4.7 | 0.5 | 5.2 | 3.5 | 2.1 | 9.2 |
| | | | | | 3.8 | (2.2) | 6.0 | | | |
| | | | | | 3.4 | 3.4 | 6.8 | | | |
| | | | | | 3.0 | (4.2) | 7.2 | | | |
| Infants | 90 | – | 90 | 90§ | 85 | 0 | 85 | 60 | 30 | 85 |
| | | | | | 65 | Present | – | | | |

*15.9 mg tyrosine per kilogram; ratio of tyrosine to tryptophan equals 5.5.
†No tyrosine.
‡15.6 mg tyrosine per kilogram; ratio of tyrosine to tryptophan equals 7.4.
§Tyrosine present.

TABLE 6-3

PATTERN OF ESSENTIAL AMINO ACIDS WHEN REQUIREMENTS ARE EXPRESSED IN RELATION TO TRYPTOPHAN5

Amino Acid Requirements
(Milligrams per kilogram of body weight)

| Subjects | Isoleucine | Leucine | Lysine | Phenyl-alanine | Sulfur-containing acids | | | Threonine | Tryptophan | Valine |
|---|---|---|---|---|---|---|---|---|---|---|
| | | | | | Methionine | Cystine | Total | | | |
| Men | 3.6 | 3.4 | 3.0 | (1.5* <br> (4.6† | 0.5 <br> 4.6 | 4.0 <br> 0 | 4.5) <br> 4.6) | 2.2 | 1.0 | 3.0 |
| Women | 2.5 | 3.3 | 1.6 | 1.5‡ | (2.2 <br> (1.8 <br> (1.6 <br> (1.4 | 0.3 <br> [1.0] <br> 1.7 <br> 2.0 | 2.5) <br> 2.8) <br> 3.3) <br> 3.4) | 1.7 | 1.0 | 4.4 |
| Infants | 3.0 | – | 3.0 | 3.0§ | (2.8 | 0 | 2.8) | 2.0 | 1.0 | 2.8 |
| Provisional Pattern | 3.0 | 3.4 | 3.0 | 2.0 | 1.6 | 1.4 | 3.0 | 2.0 | 1.0 | 3.0 |

*15.9 mg tyrosine per kilogram; ratio of tyrosine to tryptophan equals 5.5.
†No tyrosine.
‡15.6 mg, tyrosine per kilogram; ratio of tyrosine to tryptophan equals 7.4
§Tyrosine present.
Assumes about 5.0 mg per kilogram of tyrosine; ratio of tyrosine to tryptophan equals about 2.0.

proteins found to be the most efficient at fulfilling human requirements.

It thus appeared reasonable to the members of the FAO committee to express amino acid requirements in terms of an ideal proportion of essential amino acids, using their collective judgment to evolve such a provisional pattern on the basis of results of determinations of amino acid requirements in man. Table 6-4 describes this provisional pattern in terms of grams of the essential amino acids per 100 gm of protein and of milligrams of essential amino acids per gram of nitrogen. In both cases, a balance between essential and nonessential amino acids in the total protein has been arrived at by determining arbitrarily that the proportion of tryptophan is the same for the protein corresponding to the provisional pattern as it is for cow's milk. Table 6-4 also gives, in addition to the proportions of essential amino acids in the provisional pattern and in cow's milk, the proportions in human milk and eggs, two other superior sources of protein. It is readily seen that the relative requirements estimated by the FAO committee were somewhat below the proportion of essential amino acids in human milk and eggs. The relative need for sulfur-containing amino acids was judged to be somewhat higher than their relative content in cow's milk.

## PRACTICAL APPLICATIONS OF THESE CONCEPTS

The provisional amino acid pattern is being used by FAO and other international agencies concerned with the feeding of populations as a guide for supplementing protein-poor diets. For example, Table 6-5 was used by the FAO committee to show how the pattern can be utilized to plan supplementation of an all-vegetable diet. If 80 per cent of the protein of the diet is provided by corn and 20 per cent by navy beans, the diet is markedly deficient in tryptophan and somewhat deficient in sulfur-containing amino acids and lysine. Increasing the proportion of beans improves the lysine content but does little to increase tryptophan and reduce the sulfur-containing amino acids. If sesame seed is added, however, the pattern is considerably improved. The lysine and sulfur-containing amino acids contents

TABLE 6-4

ESSENTIAL AMINO ACIDS IN PROVISIONAL PATTERN AND MILK AND EGG PROTEINS[5]

| Amino Acids | Provisional Pattern | | Cow's Milk | | Human Milk | | Egg | |
|---|---|---|---|---|---|---|---|---|
| | Per 100 gm protein | Mg per gm nitrogen | Per 100 gm protein | Mg per gm nitrogen | Per 100 gm protein | Mg per gm nitrogen | Per 100 gm protein | Mg per gm nitrogen |
| Isoleucine | 4.2 | 270 | 6.4 | 407 | 6.4 | 411 | 6.8 | 428 |
| Leucine | 4.8 | 306 | 9.9 | 630 | 8.9 | 572 | 9.0 | 565 |
| Lysine | 4.2 | 270 | 7.8 | 496 | 6.3 | 402 | 6.3 | 396 |
| Phenylalanine | 2.8 | 180 | 4.9 | 311 | 4.6 | 297 | 6.0 | 368 |
| Tyrosine | 2.8 | 180 | 5.1 | 323 | 5.5 | 355 | 4.4 | 274 |
| Sulfur-containing acids | | | | | | | | |
| Total | 4.2 | 270 | 3.3 | 211 | 4.3 | 274 | 5.4 | 342 |
| Methionine | 2.2 | 144 | 2.4 | 154 | 2.2 | 140 | 3.1 | 196 |
| Threonine | 2.8 | 180 | 4.6 | 292 | 4.6 | 290 | 5.0 | 310 |
| Tryptophan | 1.4 | 90 | 1.4 | 90 | 1.6 | 106 | 1.7 | 106 |
| Valine | 4.2 | 270 | 6.9 | 440 | 6.6 | 420 | 7.4 | 460 |

## TABLE 6-5

### AMINO ACID PATTERN AS A GUIDE TO SUPPLEMENTATION[5]

| Amino Acid | Provisional Pattern | Corn Protein | | Navy Bean Protein | | Sesame Seed Protein | | 80% Corn Protein + 20% Navy Bean Protein | | 50% Corn Protein + 50% Navy Bean Protein | | 40% Corn Protein + 30% Navy Bean Protein + 30% Sesame Protein | |
|---|---|---|---|---|---|---|---|---|---|---|---|---|---|
| | | Quantity | Per cent | Quantity | Per cent | Quantity | Per cent | Quantity | Per cent | Quantity | Per cent | Quantity | Per cent |
| Isoleucine | 270 | 293 | | 358 | | 300 | | 306 | | 325 | | 315 | |
| Leucine | 306 | 827 | | 541 | | 500 | | 770 | | 684 | | 643 | |
| Lysine | 270 | 179 | 66 | 460 | | 159 | 59 | 235 | 87 | 320 | | 257 | 95 |
| Phenylalanine | 180 | 284 | | 347 | | 460 | | 297 | | 316 | | 356 | |
| Tyrosine | 180 | 385 | | 245 | | 244 | | 357 | | 316 | | 301 | |
| Sulfur-containing acids | | | | | | | | | | | | | |
| Total | 270 | 197 | 73 | 126 | 47 | 317 | | 183 | 68 | 162 | 60 | 212 | 79 |
| Methionine | 144 | 117 | 81 | 64 | 44 | 181 | | 106 | 74 | 91 | 63 | 120 | 83 |
| Threonine | 180 | 249 | | 274 | | 182 | | 254 | | 262 | | 236 | |
| Tryptophan | 90 | 38 | 42 | 58 | 64 | 93 | | 42 | 47 | 48 | 53 | 60 | 67 |
| Valine | 270 | 327 | | 379 | | 216 | 80 | 337 | | 353 | | 309 | |

Quantities are given as milligrams of amino acids per gram of nitrogen; also shown are the percentages by which the individual foods and mixtures of these foods fail to meet the levels of amino acids in the provisional pattern.

are satisfactory by then, and the tryptophan content is considerably increased. In practice, before such supplementations are recommended on a mass basis, the results of such calculations should be tested by determinations of the resultant biologic value in experimental animals and, if possible, in human subjects.

The United States Department of Agriculture (16) has compiled tables giving the amino acid content of foods. These were established for 316 items and expressed in amino acids per gram of total nitrogen in edible proteins of foods and in amino acid content per 100 gm of edible protein. The amino acids determined were: tryptophan, threonine, isoleucine, leucine, lysine, methionine, cystine, phenylalanine, tyrosine, valine, arginine, histidine, alanine, aspartic acid, glutamic acid, glycine, proline and serine. The tables give the values found for the maximal, minimal and average contents in samples of each item.

The Commonwealth Bureau of Animal Nutrition (Great Britain) (17) also published a compilation of amino acid contents of foods and foodstuffs. The availability of such tables makes it possible to calculate the protein score of a given foodstuff or diet. This protein score is the percentage of relative requirement furnished by the food material for the amino acid found to be most deficient in that particular food or diet when compared with the provisional pattern. In other words, the protein score measures the extent to which a food or food combination supplies the limiting amino acid as compared with the provisional pattern. For example, in Table 6-5, navy beans are seen to contain 126 mg of sulfur-containing amino acids per gram of nitrogen, while the provisional pattern provides 270 mg per gram of nitrogen. The protein score for navy beans is therefore $126/270 \times 100 = 47$. Actually, biologic values of 46 have been reported for navy beans with human test subjects. That such precise concordance cannot be expected for each food is due to the inaccuracy of our knowledge of the amino acid requirements in man and of the amino acid composition of foods and to the partial unavailability of amino acids in certain poorly digested foods. Results are good enough to suggest, as a rough guide, that foods and food mixtures with a protein score or a biologic value of 60 or less are unsatisfactory for growth and maintenance, and that a protein score of 70 or more is required for growth.

In the United States, the chances are small that any adult who is receiving a calorically adequate diet could be deficient in protein or in specific amino acids. Certain groups, however, are vulnerable: chronic alcoholics, who receive much of their caloric intake from alcohol and are thus on a low vitamin, low mineral and low protein diet; aged persons who are poor and live alone, some living on a simplified diet of bread and tea; and, as mentioned previously, young women and adolescent girls on faddish reducing diets, some of which have entailed subsisting on a protein intake as low as 15 or 20 gm a day. Children of various ages who, due to economic circumstances and lack of proper supervision, may elect to subsist on such foodstuffs as dry cereal and pop are another vulnerable group. As a result, such groups not only are on low protein diets but also are generally on diets of low protein quality. An example of imbalanced amino acid composition is found in corn protein, which is notoriously low in lysine and tryptophan and too high in isoleucine. The heat treatment to which corn is submitted in the production of breakfast cereals further lowers the lysine content. The fact that the combination of corn cereals and milk has an acceptable protein value is of little help in the case of small children who eat such cereals by the handful and who either do not drink milk or drink it at an altogether different period of the day. Only children with an otherwise quite deficient diet are likely to be seriously injured by such practices.

The fact that, small as they may be, there are groups of people even in this country who may be adversely affected by an unfavorable amino acid balance makes it not unreasonable to consider enriching deficient foodstuffs with synthetic amino acids; in any case we should use the mutually supplementary effect of proteins of different sources to achieve a balanced amino acid ration at each meal. There may well be situations in poor countries where supplementation of the staple foods with synthetic amino acids (e.g. corn with lysine) would be a useful short-term solution. On the other hand, at least so far, the use of large amounts of single amino acids as a nutritional adjunct in certain diseases has not proved of any value. Specific examples of such failures are the use of methionine in cirrhosis (18) and of glutamic acid in mental retardation (19). Whether certain single amino acids turn out to be of use as pharmacologic agents in acute conditions, e.g. cystine in recovery from irradiation (20) or glutamic acid (21) and arginine (22, 23) in lowering ammonia in the blood in acute hepatic requires further evaluation.

## REFERENCES

1. Mayer J.: Kwashiorkor. Postgrad. Med., 26:98 (July) 1959.
2. Lynch, H. D. and Snively, W. D., Jr.: Hypoproteinosis in childhood. J.A.M.A., 147:115, 1951.
3. Food and Nutrition Board, National Research Council: Recommended Dietary Allowances. Publication 589. Washington D. C., National Academy of Sciences, 1958.
4. Rose, W. C.: Amino acid requirements of man. Fed. Proc., 8:546, 1949.
5. Committee, Food and Agriculture Organization of the United Nations, Rome, Italy, 1957: Protein Requirements. FAO Nutritional Studies No. 16. New York, Columbia University Press International Documents Service, 1957.
6. McCoy, R. H., Mayer, C. E. and Rose, W. C.: Feeding experiments with mixtures of highly purified amino acids. J. Biol. Chem., 112:283, 1935.
7. Rose, W. C., Oesterling, M. J. and Womack, M.: Comparative growth on diets containing ten and nineteen amino acids with further observations upon the role of glutamic and aspartic acids. J. Biol. Chem., 176:753, 1948.
8. Rose, W. C., Wixom, R. L., Lockhart, H. B. and Lambert, G. F.: The amino acid requirements of man; valine requirement; summary and final observations. J. Biol. Chem., 217:987, 1955.
9. Rose, W. C. and Wixom, R. L.: The amino acid requirements of man; the role of the nitrogen intake. *Ibid.*, p. 997.
10. Holt, L. E., Jr. and Snyderman, S. E.: In Cole, W. H. (ed.): Some Aspects of Amino Acid Supplementation. New Brunswick, New Jersey, Rutgers University Press, 1956.
11. Leverton, R. M.: The quantitative amino acid requirements of young women. I. Threonine. J. Nutrition, 58:59, 83, 219, 341, 355, 1956.
12. Jones, E. M., Bauman, C. A. and Reynolds, M. S.: Nitrogen balances of women maintained on various levels of lysine. J. Nutrition, 60:549, 1956.
13. Swenseid, M. E., Williams, I. and Dunn, M. S.: Amino acid requirements of young women based on nitrogen balance data. I. The sulfur-containing amino acids. J. Nutrition, 58:495, 1956.
14. Swenseid, M. E. and Dunn, M. S.: Amino acid requirements of young women based on nitrogen balance data. II. Studies on isoleucine and on minimum amounts of the eight essential amino acids fed simultaneously. *Ibid.*, p. 507.

15. Harper, A. E., Benton, D. A., Winje, M. E. and Elvehjem, C. A.: Leucine-isoleucine antagonism in the rat. Arch. Biochem., 51:523, 1954.
16. U. S. Department of Agriculture: Amino Acid of Foods. Home Economics Research Report No. 4. Washington, D. C., U. S. Government Printing Office, 1957.
17. Commonwealth Bureau of Animal Nutrition: Tables of the Amino Acids in Foods and Feeding Stuffs. Technical communication No. 19. Aberdeen, Scotland, Rowett Research Institute, 1956.
18. Phear, E. A., Ruebner, P., Sherlock, S. and Summerskill, W. H. J.: Toxicity of methionine in liver disease. Clin. Sc., 15:93, 1956.
19. Review: Glutamic acid in hepatic disease. Nutrition Rev., 9:113, 1951.
20. Smith, D. E. and Tyree, E. B.: Attempts to provide the rat with nutrition during post-irradiation anorexia. Radiation Res., 4:435, 1956.
21. McDermott, W. V. *et al.*: Glutamic acid in hepatic disease. New England J. Med., 253:1093, 1955.
22. Najarian, J. S. and Harper, H. A.: Arginine. A clinical study of the effect of arginine on blood ammonia. Am. J. Med., 21:832, 1956.
23. Bessman, S. P., Shear, S. and Fitzgerald, J.: Effect of arginine and glutamate on the removal of ammonia from the blood in normal and cirrhotic patients. New England J. Med., 256:991, 1957.

## Chapter 7

# KWASHIORKOR

THE physician practicing in the United States will probably never see some of the great infectious diseases of mankind — bubonic plague, typhus, schistosomiasis, leprosy. Yet, some knowledge of the diagnosis, treatment and prevention of such diseases is part of his medical culture. Similarly, it is highly unlikely that most readers will ever see a single case of what are probably the most common and most malignant of all nutritional deficiencies — kwashiorkor and marasmus, the protein deficiency diseases of young children. Even the name "kwashiorkor" is probably unknown to most medical men who studied nutrition before 1950. It is a Gold Coast term, the meaning of which is yet unclear. Some say it denotes the disease of the second or displaced child and marks its association with weaning; some say the term means red child because of the associated dyspigmentation (1). The syndrome was identified just before World War II and recognized in the late 40's for what it is; one of the most widespread scourges of mankind. Because it affects tens of millions of children throughout the world, some knowledge of this disease has thus also become part of the culture of the well-rounded practitioner. Because it is the result of too low a protein level in the diet, it is relevant to the knowledge of any physician concerned with the growth and nutrition of children, even if it corresponds to malnutrition that is so extreme that it is almost never seen in the United States. (Kark (2) observed one or two cases in Chicago, and the possibility that some cases may occur among depressed groups in large cities, e.g. Puerto Ricans in New York, cannot be excluded.)

Reprinted from *Postgraduate Medicine*, 26 (No. 1), July, 1959.

## SYNONYMS

The multiplicity of names by which kwashiorkor has been called testifies to its worldwide distribution. Some of the synonyms which have been used are as follows: malignant malnutrition (South Africa), which emphasizes the lethal aspects of the disease if untreated; *bouffissure d'Annam* (Indochina), which means "Vietnamese swelling" and singles out the symptom of edema; "fatty liver of Brahman children" (India), which accents another aspect of the pathology; and *sindrome policarencial infantil* (Central America), which illustrates the fact that the protein deficiency is usually accompanied by low intakes of the water-soluble vitamins. Kwashiorkor merges with other nutritional syndromes such as mehlnahrschaden and marasmus, in which calories and protein are lacking in the diet (3).

## DEFINITION

Kwashiorkor is perhaps best defined as a nutritional syndrome (or syndromes) in which a deficiency of good-quality protein appears to be a dominant factor. It is found among many poor populations, especially among young children. Symptoms characteristic of this disease are retarded growth and maturation; apathy and sometimes also irritability; anorexia; diarrhea and sometimes vomiting; alteration in color and texture of the hair and sometimes the nails; lesions of the skin marking varying degrees of hyperkeratosis, dyspigmentation and desquamation; edema; marked fatty infiltration of the liver; and a heavy mortality in the absence of proper treatment.

## DISTRIBUTION

We have already noted that the various synonyms for the name "kwashiorkor" (which has become the accepted name since it was endorsed by the World Health Organization and the Food and Agriculture Organization of the United Nations) testify to its widespread incidence. It is found wherever tropical peoples subsist on starchy staple foods without adequate protein supplements. It has been studied particularly thoroughly in Mexico and Central America (4), South America (5), Jamaica (6), India (7), and Central and South Africa (8-10); but it is found as well in North Africa, the Near East and in many areas of Asia in addition to India. Its prevalence within populations can be extremely high. It has been claimed that practically every child in certain African and Central American regions, for example, has or has had some degree of protein malnutrition bordering on kwashiorkor.

## ETIOLOGY

Lack of proteins, particularly complete proteins, seems to be principally responsible for the constant pathologic changes in kwashiorkor. These appear to be the result of a deficiency of good-quality protein in general rather than a deficiency of a single amino acid. The disease is rarely observed during the period of breast feeding as long as the supply of maternal milk is adequate. It closely follows weaning and transfer of the child to starch gruels when maternal milk is replaced by low-grade foodstuffs.

## PATHOLOGIC AND CLINICAL CHARACTERISTICS

The following signs, symptoms and pathologic findings are observed:

1. Retardation of growth, beginning at the late breast feeding, weaning and postweaning ages. This symptom is fundamental to kwashiorkor but also common to other conditions, such as undernutrition due to lack of available calories or to anorexia, marasmus and atrophy. In spite of the serious growth retardation, the infant with kwashiorkor does not always look emaciated or starved. If he has been provided with considerable starch or sugar while being deprived of protein, his subcutaneous fat may be appreciable, and, particularly if mild edema is present and there is no dermatosis, the infant may superficially appear to be well nourished.

2. Edema. Serum albumin is generally reduced in kwashiorkor and is almost universally reduced to a marked degree in edematous kwashiorkor. Relative hyperglobulinemia is often present, whether

as a compensatory reaction, as a result of parasitic infestation, or secondary to liver damage.

3. Fatty infiltration of liver. The liver is usually not palpable but is universally found to be extrememly infiltrated with fat, frequently to such an extent that the normal lobulation is hardly recognizable.

4. Dyspigmentation and dermatoses. There may be both a reduction of the quantity of hair and skin pigment and qualitative alternation. This must be distinguished from hypopigmentation due to admixture with people of lighter color or inborn mutations ("half albinos"). Skin dyspigmentation due to kwashiorkor can be patchy or diffuse; in some cases it may cover the entire body. Hyperpigmentation is also frequently observed.

Properly speaking, dermatoses in kwashiorkor do not appear to be the same in various regions of the world and, therefore, probably have several different origins. A very common form is an eruption of sharply defined, black, varnished patches on areas exposed to irritation (diaper area, buttocks, back, etc.). These are not confined to areas exposed to sunlight (hand and face), thus permitting differentiation from pellagra. The hyperpigmented areas may become dry, cracked and scaled and may peel. In extreme cases, they may blister and resemble second-degree burns.

Vascular fragility, ischemia and necrotic lesions are also seen in extreme cases in many areas of the world.

5. Gastrointestinal disorders and reduction of pancreatic and duodenal enzymes. Mucosal lesions and atrophy, diarrhea and deficient intake may be all part of a vicious circle. Pancreatic fibrosis is observed but is by no means a constant finding. Drastically reduced lipase, trypsin and amylase may be a result of the atrophy of the pancreas and duodenal mucosa.

6. Psychic changes. Children with kwashiorkor are usually apathetic and anoretic. They appear extremely miserable and may be irritable, but they rarely cry.

7. Mortality in untreated cases. The mortality in the untreated syndrome is very high. Recent studies suggest that the high mortality is associated with irreversible biochemical changes. In the absence of proper treatment, the mortality is never less than 30 per cent, and in some areas it is 100 per cent.

## TREATMENT

Well-planned treatment is based on our understanding of the primary factor in the etiology of kwashiorkor, i.e. primary deficiency of good-quality proteins often associated with vitamin deficiency, diarrhea and parasites. Other factors taken into account are the degree of severity of the case, the nature and extent of dehydration and electrolyte imbalance, and the presence and nature of intestinal parasitosis and other infections.

The main treatment is dietary. In children more than three years old whose general condition is fair, a complete and balanced dict is given from the outset. It is adjusted to the age of the child but consists largely of skim milk and animal protein (2 gm per kilogram of body weight per day at the start, building up to 5 to 7 gm as soon as possible — usually in a week to 10 days), fresh vegetables and bananas. Some fat can be included as a source of calories after the first few days of treatment. In younger children in whom the digestive troubles are slight, milk in the dilution of two parts of fresh milk to one part of water or rice water may be given. In more severe cases, increasing amounts of diluted skim milk should be administered, with due caution exercised in the process. Skim milk is sometimed acidified as well as diluted to facilitate digestion by producing smaller coagulation clots. Treatment starts with 2 to 3 gm of protein and 60 calories per kilogram of body weight. Concentration is progressively increased, so that as soon as possible 6 to 7 gm of protein per kilogram of body weight may be reached. Within two weeks, the caloric intake should be built up to 100 to 120 calories per kilogram of body weight.

If anorexia is intense at the beginning of treatment, a nasal tube is used. Loss of weight indicates the disappearance of edema and marks the time to change very progressively to a more varied diet. Clinical experience has shown that the administration of vitamin B complex in large doses not only is useless but sometimes makes the condition worse. Vitamins C and A, in physiologic doses (the water-emulsified form of synthetic vitamin A is preferable), are often given in the early treatment, as these are the two vitamins lacking in the diet based on skim milk. Results of use of lipotropic agents have been poor. Vitamin $B_{12}$ and folic acid have been used when anemia is present and the diet is poor in these nutrients. Ferrous sulfate (300 to 600 mg orally per day) may be introduced in the course of the first or second week of treatment. Penicillin may be given from the outset as a routine precaution against possible infection, which in children with kwashiorkor, may not manifest itself by fever or by an elevated white blood cell count. Children do better if they receive personal attention and affection throughout treatment.

The following emergency treatments have given good results in severe cases: (1) appropriate intravenously administered electrolyte solutions in marked dehydration following diarrhea and vomiting (with or without edema); (2) blood transfusions in the presence of shock or extreme anemia; and (3) less toxic drugs from the outset in treatment of specific diseases such as malaria. The treatment of intestinal parasitosis is not undertaken until the child has recovered sufficiently to start treatment without danger.

## PROGNOSIS IN TREATED CASES

The short-term prognosis of mild cases given full treatment is good. The frequency of multiple episodes is high when home conditions are unfavorable. The disease recurs not only in children taken home by the parents before the cure is complete but also, less usually, in the children who leave the hospital "clinically cured." Relapse usually occurs three to six months after the child has left the hospital. The clinical state during relapse is usually similar to and often more serious than that at first admission. Mortality in such cases continues high.

The prognosis of apparently successfully treated cases over a longer period of life span is not known. It is unlikely, from the worldwide distribution of cases, that there is any direct cause-and-effect relationship between cirrhosis and primary carcinoma of the liver on the one hand and kwashiorkor on the other. Adult cirrhosis may well result from the effects of continued protein deficiency and parasitosis, infection and toxic factors on liver already damaged in childhood by kwashiorkor: A similar situation probably exists in respect to a primary carcinoma of the liver.

## PREVENTION

Proper prevention is based on:

1. Increasing the supply of animal proteins. This entails development, in particular, of milk-producing livestock — cattle, sheep and goats — and of proper veterinary and processing facilities. The expansion of fisheries and of fish farming offers considerable promise.

2. Developing proper mixtures of adequate vegetable protein, particularly by increasing availability of pulses, nuts and green vegetables.

3. Eliminating the "hungry months," during which incidence of kwashiorkor increases, by developing cash crops and other additional sources of income.

4. Supplementary feeding programs directed toward infants and young children, with emphasis on foods providing adequate amounts of good-quality protein.

5. Education. With the best intentions, young mothers in poor tropical countries commit many grave faults in the nutrition of their children. When proper nutrition education programs are in effect, it is usually found that changes in traditional patterns of infant and small child feeding can be introduced fairly rapidly. Maternity and child health centers have had considerable influence on nutrition habits. Family dietary habits also can be influenced through schools; however, in underdeveloped areas, girls often constitute a minority in school attendance.

6. Social welfare. In poor areas there are usually substantial numbers of small children who suffer from plain neglect. This situation can be remedied only through the work of strong social agencies, which in turn have to be educated in regard to nutritional requirements of this age group.


## SUMMARY

The continued existence of the widespread syndrome of kwashiorkor is a challenge to physicians and nutritionists everywhere. Perhaps the most meaningful yardstick of the success of our foreign aid programs — at least as far as members of the therapeutic professions are concerned — could well be regression of kwashiorkor.

## REFERENCES

1. Williams, C. D.: A nutritional disease of childhood associated with a maize diet. Arch. Dis. Childhood, 8:1423, 1933.
2. Kark, R. M.: Personal communication.
3. Mayer, J.: Ghana: A challenge to nutritionists. Nutrition Rev., 17:193, 1959.
4. Autret, M, and Behar, M.: Sindrome policarencial infantil (kwashiorkor) and its prevention in Central America. FAO Nutritional Studies, No. 13. Rome, Italy, Food and Agriculture Organization of United Nations, 1954.
5. Waterlow, J. C. and Vergara, A.: Protein malnutrition in Brazil. FAO Nutritional Studies, No. 14. Rome, Italy, Food and Agriculture Organization of the United Nations, 1956.
6. Waterlow, J. C.: Fatty liver disease in infants in the British West Indies. Special Reports Series, Medical Research Council, London, H. M. Stationery Office, 1948.
7. Goplan, C.: In Waterlow, J. C. (ed.): Protein Malnutrition. Preceedings of the Conference in Jamaica. Cambridge, England, Cambridge University press, 1955.
8. Brock, J. F. and Autret, M.: Kwashiorkor in Africa. WHO Monograph Series, No. 8. Geneva, 1952.
9. Trowel, M. C., Davies, J. N. P. and Dean, R. F. A.: Kwashiorkor. London, Edward Arnold, 1954.
10. Brock, J. F., Hansen, J. D. C., Howe, E. E., Pretorius. P. J., Davel, J. G. A. and Hendrickse, R. G.: Kwashiorkor and protein malnutrition. A dietary therapeutic trial. Lancet, 2:355, 1955.

*Chapter 8*

# TROPICAL MALNUTRITION: FOOD REQUIREMENTS AND NUTRITIONAL SYNDROMES; BERIBERI

Tropical climates, whether dry (arid zones) or humid (tropical rain forest zones), are often thought to cause unusual changes in nutritional requirements. Except for the amounts of calories and water, however, little evidence supports this view. The widely prevalent malnutrition in the tropics largely reflects insufficient supplies of protective foods, selectivity of diet determined by cultural and religious backgrounds, and the direct and indirect effects of infection. Many people in tropical climates are unable to obtain the basic foods essential for a good diet. Their problems are fundamentally agricultural and economic, not climatic. Other groups, because of religious beliefs or social practices, avoid animal protein. Still others prefer polished to unpolished rice. Parasitic or other gastrointestinal infections may interfere with the absorption of specific food factors or utilize those available for their own economy at the expense of the host. Systemic infections, by their effect on the metabolism or tissues, may increase significantly the daily requirements for certain nutrients. Thus the essential problem varies from region to region, depending on the practices of man and only secondarily on the effects of climate.

## NUTRITIONAL REQUIREMENTS IN VARYING CLIMATES

Energy requirements are decreased in the tropics since the higher environmental temperatures diminish the need for heat production. The relative importance of temperature has, however,

---

Reprinted from *Postgraduate Medicine, 39* (No. 3), March, 1966.

often been overemphasized. Observers have been unduly impressed by the temporary anorexia which frequently follows sudden passage from a temperate to a tropical climate. An investigation of calorie requirements was conducted during World War II using United States and Canadian troops stationed in various parts of the world. All groups retained their usual food habits and engaged in the same type of duty. Under these conditions a linear correlation was observed between voluntary calorie intake and climatic environment; the daily intake decreased by 16 calories for each degree of increase in mean Fahrenheit temperature, or 29 calories for each degree centigrade.

Additional evidence relating the voluntary intake of troops to mean annual temperature has been obtained, particularly in studies by the Royal Air Force. On the basis of these observations and national averages of caloric intake in various climates, the Second Calorie Requirement Committee of the United Nations Food and Agricultural Organization estimated that caloric requirements decreased 3 per cent for every 10° C of mean annual temperature exceeding the reference point of 10° C.

However, available evidence indicates that high environmental temperatures introduce no change of practical importance in human protein requirements. The First Protein Requirement Committee of the United Nations Food and Agricultural Organization discussed this problem in detail, and its report was especially relevant for tropical countries because these areas often lack foods containing sufficient protein of high biologic value. The report gave requirements for "reference protein," defined by the amino acid composition which most closely fulfills the pattern of human amino acid requirements, stated in grams per kilogram of body weight. The requirement for infants was estimated at 2 gm per kilogram. The requirement per kilogram then decreases in conformity with the rate of growth until puberty imposes special needs. Adult reference requirements were assessed at 0.35 gm per kilogram of body weight, although these requirements are substantially increased during pregnancy and particularly during lactation. Brief reference was made to protein requirements during old age, in pathologic states, and for those performing heavy work. To allow for individual variation, an arbitrary increment of 50 per cent over the average minimum protein requirement was recommended.

To establish safe practical allowances, a correction factor is needed to relate the quality of the dietary protein to requirements expressed in terms of the reference protein. For this purpose conversion coefficients based on "protein scores" may be applied. Conversion factors are given for various diets, particularly those based largely on cassava, maize and rice. However, this method applies mainly within a certain range of protein intake, with respect to quantity and quality. With certain diets of low-quality protein, the problem is to supplement the diet appropriately in order to improve protein quality rather than to furnish more protein within the existing diet pattern. This applies particularly to requirements during the period of growth.

The low-fat consumption in many tropical areas has received some attention. This appears to be due essentially to local economic conditions. A low-fat diet has been claimed repeatedly to be valuable where conditions causing impaired liver function are widespread.

No convincing evidence has been produced to support the claim that heat increases the requirements for thiamine and ascorbic acid. Similarly, claims that tropical climates per se predispose to rickets are obscured because other factors, such as the availability of calcium and phosphorus, are not controlled. Whenever people are regularly exposed to sunshine, rickets does not appear. This probably explains the infrequent occurrence of rickets in the tropics, despite low calcium intake and the possible "predisposing" effect of heat. The great preponderance of evidence indicates that vitamin requirements of healthy persons are essentially the same in temperate and tropical climates.

Water requirements increase roughly in proportion to the amount of sweat secreted, from 2 to 3 liters per day in a temperated climate to 13 liters or more during work in a hot environment. Under extreme conditions the need for water may actually outstrip thirst. Wartime studies demonstrated that the best level of performance is obtained when the loss of water in sweat is replaced hour by hour. Loss of minerals, sodium chloride in particular, increases in individuals on initial exposure to a hot climate, but acclimatization is accompanied by decreased concentration of salt in the sweat. Thus salt requirements are increased only slightly. The trend in recent practice has been against providing salt tablets or salinized drinking water to men working in heat, except possibly when activity and temperature are unusually extreme or the men are unacclimatized.

Thus with the exception of water and calories, no striking deviation from requirements in a temperate zone is characteristic in the tropics. The tropical climate itself may play a secondary role in the evolution of certain nutritional diseases in that such climatic factors as wind, exposure to sun, and extreme heat may influence nutritional dermatoses. The effect of sunlight on skin appearance in pellagra is well known. Local climatic conditions may contribute to the differences in skin abnormalities associated with kwashiorkor in various regions of the world. The essential significancance of tropical nutritional diseases, however, lies in fields other than human physiology. An obvious and well-known factor is the prevalence of parasitic and infectious diseases, which often contribute to decreased intestinal absorption, sometimes to increased nutritional requirements, and usually to some degree of anorexia.

A more important factor is the agricultural, economic and social status of many tropical populations. Many such peoples subsist on a diet based exclusively on one starchy staple food — rice, millet or corn, for example. The classic deficiency diseases characteristic of such diets could perhaps best be termed "diseases of society" rather than "tropical diseases," despite their geographic localization.

Pathologic conditions associated with malnutrition and found in the tropics may be placed in four categories:

1. Syndromes which are essentially of dietary origin, such as beriberi, pellagra and kwashiorkor, even though they may be complicated by parasitic and infectious conditions.

2. Conditions which probably are of nutritional origin, as tropical ulcer, sprue, pernicious anemia and certain urolithiases.

3. Conditions of unknown cause in which nutritional factors appear to be important, such as primary carcinoma of the liver and certain pancreatic fibroses.

4. Diseases of which the primary causes are non-nutritional but in which nutritional factors directly affect the response to the pathogenic agent or contribute indirectly to the development of complicating malnutrition.

Important examples of only the first two categories will be considered in this chapter. The recognized clinical syndromes present one part of the picture of malnutrition. Nutritional diseases characteristically develop as multiple deficiencies, and the signs and symptoms characteristic of several nutritional syndromes commonly appear simultaneously or successively.

## BERIBERI

Beriberi is due to deficiency of vitamin $B_1$ (thiamine) and other vitamins. It occurs in acute and chronic forms characterized by peripheral neuritis and in severe cases by congestive heart failure. It may occur in all age groups.

In the past beriberi has been widespread in the Orient and in areas of the tropics where polished rice is an important dietary staple. It has also been prevalent in Labrador, Newfoundland and Iceland, where the winter diet is restricted largely to white flour and other nonvitamin-bearing foods.

Primary beriberi results from prolonged subsistence on a deficient diet. Secondary beriberi may occur as a complication of other disease states attended by deficient absorption, incomplete utilization, or unusual requirements for thiamine such as occur with elevated levels of metabolism.

The incidence of beriberi varies with dietary habits and availability of foods providing adequate amounts of essential nutrients. It is seen most commonly in men, and evidence indicates that hard physical labor is a precipitating factor. Women most frequently contract the disease during pregnancy and lactation. Infantile beriberi is a frequent cause of death among breast-fed infants in endemic areas. Although beriberi is not infectious, "epidemics" have occurred in populations subsisting on borderline diets, since diarrhea increases the individual's physiologic requirements and diminishes his utilization of specific food factors.

The heart and nervous system are primarily involved. The cardiac changes are predominantly hypertrophy, subsequent dilatation, and a considerable increase in the weight of the heart. No specific lesions have been identified, and the pathologic changes observed are often insufficient to account for the deaths from cardiac failure. The effect on tissues other than those of the nervous system are due to congestive heart failure.

Degenerative lesions without evidence of inflammation may be found throughout the nervous system — in the peripheral nerves, spinal cord, spinal ganglia, nuclei of the medulla and pons, and structures of the autonomic nervous system. The changes in the spinal cord predominate in the posterior columns and the anterior and posterior nerve roots. Destruction of myelin sheaths may be accompanied by fragmentation of the nerve fibers and atrophy of the nerve cells. Usually these changes affect only part of the fibers constituting a nerve trunk, and their extent depends on the duration and severity of the disease. Of the peripheral nerves the sciatic is most frequently involved, and evidence of this appears early. Of the cranial nerves the vagus and phrenic nerves are most frequently affected. Secondary atrophy of the muscles accompanies the disturbance of innervation.

Four clinical types of beriberi are recognized: dry, wet, infantile and atypical. No specific phenomena are necessarily common to all. The clinical manifestations of the disease may result from cardiac hypertrophy and dilatation or from secondary effects of edema and anasarca. The onset may be rapid or gradual, and the condition may become chronic with frequent recurrences of the acute form. Early manifestations usually are muscle weakness, anorexia, neurasthenia, tachycardia and cardiac enlargement. Often slight anemia develops and, as the disease becomes established, progressive peripheral nerve palsies appear.

## Dry Beriberi

The onset of dry beriberi is usually gradual, and the outstanding symptom is progressive weakness of the muscle groups used most. The extensor muscles of the thighs are most commonly affected, and a significant early symptom in many instances is inability to rise from a squatting position. Atrophy accompanies muscle weakness. Sensory disturbances in the form of paresthesias, hyperesthesias or hypoesthesias appear at the same time but usually are less prominent. In severe cases many muscle groups may be affected, producing a clinical picture of flaccid paralysis, muscular atrophy with or without cardiac enlargement, and tachycardia.

## Wet Beriberi

The clinical picture of wet beriberi is predominantly that of acute congestive heart failure with relatively little evidence of nervous system involvement. Signs of neuropathy, however, can be elicited in most instances. The onset is frequently rapid and acute, and the marked edema may mask the presence of significant muscle atrophy.

Electrocardiographic changes are common and characteristically consist of alterations in the T waves and prolongation of the electric systole (Q-T interval). Sudden collapse is not infrequent. The exact mechanism of this form of the disease is uncertain, but it seems probable that both the heart and the peripheral vascular system are concerned.

## Infantile Beriberi

In breast-fed infants of mothers subsisting on a thiamine-deficient diet, an acute condition develops which is markedly different from the disease in adults. Usually a period of diminished urine secretion and progressively increasing edema precedes the onset. If treatment is withheld, acute cardiac failure suddenly supervenes and death may follow rapidly. With the appearance of the acute phenomena the child cries constantly, and meningismus and convulsions may occur.

In the more uncommon dry infantile beriberi, edema and circulatory disturbances are not prominent, but vomiting, constipation, anorexia, loss of weight, pallor, fretfulness and a characteristic plaintive cry of aphonia may be present. The muscles are hypersensitive, but usually little definite evidence of nervous system disease is found.

## Atypical Beriberi

The clinical picture of the disease may be modified by other nutritional disorders such as scurvy, pellagra or nutritional edema. So-called ship beriberi, land scurvy, and the polyneuritis of alcoholic beriberi fall into the category of atypical beriberi.

The essential diagnostic features are signs and symptoms of peripheral neuritis with weakness of the muscle groups used most. Hyperesthesia of muscles, especially the plantar and gastrocnemius muscles, is common and significant. An important and early physical sign is reduction or loss of vibratory sensation over the affected distal portions of the extremities, with diminution or loss of distal proprioceptive sense and later of tendon reflexes. In severe cases marked muscle atrophy occurs. Measurement of thiamine excretion in the urine may confirm the diagnosis. The normal range of 100 to 200 mcg daily is significantly reduced in clinical beriberi.

## Differential Diagnosis

Beriberi must be differentiated from other types of peripheral neuritis, tabes dorsalis, postdiphtheritic paralysis, and acute heart failure due to other causes. The following criteria have been suggested to differentiate cardiac disease due to beriberi from that due to other causes: (1) enlarged heart with normal sino-atrial rhythm, (2) dependent edema, (3) elevated venous pressure, (4) peripheral neuritis, (5) nonspecific electrocardiographic changes, (6) lack of other recognizable cause of heart failure, (7) grossly deficient diet for at least three months, and (8) clinical improvement and reduction of heart size after treatment.

## Treatment

The recommended therapy consists of thiamine chloride, 5 to 10 mg administered parenterally twice daily, and a high-vitamin diet supplemented by rich sources of the B complex, such as vitamin preparations. If these are not available, 180 gm brewer's yeast or 90 gm tikitiki (extract of rice polishings) daily can be substituted.

The treatment of wet beriberi requires absolute rest and heavy doses of thiamine, administered both intravenously and sub-cutaneously. Appropriate measures for managing acute congestive heart failure should be instituted as needed. Infantile beriberi should be treated by appropriate alternation of the mother's diet. The infant should be given heavy doses of thiamine parenterally.

Deaths from acute wet beriberi are not infrequent. The chronic form may leave permanent disability, including muscle weakness or flaccid paralysis due to degeneration of the nerve cells. Adults recover from the disease slowly; the muscle weakness and neuritis frequently persist for months. Infantile beriberi on the other hand, responds rapidly and completely to adequate treatment.

## Chapter 9

# TROPICAL MALNUTRITION: SPRUE AND KWASHIORKOR

## SPRUE

SPRUE is a chronic afebrile relapsing disease characterized by sore tongue, flatulence, steatorrhea, progressive emanciation, cachexia and hypochromic anemia which, in untreated cases, may become hyperchromic and occasionally, in terminal stages, aplastic.

Sprue occurs predominantly in the Far East in India and Ceylon and in the Western Hemisphere in Puerto Rico. It occurs sporadically in the United States and other parts of the world except Africa, where it is extremely rare. The geographic distribution of the disease has not yet been adequately explained. Its incidence is not associated with any particular diet or dietary dificiency. The disease is characteristic of the white race, affecting especially persons in upper economic levels or with long residence in endemic areas.

Although the exact cause is unknown the fully developed syndrome reflects mixed multiple nutritional deficiencies, of which folic acid deficiency appears to play the dominant role. The fact that daily administration of pteroylglutamic (folic) acid relieve the symptoms of sprue might be interpreted to indicate that sprue is a specific deficiency disease. However, although nutritional considerations dominated both the etiologic and therapeutic aspects of the disease, some epidemiologic data have suggested that the primary mechanism may be of infectious origin.

Digestion of protein, carbohydrate and fat is normal in patients with sprue, but fatty acids and glucose are incompletely absorbed, resulting in flatulence and bulky, gaseous, acid stools which

Reprinted from *Postgraduate Medicine, 39* (No. 4), April, 1966.

contain large amounts of unabsorbed fatty acid crystals. Likewise, excessive amounts of calcium are lost in the feces as insoluble calcium soaps. Hypochlorhydria is the rule and achlorhydria occurs occasionally. It has been suggested that the basic defect — loss of ability to absorb fatty acids, glycerol and glucose — is due to failure of phosphorylation and loss of phosphorus following failure of phospholipid formation.

No specific or characteristic pathologic process is known. Postmortem findings are limited essentially to wasting and atrophy of the various organs and of the body as a whole. When macrocytic anemia appears in the advances stage, the bone marrow is characteristically hyperplastic, as in pernicious anemia. In still more advanced cases the marrow may become aplastic and contain little active hematopoietic tissue.

The clinical picture varies greatly, and the onset is gradual and insidious. In the majority of cases, however, sore tongue and mouth, flatulent indigestion and diarrhea are the cardinal symptoms of the fully established disease. These features appear simultaneously or successively in any order.

Lesions of the mouth are prominent in most cases and usually precede the appearance of diarrhea. At first they consist of small, painful aphthous ulcers on the tongue and buccal mucosa. Later the tongue becomes acutely inflamed and denuded. Extension of the lesions into the pharynx and esophagus may cause severe dysphagia, and salivation may be troublesome.

Flatulence, at first mild and intermittent and frequently relieved by evacuation, gradually becomes continuous and more severe. Eventually extreme and persistent abdominal distention causes the patient much distress.

In the early stages the diarrhea is usually intermittent, mild and urgent and occurs in the early morning. Gradually the stools become increasingly voluminous, gassy, foul, and light yellow or gray in color. At first there may be only one evacuation each day; later the number increases and the stools become more fluid and irritating.

Spontaneous remissions of symptoms are characteristically followed by increasingly severe relapses, resulting in progressive papillary atrophy of the tongue, loss of weight, and increasing asthenia. In the early stages of the disease moderate microcytic anemia is commonly present.

In advanced cases the anemia is macrocytic and may be severe. The tongue is characteristically smooth, firery red, painful and extremely sensitive to heat and condiments. Extreme emaciation, marked mental depression, severe anorexia, paresthesias of the extremities, epigastric distress and flatulence are other characteristic features. The skin, expecially of the face and flanks, frequently exhibits muddy pigmentation. The abdomen is markedly distended, and individual coils of intestine are visible. Stools are frequent, liquid, white or yellowish-white in color and abnormally bulky and gassy. Excoriation of the anus may cause painful evacuation. In some patients subacute combined degeneration of the spinal cord, severe tetany, and bleeding due to lack of vitamin K may occur.

Gastric analysis reveals hypoacidity or anacidity but no achylia. The stools contain a large excess of fat and fatty acids, but there is no evidence of failure of fat splitting or of incomplete digestion of starch and protein. The fecal nitrogen is not elevated. Serum calcium is frequently low and serum phosphorus is normal or somewhat low. Hypoproteinemia is common in severe cases. A glucose tolerance test after the ingestion of 1.5 gm glucose per kilogram of body weight reveals a flat blood sugar curve; the maximum rise seldom exceeds 40 mg per 100 ml Intravenous administration of 0.2 gm glucose per kilogram of body weight, however, reveals a normal blood sugar curve. Tolerance tests for vitamin A show a flat curve, indicative of poor fat absorption.

Roentgenographic examination of the small intestine demonstrates characteristic functional disturbances. The barium tends to accumulate in the dilated coils. The mucosal pattern is much coarser than normal, and the progress of the opaque meal is slow and intermittent. Barium enema may reveal a markedly dilated and atonic colon.

## Differential Diagnosis

The characteristic case of sprue with glossitis, hyperchromic anemia and steatorrhea presents little diagnostic difficulty. The typical clinical phenomena, however, may not all be present; this has led to the clinical classification of "complete" and "incomplete" sprue. Sprue must be differentiated from chronic pancreatitis, carcinoma of the pancreas, pernicious anemia, gastrojejunocolic fistula, and regional enteritis. The following findings are characteristic of sprue:

1. Steatorrhea with normal splitting of fat and normal digestion of starch and protein.

2. Flat glucose tolerance curve on oral administration.

3. Normal Glucose tolerance curve on intravenous administration.

4. Macrocytic anemia with megaloblastic arrest of the bone marrow in severe cases.

### Treatment

The best therapy is high-protein, high-vitamin, low-fat diet with possible restriction of starches and sugars in patients having severe flatulence. Folic acid, 15 mg intramuscularly, should be given daily at the outset, followed by a maintenance dosage of 5 mg orally per day when the patient's condition permits. If folic acid is not available, 60 gm brewers' yeast or 30 gm tikitiki should be given daily by mouth, supplemented by daily intramuscular injections of 5 ml concentrated aqueous liver extract. Parenteral administration of vitamin K or oral administration of a water-soluble vitamin K preparation completes the regimen.

Effective treatment is followed by rapid healing of the lesions in the mouth and progressive intestinal improvement. Stools become less frequent, the volume is diminished and consistency improved, the color returns to normal, and the amount of unabsorbed fatty acids decreases. If no gastrointestinal and hematologic response to folic acid occurs, the diagnosis is doubtful, and the response to vitamin $B_{12}$ should then be tested.

The prognosis depends to a large extent on the duration and severity of the disease before institution of adequate therapy. Patients with mild cases may ultimately be able to resume a normal diet without medication. More commonly, fats must be restricted permanently and parenteral injections of liver continued at intervals of one to two weeks. The character of the stools, the amount of unabsorbed fatty acids in the feces, and the presence or absence of flatulence provide satisfactory guides to therapy.

## KWASHIORKOR

The multiplicity of names for kwashiorkor testifies to its worldwide distribution. Among the synonyms are "malignant malnutrition" (South Africa), which emphasizes the lethal aspects of the untreated disease; *bouffissure d' Annam* (Vietnam), which means "Vietnamese swelling" and emphasizes the edema; "fatty liver of Brahman children" (India), which accents another aspect of the pathologic findings: and *sindrome policarencial infantil* (Central America), which illustrates that protein deficiency is usually accompanied by low intake of the water-soluble vitamins. Kwashiorkor, the name endorsed by the United Nations World Health Organization and the Food and Agricultural Organization, merges with other nutritional syndromes such as *Mehlnahrschaden* and marasmus, in which the diet lacks calories and protein.

Kwashiorkor is found wherever tropical peoples subsist on starchy staple foods without adequate protein supplements. It has been studied particularly thoroughly in Mexico and Central America, South America, Jamaica, India, Central Africa and South Africa. It also is found in North Africa, the Near East, and other areas of Asia. Kwashiorkor can be extremely prevalent within a population. It has been claimed that practically every child in certain African and Central American regions at one time in his life has some degree of protein malnutrition bordering on kwashiorkor.

Lack of proteins, especially complete proteins, seems to be principally responsible for the constant pathologic changes in this nutritional syndrome. The deficiency is of good-quality protein in general rather than of a single amino acid. The disease is rarely observed in a breast-fed child as long as the supply of maternal milk is adequate. The onset closely follows the weaning and transfer of the child from maternal milk to low-grade foodstuffs such as starch gruels.

Retardation of growth, beginning about the time the child is weaned, is a fundamental characteristic of kwashiorkor, although it is also common to other conditions, including undernutrition due to lack of adequate calories, anorexia, marasmus or atrophy, However, even when growth reatardation is severe, the infant with kwashiorkor does not always look emaciated or starved. If considerable starch or sugar is provided while protein is lacking, the child's subcutaneous fat may be appreciable and, especially if milk edema is present without dermatosis, the infant may superfically appear to be well nourished.

The serum albumin is generally reduced in kwashiorkor and is almost universally reduced to a marked degree in edematous kwashiorkor. Relative hyperglobulinemia is often present as a compensatory reaction, as a result of parasitic infestation, or secondary to liver damage.

The liver usually is not palpable but universally shows extreme fatty infiltration, frequently to such extent that the normal lobulation is hardly recognizable.

Dyspigmentation and dermatoses are common sypmptoms of kwashiorkor. Both reduction in the quantity of hair and skin pigment and qualitative alteration may be present. The reduction in skin pigment must be distinguished from hypopigmentation due to admixture with peoples of lighter color or to inborn mutations (so-called half-albinos). Skin dyspigmentation due to kwashiorkor can be patchy or diffuse or may cover the entire body. Hyperpigmentation is also a frequent finding.

Dermatoses in kwashiorkor appear to differ in various regions of the world and therefore probably have several different origins. A very common form is an eruption of sharply defined black varnished patches on areas exposed to irritation, such as the diaper area, buttocks and back. These eruptions are not confined to areas exposed to sunlight (the hands and face), permitting differentiation from pellagra. The hyperpigmented areas may become dry, cracked and scaled and may peel. In extreme cases they may blister and resemble second-degree burns. Vascular fragility, ischemia and necrotic lesions are also seen in extreme cases in many areas of the world.

Gastrointestinal disorders and reduction of pancreatic and duodenal enzymes are common. Mucosal lesions and atrophy, diarrhea and deficient intake may produce a vicious circle. Pancreatic fibrosis is observed but is by no means a constant finding. Atrophy of the pancreas and duodenal mucosa may drastically reduce lipase, trypsin and amylase.

Children with kwashiorkor may show psychic changes. Usually they appear apathetic, anoretic and extremely miserable; they may be irritable but rarely cry.

The mortality in untreated cases is very high. Recent studies have suggested that the high mortality is associated with irreversible biochemical changes. When proper treatment is not instituted, the mortality is never less than 30 per cent and in some areas is 100 per cent.

## Treatment

Well planned treatment is based on our understanding of the primary cause of kwashiorkor, i.e. deficiency of good-quality proteins often associated with vitamin deficiency, diarrhea and parasitic infestation. Other factors to be considered are the severity of the case, nature and extent of dehydration and electrolyte imbalance, and presence and nature of intestinal parasitosis and of other infections.

The main treatment is dietary. In children more than three years old whose general condition is fair, a complete and balanced diet is given from the outset. The diet is adjusted to the age of the child and consists largely of skim milk, animal protein, fresh vegetables and bananas. About 2 gm of protein per kilogram of body weight is given each day at the outset; this is increased to 7 gm as soon as possible, usually in a week to 10 days. Some fat can be included as a source of calories after the first few days of treatment. In younger children with only slight digestive trouble, a dilution of two parts fresh milk to one part water or rice water may be given. In more severe cases increasing amounts of diluted skim milk should be administered with care. Skim milk may be acidified as well as diluted to facilitate digestion by producing smaller coagulation clots. Treatment starts with 2 to 3 gm of protein and 60 calories per kilogram of body weight.

If anorexia is intense when treatment is begun, a nasal tube is used for feeding. Loss of weight indicates the disappearance of edema and signals the time to change to a more varied diet. Clinical experience has shown that the administration of vitamin B complex in large doses not only is useless but also has aggravated the condition at times. Vitamins C and A (preferably the water-emulsified form of synthetic vitamin A) in the physiologic doses are often given early in a diet based on skim milk. Use of lipotropic agents has given poor results. Vitamin $B_{12}$ and folic acid have been used when anemia is present and the diet is poor in these nutrients. Ferrous sulfate, 300 to 600 mg orally daily, may be introduced during the first or second week of treatment. Pennicillin may be given from the outset as a routine precaution against possible infection which, in children with kwashiorkor, may not manifest itself by fever or an elevated white blood cell count. Children improve more rapidly if they receive personal attention and affection throughout therapy.

The following emergency treatments have given good results in severe cases: (1) appropriate intravenous electrolyte solutions in marked dehydration following diarrhea and vomiting, with or without edema; (2) blood transfusions in the presence of shock or extreme anemia, and (3) less toxic drugs from the outset for treating specific diseases such as malaria. The treatment of intestinal parasitosis is not undertaken until the child has recovered suffcently to undergo treatment without danger.

The short-term prognosis is good for patients with mild cases given full treatment. The frequency of multiple episodes is high when home conditions are unfavorable. The disease recurs not only in children taken home by the parents before they are cured but also, although less often, in children who leave the hospital clinically cured. If relapse occurs, it is usually three to six months after the child has left the hospital. The clinical state during relapse is usually similar to that at first admission; often it is more severe. Mortality in such cases continues high.

The prognosis of apparently successfully treated cases over a longer period or life-span is unknown. It is unlikely, considering the worldwide distribution of cases, that any direct cause-and-effect relationship exists between cirrhosis and primary carcinoma of the liver on the one hand and kwashiorkor on the other.

Cirrhosis in adulthood may well result from the effect of continued protein deficiency, parasitosis, infection and toxic factors on a liver already damaged in childhood by kwashiorkor. A similar situation probably exists in respect to primary carcinoma of the liver.

## Prevention

Kwashiorkor is best prevented by the following measures:

1. Increased supply of animal proteins. This entails development, in particular, of milk-producing livestock — cattle, sheep and goats — and of proper veterinary and processing facilities. Expansion of fisheries and fish farming offers considerable promise.

2. Proper mixtures of adequate vegetable protein, particularly by increasing availability of pulses, nuts and green vegetables.

3. Elimination of the "hungry months" during which the incidence of kwashiorkor increases, by developing cash crops and other additional sources of income.

4. Supplementary feeding programs for infants and young children, with emphasis on foods providing adequate amounts of good-quality protein.

5. Education. With the best intentions young mothers in poor tropical countries commit many grave faults in the nutrition of their children. When proper nutrition education programs are in effect, changes in traditional patterns of feeding infants and small children usually can be introduced fairly rapidly. Maternity and child health centers have had considerable influence on nutrition habits. Family dietary habits also can be influenced through schools; however in underdeveloped areas girls often constitute a minority in school attendance.

6. Social welfare. In poor areas substantial numbers of small children usually suffer from plain neglect. This situation can be regarded only through the work of strong social agencies, which in turn must be educated in regard to the requirements for good nutrition in this age group.

*Chapter 10*

# TROPICAL MALNUTRITION:
# PELLAGRA AND OTHER SYNDROMES
# OF MALNUTRITION

## PELLAGRA

PELLAGRA is the principal manifestiation of a severe deficiency of niacin, generally complicated by deficiencies of other B vitamins. It is characterized clinically by a sore red tongue, disturbances of the alimentary tract, symmetrical dermatitis, and changes in the central and peripheral nervous systems.

The disease has a worldwide distribution and is generally associated with diets containing an excessive proportion of corn (maize). The disease is more prevalent during the spring than in any other season.

Endemic pellagra is due to prolonged ingestion of a low-protein diet containing small amounts of nicotinic acid. The human organism can convert the amino acid tryptophan to niacin, so that both nutrients must generally be insufficient for pellagra to appear. Diets high in corn and containing little or no meat, milk, fish or other good sources of protein are pellagragenic. The importance of the amino acid composition of the diet is illustrated by the fact that wheat diets are not pellagragenic in spite of a niacin content often lower than that of corn diets.

Niacin deficiency interferes with the formation and function of two essential respiratory enzymes, the diphosphopyridine and triphosphopyridine nucleotides. The effects of this deficiency can therefore be expected to be widespread. Less severe deficiencies of niacin produce milder symptoms.

While lack of nicotinic acid and tryptophan in the diet is an

Reprinted from *Postgraduate Medicine, 39* (No. 5), May, 1966.

essential etiologic factor of edemic pellagra, certain organic diseases which interfere with the ingestion, assimilation or utilization of pellagra-preventing food factors contribute to the prevalence of pellagra. Amebic dysentery, hookworm, malaria and cirrhosis of the liver are of particular importance in tropical regions. Secondary pellagra is sometimes associated with chronic alcoholism.

As in other deficiency diseases, the phenomena characteristic of pellagra are usually accompanied by a relative lack of other essential nutrients. Cheilosis responding to riboflavin administration and peripheral neuritis responding to thiamine treatment are frequent complications.

The clinical picture is variable and the disease may be acute, subacute or chronic. The onset is usually gradual, with asthenia, loss of weight, mental depression, and a sore red tongue. No characteristic or constant pathologic changes are observed. In acute cases certain areas of the skin and mucosa, particularly of the mouth and pharynx, are actively inflamed. Repeated attacks lead to atrophy and pigmentation of the affected skin regions.

Dermatitis also may occur, symmetrically distributed and affecting areas which are exposed to the sun or to irritation, such as the dorsa of the hands, wrists and feet, elbows, face, neck, skin beneath the breasts, perineal region, and patellar areas. In the early age erythema resembling sunburn appears, followed by vesculation and bulla formation. The skin becomes thick and rough and as the acute imflammation subsides brownish pigmentation remains. Repeated attacks lead to marked atrophy of the skin.

Lesions of the tongue and mouth are usual. Acute glossitis and stomatitis may progress to extensive ulceration. Simultaneously fissuring occurs at the angles of the mouth. The tongue is swollen, denuded of papillae, extremely sensitive, and often painful. Hypochlorhydria or achlorhydria is common, and diarrhea or alternating diarrhea and constipation may occur. The stools are abnormal in color and contain no excess fat.

A variety of symptoms referable to the nervous system accompanies the disease. In the early stages the picture is that of neurasthenia, which increases in severity as the disease progresses. True psychoses appear in patients with advanced and long-standing disease. Peripheral neuritis, spastic gait and other indications of organic involvement are not uncommon.

The cardinal symptoms — dermatitis, glossitis, gastrointestinal symptoms and psychic disturbances — are characteristic in patients with a well-developed acute pellagra.

Diagnostic difficulties may be encountered in the early stages or in advanced chronic cases in which the characteristic acute phenomena are lacking. The combination of pigmentation and atrophy of exposed skin areas, smooth atrophy of the tongue, and neurasthenia should arouse suspicion. Analysis of the urine for $N^1$-methylnicotinamide content may be helpful. Normal excretion is usually more than 3 mg per day. Levels of excretion below 1 mg reinforce the presumption of pellagra or a prepellagrous state.

## Treatment

A high-protein, high-vitamin diet is recommended for treatment, with nicotinic acid or nicotinic amide, 300 to 500 mg daily in divided doses, and therapeutic doses of the B complex vitamins, especially thiamine chloride, 5 to 10 mg daily as indicated. An adequate diet is essential to the prophylaxis of pellagra.

## NUTRITIONAL EDEMA

This disorder follows long-continued subsistence on a diet deficient in biologically complete protein. It is characterized by changes in the concentration of the plasma proteins, altered osmotic tension of the blood, edema and anasarca. Nutritional edema occurs particularly in famine areas. It was prevalent in central Europe during and immediately after World War I and in Spain during the Spanish Civil War. It also has occurred in India, Mauritius, Fiji and Java and endemically as a complication of other nutritional diseases.

Nurtitional edema develops when the diet is limited in total calories and the average protein content is less than 50 gm per day. The appearance of the clinical syndrome is preceded by a prolonged period of negative nitrogen balance. In the early stages the total plasma protein is unchanged while the albumin-globulin ratio is accompanied by disturbances of osmotic relationships and water retention in the tissues. The normal values for the plasma proteins are: total protein, 6.5 to 8.5 gm per 100 ml; albumin, 4.2 to 5.7 gm and globulin, 1.3 to 3.0 gm.

Progressive weight loss due to the limited caloric intake usually precedes the onset of the syndrome. As the chemical imbalance is established, further weight loss is checked by water retention and may be followed by an actual gain in weight. The marked pitting edema of the lower extremities in the early stages later becomes generalized and, if progressive, leads to general anasarca.

The occurrence of edema in individuals subjected to famine conditions suggests this syndrome. The diagnosis is based on fluid retention in the absence of congestive heart failure or significant renal disease and is confirmed by determination of the plasma proteins and demonstration of inversion of the albumin-globulin ratio.

## *Treatment*

Nutritional edema is treated with a high-protein, high-vitamin diet providing 120 to 150 gm of animal protein per day and restriction of salt and fluids.

## EPIDEMIC DROPSY

Epidemic dropsy is believed to be nutritional edema complicating other nutritional disorders such as pellagra and beriberi. It has appeared in mass outbreaks, especially in India, and is often accompanied by the neurologic symptoms and signs of beriberi and by erythematous skin lesions, followed by pigmentation of exposed areas suggestive of endemic pellagra.

## OSTEOMALACIA

Osteomalacia is caused by a deficiency of calcium and phosphorus. It is characterized by a negative balance of the nutrients and deficient calcification of all osteoid tissue. It occurs primarily in women, particularly during pregnancy and lactation, and becomes more severe with each succeeding pregnancy. It is widely endemic in northern India, China and Japan and occurs sporadically in central Europe.

Osteomalacia and rickets are the same disease. Continuous resorption and formation of new bone occur, but the newly formed osteoid tissue fails to calcify because of insufficient absorption of calcium and phosphorus from the diet. This malabsorption may be due to dietary deficiency, abnormal dietary ratio of calcium to phosphorus, steatorrhea, or deficiency of vitamin D. Usually several of these factors are involved, most commonly lack of calcium and phosphorus in the diet and insufficient vitamin D. The evaluated mineral demands of pregnancy and lactation on the maternal organism are important in the progression of the disease.

The abnormal ossification produces gross progressive skeletal deformities, especially of the pelvis, thorax, spine and long bones. The bones become soft and flexible, and the deformities are more frequently caused by bending than a fracture. The bone cortex is thin, and the trabeculae are greatly reduced or absent. Microscopic examination reveals deficient calcification. Osteoclasts are present in normal number whereas osteoblasts are numerous.

Weakness, bone pains and often generalized aching are dominant symptoms. Bony tenderness is common and severe tetany may occur. Symptoms are particularly acute during pregnancy and lactation, and the process characteristically remains relatively stationary in intervals between pregnancies. Progression of the disease leads to great deformity and disability. Distortion of the bony pelvis either causes difficult labor or makes parturition impossible.

The marked deformities, particularly of the lower extremities, thorax and spine, are suggestive in endemic areas. X-ray examination of the skeletal reveals generalized osteoporosis, and the vertebrae often show biconcave deformity, the so-called fish vertebrae. The diagnosis is established by findings in the blood chemistry. In severe cases the serum alkaline phosphatase is increased. In mild cases the calcium may be normal or only slightly reduced, whereas the phosphorus is below normal levels and the phosphatase slightly increased.

Osteomalacia must be differentiated from other osteoporotic diseases; particular difficulty is encountered with the osteoporotic form of hyperparathyroidism. The blood chemistry findings in the latter condition are distinctive, however; the serum calcium is elevated, the phosphorus low, and the alkaline phosphatase above normal.

## Treatment

Treatment of osteomalacia can protect only against further deformities and consists of a diet high in calcium and phosphorus and the administration of 10,000 to 50,000 units of vitamin D daily.

## VITAMIN A DEFICIENCY

Vitamin A deficiency is widely prevalent in the tropics, especially where other nutritional deficiency conditions are common. It usually occurs as a primary response to a diet insufficient in vitamin A or, less frequently, as a secondary complication of diseases associated with defective absorption of fats.

Vitamin A deficiency is characterized by skin changes, reduced adaptability to darkness, and lesions of the eye and nervous system. In many regions of Africa and India a majority of children present skin changes which respond to administration of vitamin A, and many hospitalized patients show evidence of xerophthalmia.

The skin changes associated with vitamin A deficiency have been variously called toadskin, phrynoderma, sharkskin, keratosis pilaris, lichen spinulosus and Darier's disease. The usual changes in the skin include dryness and roughness, followed by eruption of hyperkeratotic papillae. Some hyperkeratotic changes associated with vitamin A deficiency do not respond to treatment with vitamin A and presumably have a different origin in spite of their clinical similarity. The hair becomes dry and brittle, and the nails develop transverse or longitudinal ridges.

Adaptability of the eye to darkness is impaired, producing

so-called night blindness. Photophobia, xerosis and Bitot's spots may be present, and in extreme cases keratomalacia may lead to corneal ulceration, panophthalmitis, and loss of the eye.

The susceptibility of the nervous system to vetches of the genus *Lathyrus* is increased by a deficiency of vitamin A. The clinical syndrome lathyrism, characterized by a spastic paraplegia, is common in parts of India and has been reported elsewhere in the world.

## Treatment

Effective treatment of conditions due to vitamin A deficiency requires daily administration of large doses of vitamin A, 50,000 to 100,000 IU.

## TROPICAL MACROCYTIC ANEMIA

Tropical macrocytic anemia appears to be a response of the hematopoietic system to a nutritional deficiency. Although this entity may resemble certain aspects of sprue, it does not interfere with intestinal absorption. Like sprue, it responds satisfactorily to folic acid.

## COMMENT

One of the main characteristics of many parts of the tropical world is the seasonal variation in climate and, more specifically, in rainfall. Since the people in many of these regions are very poor, such variations profoundly affect the nutritional status of the population. Lack of rainfall can bring about partial starvation for adults, and even a hitherto obtainable source of calories (although poor in good-quality protein), such as corn, millet or a starchy root, may become unavailable to children. The resulting clinical picture may change from prevalence of kwashiorkor to that of marasmus. Shortages in vitamins C and B may also be seasonal, so that latent deficiencies – scurvy, beriberi or pellagra – may appear at certain times of the year. Because vitamin A is much better stored in the body than the water-souluble vitamins, vitamin A deficiency is more likely to be constantly present than deficiencies due to shortages in the vitamins B and C; however, even the incidence of vitamin A deficiency may show seasonal variation, particularly in small children. Thus the seasonal vulnerability of the food supply, in both quantity and nature, should lead to special emphasis on maintaining sufficient stores of food and on the qualitative aspects of food conservation, particularly preservation of the vitamin content.

The existence of a satisfactory physiologic adaptation to undernutrition and malnutrition has never been demonstrated. Caloric undernutrition leads to excessive loss of weight, decreased work efficiency, and cessation of physical effort. It thus initiates a vicious circle in which the reduction in income and food production increases the risk of continued undernutrition. Malnutrition, resulting in decreased stores of nutrients in the body, makes the organism more and more vulnerable to extreme nutritional shortages, infection and trauma.

Far from encouraging the belief that populations hitherto malnourished are capable of coping physiologically with continued nutritional shortages, all available evidence confirms that only prolonged good nutrition prepares a man for a period of temporary deprivation without lasting damage.

*Chapter 11*

# VITAMIN D IN RICKETS
# AND HYPOPHOSPHATEMIA

RICKETS, properly speaking, is a nutritional
disease that occurs in infancy and early childhood and is caused by
a deficiency of vitamin D. The deficiency is characterized by
insufficient calcium in the body due to impaired absorption of
calcium from the intestine. Lack of calcium affects the nerves,
muscles, and especially the bones, which become deformed. Severe
cases of rickets can result in pigeon breast, contracted pelvis,
knock knees, and bow legs.

Deformities develop when the normal degeneration of the
growing epiphyseal cartilage becomes defective, resulting in
widening of the zone between diaphysis and epiphysis. At the
diaphyseal end, the cartilage is irregualarly invaded by osteoid
tissue in which little calcification occurs. Calcification is also
limited under the periosteum.

## CLINICAL RICKETS

Chemically, the blood calcium level tends to fall below the
normal level of about 10 mg per 100 ml. Tetany usually occurs
when the level drops to about 5 mg per 100 ml. The serum
inorganic phosphate also falls from a normal level of 3.5 mg to 3
mg per 100 ml or less, a phenomenon probably due to the
response of the parathyroid glands to the decreased serum calcium.
The combination of a normal serum calcium and a low phosphorus
level suggests full response of the parathyroid glands, with
consequent rapid decalcification of the bones. A low calcium level
and an adequate phosphorus level suggest poor response of the
parathyroid glands, and unless corrected, will lead to hyper-

Reprinted from *Postgraduate Medicine, 48,* November, 1970.© McGraw-Hill, Inc.

excitability of the neuromuscular conducting mechanism and tetany.

Another major biochemical finding is an increase in serum alkaline phosphatase, which occurs even when the serum levels of calcium and phosphorus are within normal limits. This enzyme is generally considered to be formed by the large numbers of osteoblasts that accumulate in the osteoid tissue at the growing points in the bones. However, the osteoblasts cannot make bone without an adequate supply of calcium, and the excess alkaline phosphatase is liberated into the plasma. Even in mild cases of rickets, the number of King-Armstrong units of alkaline phosphatase climbs to 30 from a normal of 10.

The precise ways in which vitamin D acts in the body are still unknown, but its effectiveness in ordinary rickets is established. Recent evidence indicates that in the intestine, vitamin D promotes the synthesis of proteins involved in calcium transport, but it has not yet been shown that vitamin D can mobilize bone mineral or that the pathology of vitamin D deficiency differs from that of calcium deficiency in a number of species.

Calcification at the end of the bones will become evident with the following regimen: vitamin D in a dosage of 1000 to 5000 IU daily, depending on the severity of the disease; a diet rich in calcium (including at least 1 pt or preferably 1 qt of milk daily, supplemented with calcium glutamate if necessary) and adequate in other nutrients (particularly iron and ascorbic acid); and good general hygiene, with proper feeding practices and exposure to sunlight. Normal levels of calcium and phosphorus will follow, although the pattern of improvement is inconstant. The serum alkaline phosphatase level usually remains elevated for several weeks after treatment is initiated. During this period, therapeutic doses of vitamin D should be given; when the serum alkaline phosphatase level returns to normal, vitamin D can be gradually reduced to the prophylactic dosage of 400 IU daily.

## RESISTANT RICKETS

The classic picture of pathology, clinical chemistry, and therapy of what can be called ordinary rickets is modified in resistant rickets, a disease of somewhat greater complexity. Resistant rickets is similar to deficiency rickets that persists into late childhood (late rickets) or into adulthood, when the clinical picture is the same as rickets followed by osteomalacia. However, resistant rickets responds only to massive dosages of 150,000 IU of vitamin D daily, or more if tolerated, and 5 gm of calcium three times daily.

## HYPOPHOSPHATEMIA

Hypophosphatemia is a familial disease inherited as a sex-linked dominant trait. The skeletal deformities and roentgenographic changes are similar to those in rickets, serum phosphorus is reduced, and alkaline phosphatase is greatly increased. Serum calcium is normal.

Hypophosphatemia also has been said to "respond" to large doses of vitamin D, and dosages of 30,000 to 50,000 IU per day have been reported effective. The pathogenesis of the condition is unknown, but a number of mechanisms have been proposed: decreased renal tabular absorption of phosphate, decreased intestinal absorption of calcium with secondary hyperparathyroidism, and abnormal metabolism of vitamin D.

The syndrome has received renewed attention, and the findings are clinically disturbing in that they show roentgenographic evidence of healing after therapy, but the growth response, if it occurs, is very limited, the findings are also intellectually disturbing inasmuch as enormous doses of vitamin D correct bone and other defects but do not cause resumption of growth, suggesting that our attempted explanations of the role of vitamin D therapy have been far too simplistic.

In a survey of hypophosphatemia in nine patients, Stickler (1) noted that body length at birth was normal, the length of the various segments was normal, and growth retardation was not apparent until after the first year. By the end of the third year, all but one patient were below the tenth percentile in height, and therapy even when it had been started in the first year had little, if any, effect. Serum phosphorus was low in all patients tested in the first three months, alkaline phosphatase was elevated in two, and serum calcium was atypically increased in another.

In a second survey of the disease in 36 patients seen in the past 30 years, McNair and Strickler (2) reported the same dismal picture of total failure of growth response to vitamin D therapy whether or not osteotomy had been performed. Serum phosphorus levels were equally unaffected. Alkaline phosphatase levels decreased but remained higher than normal. As had been noted before in patients with hypophosphatemia, the trunk length (from crown to pubis) and arm span were normal. Loss of stature was essentially confined to the lower segment, from pubis to heel, and cannot be accounted for by any deformities of this weight-bearing area. Thus regional inhibition of skeletal growth in length must be accepted.

In more than 30 years of vitamin D therapy its failure to renew growth has been given little acknowledgment in clinical and nutritional literature. Even the best textbooks of clinical nutrition simply imply that with sufficiently high vitamin D dosage, a normal pattern of growth will resume. Vitamin D therapy should not be abandoned in hypophosphatemia, for it promotes healing, decreases deformities, and relieves bone pain. However, normal height apparently should not be expected.

Increasing therapeutic doses of vitamin D to even higher levels than those used in the past to overcome dwarfism is likely to lead to toxic reactions, of which renal damage is the most dangerous. Much more knowledge is needed regarding the interaction of calcium, phosphate, protein, and vitamin D metabolism.

## REFERENCES

1. Stickler, G. B.: Familial hypophosphatemic vitamin D resistant rickets. The neonatal period and infancy. Acta. Paediat. Scand., 58:213 (May) 1969.
2. McNair, S. L. and Stickler, G. B.: Growth in familial hypophosphatemic vitamin-D-resistant rickets. New Eng. J. Med., 281:511, 1969.

*Chapter 12*

# IRON DEFICIENCY, MENSTRUATION AND DIET

THAT iron deficiency is much more common in women than in men is well known. It is universally recognized that this is because women need more iron to cover their menstrual losses of this mineral, while at the same time their generally smaller food intake provides a smaller supply in the diet. The demands of pregnancy and lactation, although associated with an interruption of menstrual losses, may further aggravate already unsatisfactory conditions. The considerable variability of iron loss among women is less well known and, when viewed in conjunction with the variability in iron intake, goes a long way toward explaining why certain otherwise healthy women may become anemic on a "normal diet" in the absence of any detectable pathologic condition. A series of Swedish studies provides numerical data underlying this phenomenon and enables us to draw practical conclusions on the treatment and prevention of iron deficiency (1).

In a series of research reports, Hallberg and his collaborators in Göteborg (2, 3) have illustrated the variability of menstrual iron losses. In one investigation they studied 12 nurses for 12 consecutive menstrual periods. In a second study they examined 117 female industrial workers during two consecutive periods. Finally, in an effort to see whether menstrual blood loss was genetically controlled, they measured the loss for two menstrual periods in 18 monozygotic (identical) and 24 dizygotic (nonidentical) twin pairs.

Results of these studies clearly showed that the individual variation in menstrual blood loss was small from one period to another but that differences between various women were great.

Reprinted from *Postgraduate Medicine, 44* (No. 5), November, 1968.© McGraw-Hill, Inc.

There appeared to be little difference with age, suggesting that once an individual pattern is established it remains reasonably constant during the fertile period of the life span. Identical twins had a much greater similarity of menstrual losses than nonidentical twins. Such a finding is classically considered to indicate that genetic determination is paramount over the influence of environmental factors.

Hallberg and associates also studied menstrual blood loss in a randomly selected sample of 476 women from Göteborg. They found that the average menstrual blood loss was 43.4 ml, with a range from 0 to 542 ml. The average daily iron loss corresponding to the average monthly blood loss was 0.6 mg per day. This is roughly the same amount as the sum of the other losses of body iron in women (chiefly by desquamation of epithelial and endothelial cells). The variability of iron losses is illustrated by the fact that the daily total iron loss exceeded 1.1 mg in 50 per cent of the women, 1.5 mg in 25 per cent, and 2 mg in 10 per cent.

The relationship of menstrual blood losses to the state of iron nutrition and the etiology of iron-deficiency anemia was clearly demonstrated by the fact that subjects whose menstrual blood losses exceeded 60 ml showed a statistically significant decrease in hemoglobin concentration, mean corpuscular hemoglobin concentration (MCHC), and plasma iron. They also showed a marked increase of the total iron-binding capacity and no stainable iron in the bone marrow. (The few women who had stainable iron in marrow smears with blood losses over 60 ml were 45 years of age, and it was hypothesized that the measured losses were larger than they had been during most of the fertile life span and were subjected to a premenopausal increase). Incidentally, Hallberg and colleagues interpreted the lack of difference in iron intake between individuals with and without stainable iron in the marrow as indicating that iron loss is the main differentiating factor influencing iron balance.

The investigators concluded from their interesting and careful studies that 60 ml is the largest amount of menstrual blood loss which on the average will not induce signs of iron depletion. If one disregards the effect of pregnancies, one would expect, from the distribution of menstrual losses data, that 25 to 35 per cent of adult women would show some signs of iron deficiency, a value which agrees closely with observed data. The investigators further concluded that inasmuch as the average intake of the women studied was of the order of 10 mg, only about 12 to 16 per cent of ingested dietary iron was absorbed by adult women with low stores. Intakes in the United States are probably somewhat higher because flour (and hence bread) is enriched with iron. The fear of weight gain and the general belief that avoidance of bread and other baked goods is the *sine qua non* condition of weight control do much to reduce the effectiveness of bread enrichment as far as iron supplementation of the diet of American women is concerned. Thus, conclusions from the Swedish studies are essentially applicable to this country.

What practical conclusions can we derive from these results: Basically, while nutrition education leading to the consumption of a diet richer in iron is likely to be effective in the prophylaxis of iron deficiency of women with moderate menstrual losses, iron supplementation is absolutely necessary for women with menstrual losses greater than 60 ml and for most women during pregnancy and lactation. The loss of iron involved in a normal pregnancy (iron content of fetus, 400mg), delivery (iron content of placenta, uterus and blood loss, 325 mg), and lactation (iron content of milk during three months of lactation, 75 mg) may total 800 mg. This in turn represents an increase in iron requirements of 2 mg per day for 400 days. Adding this value to the 0.6 mg (basal) required for nonmenstruating women, it is readily seen that with a 12 per cent efficiency of absorption, the intake has to be in the vicinity of 25 mg per day – completely outside the usual range for most American women, many of whom get no more than 10 to 15 mg a day of iron in their diet and some of whom get less than 10 mg.

The average iron loss of 1.2 mg a day of menstruating women can be covered by an average diet. It is obvious that most "normal" diets are inadequate for women with 1.5 mg a day iron loss (25% of the Swedish sample) and are grossly inadequate for women with 2 mg loss a day (10% of the Swedish sample). Iron-deficiency anemia in males in the United States is seldom primarily due to nutritional causes, and the diagnosis of chronic nutritional hypochromic anemia should never be made in men unless all sources of pathologic blood loss and organic disease have been excluded. The situation is obviously different in women.

As a nutritionist, I would be the last to minimize the importance of a good diet in preventing iron-deficiency anemia. This is all the more important at a time when iron cooking utensils have been eliminated (thus eliminating an appreciable source of iron in the diet), when fat represents over 40 per cent of the American diet, and when dairy products (extremely low in iron) are consumed in large amounts. The U.S. diet is often much lower in iron than are the diets of poorer populations, which are high in partially milled cereals prepared in primitive pots and pans. On the other hand, it must be noted that in practice, for an appreciable proportion of menstruating women, iron supplements on a periodic or chronic basis are indispensable if progressive iron depletion is to be avoided. While we can hope that women will eat some meat, fish, eggs and green vegetables, it is unrealistic to hope that they will eat the frequent portions of liver which women with copious menstrual losses require. Once anemia has set in, it is unrealistic to think it can be cured by diet alone.

## REFERENCES

1. Swedish Nutrition Foundation. Blix, G. (Ed.): Occurrence, causes and prevention of Nutritional anaemias. Almqvist and Wiksells, Uppsala, 1968.
2. Hallberg, L., Hallgren, J., Hollender, A., Hogdahl, A.-M. and Tibblin, G.: Occurrence of iron deficiency anaemia in Sweden. Ibid., p. 19.
3. Hallberg, L., Hogdahl, A.-M., Nilson, L. and Rybo, G.: Variation of iron loss in women. Ibid., p. 115.

*Chapter 13*

# ZINC DEFICIENCY:
# A CAUSE OF GROWTH RETARDATION?

THE role of zinc as an important element in biochemistry was recognized as early as 1869, when Raulin showed it to be necessary for the growth of molds. It was found in human liver in 1877. However, not until 1934 did Gabriel Bertrand, Paris, show that this metal was essential for the growth of the mouse, thus opening the chapter of zinc in mammalian physiology. The following year Stirn, Elvejehm and Hart showed zinc to be essential for the growth of the rat. The next milestone was reached in 1944, when Keilin and Mann demonstrated that the enzyme carbonic anhydrase contains 0.33 per cent of zinc and showed that the presence of this metal was thus essential to the elimination and incorporation of carbon dioxide. Since this time a considerable amount of work, well reviewed up to 1959 by Vallee (1), has ascribed to this metal a fundamental role in biology. Recent and important work on the effect of zinc deficiency in man makes a brief summary of these findings of topical interest.

## OCCURRENCE OF ZINC IN ENZYMES

It would be tedious to attempt to give a complete list of the many enzymes which, following Keilin and Mann's work, were found to contain or to be activated by zinc. Zinc metalloenzymes of known metal content include carboxypeptidase, alcohol dehydrogenase, glutamic acid dehydrogenase, muscle lactic dehydrogenase, and kidney alkaline phosphatase. In addition, zinc activates a number of enzymes important in the metabolism of protein, including glycylglycine dipeptidase, arginase, dehydropeptidase, tripeptidase, carnosinase, histidine deaminase, etc., as

Reprinted from *Postgraduate Medicine, 35* (No. 2), February, 1964.

well as oxaloacetic carboxylase and some lecithinases and enolases among others. The fact that such enzymes are present in plants as well as in animals explains the great importance of zinc in agriculture as well as in husbandry. Entire sections of California, Texas and Australia have been reclaimed and made productive by the addition of zinc to the soil.

## OCCURRENCE OF ZINC IN MAMMALIAN TISSUES

The occurrence of zinc is widespread in mammalian tissues. Injection of the radioisotope zinc[65] permits following the distribution of the metal in tissues. The liver contains the largest initial fraction of the injected dose. The pancreas, kidneys and pituitary also show rapid uptake. Least activity is found in the

TABLE 13-1

EXAMPLES OF DIETARY SOURCES OF ZINC

| Food | Zinc Content (Mg/100 Gm Edible Portion) |
|---|---|
| Beef | 2-5 |
| Bread (whole-wheat) | 2.5-3.5 |
| Butter | 0.3 |
| Carrots | 0.5-4 |
| Corn | 2.5 |
| Egg yolk | 2.6-4 |
| Herring | 70-140 |
| Lettuce | 0.1-0.7 |
| Liver (beef) | 3-8.5 |
| Liver (pork) | 3-15 |
| Milk | 0.4-3 |
| Oatmeal | 15 |
| Orange | 0.1 |
| Oyster | 160 |
| Peas | 3-5 |
| Potatoes | 0.2 |
| Rice | 1.5 |
| Wheat | 2.5-8.5 |
| Yeast (dry) | 8 |

erthrocytes, skeletal muscles and skin, with the spleen, gastrointestinal tract, adrenals, lungs, lymph nodes, brain, heart and thymus showing an intermediate degree of the uptake. Of particular interest is the content in the male genital organs, pancreas, eyes, blood and human milk. There is no explanation for the high zinc concentrations found in the male mammalian genital tract, particularly in animal and human semen as well as in the epididymis and prostate. Carbonic anhydrase accounts for only a small part of this content. The level of zinc is high in the pancreas, and early studies suggesting a decreased content in the presence of diabetes led to a voluminous amount of work. Contrary to early hypotheses, it was found that both insulin and glucagon can be obtained free of zinc; yet both are fully active in vivo. While it has been proposed that the zinc-free hormones will associate with zinc in the organism for certain actions, definite evidence supporting this hypothesis is still lacking. Zinc is seen in large amounts in certain areas of the eye, particularly in the tapetum cellulosum, where a zinc-cysteine complex has been isolated. The zinc content of the retina is substantial. Retinene reductase, which catalyzes the redox conversion of vitamin A, alcohol and aldehyde, is apparently identical with alcohol dehydrogenase.

Zinc is distributed in various fractions in the blood, with 12 per cent in the serum, 3 per cent in the leukocytes, and 85 per cent in the erthrocytes. The serum concentrations are decreased in chronic infections, untreated pernicious anemia, Laennec's cirrhosis, and myocardial infarction and increased in hyperthyroidism, hypertension and polycythemia vera. There are similar increases or decreases in the zinc concentration in blood cells in a variety of pathologic conditions. Vallee's comprehensive review (1) gives a more complete list.

The concentration of zinc in cow's milk (3 to 5 mg per liter) is 10 times that of iron and 100 times that of copper. Human milk, like cow's milk, starts from a high level in colostrum, as high as 20 mg per liter at the time of delivery. However, in human milk the level falls slowly to 650 mcg at the end of six months. Feeding zinc increases the zinc content of milk.

## ZINC DEFICIENCY IN ANIMALS

In the mouse, zinc deficiency retards growth and ossification and accelerates separation of the eyelids and eruption of the incisors. In the rat, growth is extremely depressed by zinc deficiency; it may be noted that at a critical level growth responds strikingly to minute additions of zinc. Hyperkeratinization, thickening of the epidermis, and intracellular and intercellular edema of the skin and mucous membranes of the esophagus and mouth are observed. Loss of hair follicles occurs. Testicular atrophy and decreased size of the accessory sex organs are seen. (This group of findings will take on added significance in the light of the human syndrome described subsequently.) In addition, a number of congenital malformations have been observed, such as rosary tail, clubbed digits and deformed nails. Corneal vascularization also occurs.

Porcine parakeratosis may be essentially zinc deficiency. The disease, characterized by dermatitis, diarrhea, vomiting, anorexia, severe weight loss, and death, responds well to administration of zinc.

The problem of zinc requirements has, incidentally, important economic aspects. Two recent studies (2, 3) indicate that practical turkey rations often do not contain sufficient zinc to meet the needs of a rapidly developing poult. Adding zinc to such rations leads particularly to an increase in the length of the long bones. Other work (4) has suggested that all zinc compounds do not make the metal equally available. Similarly, a number of recent papers on the nutrition of growing pullets and laying hens suggest that zinc may be a critical element in these aspects of animal production. A series of reports, beginning in 1961, suggest that this work in experimental and farm animals may have an important bearing in human nutrition.

## POSTALCOHOLIC HUMAN CIRRHOSIS

Postalcoholic cirrhosis is one area in which a clinical role of zinc has been suggested. Marked abnormalities of zinc metabolism are seen in patients with this condition. Zinc serum levels are markedly depressed — to 70 mcg or less instead of the normal 120 mcg per 100 ml. Comatose patients may show concentrations of 30 mcg per 100 ml. Excretion in the urine is high. Orally administered zinc sulfate tends to restore normal excretory patterns and produce a tendency toward normal liver function. Inasmuch as liver alcohol dehydrogenase is a zinc-containing enzyme, it appears possible that the disorders in zinc metabolism bear a direct relationship to the alcoholic condition.

## DWARFISM AND HYPOGONADISM IN MAN

An initial report by Prasad, Halstead and Nadimi (5), published in 1961, described a syndrome of dwarfism and hypogonadism associated with severe anemia, geophagia and hepatosplenomegaly in male Iranians. None of these subjects had schistosomiasis or hookworms. Prasad and co-workers (6), among them William J. Darby, Vanderbilt University, described similar clinical manifestations in a group of persons living near Cairo, Egypt. None of these Egyptians showed geophagia, but almost all of them had schistosomiasis or hookworm infections.

The suggestion that the syndromes of both dwarfism and anemia might be related to zinc (and iron) deficiencies was strongly documented in a remarkable series of publications by Prasad and co-workers.

The patients living near Cairo were 16 to 19 years old and were free of acute or chronic febrile illness. They were anemic (hypochrome or microcytic anemia); their growth was markedly retarded; their external genitalia were remarkably small, with both atrophic testes and small penises; and they had no facial, pubic or axillary hair. The patients appeared much younger than their chronologic age. Bone age was retarded. Their skin was rough and hyperpigmented. Pallor and hepatosplenomegaly were present. Two patients were edematous. The diet of these subjects consisted of wheat or corn bread, beans, occasionally white cheese, and only rarely meat or animal protein other than cheese. Analytic data were compared with the values obtained in a control group of normal Egyptians. Serum iron levels were low and mean plasma copper values were greater than normal. Total iron-binding capacity was greater in dwarfs than in normal subjects. Deficiencies in magnesium,. vitamin $B_{12}$, ascorbic acid, carotene, vitamin A, folic acid and pyridoxine were ruled out. A large number of enzyme determinations and endocrine function tests were also conducted. Results of gastrointestinal series, chest x-rays and electrocardiograms were not remarkable. Prasad and co-workers determined the zinc content of plasma, red blood cells and hair. These values were consistently decreased in the dwarf, compared with a group of normal Egyptian controls. Plasma zinc[65] disappearance curves were established and resolved into five phases: phase 1,0 to 30 minutes; phase 2, 30 to 60 minutes; phase 3, 60 minutes to 10 hours; phase 4, 10 hours to seven days; phase 5, more than seven days.

During the second and third phases of the zinc[65] plasma disappearance curve, the half-life was shorter in dwarfs than in the normal controls. This significantly increases plasma zinc turnover supports the concept of zinc deficiency, a finding obviously compatible with an increased migration of plasma zinc to the tissues. Similarly, the decreased excretion of zinc[65] in the urine and stools of dwarfs, compared with that of normal subjects for a period of 13 days, on the average indicated that these subjects conserved zinc. This zinc retention occurred in spite of the fact that the dwarfs lost red blood cells in their urine and stools because of their parasitic infections. Alkaline phosphatase, a zinc-containing enzyme, was decreased.

The interpretation of these findings was complicated by the severe parasitic infections in the subjects in the study just summarized. Inasmuch as severe anemia may retard growth and since in Egypt schistosomiasis is commonly considered the cause of dwarfism, it appeared possible that either directly or through its effect on the blood, schistosomiasis might be considered the cause of dwarfism. To rule out this possiblity, Prasad and co-workers (7) examined the populations of Khârga and Bulaq, two desert oases where the diet was similar to that consumed by the subjects of the previous study but where schistosomiasis and hookworm infection were absent. In Khârga, it was found that five of 109 males subjects between the ages of 14 and 19 had hypogonadism and markedly retarded growth. These subjects also appeared much younger than their stated ages. They had no facial, pubic or axillary hair; their penises were small and their testes atrophic. Three subjects had liver enlargement. In Bulaq, five of 50 patients between 15 and 19 years of age showed growth retardation and hypogonadism; one of these subjects had a palpable liver and spleen.

The iron content in the water supply of the oasis of Khârga was appreciable, but only negligible amounts of zinc were present. The Khârga dwarfs had only mild anemia, a fact probably due to the combination of the higher iron content of the water and the absence of parasites. This important difference along with the findings of the previous studies suggested to Prasad and co-workers that anemia and iron deficiency do not seem to be necessary for dwarfism and hypogonadism.

These important studies certainly strongly suggest and may perhaps be taken to demonstrate that dietary zinc deficiency in man, as well as in experimental animals, can cause extreme retardation of growth and of gonadal development. The possibility that degrees of retardation of physical development in the United States are related to a relative deficiency of zinc in the diet or to a defect in the absorption or utilization of this essential trace element deserves careful consideration.

## REFERENCES

1. Vallee, B. L.: Biochemistry, physiology and pathology of zinc. Physiol. Rev., 39:443, 1959.
2. Supplee, W. C., Creek, R. D., Combs, G. F. and Blamberg, D. L.: Zinc requirements of poults receiving practical diets. Poultry Sc., 40:171, 1961.
3. Sullivan, T. W.: Zinc requirement of broad-breasted bronze poults. *Ibid.,* p. 334.
4. ——: Availability of zinc in various compounds of broad-breasted bronze poults. *Ibid.,* p. 340.
5. Prasad, A. S., Halsted, J. A. and Nadimi, M.: Syndrome of iron deficiency anemia, hepatosplenomegaly, hypogonadism, dwarfism, and geophagia. Am. J. Med., 31:532, 1961.
6. Prasad, A. S., Miale, A., Jr., Farid, Z., Sandstead, H. H., Schulert, A. R. and Darby, W. J.: Biochemical studies on dwarfism, hypogondism and anemia. Arch. Int. Med., 111:65, 1963.
7. Prasad, A. S., Schulert, A. R., Miale, A., Jr., Farid, Z. and Sandstead, H. H.: Zinc and iron deficiencies in male subjects with dwarfism and

hypogonadism but without anacylostomiasis, schistosomiasis or severe anemia. Am. J. Clin. Nutrition, 12:437, 1963.

*Chapter 14*

# CHROMIUM IN MEDICINE

I BELIEVE that the interest in trace elements in nutrition and medicine will increase in the immediate future and that the role of some hitherto neglected trace nutrients (vanadium, chromium, manganese, zinc, nolybedenum and, perhaps, nickel among metals and selenium and, perhaps, bromine among nonmetals) will become increasingly clear. These elements, which are known to have biologic functions, may be complemented by others, such as boron, silicon, arsenic and tellurium, which are detectable in biologic material but as yet have no known function in mammalian physiology.

Diseases such as atherosclerosis and diabetes may be related to partial deficiency of these elements. Conversely, the toxicity of trace doses of metals such as lead, mercury and cadminim is beginning to be appreciated and is the basis of far-reaching government measures to decrease their prevalence among man-made pollutants.

## ESSENTIALITY OF TRACE METALS

In considering the trace elements that man appears to need, one must realize that the old, simplistic definition of essentiality — a nutrient is essential if its absence is incompatible with life — must be modified in practice when dealing with omnipresent elements, even in microscopic amounts. Mertz has pointed out that even in animals, the criterion of life or death calls for the production of a severe deficiency of these metals, a state that for most of these elements is extremely difficult to effect at present.

Reprinted from *Postgraduate Medicine, 49* (No. 1), January, 1971.© McGraw-Hill, Inc.

141

A pure or complete deficiency of trace elements in man is obviously unlikely. Mertz emphasizes that something less than this all-or-none approach is needed, and he has substituted the following criteria as a working definition of the essentiality of a trace element (1, 2).

1. An essential element must be present in the tissue of healthy individuals. Presence of the element in fetal or newborn tissue reinforces the presumption of essentiality.

2. The essentiality of an element is more likely if a homeostatic regulation can be shown; such regulations work through control of absorption or excretion.

3. The demonstration of reproducible changes in blood levels or tissue distributions after a physiologic event is good presumptive evidence of the essentiality of a mineral.

4. The identification of metalloenzymes of which the metal is a part, the demonstration of a specific role for a metal as an activator of a given enzyme, and the constant presence of a metal in definite amounts in an important body constituent are additional proof of essentiality.

5. When total or partial absence of a metal from the diet of animals can be shown to impair function or morphogenesis, the metal is very likely essential to man. When absolute deficiency cannot be produced, symptoms often can be precipitated by stresses such as repeated pregnancy (of portentuous clinical significance or by competing minerals, or the experiments can be carried out for several generations.

The fact that a supplement of a metal, as opposed to a deficiency, has an effect on an organism suggests its essentiality only if the effect is favorable and is obtained with doses of physiologic significance.

## CHROMIUM CONTENT IN MAN

All the aforementioned criteria can be applied to chromium, which not only appears essential to man but also may be in somewhat short supply in the diet of many Americans, with important clinical consequences.

Chromium is present in the trivalent state in all plants and animals. Elucidation of its role in maintaining normal glucose metabolism and preventing atherosclerosis could be an important contribution to medicine and public health in the next decade. Chromium concentrations depend on its content in soil and water, and each species has a certain range of concentration. In general, meat is a much better source of chromium than fish. In man, the chromium content is low in the heart and very high in various parts of the brain. It is also high in the hair, skin and fat, and particularly high in the omentum.

Age is an important influence on the chromium content of human tissue. Unlike the levels of iron and copper, which are essentially constant throughout life, or of lead and cadmium, which increase with age as pollution exceeds excretion capabilities, the level of chromium in most organs decreases with age. The chromium level is highest in newborn tissue and thus is higher in children than in adults. It seems to be the only mineral element to evolve in this way. Levels in the United States are lower than in most countries.

Biochemically, chromium is an active compound that forms many complexes with proteins, stimulates several enzyme systems, and may stabilize certain nucleic acid structures. The presence of exceptionally high concentrations of chromium in brain tissue, particularly in the caudate nuclei, is intriguing. More readily interpretable, however, are the low-chromium states associated with a diabeteslike syndrome and increased aortic lesions in animals and, perhaps, with similar pathology in man.

A moderate degree of chromium depletion is associated with normal plasma glucose, but in animals as the depletion becomes more severe, glucose tolerance becomes increasingly impaired. Glucose tolerance improves when trivalent chromium (as chromium acetate) is added to the drinking water. Response to tolbutamide also is impaired by low chromium levels and improves with trivalent chromium therapy.

The impaired glucose tolerance in low-chromium states appears closely related to the reduced hypoglycemic action of insulin caused by low chromium. Chromium supplementation restores the normal sensitivity to insulin. In animals, severe chromium depletion produces a degree of impaired glucose tolerance that stimulates diabetes mellitus, and rigorous chromium exclusion produces fasting hyperglycemia and glucosuria.

Small amounts of chromium, alone or with germanium, nickel or noibium, have decreased the circulating cholesterol in rats. Of particular interest is the apparently specific effect of chromium in inhibiting the development of aortic plaques. In animals a diet very low in chromium causes a syndrome resembling human atherosclerosis and decreases their life span. A diet low in chromium and protein causes opacity and neovascularization of the cornea.

Human findings suggest that the aforementioned experiments are highly relevant to man. Schroeder and co-workers, Dartmouth Medical School, Hanover, New Hampshire (3), found that the chromium content of the aorta was significantly lower in subjects who died of a coronary occlusion than in those who died of an accident. They also found that older human subjects who had impaired glucose tolerance greatly improved with daily low doses (150 mcg) of chromic salts for a long period and recovered more rapidly with larger doses (2 to 10 mg). However, the response in patients with overt diabetes mellitus requiring insulin was erratic. A small group of hypercholesterolemic patients responded slowly but favorably to chromic salts.

While evidence to date does not indicate routine therapeutic use of chromic salts, the finding that chromium may favorably affect the interrelated impairment of glucose metabolism and athero-sclerosis warrants intensive clinical investigation and careful monitoring of our food supply to insure against a decreasing content of trace metals.

Substituting brown sugar for white sugar and eating whole wheat bread are partial but possibly useful measures. Studies on fortifying flour and other foods with an absorbable chromium complex or on adding chromium to chemical fertilizers to increase its content in food plants and animal feeds may be advisable.

## REFERENCES

1. Mertz, W.: Biological role of chromium. Fed. Proc., 26:186, 1967.
2. Mertz, W.: Some aspects of nutritional trace element research. Fed. Proc., 29:1482, 1970.
3. Schroeder, H. A.: The role of chromium in mammalian nutrition. Am. J. Clin. Nutr., 21:23, 1968.

# PART III
## The Seven Ages of Man: From Infancy to Old Age

*Chapter 15*

# THE FAT BABY

P RECISE knowledge of energy requirements would seem more useful in infants than in any other category of human beings, for usually infants are the only persons who eat what they are given and have no opportunity to supplement their diet. A baby can refuse to eat or spit out the food placed in his mouth, but he cannot get up at night, open the refrigerator, and add a substantial snack to the day's ration. It would appear that if one knows a healthy baby's size and rate of growth one can determine with a high degree of approximation what his calorie intake should be. Conversely, if his size and intake are known, the rate of growth or fat deposition, or both, should follow ineluctably. At a time when it is thought that the fat baby might become the obese adult, it seems possible that feeding the energy equivalent of maintenance plus just that necessary for optimal growth should permit ideal development. In fact, published tables of allowances for infants reflect this simplistic view.

Basically, all sets of allowances or requirements issued by FAO-WHO Committees on Calorie Requirements and the Subcommittee on Calories of the National Research Council have assumed that one could define an average and a range of variation (115 ± 15 cal per kilogram) for the calorie requirements of babies up to one year old. Statements in the Recommended Dietary Allowances of the National Academy of Sciences-National Research Council further qualify the figures and range: "The calorie and protein allowances per kilogram for infants are considered to decrease progressively from birth," and, more obscurely, "Allowances for calcium, thiamine, riboflavin and niacin increase proportionally with calories to the maximum values shown." The first statement leaves the impression that the

Reprinted from *Postgraduate Medicine, 44* (No. 4), October, 1968.© McGraw-Hill, Inc.

set of figures given in the tables corresponds to an average for the period (values at six months?), while the second statement makes it appear that the "maximum values" per kilogram must apply to the newborn infant, with smaller recommendations for older infants. Actually, whatever the exact meaning of the statement, the range indicated probably does cover the calorie intake of healthy infants growing normally. Regrettably, nowhere in the text accompanying the tables is there any suggestion that variability in recommended intakes for infants is closely related to variability in physical activity rather than to difference in size and rates of weight gain.

Let us first examine the magnitude of the variability. Two careful studies, by Beale in Denver (1) and Rueda-Williamson and Rose in Boston (2), gave respective ranges of 525 to 975 (median 725) cal and 530 to 1,035 (median 806) cal per day for infants five months old. Similar variability was noted throughout the infancy (2 to 15 months) of these babies.

Can differences in size or rate of growth explain the variability; Widdowson (3), the noted British nutritionist, found that only 8 to 10 per cent of the total calories consumed by a baby are used for new tissue growth, even at that stage of postnatal life when growth is probably greater than ever again. Her estimate approximates Hegsted's 1.8 per cent of the mean calorie intake deposited as new tissue protein (4) and Rose and Mayer's 5 per cent of the total intake deposited as fat (5), which combined give a total of about 7 per cent for growth.

Even though it could appear initially that an infant too young to walk would not expend a major fraction of his energy intake each day in exercise, determination of the various components of energy expenditure suggests that infant activity does consume a great deal of energy. Methods traditionally used to calculate basal calorie expenditure in infants, exemplified by Talbot's standards (6), show that about 42 percent of calories ingested are basal calories.

Inasmuch as basal expenditures were measured by Talbot and Benedict's method (7), i.e. shortly after a small feeding, it would appear that half of the specific dynamic action is included in the "basal" value. Adding 3 per cent for the remainder, about 45 per cent of the daily energy requirement is accounted for by "resting metabolism'" Our data show that about 9 per cent of the calories ingested are found in the feces, a higher value than in adults. Thus, growth, fecal excretion and resting metabolism account for about 62 per cent of the calories, leaving 38 per cent for physical activity, a percentage far from inconsiderable and much in excess of that devoted to growth.

In a study of 31 infants living in normal home environments in Boston (5), Dr. Hedwig Rose and I uncovered a number of additional facts which bear directly on the question of who the fat babies are, why they are fat, and what we can do about it. All babies studied were under two months of age and were followed for six months or more. Recumbent length, weight, triceps skinfold thickness, and diet histories were recorded twice a month. Activity was measured by the use of "Actometers," modified automatically-winding, calendar watches which measure movements in two planes and which babies can wear on the wrist and ankle without discomfort. Fecal losses were determined and alalyzed at intervals.

Data clearly showed that there was no correlation between total calories consumed and weight. By contrast, there was a strong correlation between food intake and activity, and only when activity had been accounted for was there any correlation between food intake and basal expenditure. Particularly interesting was the strong negative correlation between activity and triceps skinfold thickness. In other words, the fatter the baby, the less active it was; the thinner the baby, the more active it was. This relationship, which held true for all infants, was particularly striking in those infants, fat or thin, who had skinfold thicknesses more than one standard deviation above or below the mean. In fact, the extremely thin infants moved more and ate more than the normal babies, while the extremely fat ones moved less and ate less. Their respective hyperactivities and hypoactivities were such that the thin babies remained thin despite unusually high calorie intakes, while the fat babies remained fat despite unusually low calorie intakes. The highest infant activity rating was more than twice as high as the lowest.

A number of studies, particularly ours, have shown that obesity in older children and adolescents is often, even generally, associated with a very moderated food intake but an extremely low rate of activity. The question has inevitably arisen: Which came first, the obesity or the inactivity? This study suggests that the question is meaningless. Fatness and inactivity may exist at birth. Both may be associated with the predominantly endomorphic, mesomorphic and ectopenic body types characteristic of obesity. The fact that there is a strong correlation between body weight and obesity in parents and children, but not between parents and children adopted at birth, also emphasizes the importance of constitutional factors. Our results also cast some doubt on the often-repeated assertion that "over-feeding" with solid foods in infancy causes obesity in children.

From a practical viewpoint, it is important to realize that if the fat baby does not have a larger-than-normal intake, great caution must be used in cutting down on how much he eats. First, there is a risk of diminishing growth rather than fat accumulation. Second, it may well be that any curtailment of a moderate intake will cause hunger, and with it a great increase in crying, muscle tone and (rage) activity, which will magnify the size of the calorie correction to a level much above that anticipated and again compromise growth. Although decreasing excessive fatness in babies is probably very useful, the "dieting" prescription should be determined with caution and accompanied by frequent checks on the maintenance of growth in length, health and a reasonably happy disposition.

## REFERENCES

1. Beale, V. A.: Nutritional intake of children: I. Calories, carbohydrate, fat and protein. J. Nutr., 50:223, 1953.
2. Rueda-Williamson, R. and Rose, H. E.: Growth and nutrition of infants: The influence of diet and other factors on growth. Pediatrics, 30:639, 1962.
3. Widdowson, E. M.: Energy balance in early life. Proc. Nutr. Soc., 20:83, 1961.
4. Hegsted, D. M.: Theoretical estimates of protein requirements of children. J. Amer. Diet. Ass., 33:225, 1957.
5. Rose, H. E. and Mayer, J.: Activity, Calorie intake, fat storage, and the energy balance of infants. Pediatrics, 41:18, 1968.
6. Talbot, E. B.: Twenty-four metabolism of two normal infants with special reference to the total energy requirements of infants. Amer. J. Dis. Child., 14:25, 1917.
7. Rose, H. E.: Food intake and fecal excretion of four-to-six month old infants. Unpublished manuscript.

## Chapter 16

# HYPERTENSION, SALT INTAKE, AND THE INFANT

A GROWING number of pediatricians, nutritionists and internists are becoming worried over the high salt intake of infants — and with good reason, I believe. Breast milk has a very low sodium content (7 mEq per liter, a concentration lower than that of tap water in many cities). The total sodium intake of the infant who is entirely breast-fed is thus rarely above 10 mEq per day. Thousands of generations have shown that this small amount of sodium is entirely adequate to support healthy growth.

Cow's milk is much higher in sodium — about 30 mEq per liter. An infant reared on cow's milk is thus on a diet very high in sodium, compared with a breast-fed baby. The sodium content of the diet is further increased when solid baby foods are introduced in the diet. When the infant is six months old, milk usually contributes, at most, half the total daily sodium intake; at one year milk contributes normally less than a quarter of the total sodium, with 60 per cent of the total coming from processed meats and vegetables. As prepared by U.S. manufacturers, these foods are copiously salted apparently to make them palatable — to the mothers! Whereas the breast-fed infant receives about 1 mEq sodium per kilogram, the infant fed cow's milk exclusively receives about 3.5 mEq per kilogram.

A recent study on a large group of healthy American term babies fed cow's milk and ranging in age from 1 to 14 months showed that at one month of age the average daily intake of sodium was 4.6 mEq per kilogram, with the highest value 8 mEq per kilogram. By one year of age, the average had risen to 6.3 mEq per kilogram. The highest value recorded was 10.9 mEq per

Reprinted from *Postgraduate Medicine*, 45 (No. 1), January, 1969.© McGraw-Hill, Inc.

kilogram in a three-month-old infant — 10 times the intake of a breast-fed infant of the same age! (The intake of 1 mEq per kilogram, incidentally, agrees well with calculated requirements for infants from birth to one year, with the requirements for growth decreasing and the insensible and fecal losses increasing during that period, leaving the overall requirement per kilogram essentially constant.)

Some manufacturers appear to have been stung by the criticism that they were selling "baby foods" on the basis of their being palatable to the mothers (who are used to a high-salt diet), rather than conforming to the infant's requirements. One of their advocates has pointed out that while it is true that the salt intake of infants fed processed baby food is enormous if related to a body weight basis, so are water, calorie and protein intake. He pointed out that "the year old infant takes in 120 to 135 ml of water per kilogram per day, which is equivalent to 8.40 to 9.45 L of water per day for the 70-kg adult." He went on to show that for a 70-kg man the calorie and protein intake equivalent ot that of a baby would be 7700 calories and 140 to 245 gm of protein, and suggested that "the restriction of salt to levels of impalatability might do more harm than good."

This, of course, is a meaningless argument. The requirements for the infants have been calculated and agree well with the historically adequate intake of the breast-fed infant. There is no indication that highly salted food is particularly palatable to the infant, or that bland food — like essentially tasteless milk — is not the preferred food at that age. Furthermore, there are a great deal of experimental evidence, quite a lot of clinical material, and some epidemiologic data pointing to the dangers of high-salt diets.

Epidemiologic studies have shown that primitive peoples, by and large, have low intakes of salt and, generally speaking, no hypertension. By contrast, West Indian Negroes, who have a high intake of salt (salt pork and salt fish), have a much higher prevalence of hypertension than do white inhabitants and Indians in the same area. Lewis K. Dahl, the well-known chief of the medical service in the Medical Center at Brookhaven National Laboratory, divided a large number of adults into three groups, according to low, average and high sodium intakes. He found that over 10 per cent of the group with high intakes had hypertension, compared with 7 per cent of the average group and less than 1 per cent in the low group. Conversely, in another study hypertensive subjects were found to have a higher salt intake than those who were normotensive.

A number of populations do live on very low salt intake with no evidence of harmful effect. Among such peoples who have been investigated are the Eskimo, certain Chinese groups, American Indians of the Northwest, Lapps and the Masai of Africa (a warring people of particularly splendid physique who live essentially on meat, milk and blood and have an average intake of 1.8 gm of salt per day).

Experimental work shows that a high dietary concentration of salt induces permanent hypertension in rats. Some strains of rats are much more sensitive than others, but basically there is a dietary concentration, characteristic of each strain, which will induce this condition. In an experiment involving 30 different varieties of baby foods (all of which showed a sodium content greatly in excess of the unprocessed meats and vegetables from which they were made), Dahl and co-workers found that hypertension developed within four months in most rats predisposed to hypertension that were fed these foods. Dahl also found that very young rats are more immediately sensitive to the effect of high-salt diets than are older animals.

Clinically, it is well known that the tendency for edema to develop in prematurely born infants is a function of the sodium content of the diet. It has also been demonstrated that a high salt content of the diet increases the likelihood of renal cast formation in these infants. We do not need to be reminded of the therapeutic effects of low-salt diets in hypertension.

What can we conclude from this evidence? Certainly that there is a very definite risk that salted baby foods may be harmful. Cigarette smoking, radiation and some poisons are also harmful, but their cumulative effect is slow enough to hide the toxicity for many years, similarly, we may be just becoming aware of the role of excessive dietary intake of sodium chloride in the etiology of hypertension. It seems particularly dangerous to expose infants to the intakes that are proportionally higher than those of adults and enormously higher than those resulting from breast feeding. By contrast, there appears to be no risk whatsoever in low sodium intake.

A reasonable policy would seem to be to instruct mothers not to add any salt to eggs, cereals or other dishes they prepare for their infants. Pediatricians and their professional societies should try to influence manufacturers of baby foods — who in other respects have tried to conform with sound nutritional concepts — to stop adding so much salt (or for that matter, to stop adding any salt) to the foods they prepare. Manufacturers should be invited to participate in educational campaigns directed at the mothers to teach them not to use the same criterion in judging the "salt taste" of food for their infants as for adults.

We should remember that basically prepared baby foods add very little to the diet of milk-fed infants given vitamins. The very young infant spits out most of what is fed to him. What is ingested and absorbed does make a small contribution of iron to the baby's nutrition, at some cost (10% of allergic reactions in very young infants). It is perhaps too much to say that solid foods fed to small infants are really a status symbol for the mother, but it is legitimate to question whether for infants of less than three months, at any rate, they serve any useful purpose.

## REFERENCES

1. Dahl, L. K., Knudsen, K. D., Heine, M. A. and Leitl, G. J.: Effects of chronic excess salt ingestion: Modification of experimental hypertension in the rat by variations in the diet. Circ. Res., 22:11, 1968.
2. Knudsen, K. D. and Dahl, L. K.: Essential hypertension: Inborn error of sodium metabolism? Postgrad. Med. J., 42:148, 1966.
3. Dahl, L. K., Heine, M. A. and Tassinari, L.: High salt content of Western infant's diet: Possible relationship of hypertension in the adult. Nature, 198:1204, 1963.

*Chapter 17*

# FEEDING THE PRESCHOOL CHILD

Written in collaboration with
Frances M. Dwyer and Johanna T. Dwyer

MANY mothers and other caretakers regard the feeding of the preschool child as demanding and exasperating, and often seek advice from the physician. This discussion will highlight the major findings of one of us (F.M.D.) in an extensive series of experimental studies of children's eating habits. The basic rule of good eating habits is to invite good nutrition by providing wholesome food. The mother does this primarily by making available to the child nutritionally well-balanced foods.

From two to five years of age, the child grows rather slowly compared with the rapid gains he makes in height and weight in his first few years. His activity level varies far more than does that of an adult, which may lead to rather dramatic fluctuations in appetite. The mother may notice that the child's appetite seems to be "falling off," and worry unnecessarily because he does not eat all he is served. If he is her first child, she may not realize how much less small children eat than adults. This becomes crucial when the child switches from baby food to adult food (food prepared for everyone in the family). When the mother fed the child baby food, she took cues from the size of the container, which reassured her that the child was eating enough even if it did not seem so from her standpoint. She did not expect the baby to conform to adult standards. However, when it is time for the child to make the transition to adult food, the mother may tend to use her own or her husband's average portion sizes as a guide, giving the child perhaps two-thirds as much. This may far exceed what the child could possibly eat. At this point many mothers become desperate because the child who had been "doing so well"

Reprinted from *Postgraduate Medicine, 47* (No. 3), March, 1970.© McGraw-Hill, Inc.

suddenly starts to "eat like a bird," and they panic at the thought that he may starve. In our clinical experience, no healthy child has ever become ill or has starved because he skipped an occasional meal or did not finish everything on his plate, but at this juncture mothers often call frantically for help from the family physician.

It is important to recognize that a child's sense of taste is more acute than an adult's. The adult fare in the family may be too highly seasoned for his taste. However, a great deal of taste tolerance for different foods is determined culturally. An Italian--American preschooler may relish the sausage that he has been eating from babyhood, while an Irish-American child of the same age might find it too hot at first because of lack of experience. Adults often encounter the same phenomenon when they first taste real Mexican or East Indian cuisine, which usually is much more highly seasoned than American food.

## SNACKS

Human beings are not born with the ability to become hungry only three times a day. It is almost second nature for American adults to concentrate the bulk of their eating in three meals and perhaps a snack or two a day. These habits are not inborn; rather, they develop as a practical compromise between the physiologic need for food and convenient times to eat from the standpoint of work and social life. Mothers often become annoyed by the seemingly constant hunger of the preschool child who often wishes to be fed several times between each meal but shows little interest in eating at the family's mealtime. No law of nutrition states that one must not eat between meals to be well nourished or that eating at one time of day is better than eating at another. However, if the family eats together, it certainly is less trouble for the mother. *What* they eat is far more important than *when* they eat. The preschooler's tremendous physical activity often generates a hearty appetite at what the adult may consider a strange time of day. Within the limits of the mother's time and patience, the preschool child may be fed when he is hungry. However, the child should realize that he is also expected to join the family for meals, even if he eats only a small amount.

If the child wants a simple snack at 10 or 3 o'clock, a warmed-up hot dog, a peanut butter sandwich, an apple, or similar foods will satisfy his hunger and also contribute nutritious food to his diet. To prevent the mother from degenerating into a short-order cook on duty 24 hours a day, the child should be encouraged very early in life to satisfy his between-meal hunger pangs himself with easily obtained, nutritionally well-balanced foods. Snack foods that contain calories and little else, such as soft drinks and cookies, should be kept to a minimum, not because they are intrinsically bad but because they may satisfy the child's hunger but not give him the daily requirement of other nutrients such as protein, minerals and vitamins.

## PLATE WASTE

Allowing a child to select his own portion sizes is one way of helping him to meter his own food intake. Children's eyes are often bigger than their stomach and they may tend to over-estimate what they can eat, leaving food on the plate. Patience is necessary to remind the child not to take too much when he is serving himself. Gradually he will learn to adequately assess his appetite. It is not good to force the child to eat everything on his plate, even if he does take too much.

It never ceases to amaze us that while few people force a pet to eat everything in its dish, many insist that their children do so at every meal. A gentle suggestion to the child to eat all he can and an offer of some physical help in collecting the scattered food on the plate so he can get it on the fork or into his mouth may be in order, but desperated pleas and peremptory commands are not. If food still is left, a verbal reminder to take less next time will suffice. In feeding the preschool child, a certain amount of plate waste probably is inevitable. Adult food is more difficult and challenging to eat than the semifluid baby food mixtures that can be handled easily with a spoon. Applying these maxims will minimize waste and prevent it from becoming an emotionally charged moral issue. At the same time the child learns to become his own judge.

## DESSERTS

Whether to allow a child to eat dessert if he has not finished everything on his plate often plagues mothers. Their fears about desserts are not completely irrational, since many consist of "empty" calories, i.e. calories and no other nutrients. The reward aspect of dessert should be underplayed, since overemphasis may give the child the idea that dessert is the best part of the meal nutritionally as well as socially. Generally the mother can work this out by controlling the type of dessert served. Fruit, fruit cup, and ice cream are pleasant desserts that contain nutrients as well as provide calories. They should be served regularly, and desserts such as cake, cookies or pie, which contribute calories and little else, should be saved for special occasions. This obviates the need for withholding dessert on the basis that the child will fill up on this high-calorie food without getting the other required nutrients. The right dessert will still supply these nutrients. Furthermore, it will prevent undue emphasis on dessert as the only pleasant part of the meal.

## FOOD DISLIKES

Mothers often worry because a child has food dislikes. They forget that the adults in the family also prefer not to eat certain foods and these never appear in the house because the mother does not buy them. Food dislikes are not inherited. Therefore, it is no surprise that the favored foods of the mother and father are not always those of the children. If a child's dislikes are confined to a few specific foods, such as fried eggs or pears, there is no need to worry. The child can get all the nutrients he needs from other foods. The disliked food should be offered to the child if it is served at the table, leaving to him the option of accepting or rejecting it. Usually these food dislikes gradually disappear, and the less attention called to them, the better.

If the child dislikes whole categories of food, such as all fruits or all meats, the situation presents more of a problem, since this may lead to inadequate consumption of certain nutrients. Such a problem is relatively rare, and when it does occur, usually is of short duration. When a preschooler expresses a categorical dislike, it is best to say nothing for a few weeks and continue to offer the food but not force him to eat it. No child will become ill or die of malnutrition in a few weeks from eliminating only one type of food if that type is replaced by equivalents from the same food group, e.g. cheese or eggs for meat, fruit or fruit juice for vegetables. Maintaining a satisfactory dietary intake of all nutrients requires that the omitted foods be replaced by equivalents, using as a guide the four basic food groups (fruits and vegetables, meat and meat substitutes, dairy products, cereal and grain products).

The child should be allowed to eat all the other foods served that he wishes, but the mother should not cater unduly to his dislike by preparing special alternate foods for each meal. Substitute or equivalent foods can be given at other appropriate meals (eggs at breakfast instead of meat at dinner), keeping special orders to a minimum. The mother should not become a slavish short-order cook to serve her child's idiosyncracies, although she should exhibit a modicum of flexibility and willingness to make minimal adaptations just as she might for a dinner guest with an odd food dislike. When the child realizes the state of affairs, he may take a small portion of the disliked food, and if he eats it, he should be encouraged. If he does not, it is not wise to make excessively negative comments or to scold him. Extreme methods, such as forcing him to sit for hours until he eats the food or slapping him, should never be used. They only enrage both parties, stiffen mutual resistance, and often lead to open warfare. A comment that next time he will try the food will suffice.

If a categorical dislike continues for several months, nutritionally satisfactory equivalents should be worked into the diet as conveniently as possible for both mother and, to a lesser extent, child. The mother should consult the physician before applying more social or physical pressure on the child to eat the disliked food.

## PRESCHOOL EATING BEHAVIOR

A preschool child does not have an adult's powers of

concentration. For most adults the main business of meals is eating. They do not neglect the social amenities, but finish their food with dispatch. A small child cannot divide his attention as efficiently. When he is attracted by conversation, the actions of someone at the table, or the television set, he often forgets all about eating. If he is tired, overexcited, or coming down with an illness, he may lack interest in food or dawdle during the meal.

A small child is also at a disadvantage because he is not as efficient as an adult at the mechanics of eating. He must cope with large utensils designed for adults while sitting at a high table intended for adult comfort. The preschooler often has great trouble using a knife and may need help. In the process of acquiring eating skills, he spills, drops utensils, and makes a mess. These unavoidable imperfections in early eating should be regarded charitably. At this stage, developing wholesome attitudes toward foods is more important than the niceties of table manners that can be learned later. An extremely intolerant attitude toward any messing and holding the child to adult standards undoubtedly generate feeding problems in many children.

Children usually take a longer time to eat than adults do. This can be partially compensated by serving the preschool child first, or perhaps even a few minutes before the rest of the family sits down, so he can get a head start without the interruptions of the social interaction when the whole family sits down together.

The preschooler fidgets at the table, squirming and twisting. Part of this is due to the fact that small children find it difficult to sit still for long periods of time. Some mothers find that allowing the child to leave the table as soon as he has finished his dinner and to rejoin the others when dessert is served keeps the child more tranquil. It also allows the other family members to enjoy their meal in peace at a leisurely pace without constantly badgering the child to hurry so that they can have dessert.

When the preschool child goes to nursery school or kindergarten, regimentation and social pressure, as well as his own growth, further shape his eating behavior. The pattern of frequent snacking is modified because food is not available during many parts of the day. A pattern of three meals a day with a few snacks gradually develops of its own accord as the child adapts to the exigencies of a more scheduled life. He may be more amenable to trying disliked foods outside the home setting. He may be served, and like, many foods that have not been served in his home because of his parents' idiosyncracies or ethnically influenced eating habits. He becomes more efficient and proficient at the business of eating and can sit at the table for longer periods.

## ADVICE TO MOTHERS

The best advice the physician can give the mother about feeding preschool children is to relax. Eating should be a pleasant, natural business that depends on hunger, with only minimal dependence on arbitrary rules and special training.

A mother must be aware that the responsibility for quality control of family nutrition is primarily hers. Since she selects the food, she serves as the gatekeeper of nutritional quality for meals eaten in the home. Normal children can be trusted to a large degree to choose a balanced diet, if they select from a variety of food items. The wise mother makes available a large number of foods from the four basic food groups. She limits other foods that contribute calories but little else of nutritional value. Thus family members may freely choose from a variety of foods well balanced in all nutrients and not overloaded with calories, and she will have little to worry about.

The best policy in forming a child's eating habits is to refrain from urging and to leave him alone, gradually introducing new foods that he can take or leave, showing unconcern toward refusal of food, and being reasonably tolerant of caprices in taste and appetite. An ironclad policy of pressing the child to eat a certain food or a certain amount of food each time he is fed may lead to undue resistance to all adult attentions with regard to food. In such a situation the table becomes a battleground for a war of wills between parent and child, which does not contribute to anyone's enjoyment of eating, and probably has negligible effects on nutritional status, no matter who "wins."

The average preschool child will show a good deal more sense in eating "what is good for him" than he is sometimes credited with, even though his choices of food at a given time may seem bizarre and his intake of food on occasion may appear to be decidedly inadequate in quantity or amazingly in excess of normal. Eating is one of the great pleasures of life and the mother should direct her efforts toward making it an enjoyable experience for her family.

*Chapter 18*

# VARIATIONS IN PHYSICAL APPEARANCE DURING ADOLESCENCE: BOYS

Written in collaboration with Johanna T. Dwyer

P<small>HYSICAL</small> differences in adolescence are commonly assessed by a variety of objective measurements which are then compared with standards. It can be arbitrarily decided that an unusual pattern of development is one occurring in 15 per cent or less of adolescents of the same chronical age. For example, a boy whose height is among the shortest 15 per cent on the charts can be said to have an unusual pattern of development with respect to height. Since these variations are within the normal range from a medical point of view, physicians tend to disregard them. However, such patterns are often perceived as abnormal by the adolescents concerned and as such may generate a great deal of anxiety and unhappiness. An awareness of the resultant social and psychologic strains is thus essential for physicians who treat adolescents.

## ADOLESCENT GROWTH

### Physical Growth

The physiologic characteristics of adolescent growth explain

The research referred to in this paper that was done in the Department of Nutrition of Harvard University School of Public Health was supported in part by grants-in-aids Nos. CD 00082 and AM 02911 from the National Institutes of Health of the United States Public Health Service and by the Fund for Research and Teaching of the Department of Nutrition, Harvard University School of Public Health, Boston, Massachusetts.
Reprinted from *Postgraduate Medicine, 41* (No. 5), May, 1967.

much of the anxiety and upset of the teen years. During adolescence the velocity of growth — the overall rate of growth — suddenly rises from the slow and steady progress characterizing the previous years. The timing of this increase varies from person to person and depends on physiologic rather than chronologic age. Normal variation for the start of accelerated growth covers a six-year span (from 8 to 14 years of age in girls and 9 to 15 years in boys). Variations in timing of maturation are natural and normal. Yet peers and parents may judge these variations less benignly than does the physician.

The total time necessary to complete growth also varies from one individual to another. Some adolescents are physically adults four to five years after the first signs of puberty, while others require seven years or more to reach the same end point.

Asynchronism or lack of coordination in development is often present. Relative rates of development of different parts of the body are dissimilar in childhood, but these differences become more obvious at puberty. Asynchronisms usually disappear after a year, but while they last they may be excruciatingly embarrassing for the adolescent. Some adolescents whose growth is temporarily out of phase may be terrified that growth will cease, leaving them deformed for the rest of their lives. Others may fear that they will never stop growing. Probably the most common type of unco-ordinated growth is short-waistedness due to growth of the legs disproportionate to that of the trunk. Other common asyn-chronisms include increase in hip width before shoulder width or vice versa, growth of one part of the face before growth of another, and increase in muscle mass before increase in muscle strength.

During adolescence the velocity of genital and sex-linked anatomic changes far outstrips the rate of growth and change in other organ systems. Obviously the maturation of the procreative function has great social and psychologic significance.

The adolescent phase of growth is also unique because of its finality. Children tend to assume that once they grow up their disabilities and problems will disappear. Teenagers are confronted with the reality of permanent differences, and some of them must come to terms with permanent defects or deficiencies in physical appearance. Furthermore, pervious differences such as those in size become more noticeable. A tall fourth-grader and a short fourth-grader differ by only a few inches; a tall man and a short man may differ by as much as a foot.

Finally, a characteristic of physical growth at adolescence which has potent social implications is that girls mature earlier than boys. Since our schools are run on the basis of chronologic rather than developmental age, boys are about two years behind girls of the same age in development throughout the adolescent period.

It is obvious that the individual physical differences in these growth patterns enormously complicate tne picture of what constitutes growth at adolescence.

### Physchologic Changes

During adolescence, psychologic changes interact with the effects of physical variations in appearance. Certain social learning occurs simultaneously for all adolescents because of the similarity of school experiences. Other social learning may come earlier or later depending on the child's experiences outside of school. Thus the levels of physical, social and emotional maturation vary in adolescents of the same age,

Adolescents are acutely aware of the entire growth process and are almost always interested in it. Many are disturbed about their own growth as well. Longitudinal studies such as that of Stolz and Stolz (1) have shown that about one-third of all boys and one-half of all girls become sufficiently concerned about at least one aspect of their growth at some point that they spontaneously express their concern to the physician-investigator. Actually, so many changes take place so fast during puberty that it is remarkable that more adolescents do not become unduly upset and worried about their development.

The adolescent has a greater sense of psychologic and physical self-exsistence than does the small child. The exaggeration of individual differences in physique during the process of individual growth appears at the same time that self-awareness increases at a psychologic level. The adolescent's sophisticated thinking allows him to invest growth with symbolic meaning so that physical maturation may come to signify growth in other areas as well.

The desire to conform grows in the early teens. Peer acceptance becomes the motive for a great deal of behavior. Being different in appearance from ones peer's often seems tantamount to being inferior.

A "sex-appropriate" appearance becomes particularly important. Every country has ideals for male and female appearance. Most Americans think that men should be tall, large-shouldered, barrel-chested and narrow-hipped, while women should be petite, slender and amply endowed in the bust. Sex-typed differences extend beyond the obvious primary and secondary sex characters to more subtle differences in manner of movement, hairiness, skin texture, and symmetry of features. Marked variations in any of these characteristics may adversely influence how a person is treated by others and how he thinks of himself.

Difficulties that arise from lack of sex-appropriateness in appearance can be put into two categories. First is the transient problem of a sex-inappropriateness phase of growth. Characteristics thought to be "girlish" may be present temporarily in the adolescent boy because of a slow change of voice, late maturation, or a feminine pattern of fat deposition. The fact that these conditions are transient makes them no less painful to the sufferer. More lasting and serious are the permanent problems arising from supposed lack of sex-appropriateness in the mature body. Such characteristics as lack of muscular strength, sparse beard, and frailness may become manifest as growth moves into the decelerating phase of later adolescence.

Adolescents are particularly sensitive to these types of nonconformity in appearance for several reasons. Doctor-patient communication is likely to be poor. Adolescents are unlikely to initiate a conversation about worries concerning maturation in the sexual area because of embarrassment. Barring the presence of a gross abnormality, the physician may fail to mention a normal but unusual pattern of primary or secondary sexual development to his worried patient. He may also fail to reassure the adolescent about some condition that varies greatly from that of his peer group because he recognizes that it is simply due to a difference in the timing of maturation.

It is also important to realize that adolescent ideals of sex-appropriate appearance tend to be quite unrealistic. Adolescent girls long to look like fashion models; boys want to look like football pros. Sexual growth is particularly vulnerable to the tyranny of the often ignorant and narrow notions of normality that other adolescents possess, since the subject is so rarely discussed with parents, let alone with the doctor.

## THE EARLY MATURER

Early and late maturers may be defined as the 15 per cent of adolescents at either end of the age distribution for the year of maximum growth. Between the ages of 12 and 16 the power of the peer group in matters of appearance is particularly strong. The peer group has definite ideas not only of how one should look but also of when one should grow up, so that the timing of maturation plays an important part in the competitive comparisons of the age.

Early maturers begin adolescence with attitudes toward their bodies that they have acquired during childhood and that differ from those of most children their age. Usually they have been larger and slightly more endomorphic or mesomorphic than their peers throughout childhood. During adolescence early and late maturers tend to have quite different social experiences. They are treated quite differently in terms of both privileges that are granted to them and behavior that is expected of them.

Most of the difficulties of the early maturer arise from the discrepancy between physiologic changes and society's expectations of these changes. He faces a rapid physical change while his friends' growth is still relatively stable. He may feel bewildered and hesitant about growing up at this point, but once he has adapted to or accepted his early spurt, he may be pleased with his maturity.

The disadvantages of early maturation stem from the fact that the adolescent has acquired an adult body but still thinks and acts like a child. Some early maturers find that their mature appearance often pushes them into social situations for which they are not ready emotionally; they are expected to live up to adult standards appropriate to their size rather than their age. Other early maturers encounter an entirely different problem. Their parents continue to treat them as small children, ignoring the fact that they look older and are treated by everyone else as though they really were older.

The early maturer is at an advantage in three areas — athletics, heterosexual activity and leadership. Early-maturing boys are temporarily bigger and stronger than others their own age and thus have a competitive advantage in sports. Latham's (2) sudy of junior high school boys called attention to the dominance of athletes in the leading crowds at school. Junior high boys who were more mature were taller, heavier and more muscular. These factors may have been the reason that they were more likely to be chosen as team captains. Patterns of association for junior high school boys tend to revolve chiefly around sports. Those who are successful in athletics have a chance to become popular and are more likely to become leaders. Coleman's (3) study of several midwestern high schools indicated that in these school athletics is the chief interest. Athletic events of many American high schools are also a focus of community interest, so that high school athletic prowess is a path to glory not only among peers but also among adults.

Timing of maturation also influences behavior and success in heterosexual areas. Early-maturing boys tend to be more interested in girls (and girls in them) than are late-maturing boys. During early adolescence, when separate groups of boys and girls begin to form heterosexual groups, the early maturer has a social advantage.

Dunphy (4) proposed that adolescents learn how to behave with peers of the opposite sex by copying the behavior of the most heterosexually advanced and sociable of their friends. We might expect that this person is more likely to be an early than a late maturer. Because of his usefulness in getting the sexes together, he emerges as a clique leader in early adolescence. By virtue of his sociability and his contacts among girls, he makes it easier for less advanced and more hesitant members of both sexes to get together by arranging parties and mixed-sex activities.

## THE LATE MATURER

The late-maturing boy is a laggard in development. Almost all of the girls and most of the boys mature physically before he does. His friends' attitudes reinforce his concern over his development. When his growth spurt finally begins, he may welcome it with relief. Later-maturing boys are probably more prepared for the physiologic changes at puberty than are early maturers since they have had a chance to observe their friends as well as to read about these changes.

Late-maturing boys often appear to compete very well with their peers until midjunior high school. They are not necessarily those who were small all through childhood; they are of average height in grammar school, but by junior high school they are smaller than their early-maturing classmates. At the age of about 13 or 14 years the early-maturing boys, with their superiority in athletics and in popularity with girls, begin to crowd them out. These early-maturing boys gain the prestige and adolescent laurels which the later maturers perhaps had in the past. For the next few years the late-maturing boys are at a disadvantage.

The late-maturing boy may lack interest in dating. If he is interested, he may find that the prettiest girls are dating older or more mature boys and they ignore him except in dire straits. When maturation finally comes, the late maturer's level of social and emotional development in the heterosexual area may be retarded in contrast with that of others of his age who have had more experience. For a while he may appear to be out of step and unsure in unfamiliar social situations. It seems that a certain amount of strain in the social area is inevitable for very latematuring adolescents. If they try to be like their physically more advanced classmates and date, they may meet with rebuffs; if they ignore girls until they have grown up, they tend to be awkward from lack of experience.

This is not to say that adolescents who are less mature than others of their age are doomed to loneliness and misery. After school hours they may gravitate toward others who are younger or closer to their own physical developmental level. At school, although they may find that they are not in the leading crowd of their grade with respect to athletics, leadership or dating, they can still find a variety of extracurricular activities such as band, student council, and activity-oriented clubs (such as math club) in which lack of physical maturity is not a major drawback if they have other talents. Late matureres can also achieve high status in recreational or institutional groups outside of school, such as the Boy Scouts or church youth groups. The effects of maturation level on leadership and status, therefore, depend largely on what groups the adolescent is trying to join. If he so choses, he can move into a comfortable social setting in which he can obtain his share of social rewards, although we suspect that many late-maturing Eagle Scouts would give up all of their badges for the higher status accorded to the junior high school football star or the class Romeo.

Immaturity in one area of development often contrasts sharply with normal or superior maturity in other areas. Late maturers are often more introspective, sensitive and insightful in dealing with the problems of others because of their own experience in coping with retarded maturation.

## MEASURABLE PSYCHOLOGIC CONSEQUENCES OF MATURATION TIME

Psychologic differences between early and late maturers are large during adolescence. Jones and Bayley (5), in their study of 13-to 15-year-old boys, assessed maturation by skeletal age of the hand and knee. They assessed social behavior by observing a large number of activities and studying peer ratings. The early maturers were the largest and strongest boys in their classes and the most advanced in skeletal age. Adults and other children treated them as being more mature. They tended to be more mesomorphic in build than later maturers, and this extra muscularity conferred an advantage in sports. They showed more mature interests, greater cleanliness, greater attractiveness in appearance, and less need to strive for status than the later-maturing boys. Many of these early maturers were student leaders. Their peers rated them as more grown-up, more assured, and more likely to have older friends than their later-maturing classmates.

Mussen and Jones (6) examined differences in social behavior and thematic apperception test (TAT) protocols* of the same boys studied by Jones and Bayley (5), but at age 17. Although the test tended to present a somewhat more favorable psychologic picture for the early-maturing than for the late maturing boys, the only statistically significant difference was that the late maturers gave responses that might indicate more feelings of inadequacy than did the early maturers. Relatively few of the physiologically advanced subjects gave TAT responses that might indicate feelings of inadequacy, rejection, dominance or rebelliousness toward their families. More of them appeared to be self-confident and independent and to play an adultlike role in interpersonal relations. Although differences in these respects were not statistically significant, later maturers showed at age 17 a trend toward possessing the following characteristics: less attractive physique, less relaxation, less assurance in class, more animation, more eagerness, more uninhibitedness, more affectation, more restlessness, more behavior of an attention-getting nature, and fewer older friends. The early and later maturers did not differ significantly in observed popularity, leadership, prestige, poise, assurance, cheer or social effects in male groups. The late maturers were at a distinct disadvantage in mixed-sex groups. The authors concluded that retarded maturation conferred a slight competitive disadvantage in the boys' world and somewhat greater disadvantage in the very early heterosexual world.

Jones (7) used interviews and a variety of psychologic tests (California Psychological Inventory and Edwards Personal Preference Schedule) to study the later careers and personalities of early-maturing and late-maturing boys. At age 33 the physical differences noted in adolescence had disappeared; the young adults who had matured early did not look more attractive or well groomed than the later-maturing group. There were no significant

---

*The TAT is a projective test that consists of a number of pictures about which the subject is asked to make up a story. Although answers are very individualistic, an objective scoring schema for classifying responses was developed, using scores for 20 needs and pressures.

differences between the two groups in marital status, family size or educational level.

Those psychologic differences that remained between early and late maturers led Jones to conclude that although the overall effect of maturation time on personality later in life was small, the early maturers still tended to exhibit earlier success patterns. They scored higher on the "good impression" scale, which was an index of interest in and capacity for creating a good impression on others. Men who had been classified as physically retarded during adolescence by use of skeletal age criteria were found through interviews to be more expressive, active, talkative, assertive and eager and less settled at age 33 than their earlier-maturing colleagues. Objective psychologic tests showed few significant differences other than the fact that late maturers did appear to be more "flexible," that is, more rebellious, touchy, impulsive, assertive, insightful and self-indulgent.

## STATURE

Stature is related to maturation, since early maturers tend to exceed other boys in height at one period of early adolescence. Final differences in stature which persist throughout life might be expected to have more lasting effects on personality than transient differences due to age at maturation.

In sharp contrast to girls, who want to be short, boys want to be tall. The importance that boys attach to height antedates adolescence. Little girls tend to be aware of their best assets — face, eyes, hair — and little boys tend to be more aware of size and weight differences between themselves and their peers.

Boys want to be tall for many reasons. It is considered sex-appropriate in our culture for men to be big and tall; hence tallness may symbolize masculinity to many boys and girls. There are also social advantages in being tall. All other things being equal, a tall boy or man has less difficulty in commanding the attention of strangers or of casual acquaintances than does a short one.

If a group of adolescents who do not know one another is asked to select a leader, the group tends to choose a large boy, and shorter adolescents are well aware of this. Shortness can be a real handicap in achieving prestige through athletic prowess in many of the more popular team sports. This does not mean that the short, wiry basketball or football player has no place, but it is true that in these sports height and weight are advantageous and shortness is disadvantageous. Short or late-maturing boys may be superb athletes, but they often excel in minor sports in the adolescent prestige hierarchy such as golf, tennis, gymnastics, etc. This helps to enhance their reputation as "regular guys" but does not bring them the adulation accorded basketball or football heroes. Stolz and Stolz (1) claim that short boys do not achieve representation proportionate to their percentage in the grade in any of the sports that are most popular among adolescents.

Size is also often an excruciating embarrassing problem for adolescent boys in social relation with girls. The short, mature boy is better off socially than the short, immature boy, but both often feel handicapped. In social dancing both sexes want the boy to be at least as tall as and preferably taller than the girl. Personality and all other attributes being equal, most girls probably prefer tall and handsome boys to those who are short and handsome.

Adolescent boys rarely worry about being too tall. The only boys who were upset about their tallness in the Stolz study were extremely thin boys over 6 feet 3 inches and transiently tall early maturers, who were disturbed because they were growing while nobody else was growing.

## MASCULINITY OF PHYSIQUE

The adolescent growth spurt in males begins with changes in size of the genitals, followed by the appearance of axillary hair, the beginnings of a beard, deepening of the voice, increase in muscle strength, and development of other secondary sex characters. Men also differ from women in having generally broader shoulders, narrower hips, and longer legs and arms, especially forearms.

Differences in genital changes in boys are visible and are obvious both to the boy himself and to other boys when they see each other in men's rooms and showers. (Female genital development is far less visible to the girl herself or to others because of the social strictures concerning modesty for girls.)

The Stolzes (1) coined the term "sex-inappropriate physique" to describe a particular syndrome which gives rise to malaise in many teen-age boys. This syndrome is most likely to occur early in puberty, especially in boys whose development is slow, and it usually passes quite rapidly. These boys tend to deposit a girdle of fat around the hips and thighs. This characteristic, together with small and slowly developing primary sex characters and the slight development of subcutaneous tissue around the nipples, makes these adolescents feel not only that they are deficient in acceptable male development but also that they are following a feminine pattern of growth. Certainly it is important for the physician to reassure these patients, since such growth is likely to be a topic of attention and ridicule from peers whose growth is more rapid and sex-appropriate.

Gynecomastia or pubertal hyperplasia of the breast area consists of slight and temporary enlargement or development of small nodules and tenderness about the nipples. Tanner (8) stated that gynecomastia usually occurs after genital growth has started but before many other secondary sex characters have become very pronounced. Mild gynecomastia is fairly common, although more noticeable enlargement is rare.

Both boys and girls worry about sex-inappropriateness of facial characteristics, but girls are able to do more about defects by using cosmetics. Among the characteristics which boys complained about as being unmasculine in the Stolz (1) study were the following: eyeglasses, turned-up nose, dimples, receding chin, small rosebud mouth, lack of beard, protruding ears, tooth defects, hair problems such as cowlicks or early baldness, and acne. Acne is very common in boys during puberty. More than three-fourths of the sample in the Stolz study had skin trouble, and many of the boys had quite severe cases causing considerable upset and discomfort.

It goes without saying that physical competence in using the body for physical work is as important for the boy in defining his maleness as are some of the physical characteristics. Athletics, fistfights and performance of "men's jobs" give him a chance to show his maleness. Coordination, muscularity, strength and endurance all enter into the adolescent boy's definition of physical competence. Supposed or actual lack of these attributes may be upsetting.

## OBESITY AND LEANNESS

In sharp contrast to adolescent girls, who continually worry about being fat, adolescent boys rarely worry about obesity unless it is very marked or inspires adverse comments. Overweight, whether it is due to massiveness of frame, muscularity or fat, may be a definite advantage in some sports such as football or wrestling in which sheer crushing power is important. Male fashions do not encourage weight control since they are shapeless enough to hide fairly large amounts of extra weight.

Unless the obesity is very marked, those disturbances that do exist over body weight and fatness in adolescence generally occur in early puberty and concern body fat laid down in what the boys consider to be a sex-inappropriate manner. The girdlelike type of fat distribution around the hips, buttocks, thighs and occasionally the chest may embarrass a boy who has this growth pattern. In extremely obese adolescents the suprapubic fat may make the genitalia appear abnormally small. In the 1920's and 1930's this obesity was commonly attributed to pituitary malfunction (Frohlich's syndrome). Many perfectly normal obese adolescent boys were treated with sex hormones to correct the condition, and a great deal of unnecessary worry about genital growth was created in the patients and their parents. Hormone treatments did little good, and current practice is to let the patient outgrow the condition.

## COMMENT

We have seen that adolescent growth patterns are extremely heterogeneous, whereas social and cultural pressures stress homogeneity and conformity in patterns of appearance. We can expect that boys who have uncommon patterns of development or appearance will suffer because of this contradiction. The weight of evidence shows that persons in this country are biased against tortoises and in favor of hares as far as physical development is concerned. It is most advantageous for a boy to grow up early and to end up tall because of athletic and social advantages.

Being different from other adolescents in timing of maturation or in more lasting physical characteristics is a potential source of worry during adolescence, but happily it seems to leave few permanent scars in adult life. However, the fact that the patient's anxiety may be extremely acute justifies the expenditure of time by the physician to probe the existence of such syndromes and to give the needed reassurance.

## REFERENCES

1. Stolz, H. R. and Stolz, L. M.: Adolescent problems related to somatic variation. In Henry, N. B. (Editor): Adolescence: Forty-Third Yearbook of the National Committee for the Study of Education. Chicago, Department of Education, University of Chicago, 1944, pp 80-99.
2. Latham, A. J.: The relationship between pubertal status and leadership in junior high school boys. J. Genet. Psychol., 78:185, 1951.
3. Coleman, J. S.: The Adolescent Society: Social Life of the Teenager and Its Impact on Education. New York, The Free Press, a division of The Macmillan Company, 1962.
4. Dunphy, D. C.: Social Structure of adolescent peer groups. Sociometry, 26:230, 1963.
5. Jones, M. C. and Bayley, N.: Physical maturing among boys as related to behavior. J. Educ. Psychol., 30:129, 1950.
6. Mussen, P. H. and Jones, M. C.: Self-conceptions, motivations, and imterpersonal attitudes of late and early maturing boys. Child Develop., 28:243, 1957.
7. Jones, M. C.: The later careers of boys who were early or late maturing. *Ibid.*, P 113.
8. Tanner, J. M.: Growth at Adolescence. Springfield, Illinois, Charles C Thomas, 1962, p 191.

*Chapter 19*

# VARIATIONS IN PHYSICAL
# APPEARANCE DURING ADOLESCENCE:
# GIRLS

Written in collaboration with Johanna T. Dwyer

In our society most physicians are men, and it is relatively easy for them to establish rapport with their adolescent male patients. However, a number of conscious or subconscious factors make it more difficult for the male physician to empathize with his adolescent female patients. A careful case history is particularly important in successfully indentifying and treating anxiety arising from unusual appearance in girls. It may be necessary for the physician to bring up matters of appearance when treating adolescent females since shyness and embarrassment may prevent their mentioning such topics to the physician themselves.

Adolescent girls are usually more harsh and less guarded in judging their physical attributes than are adult women, who tend to be charitable and rather cautious. Although Jane and June may have the same height and weight, they may have entirely different and unrealistic ideas of how they look.

Girls express dissatisfaction with their appearance in many ways. One pattern is to fix anxiety stemming from many aspects of life on their looks. A fixed anxiety about appearance seems to

The research referred to in this paper that was done in the Department of Nutrition of Harvard University School of Public Health was supported in part by grants-in-aid Nos. CD 00082 and AM 02911 from the National Institutes of Health of the United States Public Health Service and by the Fund for Research and Teaching of the Department of Nutrition, Harvard University School of Public Health, Boston, Massachusetts.
Reprinted from *Postgraduate Medicine, 41* (No. 6), June, 1967.

be less annoying than a floating anxiety about many aspects of life. Another pattern is to blame the wrong characteristics; they may either generalize or particularize too much about the cause of their dissatisfaction. For example, an adolescent girl who claims she hates everything about her slender ectomorphic build may actually only be dissatisfied with her thin upper arms or flat chest.

The physician can best assess the personal importance of variations in appearance in an adolescent girl and determine the best way to cope with the resultant difficulties by asking a number of questions. What does she think other persons significant in her life think of her appearance? Much of her anxiety stems from the importance she places on the real or imagined attitudes of others about her appearance. It is also important to find out to what the girl attributes her unusual appearance. Does she blame herself, attribute it to heredity, or blame others? Finally, it is useful to ask whether the girl has tried to change her appearance and, if the disturbing aspect is something that can be changed, what she thinks a successful change in appearance would mean in her life.

The physician can be more helpful to the patient by making specific suggestions about specific aspects of appearance that are causing discontent that he can by making general positive statements about her normality. The more noticeably the patient differs from her peers — especially the girls with whom she has the highest regard — the greater is the likelihood that the variation will be disturbing. The physician should obtain a view of the ideal toward which his patient is striving before he can understand the anxiety of a girl of seemingly normal weight who is dissatisfied with her figure because she does not look like a fashion model. Unattainable ideals such as this cause a great deal of needless frustration. The relationship of one feature of physical variation (such as tallness) to other aspects of development (such as early maturation) and to problems of social adjustment explains the dissatisfaction over their appearance that many early-maturing girls experience.

## VARIATIONS IN ADOLESCENT GIRLS

Teen-age girls are even more interested in and concerned about their physical development than are boys for several reasons. Outward appearance and the inward self are more closely bound together in females than in males. Women tend to interpret objective remarks about appearance, such as "You look awful " to mean "You are awful." Body awareness in men is more stable and less sensitive to chance remarks. Therefore they can pass off remarks on dress or looks much more easily. Men seem to be more sensitive to remarks about physical performance and competence in using their bodies. They are more likely than women to resent criticism on the quality of their driving, for example.

Status in girls' groups and popularity with boys are two other reasons for the great amount of attention that adolescent girls devote to their appearance. Popularity with boys has for girls many of the competitive aspects that success in athletics has for boys. A common route to upward social mobility for a woman is to marry a man of higher social rank. Any positive attribute such as pleasing appearance, a good voice or intelligence increases the chances of this happening.

The vulnerability of adolescent girls to worries about appearance makes wide variations in development potentially anxiety-provoking. Angelino and Mech (1) found that retrospective essays by 32 women 20 years of age on aspects of development causing the most anxiety mentioned tallness and overweight most frequently. The Stolzes (2), in their longitudinal study of 83 girls examined every six months for eight years, found that almost half of the subjects were disturbed about their development. Tallness and fatness accounted for the largest share of worries. Facial features and general physical appearance accounted for the next highest number of complaints. The combination of tallness or shortness with heaviness bothered several subjects. Glasses, thinness with flat chest, late development, acne, and tallness with thinness accounted for the rest of the difficulties.

## EARLY MATURERS

Early-maturing girls are faced with the problem that few of the other girls and almost none of the boys are growing at a comparable rate. Therefore their physical changes stand out.

Embarrassment among early-maturing girls in the Stolz (2) longitudinal study centered about conspicuousness, bigness, tallness, complexion and menstruation.

Peers of both sexes are often wary of early-maturing girls because they are bigger and different from them physically. Older boys may befriend them since boys usually date girls who are younger. The lack of social and intellectual maturity in early-maturing girls and their potential competition in dating may preclude friendship with older girls who are closer to their physiologic age.

Stone and Barker (3,4) were among the first to study the differences in certain aspects of behavior and personality between early-maturing and later-maturing adolescent girls. They studied 1000 junior high school girls 13 and 14 years of age, all white Anglo-Saxon, second-generation Californians. The criterion of maturity was taken as the menarche. Admittedly the menarche is rather ambiguous measure since feminizing changes in body-build begin long before and continue long after the first menses. However, the postmenarcheal sample undoubtedly was older in physiologic age than the premanarcheal sample. The same questionnaire had been tested on older and younger subjects so that the maturity level of the responses could be scored.

The postmenarcheal group was made up of girls who matured early or at a normal rate. These girls favored responses indicating heterosexual interests, adornment or display of the person, disinterest in participating in games or activities requiring vigorous or strenuous physical effort, and greater interest in imaginary or daydreaming activities. The two groups did not differ in attitudes toward the presence of family friction or revolt against family discipline.

More (5) studied the social behavior of early-maturing and late-maturing adolescent girls. Unfortuately, half of the sample was purposefully selected to include maladjusted adolescents, and it is difficult to know how many of the differences he reported were due to time of maturation and how many to unequal distribution of maladjusted subjects obetween early-maturing and late-maturing groups. Early-maturing girls were judged by their peers to have a lower degree of motor activity and to be less quarrelsome, less demanding of attention, and less argumentative than late-maturing girls. Early-maturing girls were also regarded by their peers as participating more in peer life than late-maturing girls, and apparently their greater participation had contributed to their reputation for being bossy, assertive and more forceful. They tended to be better groomed, more calm and more physically integrated.

## LATE MATURATION

In contrast to the large amount of attention that has been directed to late maturation in boys, little has been written about this in girls. Perhaps the girls have less pronounced problems because of their two-year edge in physiologic development, so that even the late-maturing girl grows up long before the last of the late-maturing boys. Since success in heterosexual area is based partially on the appearance of sexual maturity, later-maturing girls may be at a slight disadvantage either because they are less interested in boys or less likely to be attractive to boys than are their early-maturing peers.

## OVERWEIGHT AND OBESITY

Disturbance about overweight is much more widespread and pronounced among adolescent girls than among adolescent boys.

It has been shown that body types do not have equal tendency toward obesity (6). Obese adolescents show greater mesomorphy and endomorphy than do their nonobese peers: they have larger bones, different skeletal shape, and more muscle mass. Obesity and body type may be inherited together. Because obesity is often present in conjunction with other aspects of appearance, such as a large frame, that also deviate from the ideal, it has become a convenient catchall for expressing many diverse complaints about the body. Adolescent girls tend to label as obesity a whole spectrum of dissatisfactions with their appearance; most of these dissatisfactions have little to do with excess fat. Dietary modifications are used to treat a number of different conditions, such as skin problems, in addition to obesity. Therefore it is not surprising that adolescent girls think they can change their body-build by dieting.

Huenemann and associates (7) studied gross body composition and conformation in high school students. Over a four-year period answers to yearly questionnaires on views of body size and shape showed that adolescents had a high degree of interest in body-build throughout high school. They were generally dissatisfied with their size and shape. Boys generally wanted to gain weight and size, whereas girls wanted to lose weight and reduce certain dimensions. Boys preferred exercise to change their body appearance; girls preferred dieting. However, few of the girls who had changed their diets to lose weight had been successful.

Of all the variations is appearance during adolescence, obesity is unique in that it is often linked, by the obese person himself and by others, not only with unattractiveness in terms of current cultural ideals but also with guilt and lack of willpower. No group values obesity as a body-build characteristic; its opposite, slenderness, seems to approximate the ideal of most adolescent girls. Indeed, the adolescent female's ideals with regard to body fattness are extremely unrealistic. The ideal is slenderness almost to the point of emaciation. Concern about overweight is not confined to those who really have a weight problem. Many adolescents in the Huenemann study revealed unrealistic views toward their obesity. Their evaluation of their own excessive fatness differed considerable from their actual measurements.

Obese adolescent girls seem to accept more blame and feel more guilty about their different appearance than do adolescents with other unusual variations in appearance, such as extreme tallness. In a study of 100 obese and 65 nonobese adolescent girls, Monello and Mayer (8) found that the obese girls tended to show personality characteristics strikingly similar to the traits of ethnic and racial minority groups who are the victims of intense prejudice. They showed obsessive concern, heightened sensitivity, and preoccupation with their status in projective test responses to words such as diet, reducing, overweight, calories and fat. They gave more passive responses in picture description tests. These responses tended to illustrate the obese group's isolation and feeling of rejection by their peers. Obese girls also showed acceptance of dominant values toward obesity in a sentence completion test in which they tended to consider their own bodies as being undesirable.

In another study, Bullen and co-workers (9) distributed questionnaires to similar groups of obese and nonobese girls. The answers of the obese adolescent girls reflected popular ideas of obesity. They said that they ate more than the average girl and considered this to be the cause of their obesity. However, these girls were generally characterized not by abnormally high intake of food by rather by an extremely low level of physical activity. The answers of the obese girls also depicted less unified families which they were afraid to leave.

Obesity with onset in childhood or adolescence seems to cause more sensitivity about the condition than does obesity of adult onset. Stunkard and Mendelson (10) found that subjects who had been obese since childhood or adolescence had a more exaggerated preoccupation with weight. They judged people in terms of weight, felt contempt for fat persons, and admired slender persons. They considered their obesity a handicap and believed it to be responsible for all disappointments. Subjects who had become obese in adulthood did not display such extreme attitudes.

In short, the obese adolescent girl is self-conscious about her condition, and her obesity may place her at a disadvantage, particularly in certain situations. Canning and Mayer (11) recently showed that although application rates to high-ranking colleges and academic qualifications did not vary between obese and nonobese seniors in an excellent suburban high school system, the obese students and particularly the obese girls were not accepted in as great a number as nonobese seniors. Attitudes of family, friends and society are apt to be negative and moralistic toward the obese adolescent. It is important for the physician to assure the obese patient that her problem is essentially one of appearance and not of morals and to reassure her of the regard in which he and others hold her. The next step should be to show her how to capitalize on her good features and assets. Only then should he discuss with her the possibility of dieting.

## SLENDERNESS AND ANOREXIA NERVOSA

The feminine stereotype of the ideal figure appears to be that of the slender, full-bosomed fashion model. Such a body-build rarely occurs in actuality. Dieting cannot change body-build. It can only reduce fat on the body, and in spite of the frantic efforts to achieve the ideal figure by dieting, it is only realizable for a small percentage of the adolescent female population.

One of us (J.M.) (12) has analyzed the syndrome of anorexia nervosa. This syndrome is limited almost entirely to females in the adolescent and young adult age group. A "triad of denials" characterizes the condition: denial of thinness, denial of hunger, and (generally) denial of fatigue, except in the terminal stages. Therefore anorexia nervosa can be considered as a disorder of self-image and body image. In many ways it is simply an exaggeration of tendencies present in many "normal" adolescent girls who see themselves as obese although they are not fat, who are obsessed with the desire to become thinner, and who periodically go on extremely rigid diets to lose weight in spite of the resultant hunger and fatigue.

The first step in treating anorexia nervosa is to correct the poor state of nutrition, by force if necessary. The syndrome is not cured until the disorder in body image has been remedied by instructing the patient as to the energy intake that is compatible with both good health and sensible aesthetic ideals. Adolescents have only the sketchiest information on the caloric content of foods and on sound nutritional practices. If any form of dietary therapy is in order, it is important to instruct the patient carefully.

The advice given to anoretic patients on diet and ideal weight is also appropriate for adolescents of normal weight who insist on periodic total fasts to control their weight. Happily these girls lack the abnormal resolution and perseverance characterizing the anoretic patient and are unable to persist for long on such regimens. However, the debilitation and irritability as well as the more severe physiologic consequences, such as hypoglycemic shock, that occasionally occur make such dieting technics potentially dangerous. Therefore the physician should discourage such diets and suggest more moderate regimens.

## STATURE

Girls seldom complain about shortness unless it is combined with heaviness so that they appear squat. They are more satisfied if they are short and petite. However, being tall bothers them very much. We have all seen early-maturing girls who have become stooped because of a self-conscious effort to compensate for their height. Many girls feel that their tallness hinders them in making friends with boys, especially in the early teens when the boys tend to be short. Even if they do manage to get short boys interested, tall girls may worry about how they look together since it is the cultural ideal for women to be shorter than men.

## FEMININITY OF PHYSIQUE

The adolescent girls in the Stolz (2) study felt that the following characteristics were sex-inappropriate: extreme tallness, squatness, large hands or feet, clumsy ankles, undeveloped or very large breasts, pigmented facial hair (especially when it formed a "moustache"), extreme thinness fatness, heavy lower jaw, hairy arms and legs and generally massive body-build. Gracefulness and coordination were considered to be assets for girls, whereas strength and physical competence were not as highly prized in girls as they were in boys.

Facial features that many girls regard as unfeminine include glasses, braces, large nose or mouth, receding chin, acne moles, birthmarks, scars, oily skin, large pores and freckles. However, for each individual who is upset about having such a characteristic, there are several other girls with the same characteristic who are not bothered at all.

A great deal of individual variation exists among adolescent girls as to which aspects of their figures they regard as being particularly invested with femininity. Early in childhood girls become aware of their prettiness as compared with that of other girls and also of their particular physical features that are expecially attractive.

Development or lack of development of the breasts is particularly worrisome to many girls because it is one of the first signs of maturity and because the breasts are objects of masculine interest. Our society and culture tend to emphasize the breasts as being the repositories of sexuality. Menstruation is also of some importance in the girl's definition of her femininity. In some societies the menarche is publicized and celebrated as the event marking passage into adulthood. In our own society, it is considered to be a private matter.

Although no studies have been reported on the subject, we would expect that facial hairiness or an extremely deep voice would be just as disturbing to adolescent girls as gynecomastia is to boys. Growing girls are sometimes very sensitive about body odors. Even when they use a deodorant, fear of body odor may be a constant source of anxiety for them, especially during the menstrual period.

## BEAUTY

The extremely attractive girl is subjected to special risks. Much older boys may exploit her youth and näiveté, especially if she matures early. She may be hurt by the discovery that boys are competing for her solely because of her glamour and sexual attractiveness. She may become used to receiving things she has not earned and would not receive if she were not so pretty. A further risk is that her parents may use her as a means of satisfying their pride and competitive ambition in the social area. They may overemphasize the importance of success in dating and under-emphasize the need to establish competence in other areas of life as well.

## CONCLUSION

Variations in appearance of any type, particularly the striking changes or differences that have been discussed in this paper, disrupt a person's views of himself. Yet physical change is inevitable during adolescence and is complicated by the adolescent's narrow and rigid ideas of what constitutes normal physical growth. A high degree of conformity in external appearance is prerequisite to full acceptance in the adolescent peer group. This attempt to impose a standardized mold on the natually varied character of adolescent growth causes a great deal of unhappiness in the children who are affected.

Perhaps a shift of social rewards to the attributes more subject to the individual's control and less growth-connected may lessen the anxiety caused by unusual patterns of maturation. There is a trend today to reward adolescent scholars in many secondary schools. A more practical approach might be to include in the life sciences curriculum of junior high schools an explanation by a physician of the broad range of normal individual variability in adolescent growth and appearance.

The physical reality of body appearance interacting with psychologic and social factors has important effects on self-esteem during adolescence. The first step in treating anxiety arising from appearance is to recognize and deal with all of the factors involved.

## REFERENCES

1. Angelino, H. and Mech, E. V.: Fear and worries concerning physical changes — a preliminary survey of 32 females. J. Psychol., 39.195, 1955.
2. Stolz, H. R. and Stolz, L. M.: Adolescent problems related to somatic variation. In Henry, N. B. (Editor): Adolescence: Forty-Third Yearbook of the National Committee for the Study of Education. Chicago, Department of Education, University of Chicago, 1944, pp 80-99.
3. Stone, G. P. and Barker, R.: Aspects of personality and intelligence in pre- and postmentrual females of the same chronological age. J. Comp. Physiol. Psychol., 23:439, 1937.
4. ——: Attitudes and interests in pre- and postmenstrual females. J. Genet. Psychol., 54:27, 1939.
5. More, D. M.: Developmental Concordance and Discordance During Puberty and Early Adolescence. Child Development Monographs, 1953, vol. 18, No. 56.
6. Seltzer, C. C. and Mayer, J.: Body build and obesity — who are the obese? J.A.M.A., 189:677, 1964.
7. Huenemann, R. L., Shapiro, L. R., Hampton, M. C. and Mitchell, B. W.: A longitudinal Study of gross body composition and body conformation and their association with food and activity in a teen-age population. Views of the teen-age subjects on body conformation, food and activity. Amer. J. Clin. Nutr., 18:325, 1966.
8. Monello, L. F. and Mayer, J.: Obese adolescent girls an unreconized "minority" group? Amer. J. Clin. Nutr., 13:35 1963.

9. Bullen, B. A., Monello, L. F., Cohen, H. and Mayer, J.: Attitudes towards physical activity, food and family in obese and nonobese adolescent girls. Amer. J. Clin. Nutr., 12:1, 1963.

10. Stuckard, A. J. and Mendelson, M.: Disturbances in body image of some obese persons. J. Amer. Diet. Ass., 38:328, 1961.

11. Canning, H. L. and Mayer, J.: Obesity: Its possible effect on college acceptance. New Eng. J. Med., 275:1172 (Novenber 24) 1966.

12. Mayer, J.: Anorexia nervosa. Postgrad. Med., 34:529, 1963.

*Chapter 20*

# NUTRITION AND ATHLETIC PERFORMANCE

Written in collaboration with Beverly Bullen

## DIET AND ATHLETIC PERFORMANCE

 $D$ IET fads are dangerous to the patient on at least three grounds: (1) Nutritional — by relying on the supposedly unique qualities of near-magic foods (e.g. blackstrap molasses, kelp, etc.) the patient often places himself on a highly unbalanced ration conducive to deficiencies. (2) Financial — the cost of health foods, special preparations, etc., is so high that it drains away resources needed for medical or dental care, education of children, etc. (3) Intellectual — by casting aspersions on "organized" medicine and "official" nutrition, the practice of diet faddism makes the patient less receptive to sound medical and hygienic advice and more prone to fall prey to even more dangerous forms of quackery.

The purpose of this discussion is not, however, to deal with the more widespread food fads, but to examine one special aspect frequently attached to competitive sports. From conversation and correspondence with a number of coaches, deans of colleges of physical education, athletic directors and team physicians, we have become convinced that the athletic variety of diet faddism is extremely widespread. In a single university, each coach may, through the agency of various training talks and team instruction, put his boys on his own idea of a "winning" diet. It may entail prolonged daily periods of avoiding fluids, ommitting whole classes of wholesome foods, ingesting large amounts of unnecessary, expensive items (royal jelly was used in a well-known

Reprinted from *Postgraduate Medicine, 26* (No. 6), December, 1959.

college), or slanting the diet toward a ration excessively high in saturated fats.

Such odd practices may not have eperimental foundation, but they do have historical precedents. For example, one of the most popular training-table practices has been the consumption of large quantities of meat, supposedly destined to replace the protein "losses" incurred during severe muscular work. This practice has been traced back to the fifth century B.C. Until that period, the diet of the Greek athletes had been mainly vegetarian, consisting of porridge, meal cakes, figs, some fresh cheese, and meat eaten only occasionally as relish. The change took place shortly after the Persian Wars, when a trainer, Dromeus of Stymphalus (who twice won the long race at Olympia, in 456 and 460) introduced the meat diet. This new diet (the appearance of which also coincided with the rise of professionalism in Greek sports) was meant mostly for wrestlers. Classification by weight was unknown and heavy-weight had a decided advantage. Such extremes in athletic training were denounced by Hippocrates as producing "a dangerous and unstable condition of body" (1).

Many of the more bizarre nutritional beliefs of coaches echo Greek, Roman or even older tribal advice. For example, a current best seller (2) attributes to honey a number of exceptional properties for "athletic nutrition." While eating honey is a pleasant way to take carbohydrates, there is no evidence presented in this book or elsewhere showing honey to be inherently superior to other carbohydrate foods from a physiologic viewpoint. Because the general practitioner in his frequent work as a school physician and hence as team physician, as well as in his private doctor-patient relationship, may have to pass judgment on some of the dietary practices of athletic departments, a review of what we do know of the effect of diet on athletic performance may be found useful.

## TIMING AND RELATIVE SIZE OF MEALS

The influence of the spacing, number and relative size of meals has been studied experimentally in relation to prolonged physical work. Haggard and Greenberg, using a bicycle ergometer, showed that frequent meals improved over all performance. They concluded a pattern of five meals a day led to a total work output greater than that obtained with three meals. Further reduction to two meals a day (by omitting breakfast) led to inferior performance, particularly during the morning. Haldi and Wynn (3) could not duplicate these results under actual working conditions. For example, they did not find a significant increase in the productivity of seamstresses given snacks or meals of various compositions and sizes at midmorning and midafternoon breaks.

Hutchinson (4) concluded that replacing a few large meals with more frequent moderate-sized snacks may lead to higher efficiency through psychologic effects. More frequent breaks in a routine are known to augment production. Hutchinson believes that "with breakfast as a possible exception, the ingestion of food is not followed by any great increase in industrial productivity or by improvement in athletic performance."

Tuttle and co-workers (5) studied exhaustively the effect of omission and variation of composition of breakfast. Ommission of breakfast (or its reduction to a cup of black coffee) caused a decrease in the maximal work output (measured on a bicycle ergometer) and increases in reaction time and muscle tremor. Orent-Keiles and Hallman (6) observed that work following no breakfast or an insufficient breakfast precipitated the onset of dizziness and nausea in nonworking subjects.

Causere (7) related an interesting "natural" experiment performed in South Africa. During the Ramadan period, Moslems there, as elsewhere in the Mohammedan world, eat only two meals a day, one early in the morning and the other at 6 P.M. During the rest of the year, they eat three meals a day. Better performances in timed races were achieved during the period when three meals were eaten than during the Ramadan.

It thus appears that data are not numerous and conclusions are in part contradictory. No detailed, controlled study conducted under actual athletic conditions seems available. Prolonged adaptation to an altered meal pattern could be successful. All in all, evidence at hand does suggest, however, that athletes should have at least three meals a day or perhaps more frequent, lighter meals. The latter pattern may be particularly valuable if the sport practiced is one requiring long hours of effort (e.g. skiing, distance running, swimming). Exercises of shorter duration should not require a drastic modification of the usual pattern of meal distribution. From the viewpoint of digestion, it makes sense that the last meal preceding an athletic contest should be eaten three hours or so prior to the event. This eliminates the drain on the circulatory system coincidental with active absorption. Conversely, emotions or nervousness felt by the performer prior to entering the contest is less likely to interfere with digestive processes if this last meal is eaten well in advance. (The care and speed with which a small sugar supplement is digested exempts it from such restrictions.)

## MEAL COMPOSITION AND ATHLETIC PERFORMANCE

### Carbohydrate and Fat

Carbohydrate is known to be oxidized preferentially for muscular work. It has been established that while carbohydrate yields only half as many calories per gram as does fat, the burning of carbohydrate yields more calories per liter of oxygen than does the burning of fat. On theoretical grounds at any rate, one might expect that in any sport in which the oxygen supply to the tissues is a limiting factor, using carbohydrate as the chief fuel might prove to be advantageous.

In practice, two main types of studies have been conducted to test the possible advantage of this or that type of distribution of physiologic fuels: (1) those in which subjects exercise following the ingestion of single meals of the desired composition and (2) those in which the subjects are fed for several days a special diet high in a given component (carbohydrate, fat, protein) and low in the others to "saturate" the body with one type of food prior to performance in the postabsorptive state (even after several hours under basal conditions).

Among studies of the first type is that of Haggard and Greenberg, who found that a high-carbohydrate meal increased efficiency by 25 per cent. Other investigators have not observed differences of this magnitude. Haldi and Wynn (3) did not find that a high-carbohydrate diet yielded superior performance as compared with isocaloric, low-carbohydrate meals for swimmers in 100-yard sprints. They concluded that for exercises of short duration readily available stores were sufficient so that muscular efficiency was not affected by the size or type of pre-exercise meals. Similarly, while Wrightington (8) observed the expected differences in respiratory quotients following ingestion of supplements of glucose or sucrose, there were no significant changes in muscular efficiency.

While the beneficial effect of sugar ingestion for short-term exercise must be considered unproved, there appears to be better evidence in favor of a high-carbohydrate diet for prolonged exercise. Marsh and Murlin found the average net effeciency of work (light exercise) to be similar on a high-carbohydrate diet, on a normal diet, and on a high-fat diet; however, there was a decline in efficiency on the high-fat diet following the fourth day. Christensen and Hansen found that a subject could continue strenuous work three times as long on a high-carbohydrate diet as on a high-fat diet. Christensen also maintained athletes for several days prior to exercise on extremely high-fat diets, on high-carbohydrate diets, and on mixed diets. He then had the athletes exercise in the postabsorptive state and again found endurance impaired on the high-fat diet; it was greatest on the high-carbohydrate diet. From determination of respiratory quotients, Christensen concluded that while trained athletes can utilize indifferently carbohydrate and fat during rest and light work, they increase the percentage of carbohydrate used when performing heavy work, if such carbohydrate is available.

Krogh and Lindhard compared in similar experiments efficiency on high-carbohydrate and high-fat diets and found the muscular efficiency 11 per cent higher on the high-carbohydrate diet. Bierring found that the net efficiency was 8.3 per cent higher. Gemmill (9) criticized the latter result as an inaccurate extrapolation. His own recalculation of Bierring's data would yield a 4.5 per cent difference between the high-fat and the high-carbohydrate diet. Such a difference would still be highly significant in competitive athletics.

When it is recalled that the average American diet contains

approximately 40 per cent fat, and usually more when the caloric intake is greater than normal (which it is on athletic diets), and when it is further remembered that the usual practice at training tables is to load athletes with high-fat foods (meat, eggs, milk), there are serious questions as to whether, quite apart from the possible dangers of atherogenesis, the current diets for athletes are even optimal for the coaches' purposes.

## Protein Intake

One of the most persistent misconceptions in nutrition is Liebig's theory that protein is the primary source of muscular energy. Voit and Pettenkofer in their memorable article in 1866 clearly refuted this theory. Many authors have since supported them in this refutation. Yet the claim that those doing heavy work (miners, construction workers) require more protein than do sedentary persons or even children was repeatedly advanced by unions in wartime. Even the British government had to compromise in its rationing scheme with this idea, which its scientific advisers unanimously denounced as erroneous. Present-day coaches in the United States and elsewhere still agree with the fifth century B.C. Greeks and Liebig in spite of nearly 100 years of experimental evidence to the contrary.

In experiments relating the level of protein intake to work performance, Chittenden claimed that low protein intakes (50 to 60 gm), on which subjects in training were maintained over a period of five months, actually improved efficiency and well-being to levels superior to the preexperimental period, in which protein intake had been in excess of 100 gm. However, the experimental controls necessary to demonstrate that the gradual improvement in strength observed by Chittenden was due to reduced protein intake and not to training were absent. At any rate, the experiments did seem to prove that a reduced protein intake did not impair physical performance in any way.

For two months, Darling and co-workers (10) studied three groups, one on a restricted protein intake (50 to 55 gm), one on a normal diet, and one on a daily protein intake of 160 gm. The subjects engaged in hard manual labor. While neither the low nor the high protein intake appeared to be harmful, neither appeared to be beneficial in regard to work efficiency.

While the performance of heavy physical labor or athletic exercise does not increase protein requirements, the increase in muscle mass associated with training and conditioning does, like all growth processes, require an adequate supply of good-quality protein. For example, Yamaji (11) noted positive nitrogen balance in subjects who formerly were sedentary and who were submitted to arduous physical training. The nitrogen retention was greater on a diet providing 2 gm of protein per kilogram of body weight daily than on a diet providing 1 to 1.5 gm. Yamaji noted significant drops in blood hemoglobin and albumin during the beginning of the training period. These he interpreted as indicating that muscle was formed in part at the expense of blood protein. The extent and the duration of the decrease in hemoglobin and even in albumin levels were less on the high-protein diet. It must be emphasized, however that the decreases in blood protein were transient and self-correcting and again were characteristic of transition between sedentary and active periods, not of the athletic period per se.

## Water-soluble Vitamins

Impairment or elimination of work performance in frank vitamin deficiencies is well known. It is often more difficult to recognize borderline deficiency states. In such cases, what may appear to be a favorable effect of vitamin "supplementation" on performance actually may be the therapeutic effect of the vitamin on a hitherto unrecognized borderline deficiency.

A number of workers have attempted to see whether the ingestion of vitamins in excess of the accepted standards might in some way be helpful in meeting the additional stress imposed by exercise. In particular, Simonson and associates (12) examined the influence of a surplus of B complex vitamins on the performance of 12 healthy subjects engaged in five different types of muscular work. No beneficial effects were observed on total output or efficiency, although it was noted that in eight of the 12 subjects flicker-fusion frequency increased, a finding often taken to indicate decreased central nervous system fatigue. Keys and Henschel (13) carried out an extensive series of tests on a group of pretrained army men receiving adequate diets, supplemented by a surplus of five B complex vitamins and ascorbic acid. There were no beneficial effects noted on endurance, resistance to fatigue, recovery from exertion, or muscular strength and dexterity. Studies conducted in the same laboratory on four healthy young men maintained on adequate diets plus vitamin B, administered at five levels ranging from 0.23 mg per 1000 calories to 0.96 mg per 1000 calories indicated no beneficial or detrimental effects on performance in muscular, cardiovascular, psychomotor and metabolic functions. These studies included four series of experiments each lasting 10 to 12 weeks. Vytchikova (14) suggested that the vitamin $B_1$ content in athletes' rations should be increased above the usual level of 1.5 to 2.0 mg per day on the basis of findings that following vigorous exercise both the thiamine and pyruvic acid content of blood are increased. Supplementation of the diet with 10 to 20 mg of vitamin $B_1$ per day reduced the level of pyruvic acid in blood to the values found in manual workers engaged in moderated exercise, and it improved reaction time before and after training.

Montoye and co-workers (15) concluded that experimental evidence does not justify recommending additional vitamin $B_{12}$ to athletes. In their experiments, vitamin $B_{12}$ supplements had no beneficial effect on strength and pulse rate recovery after work on a bicycle ergometer. These investigators also were unable to observe positive effects of supplementation in boys living in an institution and tested on running and in Harvard step test performance. The postulate of Bourne (16) based on his review of the literature was to the effect that there must be an increased demand for the B complex vitamins during exercise because of their important role in so many of the biochemical reactions which make energy available for muscular work. This theory would appear a priori to be justified only if the vitamin B content of the diet did not increase in proportion to the additional calories required by exercise and consumed by the subject.

These writers at any rate conclude that there is no evidence that athletic performance is improved by supplementing a nutritionally adequate diet with B complex vitamins or vitamin C. It goes without saying that should the bulk of additional calories required for exercise be provided by such "purified" food stuffs as overmilled rice or refined sugar, additional B complex vitamins might be helpful.

### Vitamin E and Corn Oil

Some of the more radical claims for the beneficial effect of vitamin preparations on athletic performance concern vitamin E. Cureton, (17) while recognizing that the effect of training is paramount during the first 8 to 10 weeks of a physical training program, claims that dietary supplements of vitamin E and wheat germ oil make possible even high endurance work performances (bicycle riding and treadmill running) and raise such performances above the plateau obtained after 8 to 10 weeks of training. Cureton further stated that such effects appear only in relatively strenuous training programs. In one group of older adults (26 to 65 years) who failed to make good adjustments to a short period of physical training (four to six weeks), the evidence was inconsistent and unstable. The fitness test performance of control subjects living normally was not raised by vitamin E or wheat germ oil supplements. In two matched groups of eight middle-aged subjects each, a dietary supplement of wheat germ oil was effective only in the group which took the physical training parallel with the feeding. While the control group showed little or no change, the experimental groups on wheat germ oil improved more than did the matched group (placed on placebos) in treadmill-running time, brachial pulse wave, auditory, visual and combined vertical jump reaction time, the Schneider index, and the T wave of the electrocardiogram (17).

The results achieved by Thomas (18) are in flat contradiction to those of Cureton in regard to the influence of vitamin E on athletes in training. Thomas experimented with 30 young male students. Fifteen were given 450 IU of alphatocopherol acetate daily for five weeks and then were given placebos for five weeks. The other group received the placebos first, followed by vitamin E. At the beginning of the experiment and at five and 10 weeks, measurements made of the reclining pulse rate, resting respiratory rate, speed sit-ups, vertical jump, and pulse and respiratory rates immediately after activity showed no differences between the groups during either test period. In addition, no changes were seen in temperment, in disposition, or in general feeling of well-being. It would appear that a clear demonstration of the beneficial effects of vitamin E has yet to be provided.

## Gelatin, Glycine and Creatine

It has been hypothesized by a number of authors that a diet supplemented with glycine (a precursor of creatine) might increase the concentration of creatine and thereby the potiential supply of high-energy phosphocreatine in muscles. Because of its high content of glycine (approximately 25%), gelatin has been advocated as a useful supplement.

Maison tested the effect of glycine and gelatin on endurance (finger extension) and could find no beneficial effect for either substance. Horvath and associates found that glycine supplements neither increased muscle strength nor accelerated the effect of training in hand dynamometer tests. Administration of gelatin did not unequivocally alter creatinine excretion. Robinson and Harmon studied the effects of gelatin on exhausting muscular work on the treadmill and in track exercises and reported that gelatin did not affect the oxygen debt. On the basis of their review of work done on this subject, King and co-workers (19) concluded, "Claims made for especial value of aminoacetic acid or gelatin in the treatment of fatigue or increased endurance are unfounded on theoretical grounds. . . .protein of the ordinary diet is fully capable of supplying the aminoacetic acid required by man."

## Electrolytes and Acid-Base Balance

The idea that alkalizing agents might alleviate fatigue or shorten the recovery period following strenuous exercise by neutralizing lactic acid has been advanced by some popular writers and often is cited by coaches. Johnson and Black (20) found no significant difference between the effects of glucose and various alkalizing supplements on timed performance during a season of competitive cross-country running. Embden's claim that phosphate preparations increased work output has been attributed by later workers to purely psychologic effects.

There is no evidence that exercise causes a need for salt in excess of the losses accompanying sweating. The problem of salt for athletes is therefore not different from that of workers exposed to hot climates. Salt is indicated only during a period (e.g. one week) of adapting to sudden heat or when the heat is extreme. Additional salt in the food is often better tolerated than are salt tablets.

## Alcohol and Caffeine

One of today's best-known athletes, the "four minute" miler Chris Chataway, is said to consume fairly copious amounts of beer as part of his training diet. Moderate amounts of wine were consumed by Greek athletes in training for the Olympic games. On the other hand, the majority of coaches frown on the consumption of even small amounts of alcoholic beverages. The rationale for this taboo is that small quantities of alcohol affect the finer coordination movements and larger amounts affect gross coordination.

Studies on the effect of coffee and tea on performance have yielded divergent results, which may be due to differences in reactivity to caffeine. Stimulants such as pure caffeine may tax a person beyond the safe limits of physical capacity. Thus, while they may mitigate fatigue for a while, stimulants constitute a long-range health hazard.

There appears to be no particular reason either to advocate alcohol or mild stimulants such as tea and coffee or to erect a complete taboo against them. The long-term psychologic effects of such taboos may be undesirable. There is increasing feeling among psychologists that, frequently, chronic alcoholics are persons in whom precisely this type of absolute taboo had been instilled concerning the intake of even small amounts of beverages which have low alcoholic content such as wine or beer.

## "CRASH" DIETS

In sports such as boxing and wrestling, present-day athletes, professional and amateur (the latter group frequently including high school students), often place themselves on crash diets combined with dehydration to "make" lower weight classifications. This is a practice to be strongly discouraged. The intention of these athletes is not to attain their most desirable weight from the viewpoint of health and fitness but rather to compete with an unfair advantage against an opponent who really does belong in a lower weight bracket. In a sense, this is the wheel gone full circle since the meat diet of Dromeus in times when weight classification did not exist. The weight standards have been set up to provide competition on an equitable basis. Violating them by using tricks such as sudden, self-inflicted starvation and temporary dehydration serves no more the ethics of sportsmanship than it does the health of the person involved. The practice has become so widespread that it has received increasing medical attention and has been the object of editorial condemnation by the American Medical Association (21).

## NUTRITION IMMEDIATELY PRECEDING AND DURING COMPETITION

While evidence concerning possible special nutritional requirements of athletes is at most meager, there are a number of rules which have been found useful by competent, objective physicians ministering to college teams (22), particularly those involved in long-duration events such as marathons. The essential objective is that nutrition should not interfere with competitive performance and its attendant physical and psychologic stresses.

### Water Balance

The requirements for salt can be met in a quantitative fashion by ingestion of boullion at least three hours before a competitive event. If thirst ensues, it should happen no less than one and one-half hours before the event. Ingestion of water at that time will still permit elimination of excess fluid before the competition.

## Carbohydrate Loading

There is a strong presumption that for long-distance events carbohydrate is a better fuel than is fat or protein. Increasing carbohydrate reserves can be done simultaneously by two methods. (1) Exercise should be tapered off 48 hours before competitive effort, and the athlete should rest 24 hours before the event. (2) The last meal eaten before the event should be one high in carbohydrate, such as cereal (oatmeal), toast, jam or honey, etc.

## Avoidance of Proteins, Bulky Foods

The problem of the need for urinary or bowel excretion during a competitive event can be serious or even disabling. Proteins are a source of fixed acids which can be eliminated only by urinary excretion. Protein intake is therefore best reduced to the minimum at the meal preceding the event. Similarly, bulky foods (high cellulose foods, such as lettuce, and seed-containing vegetables, such as tomatoes) are best eliminated from the diet during the 48 hours preceeding contests. Highly spiced foods also should be avoided during this period.

## Tea, Coffee, Alcohol

It has been pointed out that these writers take a moderate view concerning alcoholic beverages, tea and coffee. There is no evidence that small amounts of these in the training diet are harmful. On the other hand, there is good reason to avoid them just before a contest. Alcohol, even in small amounts, may have some effect on coordination. Coffee and tea, while stimulants, may have a depressing effect three or four hours later and thus impair performance if consumed at the meal preceding exercise.

## Nutrition During Contests

Some sugar feeding during a long and exhausting contest does improve performance. Feeding glucose pills, pieces of sugar, or honey, however, tends to draw fluid for their digestion and absorption into the gastrointestinal tract and further dehydrate the organism. The subject may be fed lightly with strongly sweetened tea with lemon, which does not cause this difficulty.

## CONCLUSIONS

The evidence presented in this article indicates clearly that the optimal diet for an athlete is not different in any major respect from that which would be recommended to any normal person. The diet should be adequate for maintenance, for growth if the person is still growing, for increase in muscle mass if necessary, and for fulfilling the energy requirements corresponding to the athletes's physical activity. Special attention might be given to the weight of the athlete in terms of desirability of possible gain or loss. When loss is indicated, crash diets should be avoided. Increased physical activity usually means that with moderated dietary controls, fat can be lost efficiently and relatively pain- lessly. If an increase in muscle mass occurs at the same time, the effect on weight of loss of fat may be counterbalanced by gain in body protein. Evolution of body composition can be followed by observation, caliper measurements, and by the determination of such indexes as waist circumference.

In general, it appears that athletes should not eat less than three meals a day. When the sports practiced are particularly protracted and exhausting, up to five lighter meals may be a preferable pattern. Available evidence indicates that the relative compostion or size of the meal preceding an athletic event of short duration has little influence on performance. (A reasonable delay should elapse between the meal and the competitive event.) However, there is also evidence showing that in sports requiring endurance and prolonged muscular work, performance is better maintained on a high-carbohydrate diet than on a high-fat diet (these are meant as the "usual" diet that is consumed for several days before an athletic event). In such cases, even the slight increase in efficiency with a high-carbohydrate diet (the minimal figure of 5% has been indicated by many investigators) may well prove decisive.

Wide variations of protein intake do not seem to influence performance. A well-balanced diet easily meets needs for maintenance and whatever muscle growth may take place. Large amounts of meat several times a day are unnecessary.

Supplementation of an adequate diet has not given clearly positive results. The multitude of problems encountered in the experimental design of studies purported to test the usefulness of supplements often has precluded ruling out the effects of motivation and progressive training. It is probable that hard muscular exercise does increase the need for some of the B complex vitamins, but in a balanced diet such increased needs should be met by the increase in food intake secondary to intense exercise.

The value of corn oil and Vitamin E has not been definitely demonstrated. The use of ergogenic supplements such as gelatin and phosphate has not given unequivocal results. Athletic performance per se does not increase the need for salt. Salt supplementation (food salting, salted bouillon, or tablets) is necessary only if considerable sweating occurs during the beginning of training, under vigorous climatic conditions, or with prolonged exertion.

The use of alcohol, coffee, tea or other beverages containing caffeine should be restricted to small amounts.

It thus appears that nutritional requirements of athletes are essentially similar to those of nonathletes, except in regard to amounts (which should be regulated normally by appetite) and in the avoidance of excessive amounts of fat, particularly in sports entailing protracted heavy physical activity. The practice of feeding athletes at training tables may have some justification of convenience. Athletes often start practice before colleges reopen; the sports schedule may be such as to necessitate different hours for mealtime. There may also be some justification for this practice from the psychologic standpoint, in that it may help to create a "team spirit." By the same token, some educators dislike the segregation of athletes which thus takes place and consider that the training tables decrease the opportunity for conversing with greater numbers of students. Certainly, there is no "nutritional" justification for training tables at present. The normal fare of schools and colleges should be wholesome and adequate for all students. Extra needs of athletes can be taken care of by second or third portions and increased bread consumption.

## REFERENCES

1. Gardiner, E. N.: Athletes of the Ancient World. Fairlawn, New Jersey, Oxford University Press, 1930.
2. Percival, L.: Experience with honey in athletic nutrition. In Jarvis, D. C.: Folk Medicine. New York, Henry Holt & Company, Inc., 1958.
3. Haldi, J. and Wynn, W.: Observations on efficiency of swimmers as related to some changes in preexercise nutriment. J. Nutrition, 31:525, 1946.
4. Hutchinson, R. C.: Meal habits and their effects on performance. Nutrition Abstr. & Rev., 22:283, 1952.
5. Tuttle, W. W., Daum, K., Imig, C. J., Martin, C. and Kisgen, R.: Effects of breakfasts of different sizes and content on physiologic response of men. J. Am. Dietet., A. 27:190, 1951.
6. Orent-Keiles, E. and Hallman, L. F.: The Breakfast Meal in Relation to Blood Sugar Values. Circular No. 827. Washington, D. C., U. S. Department of Agriculture, 1949.
7. Causeret, J.: Nutrition et capacities physiques. Bull. Soc. scient. hyg. aliment., 45:19, 1957.
8. Wrightington, M,: The effect of glucose and sucrose on the respiratory quotient and muscular efficiency of exercise. J. Nutrition, 24:307, 1942
9. Gemmill, C. L.: The fuel for muscular exercise. Physiol. Rev., 22:32, 1942.
10. Darling, R. C., Johnson, R. E., Pitts, G. C., Consolazio, F. C. and Robinson, P. F.: Effects of variations in dietary protein on the physical well-being of men doing manual work. J. Nutrition, 28:273, 1944.
11. Yamaji, R.: Studies on protein metabolism during muscular exercise. 1. Nitrogen metabolism in training for heavy muscular exercise. 2. Changes of blood properties during training for heavy muscular exercise. J. Physiol. Soc., Japan, 13:476, 483, 1951.
12. Simonson, E., Enzer, N., Baer, A. and Braun, R.: The influence of vitamin B (complex) surplus on the capacity for muscular and mental work. J. Indust. Hyg., 24:83, 1942.
13. Keys, A. and Henschel, A. F.: Vitamin supplementation of U. S. Army rations in relation to fatigue and the ability to do muscular work. J. Nutrition, 23:259, 1942.
14. Vytchikova, M. A.: Increasing the vitamin $B_1$ content in the rations of athletes. Chem. Abstr., 52:14787, 1958.
15. Montoye, H. J., Spata, P. J., Pinckney, V. and Barron, L: Effects of vitamin $B_{12}$ supplementation on physical fitness and growth of young boys. J. Appl. Physiol., 7:589, 1955.

16. Bourne, G. H.: Vitamins and muscular exercise. Brit. J. Nutrition, 2:261, 1948.
17. Cureton, T. K.: Effect of wheat germ oil and vitamin E on normal human subjects in physical training programs. Am. J. Physiol., 179:628, 1954.
18. Thomas, P.: The effects of vitamin E on some aspects of athletic efficiency. Thesis, University of Sothern California, 1957.
19. King, E. Q., McCaleb, L. B., Kennedy, H. F. and Klumpp, T. G.: Failure of aminoacetic acid to increase the work capacity of human subjects. J.A.M.A., 118:594, 1953.
20. Johnson, W. R. and Black, D. H.: Comparison of effects of certain blood alkalinizers and glucose upon competitive endurance performance. J. Appl. Physiol., 5:557, 1953.
21. Editorial: Crash diets for athletes termed dangerous, unfair. A.M.A. News, January 26, 1959.
22. Guild, W. R.: Fun, Fitness and Medicine. Personal communication.

Authors' Note: All references before 1942 have been omitted. A good review of the literature before that time is reference No. 9.

## Chapter 21

# SOME ASPECTS OF THE RELATION
# OF NUTRITION AND PREGNANCY

$R$ECENT publicity given to the teratogenic effects of certain drugs taken during the course of pregnancy has revived interest in the importance of nutrition during this "vulnerable" period and, in particular, in the possible teratogenic effect of dietary deficiencies. In this chapter, I shall review briefly some recent findings and concepts of nutrition in pregnancy and show that the available evidence is reassuring. There is no evidence that a reasonably sound diet which would insure a proper state of nutrition in the United States is not also perfectly adequate for pregnancy. The risk of diet-induced teratogenic effects under such conditions appears negligible. Conversely, and unfortunately, it does not appear that supplementing an adequate diet with minerals or vitamins will contribute significantly to avoiding eclamptic accidents, inasmuch as the relation of their incidence to wide variations in the nutrient content of adequate diets is unproved.

## SIGNIFICANCE OF EXPERIMENTAL
## CONGENITAL ABNORMALITIES

Congenital malformations have been induced in experimental animals by deficiencies of vitamins A, $B_{12}$, D or E, riboflavin, folic acid, or pantothenic acid in the maternal diet (1). Such experiments, which have received wide publicity, are delicate and have not always been reproducible from one laboratory to another. Dietary congenital malformations can be obtained only if the pregnant animal is in a "borderline" deficient state with respect to the essential nutrient studied. Total deprivation of an

---

Reprinted from *Postgraduate Medicine, 33* (No. 3), March, 1963.

essential nutrient results in sterility, resorption of the embryo, or the birth of dead or completely unviable young. The deficiency must be severe enough to damage the embryo without killing it.

While human reproduction may take place under comparable conditions, this is probably an exceptional occurrence (2). Poverty, whether individual or in a population, and concentration camp and war conditions have been imposed by man or nature, and severe states of deficiency in women have resulted. It would appear offhand that such conditions should lead to congenitally mutilated children. In man, however, mating and particularly conception are limited under such conditions. Loss of libido in man is one of the early effects of severe dietary restriction. In women, amenorrhea and sterility also result from undernutrition. Under such conditions women are more likely not to conceive or to miscarry children. The characteristics of pregnancy in man, particularly its duration, are quite different from those in the experimental animals in which congenital malformations have been produced by dietary means. The organogenetic period, in which the developing fetus is particularly vulnerable to deficiencies, is relatively short and is followed by a long period of growth, during which a continuing severe nutritional deficiency is likely to cause elimination of the fetus. Timed, short, complete interruption of the supply of a crucial nutrient while the rest of the diet is satisfactory has no dietary equivalent in man (although certain drugs, acting as inhibitors or antagonists, may stimulate it in their effects).

It is true that there may be at least one deficiency — endemic cretinism — which appears to cause effects similar to the experimental findings of Warkany and others. This disorder, once widespread in Europe and in limited areas of the United States, is usually attributed to maternal iodine deficiency. Use of iodized salt and foods imported from a variety of geographical sources has eliminated this condition in developed countries. While other examples of this type might be found, they are more likely to be seen in very poor populations on monotonous diets than in the Western Civilization.

This is not to decry the extreme importance of teratogenic experiments. The fact that various vitamin-induced experimental congenital syndromes differ from one another may permit the identification of the role of certain coenzymes in prenatal development. The resemblance of the effects of prenatal deficiencies to those of abnormal genes may permit the discovery of blocking mechanisms similar to or identical with those due to abnormal genes and give us a tool for the eventual control of some genetic abnormalities. But widespread concern among patients, primiparas in particular, that the slightest lapse in good nutrition may cause congenital malformations seems to have no foundation in fact and is a needless cause of anxiety.

## DIET AND REPRODUCTIVE PERFORMANCE

While the problem of congenital abnormalities due to poor nutrition during pregnancy does not seem to be significant in the United States at this time, the relation of pregnancy performance and nutrition continues to be controversial.

Until the relatively explosive development of our knowledge of nutrition and metabolism, obstetricians were primarily preoccupied with the mechanics of difficult labor. Not unnaturally, early concern with nutrition had to do with its possible direct effects on delivery. At the beginning of this century, Paton, on the basis of experiments with guinea pigs, and Prochownik, on the basis of clinical observation, advocated dietary restriction of the pregnant patient to facilitate parturition. Others such as Slemons in 1919, disagreed, believing that undernutrition weakened the mother more than it diminished the size of the fetus. This controversy, which was never completely resolved, had decreased in significance in recent years, because it has become relatively easy and safe to avoid a difficult vaginal delivery by employing a cesarean section.

As the vitamin story unfolded, interest shifted to the importance of the quality of the diet. A large number of studies seemed to confirm Mallanby's dictum that "When knowledge is more complete, this aspect of the problem (the vitamin and mineral content of the diet) will prove even more important than appears at the present time." A number of studies, such as those of Ebbs, Tisdall and Scott (3) in Toronto during World War II and those of Burke et al (4). in Boston, seemed to confirm this preposition by showing that there was a high degree of correlation between quality of the diet (protein, vitamin and mineral content) and course and outcome of pregnancy. These findings, popularized by vitamin manufacturers, caused a great enthusiasm for the almost routine supplementation of the diet of pregnant women with multivitamin preparations, with or without an assortment of minerals. As this period coincided with a steep rate of decline of accidents of pregnancy and stillbirths, this enthusiasm was not questioned.

## THE TORONTO STUDY

Perhaps the best known of these studies, that of Ebbs, Tisdall and Scott, dealt with a large prenatal clinic population in Toronto during World War II. A record was kept of intake for a week. Half the women had a "poor" diet: 1600 to 1700 calories per day, with 55 gm protein (recommended, 85 gm), 1.0 mg thiamine (recommended, 1.5 mg), 0.5 gm calcium (recommended, 1.5 gm), and 10 mg iron (recommended, 15 mg). Within that group, a subgroup received a supplement from the fourth month onward made up of food supplied without cost and containing 840 calories daily, with 45 gm protein 2.3 mg thiamine, 1.45 gm calcium, and 15 mg iron. The obstetricians and pediatricians who rated pregnancies, labors, postpartum periods and babies did not know to which group or subgroup the women belonged. Ratings for pregnancy were good, fair, poor and bad, depending on minor complaints or major complications such as severe anemia, preeclampsia and eclampsia, threatened miscarriage (any prenatal vaginal bleeding), accidental hemorrhage, pyelitis, streptococcal vaginitis and severe vomiting. For labors, miscarriages, premature births, postpartum hemmorrhage, excessively long labor, primary uterine inertia, and need for transfusions were tabulated; for convalescence, severe anemia, inflammation of the the pelvis or breast, cystitis or pyelitis, phlebitis, impetigo, embolism or thrombosis and streptococcal vaginitis were similarly tabulated. Thirty-six per cent of the women who had received a poor diet had a poor or bad prenatal rating, compared with only 9 per cent of the women who had received a good prenatal diet. For primiparas in the first group, duration of labor was 20.3 hours, compared with 15.2 in the group receiving the good diet. Convalescence ratings and babies' ratings showed similar differences.

Additional studies appeared to confirm these early indications. Jeans, Smith and Stearns (5), and Woodhill, van den Berg, Burke and Stare (6) found striking correlations between diet (assessed by dietary histories) and reproductive histories. The latter study, for example, dealt with the relation of diet to the incidence of accidents of pregnancy and success of lactation in a group of less than 200. Incidence of toxemia and prematurity appeared to be negatively correlated with dietary ratings and positively correlated with initiation and maintenance of successful lactation. Dieckmann and co-workers (7) found a relation between protein intake and the condition of the babies as graded by a pediatrician, although none between protein intake and the duration of labor, toxemia, prematurity and birth weight. Berry and Wiehl (8) gave dietary advice to pregnant women and reported a reduced incidence of preeclampsia and prematurity.

## NEGATIVE EVIDENCE

Negative results in studies such as those of Sontag and Wines (9), Hobson (10), Speert, Graff and Graff (11), Mack, Kelly and Macy (12), and McGanity and co-workers (13) failed to demonstrate any material correlations between diet and pregnancy history in population groups in Great Britain and the United States. In the study obviously involving many difficulties and causes of inaccuracies, Smith (14) found that birth weights in northwest Holland during the famine of 1945 were reduced by only about 10 per cent. At the height of the famine, the women took, on the average, less than 1000 calories per day, and the average total weight gain in the course of pregnancy fell to 2 kg. There was apparently little increase in fetal or neonatal mortality. Thomson's comment summed up these studies concisely and fairly. He stated: "The results of all these studies have been substantially negative even though some of the authors have made the most of minor and inexplicable correlations or have argued that their technique must have been inadequate."

## THE ABERDEEN STUDY

Thomson's (15) particularly painstaking study in Aberdeen deserves special mention. He studied a sample of all pregnant women in the city, limiting the material to primiparas who were less preoccupied with multiple household chores and more likely to cooperate in the study. The Registrar General's classification of social classes was used to characterize the various groups within this population; for example, the lower social groups (IV and V in that classification) were made up of women whose husbands were in a semiskilled or unskilled occupation. Thomson, a particularly critical scientist, chose as his dietary method one of the most exacting — a weighed dietary record kept by the women in their homes for one week during the seventh month of pregnancy. While it is conceivable that such a procedure does alter consumption levels, its major advantage is that of being a more objective determination than estimates based on recall, however carefully guided. The particular period of pregnancy was chosen because by that time the alteration in eating associated with nausea and vomiting has subsided, while the fetus is not large enough to alter the functioning of the gastrointestinal tract and thus change dietary habits. By the same token it may be argued that this seventh month may not be representative of pregnancy as a whole, but may tend to yield overestimates of intake. A few individuals were resurveyed six weeks later; agreement was good.

Acceptable dietary histories were secured from 489 of the 713 subjects. The percentage of "reliable" histories decreased from 93 in the top social group to 61 in the lowest group. Daily caloric intake went down from 2,633 for the average of the top social group to 2,354 for the average of the lowest social group. Daily protein intake decreased from 80 to 72 gm, calcium from 1.19 to 0.88 gm, and ascorbic acid from 79 to 61 mg. Some of these figures, particularly for calcium, are well below the recommended dietary allowances of the Food and Nutrition Board of the

National Research Council (2600 calories daily, with 75 gm protein, 1.5 gm calcium, 100 mg ascorbic acid). Furthermore, the range within the lowest social group embraced some much lower values. Still, all in all, it must be noted that these values are much better than those characteristic of Tisdall's poor-diet group. Normal pregnancies were defined as those in which there was no specific abnormality requiring treatment, labor was completely spontaneous within 24 hours, and the baby was in good condition and weighed 6 lb or more at birth. After a normal puerperium the mother and baby were discharged together from the hospital, with the baby being successfully and exclusively breast-fed at that time.

By these admittedly stringent criteria, 197 women were found to have experienced a normal pregnancy, 292 an abnormal one. The women in the abnormal group had greater mean caloric intakes and slightly greater intakes of all nutrients, a result which at first blush appeared weighted in part by the fact that some of the women in whom preeclampsia developed gained a little excessive weight, even after estimated allowance for the extra water retained. Actually from an extensive statistical evaluation of his results, which indicate a wide overlap of the normal as well as the preeclamptic group, Thomson suggested that "the present findings indicate that overeating may play some part in the etiology or the development of preeclampsia. But a conclusion that overeating is a major cause would probably not be warranted."

There was no relation between caloric intake and length of the gestation period. The birth weight of the baby tended to increase slowly with increase in caloric intake. This was true within each social class, but there was some evidence that social class had a greater influence on birth weight than caloric intake. Women in the upper social classes were taller and heavier; this appeared to account for the tendency of their babies to be larger. There was no evidence that birth weight was associated to a greater extent with any of the nutrients than with calories. Women whose babies were delivered by cesarean section had smaller intakes; however, as the smaller woman had a relatively high incidence of contracted pelvis, this suggests association rather than causation.

The diets of the mothers of 14 babies who were stillborn or

neonatal cases did not significantly differ from those of mothers of normal babies. Thomson rightly pointed out however, that his study may have embraced too few subjects to detect the influence of nutrition on stillbirth or newborn mortality. The stillbirth rate in England and Wales decreased from 38 per 1000 in 1940 to 28 per 1000 in 1945, perhaps partially because of improved maternal nutrition. In order to detect similar differences as a result of differences in diet, a minimum of 10,000 subjects would have had to be studied.

## A NUTRITIONAL DILEMMA?

The weight of critical evidence indicates that diet during pregnancy can vary within wide limits without demonstrably impairing the health of the mother or the baby. Classical disorders of pregnancy in this country seem unlikely at this date to be direct manifestations of classical deficiency states. Early indications of a strong correlation between variations of a passable but perhaps not really adequate diet and the presence or absence of accidents of pregnancy have not been extended by critical studies of groups on generally adequate diets. Must we conclude that sound nutrition has no relevance to the management of pregnancy? Are we in the presence of a nutritional paradox? I believe that this is not the case, and the authors of some of the most "negative" studies would be the last to suggest such an interpretation (15).

First, a possible explanation of at least some of the apparent contradictions is the fact that the various studies may not have been dealing with subjects at comparable levels of nutrition. We have studied the details of two of the best studies, those of Ebbs' group (3) in Toronto and of Thomson (15) in Aberdeen. It seems apparent that the British postwar diets were considerably better and in spite of the wide range of intake, closer to recommended allowances even in the lower social groups than the Canadian World War II diet. It may be, therefore, that the influence of nutrition on pregnancy is very marked in the lower range of quantitative and qualitative intakes, with the effect showing a rapidly diminishing return as one nears the adequate level, where "enough" is as good as (or better than) a feast. Such an interpretation is in the accordance with the observation that the wartime "feeding experiment" in Great Britain, while uncontrolled, was accompanied by the first major reduction in the stillbirth rate, which until then had been responding very slowly to the extension of maternity services (16). This result was the more striking as it was achieved under deteriorating living conditions other than dietary. Incidentally, this experiment also had the advantage of size, so that it could reveal effects perhaps not readily demonstrable on a smaller group, however well supervised.

Finally, no worker in the field would deny the most important consideration that diet in pregnancy is but the continuation of the woman's nutritional experience. Her ability to withstand this physiologic stress and that of lactation depends on her general fitness — itself very much a function of her past nutrition. Even if nutrition education seems so often to fail to prevent such accidents as prematurity and eclampsia, it has a role in managing nausea, vomiting and constipation, eliminating food faddism, and avoiding obesity — the last-mentioned having results extending far beyond the particular pregnancy. It can perhaps be concluded that while the role of nutrition in obstetric practice — at least among a relatively prosperous population — is perhaps not as dramatic as early workers imagined it, the obstetricians' contribution in the long-term health picture of the pregnant woman and her family, through his role as a nutrition educator, is growing with our advancing knowledge.

## REFERENCES

1. Warkany, J.: Etiology of congenital malformations. In Levine, S. Z., Butler, A. M., Holt, E. L., Jr. and Weech, A. A. (Editors): Advances in Pediatrics. New York, Interscience Publishers, Inc., 1947, vol. 2.
2. ——: Congenital malformations induced by maternal dietary deficiency. Nutrition Rev., 13:289, 1962.
3. Ebbs, J., Tisdall, E. F. and Scott, W. A.: The influence of prenatal diet on the mother and the child J. Nutrition, 22:515, 1941.
4. Burke, B. S., Beal, V. A., Kirkwood, S. B. and Stuart, H. C.: Nutrition studies during pregnancy. Am. J. Obst. & Gynec., 46:38, 1943.
5. Jeans, P. C., Smith, M. B. and Stearns, G.: Incidence of prematurity in relation to maternal nutrition. J. Am. Dietet. A., 31:567, 1955.
6. Woodhill, J. M., van den Berg, A. S., Burke, B. S. and Stare, F. J.:

Nutrition studies of pregnant Australian women. Am. J. Obst. & Gynec., 70:987, 1955.

7. Dieckmann, W. J., Turner, D. F., Meiller, E. J., Savage, L. J., Hill, A. J., Straube, M. T., Pottiger, R. E. and Rynkiewicz, L. M.: Observations on protein intake and the health of the mother and baby. J. Am. Dietet. A., 27:1046, 1951.

8. Berry, K. and Wiehl, D.: An experiment in diet education during pregnancy. Milbank Mem. Fund Quart., 30:119, 1952.

9. Sontag, L. W. and Wines, J.: Relation of mothers' diets to status of their infants at birth and in infancy. Am. J. Obst. & Gynec., 54:994, 1947.

10. Hobson, W.: A dietary and clinical survey of pregnant women with particular reference to toxaemia of pregnancy. J. Hyg., 46:198, 1948.

11. Speert, H., Graff, S. and Graff, A.: Nutrition and premature labor. Am. J. Obst. & Gynec., 62:1009, 1951.

12. Mack, H. C., Kelly, H. J. and Macy, I. G.: Complications of pregnancy and nutrtional status. Am. J. Obst. & Gynec., 71:577, 1956.

13. McGanity, W. J., Cannor, R. O., Bridgforth, E. B., Martin, M. P., Densen, P. M., Newbill, J. A., McClellan, G. S., Christie, A., Peterson, J. C. and Darby, W. J.: The Vanderbilt cooperative study of maternal and infant nutrition. Am. J. Obst. & Gynec., 67:501, 1954.

14. Smith, C.: Effects of maternal undernutrition upon the newborn infant in Holland (1944-1945). J. Pediat., 30:229, 1947.

15. Thomson, A.: Diet in pregnancy. Brit. J. Nutrition, 1. 12:446, 1958; 2. 13:190, 1959; 3. 13:509, 1959.

16. Duncan, E. H. L., Baird, D. and Thomson, A. M.: The causes and prevention of stillbirths and first week deaths. J. Obst. & Gynec., Brit. Emp., 59:183, 1952.

*Chapter 22*

# MANAGEMENT OF WEIGHT
# IN PREGNANCY

Written in collaboration with
Johanna T. Dwyer, Howard N. Jacobson, and Bobbie K. Huchins

$Q$UANTITY and quality of weight gain in pregnancy are matters of interest and concern to both physician and patient. For the physician, weight gain indicates the progress of fetal growth. If interpreted wisely, it may warn of physiologic deviations in the pregnancy, such as preeclampsia, or of future obstetric difficulties that can be avoided with its proper manipulation and other therapy. However, the expectant mother may have misgivings in spite of assurances that all is progressing normally. She may fear that weight gain during pregnancy will lead to obesity and ruin her figure. Thus, the doctor and the patient may fail to understand each other's concerns about weight gain during this period and, consequently, difficulties may arise.

If the physician is to obtain the cooperation necessary to manage weight gain sucessfully, he must understand some of his patient's more common worries about it and be able to explain in comprehensible language the rationale behind his advice. This chapter answers several common questions about managing weight gain in pregnancy.

## GOALS OF WEIGHT GAIN IN PREGNANCY

The primary goal of weight management during gestation is to help promote a healthy pregnancy and optimal growth and development of the fetus so that the infant will be well born at full term with the best possible chance for survival. The secondary

Reprinted from *Postgraduate Medicine, 48* (No. 1), July, 1970.© McGraw-Hill, Inc.

goal, and it is only secondary, is to keep the mother from accumulating excessive fat, so that about a month after delivery she can return to within a few pounds of what she weighed before she became pregnant.

## NORMAL WEIGHT GAIN DURING PREGNANCY

Pregnancy appears to be most successful when weight gain is 20 to 24 lb or even more over prepregnancy weight. This range covers most individual variations. At first glance, such a goal may seem a bit high. However, the best estimates for women in the United States indicated that the weight of the product of conception (fetus, placenta, amniotic fluid) and changes in the maternal body other than fat storage (increased size of uterus and breasts and increased blood volume and body water) alone acount for slightly more than 20 lb.

Much of this weight is lost immediately after delivery, and most women automatically lose several more pounds in the first few weeks of the puerperium, even without restricted food intake. Several recent studies have indicated that pregnancies and obstetric results are better with slightly large weight gains than with gains that cover only the inevitable losses at or shortly after parturition. Such results obviate the risk involved in temporarily adding a few pounds of fat. Weight gain of this order is justified experientially and, moreover, does not seem to increase greatly the likelihood of obesity occurring after delivery.

In the past, weight-gain figures in the teens were often suggested. These were derived from obstetric experiences of half a century or more ago and from early body composition studies, which involved imprecise estimates of the components of gain and rarely included studies of the infant's condition at birth or his subsequent survival. In those days, physicians often had to cope with the difficulties of vaginal delivery of patients who had various pelvic malformations due to rickets or other causes or of very obese patients whose labor was unsatisfactory. Cesarean section then entailed enormous risk. Severely limiting weight gain by means of dietary restriction of calories, sodium and fluids (often leading to maternal dehydration) was often done to produce low-birth-weight babies and to facilitate delivery. These measures may well have been justified considering the state of obstetrics at the turn of the century, but are not necessary today.

Modern obstetric technics have outdated "growing" the baby to fit the pelvis. Unfortunately, as times have changed, the conditions and supporting data for such restrictive recommendations have been forgotten, while the "magic numbers" in the teens remain firmly entrenched in the minds of many physicians and laymen as the *sine qua non* of satisfactory weight gain in pregnancy.

## PATTERN OF NORMAL GAIN

A slow, steady weight gain is a good sign that the mother and fetus are progressing normally. Some rather rough but useful bench marks are: a gain of about 2 lb in the first 10 weeks, about 10 lb by 20 weeks, about 20 lb by 30 weeks, and 25 to 30 lb by 40 weeks. Maximal rate of gain is to be expected in midpregnancy. In the second half of pregnancy, a gain of slightly more than a pound a week or slightly less until delivery. Decreased appetite and a feeling of fullness with less food intake help most women brake weight gain during the last four to six weeks of pregnancy.

## PRECONCEPTION WEIGHT MANAGEMENT

With more widespread use of contraception, planned pregnancies have become more common. Before a woman starts her family and while she is using contraceptives is an ideal time to bring weight down or up to a desireable level. Women are likely to have better obstetric experience when they enter pregnancy at a desirable weight than when they are underweight or overweight. Unfortunately treatment of these problems in the prepregnancy period is too often neglected.

## WEIGHT GAIN IN OBESE WOMEN

Weight management in the obese or slightly overweight woman who becomes pregnant is a special problem. Contrary to what most obese women and many physicians think, even obese women should gain some weight during pregnancy. However, weight gain must be carefully monitored so that deposition of fat is not over the necessary weight gain resulting from increases in nonfatty tissue. These increases are part of a healthy fetal and maternal growth. Pregnancy is not the time to launch even a grossly obese but otherwise normal woman on a strict weight-reducing diet in the hope of achieving an ideal weight. Rather, the goal in pregnancy should be to prevent excess fat from accumulating.

It is true that an obese woman's adipose tissue reserves can be used to supply some of the energy needed for fetal growth. However, if food intake is severely limited by a rigorous starvation-type diet, the intake of vitamins, minerals and protein, as well as calories, is almost invariably decreased. Heavy drains on maternal stores of these nutrients are then necessary to support growth of the fetus, because a restricted food intake does not supply these nutrients in sufficient amounts.

The obese mother may not have reserves; if she does have reserves, she can ill afford to lose them, since her intake of certain of these nutrients is apt to be lower even before pregnancy than that of the normal-weight woman. Overweight women have at some time in their lives been overnourished in calories but are often undernourished in other nutrients. Frequently overlooked is the fact  that they may not even be eating more calories than they need at the time they come to the physician. An avoidable deterioration of the nutritional status of the mother and perhaps of the fetus, as well as pregnancy and obstetric difficulties, may result if the obese pregnant woman is automatically placed on a low-calorie diet.

Even for the obese woman, a gain of 20 to 24 lb is a good goal. However, on the physician's advice or her own initiative, she may attempt to limit her weight gain to 10 to 15 lb to insure that no fat will be gained or that fat will be lost during gestation. Unfortunately this compromises the primary goal of weight management in pregnancy. The ill effects on the health of the fetus or on the mother that may result if the primary goal (i.e. optimal growth and development of the fetus) is sacrificed may not be reversible.

Postdelivery weight management should be instituted to reduce the mother to nearer her ideal weight. Temporarily shelving weight reduction for a holding effort (i.e. preventing further gains in fatty tissue) during pregnancy entails less risk to the expectant mother's health if her obesity is not complicated by other conditions and if her weight problem is attacked as soon as the pregnancy is over.

Because of social pressure, perhaps vanity, and habit, women are extremely concerned about weight gain at any period of their life and, for the most part, regard it as highly undesirable, even in pregnancy. Few nulliparas or primigravidas realize that weight gains of three or even four times the weight of the baby they will produce are perfectly normal, if not optimal, and that most of the weight gain will be lost at delivery or shortly thereafter. A brief and simple explanation of where the weight comes from and of what it consists will do much to allay a patient's fear about allowing a physician to supervise her figure during pregnancy. Such reassurance is **particularly** necessary and useful if the patient is obese and panics at the thought of gaining still more weight, or if the patient is of more normal weight but has a tendency to be unusually concerned about her weight and her figure.

Obese women must be carefully watched during pregnancy. At the first visit to the physician, they should be referred to a nutritionist or dietitian for counseling if the physician cannot spare the time to take a careful history of food habits and dietary intake. Some obese women eat enormous amounts of food during pregnancy and consequently gain weight far too rapidly. Perhaps more commonly, they gain excess weight because of extreme inactivity, which becomes even more pronounced with pregnancy than it was before.

Because of decreased energy output due to decreased activity, many women gain weight on the caloric level of their prepregnancy diet. Often they are caught in a double bind by a physician who is unaware of this fact. On the physician's advice, they continue eating the foods they ate before pregnancy plus plenty of dairy products and extra meat that he has recommended. On their next visit to the physician, he is distressed because they have gained excess weight. A better approach is to encourage the pregnant woman to substitute foods high in nutrients needed for some of the high-calorie, low-nutritive value foods she was eating prior to pregnancy. This avoids the problem of overloading the diet with excessive calories that may not be needed.

Some obese women and many other women who watch their weight closely undertake drastic reducing diets on their own at the first sign of pregnancy wieght gain, especially if they are unaware that they are pregnant. Others, realizing that they are pregnant, restrict their diet, assuming that they can transfer their excess weight to the baby and be delivered of both obesity and baby at the end of nine months. Some obese women fast or take laxatives and diuretics, if they can obtain them, for a few days before visits to the physician because they think they will be chided for an excess weight gain. The physician can discourage these practices by carefully explaining the lack of wisdom of such procedures.

## MANAGING UNDERWEIGHT WOMEN

Underweight women who become pregnant are also at a higher risk than is normal. Small, slender women often have a great deal of difficulty in gaining enough weight during pregnancy. Their activity level remains high while their already low food intake is reduced still further by the nausea and revulsion toward food generally that sometimes develop early in pregnancy. Often they are overtired as well as undernourished. Since exhaustion often contributes to lack of appetite, such women should be urged to get plenty of rest — to take short naps in the afternoon or when they come home from work and to get extra sleep every night and on the weekends.

Small, frequent meals rather than large quantities of foods at three meals are advisable, since the former are less likely to cause discomfort. Liquid diets (e.g. Metrecal®) taken between meals and before bedtime in addition to meals seem to be well tolerated and help to increase food intake. Liqueurs (e.g. Benedictine) or wine may quiet the stomach and aid relaxation. If a dietitian is available, underweight patients should be urged to see her.

## COMMENT

Weight gain in most pregnant women is a normal physiologic

process, and unless it is clearly associated with some pathologic process such as preeclampsia or galloping obesity, the physician should manage the weight gain in a relaxed and supportive manner.

## Chapter 23

# NUTRITION-RELATED PROBLEMS
# IN PREGNANCY

Written in collaboration with
Johanna T. Dwyer, Howard N. Jacobson, and Bobbie K. Huchins

SINCE so few dietitians work with patients seen in private practices, these patients often receive relatively less prenatal dietary advice and treatment than those attending outpatient clinics in hospitals and health centers. This situation can be remedied by earlier and more accurate identification of dietary problems and more widespread use of dietitians in private practices.

To improve the effectiveness of dietitians, the physician will find it helpful to separate his patients into three groups; those who require therapeutic diets, those who need lengthy nutritional counseling, and normal, healthy expectant mothers.

## PATIENTS REQUIRING THERAPEUTIC DIETS

A small group of patients need carefully supervised therapeutic dietary regimens for a comfortable, safe pregnancy.

### *Patients with Preexixting Medical Complications*

Pregnancy complicated by diseases such as diabetes, tuberculosis, cardiovascular, renal or gallbladder disorders, or ulcerative colitis requires careful dietary planning. The disease may be nonnutritional in origin, but if treatment involves a well-defined nutritional component, the patient's diet usually must be modified to meet the added requirements of the pregnancy and her progress must be closely supervised.

Reprinted from *Postgraduate Medicine, 48* (No. 4), October, 1970.© McGraw-Hill, Inc.

### Women with Poor Obstetric Histories

Many complications are associated with inadequate diets, but the mechanisms of dietary influence are poorly understood. Women with a history of toxemia, abruptio placentae, spontaneous premature labor, or repeated abortions are at high nutritional risk and should be followed carefully. Specific therapeutic regimens may not be indicated; however, nutritional problems such as fluid retention and weight gain often arise.

### Overweight or Underweight Patients

Pregnant women whose prepregnancy weight was 10 per cent below or more than 20 per cent above the desirable weight for height are at higher than normal risk and usually require dietary surveillance. Because weight gain causes these patients a great deal of anxiety, the weight-gain plan must be made clear to them. Diets of both the overweight and underweight person may be low or lacking in essential nutrients.

The most frequent mistake in treating these patients is prescribing unduly restrictive diets when only moderate modifications are necessary. Drastic restrictions, when required, should deviate as little as possible from the patient's normal diet. This helps to insure that the patient will follow the prescribed diet.

Dietary problems are more complex for patients living at home than for those in hospitals. Patients at home must interpret instructions correctly and shop for and prepare the dietary food while carrying out their normal household responsibilities. Thus the physician, nurse or dietitian must invest more time than usual in helping them. In our experience, the patient with special problems that warrant such dietary measures requires a minimum of one-half to one hour of consultation time to comprehend the dietary regimen and to achieve an acceptable degree of individualization to insure adherance to the diet.

Many busy private physicians give their patients ready-made diet sheets that are furnished by various sources. These sheets may seem helpful because the directions appear to be simple and straightforward. Unfortunately, most of them are inadequate. For example, the sheets usually present fixed menus with specific foods that must be eaten at each meal, with no regard for the patient's food preferences or eating habits, and they fail to state which modifications are crucial.

Rather than being informative and individualized guides for planning meals within the broad therapeutic limits that are deemed necessary, the diet sheets commonly assume the appearance of elaborate menu prescriptions that seldom apply to the patient's specific needs. Furthermore, the patient may be asked to deviate so far from her normal eating habits that mealtimes may become sessions in which food is regarded as medicine. In such cases, it is not surprising that failure to adhere to the diet is the rule rather than the exception.

## PATIENTS NEEDING LENGTHY NUTRITIONAL COUNSELING

Patients who need extensive advice in dietary adjustment are often overlooked early in pregnancy because their problems are sociologic rather than physiologic. Early nutritional counseling often can prevent the development of full-blown diet-related complications and, in any event, can make pregnancy more comfortable. Because these patients may be at a disadvantage due to age, education or income, pregnancy is one of the few periods in their life when they can ask for professional dietary help.

### Adolescents

Because their prepregnancy diets are of poor quality and their own growing bodies need highly nutritive foods, adolescents are often likely to be undernourished, particularly in iron and vitamins. They are particularly vulnerable to nutritional problems because they may fear that pregnancy will ruin their figure, they may not want the baby, or they may have budgetary and personal problems. Adolescents especially need vitamins, minerals and, to a lesser extent, proteins. Routine diet sheets do not meet their special needs.

## Indigent Patients

It is imperative that the physician recognize and deal with food problems related to income, as even the most destitute patient may be reluctant to tell him about a financial problem. Many of these patients do not need therapeutic regimens, but they still need extensive counseling and assistance in adjusting their diet to the demands of pregnancy. Food budgeting often becomes acute when the female wage earner in a family on a limited income must give up her job because of approaching delivery. Therapeutic regimens involving special supplements or high-protein foods are often not followed because the patient is unable to buy, store or prepare the food or perhaps to understand how to follow the prescribed diet. Management of these problems often requires full use of community resources.

## Patients with Ethnic and Language Problems

These patients may not have inadequate diet but may need counseling because routine advice based on standard American eating patterns may be incomprehensible or alien to them. They will need diets that are adjusted to their cultural background.

## Patients with Unusual Eating Habits

Vegetarians, health-food enthusiasts, and members of certain religious groups may find the routine dietary advice for pregnant women to be philosophically or morally unacceptable. However, such dietary restrictions fortunately pertain only to foods, not to nutrients, and it is usually possible to respect the patient's beliefs and still satisfy nutritional requirements.

## Women Planning a Future Family

Every woman in one of the aforementioned categories who is currently using contraception but wants to have children later should receive dietary counseling. The ideal time to treat longstanding nutritional problems is before pregnancy.

These patients need more than reassurance and cursory general advice coupled with a prescription for vitamin and mineral supplements. Although such preparations, particularly iron and folic acid, may be beneficial, one should remember that these are only supplements and are not substitutes for an adequate diet.

## NORMAL, HEALTHY EXPECTANT MOTHERS

Only minor adjustments in eating habits are needed to accommodate the physiologic demands of pregnancy in this large group of women. For the moderately sedentary homemaker, a few dietary changes in eating patterns to keep weight gain under control usually are the only suggestions needed. It is not necessary to raise caloric intake drastically; only slight increases (a few hundred calories a day) are necessary. Often these calories can be added without changing food intake because of the energy saved when physical activity decreases in late pregnancy. Active women, of course, require different guidance.

A good daily diet for healthy pregnant women includes 1 qt of milk (or an equivalent amount of cheese), at least 1/2 lb of meat or meat substitute, one egg, two servings of fruit or vegetables, and four servings of bread or cereal. Substitution rather than the addition of foods to conform with this pattern should be stressed. If the pregnant patient does not usually include these foods, she should be encouraged to substitute them for other less essential foods that she may be eating.

## TECHNICS OF DIETARY COUNSELING

Few physicians have the time necessary to carefully explain a therapeutic diet, and they may lack expertise in dealing with the home economics imposed by budgetary problems or the intricacies of ethnic eating patterns; thus, it is probably best to delegate this aspect of treatment. This is easy to do when the patient is seen in a hospital or clinic where dietitians are available, but it is more difficult in private practice where such personnel are less accessible.

Sometimes the private practitioner can solve this problem by delegating dietary counseling to his office nurse. Nurses who have had a short course in nutrition to supplement the information they received during training can handle most of the relatively simple dietary modifications that patients need during pregnancy.

Another solution to this problem is for the busy office-based physician to employ a dietitian. If space in the physician's office is limited, he may refer patients to the dietitian at her own office and telephone his instructions for management. Since most dietitians and nutritionists are married and have family responsibilities that preclude full-time hospital-based work, they are interested in part-time counseling in a physician's office. Names of available qualified dietitians can be obtained from local branches of the American Dietetic Association.

Therapeutic diets and nutritional counseling, whether directed toward correcting a physiologic deviation arising in pregnancy or toward improving long-term food habits, involve the difficult task of changing long-entrenched eating patterns. When the dietitian sees high-risk patients early in pregnancy, she can obtain baseline information for evaluating later deviations, and her dietary counseling has time to make an impact on the patient.

Finally, a skillful dietitian is often able to detect early signs of trouble, such as nausea and fatigue, that are frequently reflected in food habits. When she is brought in for consultation after problems are well developed, she may be unable to do much to remedy the situation. An even more serious handicap for the dietitian is to be used only to punish offenders for nutritional violations. Threats of "Control your weight or I'll send you to the dietitian" lessen chances for needed dietitian-patient rapport.

*Chapter 24*

# IS BREAST-FEEDING COMING BACK?

$A$T the White House Conference on Food, Nutrition and Health, the Panel on the Family as a Food Delivery System wrote in its sixth recommendation:

> The Panel recognizes that all other things being equal, "the mother who nurses her baby establishes, at an early date, an intimacy with her child which makes further relationships with him easy and natural" (H. Baldwin, M.D.). The Panel further recognizes the special benefits to the child: that breast milk is the perfect food for his nutritional needs and development; that it is the most natural way to feed babies; and that it provides a protection against infection and allergies that cannot be duplicated. Thought must be given to the fact that a nursing mother must have a good diet, in addition to enough sleep and relaxation, or she will not produce milk of . . . sufficient quality or in sufficient quantity.
>
> It is recommended:
>
> 1. That more support for the breast-feeding decision and educated assistance be given to the vast majority of women who are physically and emotionally capable of nursing their babies, by reemphasis in medical schools, schools of nursing and in all other allied health training programs including education in how to help a mother be successful in nursing her child.
>
> 2. The maternal and child health services (both federal and local) be directed to give high priority to doing all possible to assure an adequate food supply to low-income pregnant and nursing mothers and their families on inadequate diets.

The Panel that made this recommendation was headed by Dr. Effie O. Ellis, then director of the division of maternal and child health, Ohio State Department of Health, and now an official of the American Medical Association. The Panel also included a number of eminent medical and lay persons. The women's task force, representing women's organizations with a combined membership of over 60 million in the United States, commented

Reprinted from *Postgraduate Medicine, 47* (No. 4), April, 1970.© McGraw-Hill, Inc.

favorably on this recommemdation. At the Conference itself, the topic evoked intense participation from a large audience composed of all groups of society and served as a great bond between them. Women participants questioned at length the representatives from La Leche League International, an organization that promotes breast-feeding. The fact that many of those present judged the representatives' answers unsatisfactory did not seem to decrease interest in the topic. The women generally agreed that breast-feeding is desirable.

The report of this consensus led me, as chairman of the White House Conference, to explore the present status of breast-feeding in the United States to see if the recommendations were harbingers of a changed attitude among American women.

The best available data on breast-feeding in the United States are from the impressive studies of Bain (1) and Meyer (2, 3). These investigators gathered data from about 3000 hospitals with a birth incidence of over 2,700,000 babies. There are also a number of local studies, such as those of Salber in Boston in the late 1950s and the 1960s.

In 1966 breast-feeding among mothers dismissed from the hospital had declined to 18 per cent for the United States as a whole, compared with 38 per cent for 1946 and 21 per cent for 1956. The decline was precipitous in the Southwest. Arizona figures fell from 70 per cent in 1946 to 44 per cent in 1956, to 16 per cent in 1966. The decline was steep in the Southeast. Alabama percentages went from 60 in 1946, to 34 in 1956, to 23 in 1966, with Arkansas, North Carolina and Tennessee reporting even greater drops and rates in South Carolina falling from 60 per cent to 12 per cent in the same period. Only in the mountain states of Colorado, Idaho and Utah did the percentage consistently remain above 30 per cent from 1956 to 1966.

In his 1966 study (3), Meyer tried to determine what factors influenced the new mother in deciding whether or not to breast-feed. Of over 1700 hospitals whose personnel answered questionnaires on this subject, 48 per cent selected the nursing personnel as having the key influence; 40 per cent designated the obstetrician and 12 per cent the pediatrician. Hospitals obviously regarded as secondary the intentions of the mother as well as social influences unrelated to medical factors.

The educational and socioeconomic status of the infant's parent apparently influences the decision to breast-feed. While metropolitan and suburban areas showed a lower incidence of breast-feeding in 1946 than rural areas, this was no longer true in 1966, when breast-feeding was more common among suburban mothers than among mothers in other population areas. This suggested that breast-feeding was becoming more frequent in the higher socioeconomic and intellectual classes, a view supported by Boston studies in the early 1960s showing that 40 per cent of these mothers nursed, compared with 24 per cent of mothers in lower socioeconomic strata.

The same study showed that 70 per cent of women married to students (the majority of whom were professional and graduate students) breast-fed their infants. Another study found that women of professional status also exhibited a higher incidence of breast-feeding than the population as a whole. More recent studies confirm this trend. With increasing frequency, college-educated women seem to decide to nurse long before the birth of the child, and the attending physician rarely influences their choice.

While available data are too scant and the period of observation too short to conclude that there is a definite trend toward a return to breast-feeding, it may well be that we are in the midst of a slow change led by the more educated women and community leaders in general. Perhaps, as history has often shown, other social classes will slowly follow. Certainly the intense interest displayed by Conference participants in the subject of breast-feeding appears to be something new.

## REFERENCES

1. Bain, K.: The incidence of breast feeding in hospitals in the United States. Pediatrics, 2:313, 1948.
2. Meyer, H. F.: Breast Feeding in the United States: Extent and possible trend. Pediatrics, 22:116, 1958.
3. ——: Breast Feeding in the United States. Report of a 1966 national survey with comparable 1946 and 1956 data. Clin: Pediat., 7:708, 1968.

## Chapter 25

# NUTRITION AND LACTATION

I<small>T</small> is easy to justify the general principles of breast-feeding in poor countries where cheap, hygienic milk and adequate milk substitutes do not exist. In such areas the availability to the infant of an adequate supply of breast milk is a necessary element of survival. The discontinuation of breast-feeding because of the poor state of health and nutrition of the mother, and the progress of a subsequent pregnancy, or the natural course of time is often the immediate and main cause of the development of the protein deficiency syndrome in the infant. In recent years this syndrome has come to be known by the Ghanaian term "kwashiorkor" (1).

In the United States and in Western Countries generally, such a compulsory argument does not exist. Physicians anxious to justify breast-feeding on nutritional grounds point to the fact that Gyorgy (2) has shown that human milk contains an essential nutrient for the bacterium *Lactobacillus bifidus* (variant Penn.). This nutrient is not found in cow's milk. However, the biologic value of this compound to the infant has not been established, although it is interesting that the prevailing microorganism in the feces of normal breast fed infants is *L. bifidus,* sometimes to the near exclusion of all other species. By contrast the feces of infants fed cow's milk show a great variety of organisms and are usually alkaline or neutral rather than acid as in breast-fed infants. It has been suggested, although the evidence is meager, that the intestinal flora favored by human breast milk aids the efficient utilization of its protein.

Human milk differs from cow's milk in other respects. Human milk has a greater lactose content, less calcium (30 mg per 100 ml

Reprinted from *Postgraduate Medicine, 33* (No. 4), April, 1963.

versus 120 mg per 100 ml in cow's milk), less phosphorus (10 to 20 mg per 100 ml versus 100 mg per 100 ml), less thiamine, riboflavin and vitamin A, and several times as much vitamin C. Again, the biologic significance of most of these differences (vitamin C is the exception) has not been established. Actually, supplies of vitamin C, although higher in breast milk, cannot be relied on for ideal nutrition; a daily supplement of 25 mg of ascorbic acid and 400 units of vitamin D still should be administered to the breast-fed infant. Whether, as some pediatricians have suggested, the higher sodium content of cow's milk really imposes a stress on the infant's adrenals and on its elimination mechanism is also still in doubt. The old idea that the protein of cow's milk is significantly less adequate for optimal growth than that of human milk has been dispelled as better evaporated milks and infant milk preparations have become available. This old concept was embodied in the recommended dietary allowances of the National Research Council (3), which recommended a daily intake of 3.5 gm of protein per kilogram of body weight; breast-fed infants usually receive only 2 to 2.5 gm of protein per kilogram of body weight. The concept of a poor biologic value for cow's milk has been repeatedly disproved by Holt (4), who has shown that poor digestibility of non homogenized milk in early preparations was largely responsible for earlier findings. More recently Fomon and May (5) have exhaustively studied a small group of healthy full-term infants fed a cow's milk formula in which the protein concentration was similar to that found in human milk. Observations on nitrogen balance, weight and height, hemoglobin, blood urea, and serum protein over the first six months of life disclosed no outstanding advantage of human milk over cow's milk.

If purely nutritional evidence in favor of breast-feeding over medically supervised artificial feeding is thus lacking, there nevertheless remains a strong case for breast-feeding. Nursing is a satisfying emotional experience for the mother, and should be encouraged from her standpoint unless medical reasons to the contrary exist. In considering the child, this writer shares Holt's (4) view that the argument of certain psychiatrists that failure to nurse at the breast causes emotional deprivation and maladjustment has not been proved. More convincing is the argument that natural nursing is a foolproof method which can be duplicated only by intelligent, constantly careful, clinically guided — and costlier — artificial feeding. Under less than ideal conditions, morbidity and mortality are consistently greater in artificially fed infants than in the breast-fed.

Although breast-feeding is generally desirable from the standpoint of the infant's hygienic welfare and the mother's emotional satisfaction, it should not be carried out at the expense of other health considerations in the mother. Poor general health and debility, a recent history of tuberculosis, severe complications of labor, and breast infections are obvious contraindications. It is a priori obvious that maintenance of maternal health in the presence of satisfactory lactation will be insured only if maternal nutrition is adequate. All too often this is forgotten. The nutritional demands caused by lactation are greater than those of pregnacy. The infant synthesizes much more tissue each day than the fetus does. The infant has to insure his own thermoregulation; his movements are more extensive; more intermediary processes occur between the mother's food ingestion and the infant's tissue metabolism, with the result that the whole process is less efficient than during pregnancy; and the mother's metabolism itself may be less efficient than during pregnancy. The mother's spontaneous activity is always restricted at the end of pregnancy, whatever demands are made on her by the environment. In the case of a primipara not engaged in outside work, such demands are sufficiently decreased to nullify the increased in caloric requirements which the last trimester of pregnancy would otherwise create. By contrast, the postpartum woman tends to be unusually active. Whatever she did before pregnancy she probably will continue to do, and in addition she has to satisfy the demanding requirements of infant care. Yet this is a period during which diet is often neglected.

The exaggerated idea of an increase in nutritional requirement in pregnancy and the fear that the unborn child will be harmed by any but the most luxurious diet make the pregnant woman pay particular attention to her diet. She is, she feels, "eating for two." Yet during lactation, when she is actually feeding two independent organisms, she usually ceases to feel this responsibility. Obstetric care all too often ceases at this particular period or is confined to the routine observation of surgical healing. The woman wants to lose too fast whatever weight accumulation has not been eliminated by parturition, and teachings concerning the very large nutritional needs of lactation, as well as care of the breasts, possible correction of defective shape of the nipples by plastic cups, and correct position of the infant during nursing are all too often neglected in an era in which artificial feeding has been prevalent. All too often also the obstetric staff, particularly the nurses, is not prepared to spend the necessary time for initiating good breast–feeding habits, with all it implies in terms of extra care and handling. The result is that breast-feeding fails more frequently than necessary or it is done at the cost of maternal depletion in the essential nutrients which are poured into the milk.

We shall now review briefly what is known about the influence of nutritional factors on the volume and the composition of breast milk, and conclude by suggesting some generally prudent rules on nutrition during breast–feeding.

Volume of milk differs among women, between breasts of the same woman, from nursing to nursing, and from day to day. There are two methods of determining such volume, both entailing errors. The infant can be weighed before and after nursing. The milk can be extracted manually or by breast pump and weighed. Macy and co-workers (6) have given evidence that manual extraction is probably the method giving the highest yields. They also found that the greater volume is secreted by the larger breast. There is general agreement that the volume is greatest during the morning and decreases toward evening, perhaps because the overnight interval between nursings is greater than daytime intervals.Thorough studies of the variation of volume with the stage of lactation are missing except for wet nurses. The studies of Macy et al. (6) and Escudero and Pierangeli (7) show that such women can maintain a high yield for a long time. The plateau of maximal yield begins after about two months and may continue for four or five more. Ordinary women seem to show a peak between the twentieth and thirty-second weeks. There is also general agreement that the volume at the end of the colostric period exceeds the flow maintained immediately afterward.

Data on the variation of volume with parity and age are also scarce and apparently contradictory. Ström (8) determined the milk volume from the second to the seventh days of lactation in 228 primiparas and 308 multiparas. The mean values were 1900 ± 24.19 ml per day for the former and 1,243±20.7 ml per day for the latter. The difference would be more convincing if further data on the same women were included. Ström also found an inverse relation between amounts of milk during the colostric period and the mother's age. This effect was greater in primiparas than in multiparas. These results actually permit an interpretation of the contradictions found in the literature, since they suggest that the effects of parity and age on milk volume are antagonistic.

Finally it must be emphasized that while volume of milk differs considerably in normally lactating women (the average for the United States between one and four months is of the order of a liter) physiologic factors is such differences are not known.

## EFFECT OF DIET AND FLUID INTAKE ON VOLUME

The most ambitious study in the United States of the effect of diet on milk volume is the old one of Deem (9), who determined yields in five subjects fed for a week at a time on six diets: institutional, high-protein, high-protein and vitamin B, high-sugar, high-fat and low-protein. Milk yields were somewhat lower on the none-too-satisfactory institutional diet, but the one-week periods were too short to demonstrate convincingly the influence of the diet.

The common belief that milk volume is highly sensitive to fluid intake is better supported by studies of cows than by studies of women. In cows, as Leitch and Thomson (10) have shown, fluid intake increases with milk yield; metabolic water increases with the increased food intake. The water of urine and feces and vaporization water also increase at this time, since greater amounts of waste material and greater metabolic heat have to be disposed of. It would appear reasonable to assume that similar phenomena occur in women. However, Macy (in only three sujects) could find no correlation between milk volume and fluid intake in the course of 65 weeks. Olsen found that variations of fluid intake from 600 to 2,775 ml per day in 13 subjects had no effect on the breast milk supply. Lelong showed that such findings could be interpreted by the concomitant and inverse variability of other water losses, with fluid shortage resulting in drastic curtailment of urine and respiratory water. This constancy of milk volume indicates the high priority given by the organism to this function. It appears wholly reasonable not to force the body to concentrate urine excessively so as to maintain milk yields; a generous supply of fluid is thus recommended. At the same time, these results suggest the futility of attempting to push up milk production by presenting a fluid intake in excess of that required to cover normal needs plus milk volume.

## MILK COMPOSITION AND DIET

*Protein*

One point often neglected in studies of the nitrogen content of human milk is that an important part of the nitrogen is in the form of nonprotein nitrogen (20%, compared with only 5 % in cow's milk). Most of this nonprotein nitrogen is made up of urea and free amino acids. The clinical expression of the "protein" content of human milk (nitrogen determined by Kjeldahl's method x 6.38) must therefore be viewed with qualification. With this reservation, the average "protein" content of milk in this country is 1.213 ± 0.256 gm per 100 ml. The corresponding value for European women is 1.575 ± 0.322 gm per 100 ml, based largely on British and German determinations (7). The reasons for these slight but possibly significant differences are not clear. The most recent European figures seem to be closer to the American. For example Kon and Mawson (11) found an average of 1.26 ± 0.19 gm per 100 ml in their studies. There is no definite evidence of any difference in the milk from the two breasts, or a change between nursings or in the course of a given day. Nitrogen content decreases during the first 10 days (colostric period) and may continue to decline very slowly during the course of lactation. Individual variations are large. In a sample of 915 women, the range was 0.5 gm per 100 ml to 2.9 gm per 100 ml (7). There is some evidence of a decrease in total nitrogen with parity and age. The evidence regarding the effect of a diet low in protein content on milk is scanty and generally inconclusive. It appears that a diet low in protein will eventually curtail the amount of milk secreted but that it has little influence on milk composition.

## Fat

The mean fat content of milk based on appoximately 300 24-hour milk samples was 3.33 gm per 100 ml with a standard deviation of 0.57 gm. Again the range was large, with most values between 2.5 and 4.5 gm per 100 ml. Most but not all recorded data show a diurnal rhythm with a maximum in the morning. Fat content tends to increase during the course of a given feeding; there is no correlation with stage of lactation, volume of milk, age or parity. Day-to-day variations are large. The only clear evidence that diet may influence the fat content of human milk is an old experiment by Polonovski (12) showing that administration of large amounts of glucose increases the fat content and can even double it. Experiments where the diet is a whole was modified have been generally inconclusive. There are indications that the fatty acid composition of human milk fat, like that of cow's milk, can be influenced to a certain extent by modifying the fatty acid mixture in the maternal diet.

## Lactose

The mean lactose value for 1,010 samples was 7.2 ± 0.679 gm per 100 ml. Day-to-day variation is great but there is no definite evidence of any effect of diet.

## Vitamins

Again, information on the influence of diet on the vitamin content of milk is inadequate. An interesting comparison of the vitamin content of breast milk in Bantu and European women in South Africa (13) is difficult to interpret in terms of diet alone. Bantu mothers breast-feed abudantly on relatively poor diets.

Among Bantu women the induction of a flow of milk from virgins has been claimed, as well as the capacity to lactate even beyond menopause (14). The milk of Bantu women contains only 70 mg of niacin per 100 ml, compared with 150 mg per 100 in European women. The children seem unaffected by the lower concentration of this vitamin; Bantu and European babies exclusively breast-fed until the age of six months are comparable in height and weight. More surprising is the fact that the concentration of plasma vitamin C is high in Bantu babies, in spite of the mothers' low intake, a state of affairs which has led some good workers in South Africa to hypothesize that perhaps these children can synthesize some vitamin C (13). The thiamine level of breast milk is likely to be affected by the mother's thiamine intake, as suggested by the prevalence of infantile beriberi in breast-fed infants in some parts of the world.

## Minerals — Calcium

Macy (15) found a mean calcium content of 34.4 ± 0.27 mg per 100 ml for 628 samples. The fact that this United States value is much above the 29.9 ± 0.5 mg per 100 ml found by Kon and Mawson (11) in England and the 22.4 ± 0.5 mg per ml found by Uga for Japanese women might suggest a nutritional influence. State of lactation, parity, and day-to-day variations have been found to have a small and inconsistent influence. The evidence at hand suggests that elevating calcium alone in the diet of mothers is of little avail but that simultaneous administration of vitamin D and calcium can increase milk calcium by as much as 25 per cent (16) and even double it. Incidentally, the fact that cow's milk is much higher in calcium than breast milk (of the order of 120 mg per 100 ml) has been implicated in the development of idiopathic hypercalcemia in susceptible infants. It must be noted, however, that this complex and as yet little understood disease has been seen in at least one infant who was still essentially breast-fed (17).

## Other Minerals

Evidence that diet influences the content of phosphorus in breast milk may be a plus factor in that it decreases the risk of hypocalcemic tetany. The lower osmotic pressure of breast milk, due to lower sodium and potassium content, decreases the work of the kidneys of the young infant. Sodium and potassium levels in milk are not known to be influenced by the diet. Utilization of iron by the newborn is poor enough that small differences in the milk iron are probably of little significance. Breast milk levels of iodine and fluorine, on the other hand, are highly significant to the infant and are known to be influenced by the maternal diet, which must contain an adequate amount of these nutrients.

## CONCLUSION

It is obvious from this review that if the mother's diet is sound and has been adequate during pregnancy, the initiation of breast-feeding indicates no unusual qualitative nutritional requirements. Hytten, Yorston and Thomson (18) in their careful study of breast-feeding in Aberdeen found no difference in incidence of breast-feeding among social classes in similarly motivated women, in spite of marked differences in dietary habits. Once properly initiated, however, maintenance of a proper supply of breast milk without undue depletion of the mother obviously depends on provision of sufficient calories, proteins and nutrients. The efficiency of milk production has been estimated at no more than 60 per cent. To provide 700 calories of milk (1000 ml), more than 1000 additional calories are needed. (In some women, however, the appetite is not increased proportionately to the physiologic needs, and they find it difficult to eat 3000 calories per day. A slight deficit is usually not of great moment.) Similarly, 2 gm of protein of high nutritive value appears to be needed to produce 1 gm of milk protein. This means that something like 25 gm of additional protein of good quality is a minimum. In practice, addition to the normal maintenance diet of an extra liter of cow's milk, and extra serving of a high-protein food (meat, fish, cheese or beans), a large serving of citrus fruit, and 1 oz of leafy vegetable — in other words, one extra meal, with more milk throughout the day — will cover such requirements. Iodized salt and a fluorine supplement in unfluoridated areas should be used. The increases in fluid requirement can be covered by the extra milk and orange juice. While this requirement should be generously covered, it is useful to remember that as mentioned previously forcing fluid intake beyond this point has no effect on milk secretion.

## REFERENCES

1. Mayer, J.: Kwashiorkor. Postgrad. Med., 26:98, 1959.
2. Gyorgy, P.: A hitherto unrecognized biochemical difference between human milk and cow's milk. A.M.A. J. Dis. Child., 96:98, 1958.
3. Food and Nutrition Board, National Research Council: Recommended Dietary Allowances. Publication No. 302, Washington, D. C., 1953.
4. Holt, L. E., Jr.: Nutrition in infancy. In Wohl, M. G. and Goodheart, R. S. (Editors): Modern Nutrition in Health and Disease. Ed. 2. Philadelphia, Lea & Febiger, 1960.
5. Fomon, S. J. and May, C.: Nitrogen retention during the first six months of life. Nutrition Rev., 17:68, 1959.
6. Macy, I. G., Nims, B., Brown, M. and Hunscher, H. A.: Human milk studies. VII. Chemical analysis of milk representative of the entire first and last halves of the nursing period. Am. J. Dis. Child., 42:569, 1931.
7. Escudero, P. and Pierangeli, E.: In Morrison, S. D.: Human Milk. Farnham Royal, Slough, England, Commonwealth Agriculture Bureau, 1952.
8. Strom, J.: The breast feeding of mature infants during the neonatal period and the influence of some factors on the same. Acta paediat., supp. 1, 35:55, 1948.
9. Deem, H. E.: Observations on the milk of New Zealand women. Arch. Dis. Childhood, 6:53, 1931.
10. Leitch, I. and Thomson, J. S.: The water economy of farm animals. Nutrition Abstr. & Rev., 14:137, 1944-1945.
11. Kon, S. K. and Mawson, E. H.: Medical Research Council Special Report No. 269 1950.
12. Polonovski, M.: Influence de l'ingestion de glucose sur la composition du lait et du beurre de femme. Compt. rend. Soc. de biol., 112:191, 1933.
13. Walker, A. R. P.: Some aspects of nutritional research in South Africa. nutrition Rev., 14:321, 1956.
14. Greenway, P. J.: Artificially induced lactation in humans. East African M. J., 13:346, 1937.
15. Macy, I. G.: Composition of human colostrum and milk. Am. J. Dis. Child., 78:589, 1949.
16. Ritchie, B. V.: The calcium and phosphorus content of milk from Australian women. M. J. Australia, 1:331, 1942.
17. Morgan, H. G., Mitchell, R. G., Stowers, J. M. and Thomson, J. S.: Metabolic studies on two infants with idiopathic hyperdalcaemia. Lancet, 1:925, 1956.
18. Hytten, F. E., Yorston, J. C. and Thomson, A. M.: Difficulties associated with breast feeding. Brit. M. J., 1:310, 1958.

*Chapter 26*

# MIDDLE-AGED MEN MUST EXERCISE

THIS past summer I had the opportunity to participate in a symposium on "Nutrition and physical activity," held under the auspices of the Swedish Nutrition Foundation. After listening carefully to a series of excellent papers and lively discussions, I am more than ever convinced that medicine in the United States has yet to recognize the formidable health problem caused by the growing — and by now nearly total — physical inactivity of our citizens and has yet to come to grips with it. It may well be that no currently available medical measure could be as beneficial as an increase in the amount of exercise taken by our population.

The main concern is, of course, the relationship of inactivity to heart disease and to obesity, although maturity-onset diabetes and, perhaps, osteoporosis may also result in part from a sedentary life. About 30 per cent of all deaths in this country are from coronary arteriosclerosis, and the chief target is increasingly the male. In 1930 death from heart disease was about equal in men and women. Now, when all age groups are considered together, the death rate is two and a half times higher in males than in females. With our population increasingly besieged by this pandemic, little excitement or action has been generated, compared, for example, with that caused by a small epidemic of encephalitis or poliomyelitis. While cigarette smoking, high-fat diets, and unrecognized and untreated hypertension are obviously important factors in this increase in the prevalence of coronary disease, the significance of constantly decreasing physical activity, particularly among men, is still largely unrecognized. Most physicians are not convincing in

Reprinted from *Postgraduate Medicine, 40* (No. 6), December, 1966.

recommending an increase in activity, and when they do make such a recommendation, it is almost never in the form of a detailed prescription.

Before going on to practical advice, let us review briefly the evidence linking inactivity with obesity and with heart disease.

## OBESITY AND INACTIVITY

A physiologic basis for reassessment of the possibly primary contribution of inactivity as a cause of obesity was established when work done in my laboratory demonstrated that when activity is reduced to below a minimum level in experimental animals and in adult men, food intake does not decrease proportionately, and obesity develops. Actually, at very low levels of activity in experimental animals as well as in men, food intake tends to increase, a phenomenon long known by farmers who "pen up" animals they want to fatten. This phenomenon may be interpreted in the framework of a glucostatic mechanism in the regulation of food intake, as we have shown that inactivity reduces glucose utilization. It was also shown that genetically obese mice are extremely inactive and that, conversely, exercising them as well as animals with other forms of experimental obesity causes spontaneous loss of weight (1).

We also found that the onset of excessive weight gain among obese children in the public schools of Newton and Brookline (Massachusetts) generally occurred during the winter. This suggested that inactivity might be an important factor in the development of obesity. A more detailed study (3), comparing the food intake and activity schedules of 28 obese high school girls selected from this population with those of controls of normal weight and of the same height, age, scholastic standing and socioeconomic status, showed that obese girls ate less – not more – than their normal-weight controls but spent strikingly less time (two-thirds less) in activities involving any amount of exercise. In another study we examined the food intake and amount and degree of participation of obese adolescent boys and paired nonobese controls at a summer camp. We found both significantly less food intake and less participation in exercise among the obese boys. In a study conducted at a girls' camp, we found that a group of adolescent girls lost weight with increased exercise. Using a new technic developed for time-motion studies in industry and involving the taking of a number of photographs which are then used as a basis for estimating caloric expenditures based on the particular pose represented, we were able to demonstrate unequivocally that the average obese adolescent girl expends far less energy during scheduled exercise periods than does her nonobese counterpart (4).

Inactivity in youngsters, resulting from availability of school buses and individual means of transportation, the fact that physical chores are no longer required, and short, inadequate physical education programs, is of considerable importance in interpreting the prevalence of obesity in youngsters.

While inactivity is thus of paramount importance in the cause of obesity in children, it is apparently at least as important in explaining the increase in prevalence of obesity in adults, particularly in adult males. All the reliable statistics we have on food intake and on weight indicate that in Western countries, particularly in the United States, average caloric intake has decreased since 1900 while prevalence of obesity has increased.

Considering the laws of conservation of energy and matter, the only possible explanation is that expenditure ascribed to physical activity has decreased faster than food intake, with the difference accumulating as fat. In fact, what we now understand as a moderately active man, who engages in two hours of walking every day, gardening and some sport every weekend, was considered a sedentary man at the turn of the century.

## EXERCISE AND BLOOD CHOLESTEROL LEVELS

While early work on the relationship of serum cholesterol and exercise in animals yielded equivocal results, a number of studies in man have demonstrated that very hard, prolonged physical work at a level probably difficult to achieve in urbanized Western societies does lower serum cholesterol levels even in subjects consuming a high-fat diet.

Karvonen and co-workers (5) studied the food consumption of

lumberjacks in five camps in Eastern Finland. These men had an extremely large average daily intake – over 4700 calories, of which no less than 45 per cent were derived from fat. Yet their serum cholesterol levels were no higher than that of the average Finnish man with a much lower caloric intake, only 35 per cent of which is derived from fat. Gsell and I (6) compared an extremely active Swiss village population with an urban Swiss population. The village population had a high fat intake and a daily caloric intake 1000 calories higher than the urban population. However, the serum cholesterol levels of both men and women on the high physical activity and high-fat intake regimen were significantly lower than those found in their urbanized countrymen.

## EXERCISE AND MORTALITY DATA

The first documented evidence on the protective effect of exercise against heart disease was the well-known study of Morris and co-workers (7). The British investigators found that London bus drivers showed a higher incidence and a greater severity of coronary heart disease than did the bus conductors, who in the two-level London buses do a greater deal of stair climbing in the course of a day.

The nutritional habits of the two groups were essentially identical and it seemed that the two main variables differentiating the two groups were the greater exercise of the conductors and the possibly greater stress associated with driving in the London city traffic.

A later study by Morris (8) compared rural mail clerks and rural delivery mailmen. In this case, the element of stress was eliminated and the protective effect of exercise appeared clearly. Mortality from coronary disease was significantly less among the walking than among the sitting mailmen.

A study by Taylor and co-workers (9) in this country gave similar findings. They studied railroad employees, a group remarkable for its stable employment. Union rules are such that it is highly desirable for an individual to stay in his partiucular line of employment throughout his working life lest he forfeit his seniority. As a result, whatever job switching is done tends to be done early in a man's career. Taylor and associates studied three groups: clerks, switchmen and section hands. They found that mortality from arteriosclerotic heart disease was inversely correlated with the physical activity characteristic of each class of work. It was 5.7 per 1000 for clerks, 3.9 per 1000 for switchmen, and 2.8 per 1000 for section hands. The difference in mortality from arteriosclerotic heart disease among groups, in the same order and significance for all age groups, increased with age up to the 60-to 64-year-old group. Clerks showed a death rate of 10.4 per 1000, switchmen 6.7 per 1000, and section hands 4.2 per 1000. While there are minor difficulties in interpretation, such as higher death rates from violence among section hands and more rural location among section hands than among switchmen and clerks, it seems unlikely that these would invalidate the general conclusion that daily exercise of sufficient duration and intensity decreases mortality from coronary atherosclerosis.

## EXERCISE AND COLLATERAL CORONARY CIRCULATION

I am strongly convinced that the medical profession has not paid enough attention to the very basic work of Richard W. Eckstein (10) on the effect of exercise and coronary artery narrowing on coronary collateral circulation. This work, which has recently been produced and extended by Dr. Bernard Lown and his associates in our nutrition department at Harvard University School of Public Health, established clearly that exercise may favorably affect the course of coronary artery disease by one or more of several means. It may actually delay the progression of the disease or stimulate the growth of coronary collateral vessels during the disease process, or both.

Eckstein's study involved operating on 117 dogs and isolating the circumflex artery near its origin. Ligatures were tied over a probe to produce various degrees of constriction, causing T wave inversion and S-T segment depression before the probe was removed. After removal of the probe, return of the T wave and S-T segment to normal or nearly normal indicated patency of the narrowed vessel. After closing of the chest, air evacuation from the pleural cavity, and three days of rest with pennicillin therapy, the dogs were divided into two groups, both groups being kept at rest for one week to allow healing. One group was then exercised on a treadmill placed at a positive incline of 30 degrees. During the first week the speed was gradually increased from 3.2 to 4.7 mph. The animals were exercised from 15 to 20 minutes, four times daily, five days a week for six to eight weeks. During this period the second group remained at rest.

Examination of collateral function, through measurement of retrograde flow previously shown to be proportional to the anatomic development of the collateral vascular bed, showed clearly that in general the extent of collateral blood flow was proportional to the degree of constriction. It was clear that exercise increased the extent of collateral circulation by a very marked amount over and above that due to narrowing alone. The absence of electrocardiographic changes of complete circumflex occlusion, shown at the end of the experiments in exercised animals with high retrograde flow, clearly demonstrated the functional adequacy of these channels.

Significant collaterals did not develop in the rested animals with slight circumflex narrowing. The retrograde flow was low, and if complete circumflex occlusion was effected at the end of the experimental period, the electrocardiographic changes resembled those following complete circumflex occlusin in normal dogs.

The preparations from this study appeared comparable to human beings with coronary disease limited to one major artery or with severe narrowing of one major artery and limited narrowing of other arteries. Evidence obtained in the study of anastomoses in the heart of anemic patients also suggests that Eckstein's models are valid for man (11). It seems, therefore, highly likely that in man, as in dogs, under conditions of mild arterial narrowing, the myocardium is susceptible to infarction subsequent to sudden valcular occlusion because adequate collateral vessels are absent. Vascular occlusion through thrombosis or through hemorrhage into the vascular wall is more likely to develop in patients with a small degree of narrowing of a main coronary artery than in individuals with large, elastic arteries.

The experimental results reviewed here strongly suggest that during the early stage of the atherosclerotic process, exercise may be of particular value in promoting the growth of collateral vessels. Inasmuch as most middle-aged American males appear to be in this early and, at present, invisible stage of the disease, it appears imperative to encourage asympomatic middle-aged men to exercise. Through a program of exercise falling just short of anginal pain, collateral circulation may also be developed in patients who have had a recent coronary attack. While the benefits of surgical therapeutic measures may be desirable in certain cases, it would appear that a program of exercise started early enough and properly conducted might make other curative measures unnecessary in many cases.

## CLASSIFICATION OF EXERCISE

First of all, it must be recognized that "exercise" is a vague term. Different kinds, intensities and durations of exercise accomplish very different results.

1. Moderate exercise. Some type of moderate exercise, particularly walking, should be pursued every day for a sufficient time, e.g. one hour, This is essential for maintaining body weight, especially in mesomorphic or mesomorphic-endomorphic individuals.

2. Limbering, coordinating and strengthening exercises. Although useful in training young people, such types of exercise are probably of less significance as far as health is concerned.

3. Constant vigorous physical labor. This type of activity for 10 hours a day, obviously incompatible with the mode of employment of most Americans, appears to permit individuals to handle a diet high in saturated fat without the usual increase in serum cholesterol. It also appears to be beneficial in regard to elasticity and patency of the vessels of the heart and is associated with a smaller mortality from coronary athersclerosis.

4. Exercise considerably increasing work of the heart. If properly spaced, exercise of sufficient intensity to increase considerably the work of the heart will train the cardiovascular system. The intensity does not need to approach the maximum energy expenditure. Under extreme conditions, a portion of the energy breakdown comes from anaerobic processes, with little

immediate benefit as far as the cardiovascular system is concerned. While anaerobic training is of value to the athlete competing in sprint-type events, it is not indicated for the middle-aged man in need of conditioning.

The nature of this relatively intense exercise is of little importance, provided a large enough fraction of the total muscle mass is involved, The larger the muscle mass involved, the greater is the heart response. Push-ups involve essentially the muscles of the arms and shoulders, whereas running, rowing and swimming involve most larger muscles. While it is desirable for a younger man still is good condition to build up his practice of exercise to a half hour daily, with an expenditure of 500 calories (hourly rate of 1000), Swedish results show that three 15-minute periods of intense exercise a week together with the daily hour of walking, are sufficient to improve cardiovascular fitness to a considerable extent.

## PRACTICAL ADVICE

Various rules have been suggested in regard to conditioning; for example, the exercise should not be so violent as to cause a pulse rate over 110 after one minute of exercise. However, it is difficult to legislate for the masses, especially in a situation such as exists in the United States, where a patient cannot easily be referred to a reconditioning center for basic measurements of performance on the treadmill or the bicycle ergometer. It appears that in Sweden bicycle ergometers are becoming common in factories and office buildings. They not only allow individuals to know their physiologic limitations at a given time, but also serve as a powerful incentive by measuring improvement in conditioning (maximum performance and pulse rates for various levels of energy expenditure).

While tennis, golf (with vigorous walking), and other competitive sports are both good exercise and sound mental relaxation, because they require almost complete absorption and hence exclusion of the day's worries, they are often difficult to practice on a daily basis. Running is cheap and requires no partner or special equipment. Early in the morning, before breakfast, is a good time of day for running, particularly in suburban neighborhoods; however, it may be more convenient to do it at the end of the day, and this is not harmful. In fact, at this time muscles will be somewhat "warmed up" by the normal activities of the day. Exercise before supper, particularly if vigorous, will usually decrease rather than increase appetite. There are also psychologic advantages of a "break" at the end of the day. either before supper of just before going to bed. It is often advisable to tell a patient to exercise at a time when he will receive a minimum of attention, so that he will not be discouraged by inactive neighbors. Finally, the conditioning should be gradual, so that the increase in physical activity is built on previous performance, producing a steady improvement without excessive effort.

## RECONDITIONING CENTERS

It is perhaps unfortunate that we do not have in this country the equivalent of the European reconditioning centers. For example, West Germany has a number of such centers, where tens of thousands of workers are reconditioned during periods of four to six weeks. These centers are operated by insurance companies as well as by big industrial enterprises. They will accept a man on recommendation of his insurance physician at insurance expense. The centers are operated by physical educators and under medical supervision, and present a systematic program of calisthenic and endurance exercises such as swimming and running, as well as games and health lectures. The men selected for such programs are judged to be prone to heart disease.

The USSR has a program of much greater magnitude, with five million persons going through such reconditioning centers. Other Eastern European countries also have large-scale programs of this type. In the absence of such facilities in this country, it would appear reasonable that internists and general practitioners should be much more directive in regard to a patient's schedule of activity and give close periodic attention to the patient's cardiovascular function during and after exercise.

## REFERENCES

1. Mayer, J. et al.: Exercise, food intake and body weight in normal rats

and genetically obese adult mice. Amer. J. Physiol., 177:544, 1954.

2. Johnson, M. L., Burke, B. S. and Mayer, J.: Prevalence and incidence of obesity in a cross-section of elementary and secondary school children. Amer. J. Clin. Nutr., 4:231, 1956.

3. ——: Relative importance of inactivity and overeating in the energy balance of obese high school girls. *Ibid.*, p. 37.

4. Bullen, B. A., Reed, R. B. and Mayer, J.: Physical activity of obese and nonobese adolescent girls apparaised by motion picture sampling. Amer. J. Clin. Nutr., 14:211, 1964.

5. Karvonen, M. J., Pekkarinen, M., Maetsala, P. and Rautanen, V.: Diet and serum cholesterol of lumberjacks. Brit. J. Nutr., 15:157, 1961.

6. Gsell, D. and Mayer, J.: Low blood cholesterol associated with high calorie, high saturated fat intakes in a Swiss Alpine village population. Amer. J. Clin. Nutr., 10:471, 1962.

7. Morris, J. N., Heady, J. A., Raffle, P. A. B., Roberts, C. G. and Parks, J. W.: Coronary heart disease and the physical activity of work. Lancet, 2:1053, 1111, 1953.

8. Morris, J. N.: Occupation and coronary heart disease. Arch. Intern. Med., 104:903, 1959.

9. Taylor, H. L., Klepetar, E., Keys, A., Parlin, W., Blackburn, H. and Puchner, T.: Death rates among physically active and sedentary employees of the railroad industry. Amer. J. Public Health, 52:1697, 1962.

10. Eckstein, R. W.: Effect of exercise and coronary artery narrowing on coronary collateral circulation. Circ. Res., 5:230, 1957.

11. Zoll, P. M., Wessler, S. and Schlesing, M. J.: Interarterial coronary anastomoses in the human heart, with particular reference to anemia and relative cardiac anoxia. Circulation, 4:797, 1956.

## Chapter 27

# BODY MEASUREMENTS IN RELATION TO DISEASE

Written in collaboration with Carl C. Seltzer

W ITH the constant expansion of medical departments in companies, labor unions, universities, prepaid health care organizations, etc., that follow large numbers of individuals over a long period, there has been a corresponding increase in interest in the basic physical description of the recipients of this medical care. Many physicians concerned with periodic health examinations would like to be able to correlate the manifestations of degenerative diseases such as diabetes, hypertension and atherosclerosis with their patients' body-build. They are also seeking better ways to follow somatic changes in the same patient.

Physicians are constantly authors for better criteria for morphologic definition of individuals followed in large groups. Therefore, it appeared appropriate in the chapter to attempt to give an exposition of those principles of physical anthropology that are most relevant to the practicing physician and that are most easily used to characterize individuals undergoing periodic health examination.

There are many areas of contact between physical anthropology and medicine. The obstetrician constantly uses anthropometry in comparing the pelvic dimensions of a pregnant woman with the estimated dimensions of the head and shoulders of the infant about to be born. The orthopedic surgeon regularly determines the length of various bones. Growth, and object of daily concern to the pediatrician, is essentially a morphologic phenomenon. Blood grouping can be considered a legitimate part of physical

Reprinted from *Postgraduate Medicine, 40* (Nos. 4 and 5), October and November, 1966.

anthropology.

We will not attempt to consider all these aspects of physical anthropology in this chapter. Essentially we shall concern ourselves here with the anthropological description of patients as a neglected element in the collection of data by physicians interested in the relation of body-build to disease. At this point it may be useful to distinguish between three terms that are all too often used indifferently, i.e. "constitution," "inheritance" and "body-build." Constitution refers to the aggregate of physical, physiologic and mental characters that result at a given time from the effects of genes and environment and are relatively fixed and unchanging. Inheritance is the total genetic endowment of the fetus. Body-build is the phenotypic or visible morphologic component of this endowment as it has developed in a given environment.

In this chapter we shall consider the relation of both constitution and body-build to medicine.

## HISTORICAL DEVELOPMENT

The relation between body-build and disease has facinated physicians since the beginning of medicine. In his epidemiologic treatise "On Airs, Waters and Places," Hippocrates ascribed many of the obvious differences between peoples to the effect of their environment: Mountain people are tall and vigorous; thin, nervous and predominantly blond people live in dry, treeless countries; small fat people live in areas of rich pastures, etc. However, Hippocrates also recognized the paramount importance of inheritance. From a medical viewpoint, he recognized two major "temperaments," the phthistic habitus and the apoplectic habitus.

Galen's classification into four types (sanguine, phlegmatic, choleric, melancholy) based on the theory of humors dominated medicine until the Renaissance. The enthusiasm for anatomy and physiology of the sixteenth and seventeenth centuries, typified in Vesalius and Harvey, effected a decline in human typology as physicians became interested in the general aspects of both morphology and function rather than in the individual or categorical aspects.

By the end of the nineteenth century interest in body description had reawakened and many classifications were developed. The following were of special interest:

1. The dual classification of Stockard and de Giovanni divided mankind into two types — the broad type (apoplectic, lateral, pyknic) and the slender type (phthistic, linear, asthenic, lepto-somatic) — and thus was not unlike the classification of Hippocrates. Bryant's variation of the dual classification contrasted the carnivorous, slender type predisposed to hyperthyroidism, anemia, low blood pressure, and dominance of the parasympathetic system with the herbivorous or horizonatal type, robust and predisposed to obesity, pancreatic hyperactivity, and high blood pressure.

2. The three-legged classification of Bunak divided mankind into three types: the stenoplastic (vertical or slender), thin and weak with little adipose tissue; the mesoplastic (intermediate), strong with an average amount of adipose tissue; and the euryplastic (horizontal or broad), with an average musculature and considerable adipose tissue. Kretchmer similarly distinguished the asthenic, athletic (muscular) and pyknic types.

3. The four-legged classification of Rostan and particularly the French school was based entirely on outside shape and included the cerebral type (large cranium, average facial size, short, thin and feeble), the digestive type (predominantly abdomen and jaw), the respiratory type (large thorax), and the muscular type. In addition, Viola and the Italian school attemped a much more complex classification based on 10 body measurements leading to a more detailed description.

The relation of the intellect to physical features also fascinated nineteenth and early twentieth century writers. Lavater, Gall and Cabanis attempted to predict intellectual type from the appearance of the face, the shape of the skull, or general appearance. Ceasare Lombroso defined the criminal type as a person exhibiting five or more of the following stigmata: cranial or facial asymetry, Inca or interparietal bone, receding forehead, large ears, large frontal sinuses, square and projecting chin, broad cheekbones, exaggerated arm span, prehensile feet, left-handedness, deficient olfactory and taste organs, limited sensibility, and exhibitionism evidenced by an addiction to tattooing.

Modern physical anthropology, though less picturesque, has developed authoritative and descriptive methods that not only permit a more objective description of the patient but also allow for more seriously established correlations.

## GENERAL CONSIDERATIONS IN MORPHOLOGIC DESCRIPTION

It cannot be overemphasized that the practice of presenting only a subject's height and weight as the total of morphologic description is woefully inadequate. This practice contributes minimal information on the morphologic nature of individuals or series of individuals except with respect to extremely light or extremely heavy persons, and even in these cases there is only presumptive identification of body form or composition. Even when subjects are placed in specific height-weight categories, data on height and weight alone fail to provide necessary information as to body-build and its components of skeletal dimensions, muscularity, adiposity, proportions, contours, etc (1).

Thus it is clear that individuals cannot be classified into body types by the simple measurement of height and weight, and the absence of significant differences between two series in mean height and weight does not necessarily signifiy that one is dealing with populations similar in morphologic characteristics. Furthermore, this traditional reliance on height and weight has perpetuated the concept of underweight-overweight, which ignores and neglects the individuality of morphologic structure by failing to differentiate between individual variations in body form and composition and between overweight and obesity (fatness) (1, 2).

What descriptive measures should the clinician and investigator normally take as a "minimal" representation of a subject's physique: No single set of recommendations will suit all purposes and conditions. The selection of morphologic measures should be tailored to meet the demands of the problem at hand. When anthropometry is required, those parts of the body that require special emphasis should be measured in adequate detail. For example, if the subject has emphysema, it would be essential to take detailed measurements of the chest — length, breadth, depth, circumference at rest and at maximum inspiration and expiration, etc. If the investigator is interested in an objective description of genetic variation of the shape of the head and face, he should take the many craniologic and facial measurements that are refined enough to reflect genetic conditions. There is no sense in collecting 40 or 50 anthropometric measurements when the problem at hand does not call for such information. Such unnecessary measurements will leave the investigator with a large body of data that is not directly pertinent to the problem at hand and that he may find difficult to interpret.

On the other hand, in many studies the relevant questions of morphologic importance are not known in advance and cannot be predicted a priori. This may be true in broad survey studies or in general studies of chronic diseases. The investigator must then secure sufficient minimal information on body-build to estimate the significance of the morphologic variable as a host factor. We shall attempt to describe such "minimal" information later in this article.

In evaluating body-build or physique we will be concerned with two elements, body form and body composition. These two elements are not mutually exclusive in an absolute sense, but the various descriptive procedures utilized have been resulted in a tendency to separate them. Body form refers to size, shape, contour and proportion and is to a large extent external in character. Body compostion refers to the structural components — bone, muscle and fat — and is especially useful in appraising nutritional status and in studying changes in health and disease states in a given individual or in a population. More often than not in actual practice, however, no sharp distinctions are made between body form and body composition since in most cases the ultimate goal is an understanding of the subject's overall body-build or physique and since the two elements supplement and complement each other.

The most commonly used methods for describing body build are the following: (1) anthropometry, (2) anthroposcopy, (3) skin fold thickness, (4) strength tests, and (5) somatotyping. Each of these will be discussed separately.

## ANTHROPOMETRY

Anthropometry is the technic used to express quantitatively the form of the body. It consists primarily of the direct measurement, by means of the anthropometer, calipers, steel tape and scales, of various body dimensions — weight, height, segmental lengths, depths, breadths, circumferences and arcs, including detailed measurements of the head and face. Nearly 100 standardized anthropometric measurements are available. However, for an investigation in which morphology per se is not of predominant importance, only a few are recommended for ordinary usage. These are given in Table 27-1.

Of these basic measurements, height and weight are certianly minimal essentials and should be measured with the subject as nearly nude as possible. It is highly desirable to obtain a history of the subject's weight at various ages and periods in his life, including the maximal weight attained. Chest depth and arm circumference are also very important, as we shall see later, in predicting somatotype. Bi-epicondylar breath, biacromial and bi-iliac diameters, and chest dimensions are useful indicators of skeletal robustness, while arm and calf circumferences may afford some estimate of muscularity. If this limited anthropometric

TABLE 27-1

BASIC ANTHROPOMETRIC MEASUREMENTS

Height
Weight
Sitting height
Biacromial diameter
Bi-iliac diameter
Chest depth
Chest breadth
Chest circumference
Arm circumference
Waist circumference
Calf circumference
Bi-epicondylar humerous breadth

schedule were to be abbreviated still further the essential measurements should at least include height, weight, chest depth and arm circumference.

The reader is again reminded that the list of measurements in Table 27-1 would not be considered an optimal schedule if trained personnel were available and conditions were favorable. Furthermore, other measurements should be readily added as indicated by the specific problem under study.

Descriptions are available of the technics and instruments used to obtain accurate, standardized anthropometric measurements. We recommend the excellent descriptions by Hertzberg and co-workers (3), which are clear and concise, illustrated with photographs, and fully accepted as standard procedures by anthropological specialists. Other sources of reference are works by Ashley-Montagu (4) and Comas (5).

## ANTHROPOSCOPY

Anthroposcopy refers to the visual observation and description of body features that do not lend themselves readily to exact measurement. Such features include the form, character and distribution of hair, skin color, eye color, the shape of the nose, the lips, the color and distribution of striae, etc. (Many of these traits may be referable to racial origin; one may wish to use objective criteria to substantiate racial designations.)

For example, anthroposcopy with reference to striae should include observational description of the location (chest, breast, abdomen, back, buttocks), intensity or severity (absent, mild, moderate, severe), and color (white, pink, purplish, mixed). Anthroposcopy with reference to hair would include classification of hair form as straight, low waves, deep waves, curly, frizzly, or woolly; hair texture as fine, medium, coarse, or wiry; hair quantity as submedium, medium, marked, etc.

Since the collection of anthroposcopic data is usually tailored to specialized problems and investigations, no standardized procedure for epidemiologic or broad survey studies is recommended here. The most common anthroposcopic criteria and methods of categorization are described in the volumes of Ashley-Montagu (4) and Comas (5).

## SKINFOLD THICKNESS

Measurement of skinfold thickness at various sites on the body is becoming increasingly important in estimating fatness, especially when it is not possible or feasible to use more elaborate and cumbersome laboratory technics such as densitometry, hydrometry, measurement of whole body radiopotassium, or electrolyte content methods. These technics are important and accurate research tools, but they are too difficult and time-consuming to be performed by the physician who wants to make a rapid objective diagnosis of obesity. Measurement of skinfold thickness offers a reasonably accurate means of estimating the degree and distribution of fatness and following its changes. The economy of this method is all the more important in field surveys or studies involving a large number of persons. It gives not only a good indication of subcutaneous fat, which constitues about 50 per cent of the total body fat, but also a reliable estimate of the total body fat.

Skinfold measurements are obtained by applying a special caliper* to selected sites. The technic is relatively simple, and with proper directions and a minimum of demonstration by an experienced person, the physician can obtain reproducible measurements. Since standardization of skinfold calipers is necessary for universal comparability of fatfold measurements and conversion to total body fat, the accepted national recommendation is an instrument so designed as to exert a pressure on the caliper face of 10 gm per square millimeter and with a contact surface of 20 to 40 mm.

The skinfold measurement to be obtained is the (doubled) thickness of the pinched "folded" skin plus the attached subcutaneous adipose tissue. The person making the measurement pinches up a full fold of skin and subcutaneous tissue with the thumb and forefinger of his left hand at a distance of about 1 cm from the site at which the caliper is to be placed, pulling the fold away from the underlying muscle. The fold is pinched up firmly and held while the measurement is taken. The caliper is applied to

---

*The Lange Skinfold Caliper is manufactured by Cambridge Scientific Industries Inc., Cambridge, Maryland.

the fold about 1 cm below the fingers, so that the pressure on the fold at the point measured is exerted by the faces of the caliper and not by the fingers. The handle of the caliper is released to permit the full force of the caliper-arm pressure, and the dial is read in millimeters. Caliper application should be made at least twice for stable readings. If the folds are extremely thick, dial readings should be made three seconds after the caliper pressure is applied.

Various workers have used a number of measurement site, including the triceps, subscapular, abdominal, hip, pectoral and calf areas. For general purposes and for the general population, the Committee on Nutritional Anthropometry of the National Research Council has recommended the triceps and the subscapular skinfolds as good indexes of overall fatness.

The triceps skinfold is located at the back of the right upper arm midway between the acromion and olecranon processes. The midpoint should be marked with the aid of a steel tape. The arm should hang freely during the skinfold measurement. Because of the gradation of a subcutaneous fat thickness from shoulder to elbow, location of the midpoint is somewhat critical and should be carefully ascertained.

The subscapular skinfold is located just below the angle of the right scapula (shoulder and arm relaxed). The fold is picked up in a line slightly inclined in the natural cleavage of the skin. Because the subcutaneous fat is fairly uniform in this region, precision of location is less critical.

The selection of sites to be measured hinges on the nature of the study. If the problem at hand involves the relative distribution of adipose tissue on various parts of the body between two groups or the disproportionate distribution of fatty tissue in subjects, then a comprehensive series of sites covering the pertinent anatomic parts should be selected. Thus, if one were investigating the relative distribution of body fat in diabetic and nondiabetic obese subjects, then the number of sites selected for skinfold measurement should be extensive and include the cheek, triceps, subscapular, forearm, chest, abdomen, side, hip, thigh, calf, etc.

However, in most cases physicians and investigators are looking solely for an estimate of overall fatness and a means of judging whether or not the subject is obese. A good, objective criterion of obesity then becomes a highly desirable and important tool. The concept of overweight and underweight based on the life insurance tables of average and desirable weights has proved unsatisfactory and poor practice. Furthermore, the Society of Actuaries' data on height and weight are not representative of the present general population, do not take into account individual variations in body-build, and fail to clearly separate obese and nonobese persons.

This oversimplified classification of physique by the life insurance studies has tended to obscure the relation between body-build, disease and mortality. Except in extreme overweight, what does measurement of weight really represent? If the degree of fatness is being sought, skinfold thicknesses should be measured. The current and indiscriminate use of such terms as underweight and overweight in assessing obesity may be quite misleading and faulty and may bear little relation to the persons true fat status. Application of skinfold measurement and body-build typology to populations in which data are being collected on disease and mortality will considerably advance the present knowledge of the etiology of disease.

Tables of skinfold thickness appropriate to each body-build type should eventually replace the tables of "ideal" or "desirable" weight for height. In any event, criteria of obesity actually based on a measurement of fatness are superior to those based on height (6).

Our work as well as that of others leads us to believe that for distinguishing obese persons the triceps skinfold, which is the easiest to measure, is also the most representative of total body fatness. No special advantage is gained from the use of any other skinfold measurement in addition to the triceps skinfold. On this basis we have recommended the measurement of the triceps skinfold as the distinguishing criterion. For the American population, in individuals 30 years of age or over, we have further recommended the figures of 23 and 30 mm respectively for male and female Caucasians as minimums defining the presence of obesity. We have given similar minimum levels defining obesity for persons 5 to 30 years of age (2).

## SOMATOTYPING

The triceps skinfold and the handful of anthropometric measurements described earlier are not comprehensive enough to provide a fully adequate assessment of a person's physique or to classify it as a specific body type. Body typing can best be accomplished by means of the somatotype technic, which has proved to be an immensely useful descriptive tool. Devised by Sheldon (7) in 1940, this technic has been widely used by physical anthropologists and physicians who have made serious efforts to evaluate the morphologic aspects of subjects under study.

Somatotype is a body-type classification based on the rating of three primary components — endomorphy, mesomorphy and ectomorphy, in that order — on a numerical scale of 1 to 7; 1 represents the minimum expression of a component and 7 the maximum expression. Endomorphy rates the element of softness, roundness and smoothness but not necessarily the amount of fat. An endomorph can be round, soft and smooth without being frankly obese, although the extreme endomorph is usually obese. When endomorphy predominates, abdominal mass overshadows thoracic bulk the thorax tends to be round, and hamming of the upper arms, juxtaposition of the thighs, small features, and greater anteroposterior than transverse diameters are present.

Mesomorphy rates bone and muscle development. When mesomorphy predominates, the chest is massive and muscular and dominates over the abdomen. Strong muscular relief, prominent bone joints, broad hands, massive shoulder and leg muscles, and tapering from shoulder to hip characterize the mesomorph.

Ectomorphy rates the element of linearity, fragility and attenuation. When ectomorphy predominates, the individual tends to be slender, lanky, thin and delicate in bone structure and stringy in muscular development. The hands are usually long and narrow; the fingers and toes are long. These structural characteristics distinguish the extreme ectomorph from the merely emaciated person.

Somatotype ratings are determined by anthroposcopic (inspectional) study of photographs of the nude subject in the front, side and back views, all on a single 5 by 7 inch film in accordance with Sheldon's technic. The subject is carefully posed in the three standard views on a 90 degree turntable and photographed at a standard distance with a known magnification factor.

In addition to the somatotype ratings, one may use the photographs to obtain ratings of gynandropmorphy and dyplasia (also on a 1 to 7 scale) as well as reliable measurements of body diameters, planimetric determinations of body areas, evidence of hair patterns, etc.

Although the process of obtaining the somatotype rating cannot be described here in detail, some examples of the numerous criteria used may be of interest. To determine endomorphy, the observer rates the degree of body contours, the amount of fatty covering, the prominence of the shoulder-blades, spinous processes of the vertebrae, clavicles, ribs and sternum and their fatty covering, the relative predominance of abdomen as compared to the chest, the outer curve of the calf, etc. To determine mesomorphy, the observer rates the hardness, squareness and ruggedness of the body outline, the muscularity of the neck, back, chest, arms and legs, the size and prominence of the bony structure, the heaviness and massiveness of hands and fingers, the predominance of throax as compared to the abdomen, etc. To determine ectomorphy, one rates the linearity, fragility and delicacy of the various body parts, the slightness and "threadiness" of musculature, the relative shortness of trunk and length of limbs, the shortness, flatness and shallowness of abdomen, the narrowness of shoulders, the prominence of ribs, the clavicular hollows, the fragility and length of toes and fingers, and the slightness and angularity of cranial and facial features.

The actual somatotype ratings are usually made by experienced somatotypologists from careful inspection of the photographs. Ratings of the same subject by experienced observers are highly comparable. However, while this procedure is satisfactory when physical anthropologists are performing the study, it is altogether different when a physician untrained in somatotypology attempts to rate subjects. In addition, the physician may have difficulty in obtaining the necessary photographs.

Damon (8) recognized these difficulties and devised a practical objective means of deriving the somatotype ratings from a limited number of anthropometric measurements by means of predictive formulas. At present validated formulas are available only for white males 20 to 60 years of age. The technic requires seven anthropometric measurements: weight (pounds), height (inches), chest depth (millimeters), upper arm circumference (millimeters), triceps skinfold (millimeters), subscapular skinfold (millimeters), and grip (kilograms). An eighth quantity, the ponderal index, is a calculated figure representing height divided by cube root of weight.

To determine somatotype, the physician or his assistant makes the following calculations:

1. 10 (endomorphy) = 125.5245 + 0.05969 (weight) + 1.0180 (height) − 11.7750 (ponderal index) − 0.0801 (upper arm circumference) + 0.3850 (triceps skinfold) + 0.3073 (subscapular skinfold) − 0.1771 (grip).

2. 10 (mesomorphy) = 130.2032 + 0.1810 (height) − 0.0583 (chest depth) − 9.3970 (ponderal index) + 0.1073 (upper arm circumference) − 0.5003 (triceps skinfold) − 0.3241 (subscapular skinfold) + 0.1935 (grip).

3. 10 (ectomorphy) = − 151.1550 + 0.2470 (height) − 0.0288 (chest depth) + 14.8450 (ponderal index) − 0.0511 (upper arm circumference) + 0.0374 (triceps skinfold) + 0.1126 (subscapular skinfold) − 0.0114 (grip).

4. 10 (gynadromorphy) = −24.8480 +0.4042 (wieght) − 1.6950 (height) − 0.0542 (chest depth) + 10.8790 (ponderal index) − 0.1022 (upper arm circumference) + 0.4018 (triceps skinfold) − 0.1311 (grip).

## *Strength Test*

Because of its relation to muscularity, the strength of the hand grip is important in estimating somatotype. Hand grip strength is measured by the hand dynamometer.* The measurement is simple to obtain, although the physician must take care that the subject stands with his arm held away from his body while he is squeezing the dynamometer.

---

*The Narragansett and Smedley spring dynamometers give satisfactory results.

## RELATION OF BODY-BUILD TO DISEASE

There is a large body of published work — not always sound from the viewpoint of definition of disease, description of body type, or statistical treatment — linking body-build and disease. Among the better-documented associations are the following:

### *Tuberculosis*

Much evidence points to a high correlation between susceptibility to all forms of tuberculosis and the ectomorphic somatotype (tall and thin, leptosomatic, asthenic habitus). Widespread belief exists among European physicians that tuberculosis tends to follow a stormier course in redheads and persons with freckles than in those with other complexions.

### *Cardiovascular Disease*

Valvular diseases following rheumatic fever and other infectious diseases are most often seen in tall thin persons. Other cardiovascular diseases, including myocardial infarction, are most often seen in mesomorphs or endomorphic mesomorphs. Although hypertension is clearly associated with stocky rather than lean builds, accelerated primary hypertension appears to be more common in tall thin females while it is evenly distributed among males.

### *Arthritis*

Osteoarthritis appears to be associated with endomorphy (pyknic habitus) while rheumatoid arthritis is associated with predominant ectomorphy and mesomorphy.

### *Gastrointestinal Disease*

A high correlation exists between asthenic habitus and diseases of the gastrointestinal tract. Disease of the gallbladder, however appear to be closely associated with endomorphic mesomorphy. It is also claimed that gastric ulcer is conspicuously absent in gynadromorphs. Duodenal ulcer is more common in individuals of blood group O.

## Cancer

Evidence has linked blood group A to cancers arising in the body of the stomach as compared to cancers arising in the antrum or pylorus. Cancers of the uterus and breast are said to be more numerous in endomorphic mesomorphs. However, it has been reported that women with endometrial cancer, in contrast to those with breast or cervical cancer, tend to be more endomorphic than mesomorphic.

## Menière's Disease

This disease has been investigated in both males and females and has been found to be more common in mesomorphic females and in mesomorphic and endomorphic mesomorphic males.

## Obesity

Our work has shown that obesity rarely occurs in persons with a sufficient ectomorphic component and that obese persons are more mesomorphic (and obviously more endomorphic) than nonobese persons.

## COMMENT

It is hoped that interest in the relation of the body-build to disease will continue to be cultivated and that new information will be added to our present body of knowledge. The danger exists that, just as the Pasteurian revolution at first emphasized infectious diseases in the agent rather than in the host and the vitamin revolution emphasized nutrition in the diet rather than in the host, advances in genetics may emphasize single genes or chromosomal abnormalities rather than the constitution in general. Certainly we do not wish to deprecate the analytic approach; however, there is still much to be said for looking at the patient's whole body and describing it comprehensively.

# REFERENCES

1. Seltzer, C. C.: Some re-evaluations of the Build and Blood Pressure Study, 1959 as related to ponderal index, somatotype and mortality. New Eng. J. Med., 274:254 (February) 1966.
2. Seltzer, C. C. and Mayer, J.: A simple criterion of obesity. Postgrad. Med., 38:A-101 (August) 1965.
3. Hertzberg, H. T. E., Churchill, E., Dupertuis, C. W., White, R. M. and Damon, A.: Anthropometric Survey of Turkey, Greece and Italy. New York, The Macmillan Company, 1963.
4. Ashley—Montagu, M. F.: An Introduction to Physical Anthropology. Springfield, Illinois, Charles C Thomas, 1960.
5. Comas, J.: Manual of Physical Anthropology. Springfield, Illinois, Charles C Thomas, 1960.
6. Mayer, J.: Some aspects of the problem of regulation of food intake and obesity. New Eng. J. Med., 274:610, 662, 722, 1966.
7. Sheldon, W. H.: the Varieties of Hyman Physique. New York, Harper & Row, Publishers, 1940.
8. Damon, A.: Delineation of the body-build variables associated with cardiovascular diseases. Ann. N. Y. Acad. Sci., 121:711, 1965.

## Chapter 28

# NUTRITION IN THE AGED

## REQUIREMENTS IN OLD AGE

IT is difficult to generalize in regard to nutritional requirements in old age, particularly caloric requirements. The first committee on calorie requirements convened by the Food and Agriculture Organization in 1949 (1) suggested that there should be a 7.5 per cent diminution in the caloric allowance for each decade of life after 25 years. The second committee on calorie requirements, called in 1957 (2), recognized that additional facts obtained in the interval did not support the idea of a consistent and steady decrease in energy requirements with aging. The members of the committee, myself among them, felt that, provided the adult remained normally active or had an occupation requiring physical labor, the decrement in energy requirement was quite slow during the middle years, and that the energy requirements decreased only after 45 years of age at the earliest. The committee therefore suggested decreasing the caloric allowance for the decades of life from 25 to 35 and 35 to 45 years of age by only 3 per cent of the requirements at age 25, and retaining the 7.5 per cent decrement for the decades from 45 to 55 and 55 to 65 years. In the decade from 65 to 75, a further decrement of 10 per cent of the requirements at age 25 seemed justifiable, with no further decrement after 75 years of age.

More recent information, such as that collected by Durnin (3), argues for both a more progressive and a more individual basis for the caloric allowance. Durnin feels it is useful to try to classify differing degrees of aging. He calls persons between 60 and 75 years of age "elderly" (according to the concise Oxford dictionary this means "getting old") and those 75 and older "old." His main

Reprinted from *Postgraduate Medicine, 32* (No. 4):394-401, October, 1962.

concern is with the elderly. His studies as well as those of other contemporary authors (4) show that in Western countries such as Great Britain and the United States physical activity changes little between the ages of 30 and 60 to 70 years. During this same span, muscular efficiency appears to decrease, in part because of the slow loss of precision in neural-muscular coordination. Because of this decrease in strength and proficiency an older person requires more energy for a particular task than would a younger person. Finally, while there are progressive changes in body composition, these (except in "old" or excessively sedentary persons) are not quite as marked as is commonly believed. (The interesting and important demonstration by Brozek and Keys (5) of a slow replacement of muscle tissue by fat has tended to be exaggerated in magnitude in the minds of physicians concerned with aging.) Thus, the evolution of the three factors — changes in physical activity, body composition, and efficiency of muscular movement — accounts for the smallness of observed change in the total gross metabolism of large groups of men, particularly men whose work entails physical exertion, which varies little over decades. The decrease is generally more important in women; the physical task of housework usually is greatly lessened in later life.

We may conclude that if a person's caloric intake (particularly a man's) was not excessive in early middle age and if he has retained the same schedule of work and other activities, there is no call to limit the caloric intake simply because he is getting old. Obviously, if activity diminishes drastically because of chronic disease or change in occupation the caloric intake has to be decreased to prevent obesity; this is true at any age. While a decrease in physical activity is common in elderly persons, it is by no means universal.

Similarly, to my knowledge a specific increase or decrease of nutrient requirement (including protein) due to age per se has not been demonstrated. (This statement does not exclude the possibility that some such change may be found.) Consumption of a varied diet in proper amounts will usually cover requirements in old age, without the need for special supplements. Such additional recommendations as sufficient exercise for bowel evacuation and sufficient fluid intake for proper renal function are not specifically directed toward old age. At most, it may be said that neglect of long-term health practices is likely to have more catastrophic effects in old age because physiologic functions are more precarious and capacity for adaptation may be impaired.

## CALORIC RESTRICTION AND LONGEVITY

In view of comment and speculation in the professional and lay press concerning the effect of underfeeding on the life span of experimental animals, rats in particular, a short discussion of these experiments may be in order. Confusion seems to exist between (1) experiments dealing with the effect on the adult life span of avaoidance of obesity and (2) experiments dealing with the effect on over all longevity of retardation of growth and sexual maturation.

It is a very general finding that in nonexercised animals the daily restriction of calories so as to prevent obesity causes them to live longer than nonexercised animals which are fed ad libitum and become obese. Frequent intermittent restriction of calories also prolongs life by reducing early mortality. Carlson and Hoelzel (6) showed that by fasting animals one day in three they could increase the life expectancy by about 15 per cent in rats receiving an omnivorous diet; the gain was less with a vegetarian diet. Evidence is not conclusive that avoidance of obesity through exercise in animals fed ad libitum provides life spans as long as or longer than those achieved by avoidance of obesity through caloric restriction in nonexercised animals, but it points in this direction (7). Thus, the results of experimental work on the effect of prevention of obesity on the adult life span rejoin the fiindings of insurance companies in studies of the survival rate of nonobese human beings.

It is the second type of experiment dealing with the effects on over all longevity of undernutrition and growth retardation in young animals, which has most often been misunderstood. The prevention of obesity in adult animals, effective as it is, prolongs life only for a period equivalent to a few years in man; in contrast, growth retardation and delay in sexual maturation produced by drastic caloric restriction cause a tremendous increase in the total life span in many species. This early restriction produces animals whose life spans are equivalent to that of the famous and perhaps mythical Shropshire farmer, Thomas Parr, who reputedly was 153 years old when he died in 1635. The life cycle of many invertebrates, insects in particular, can be lengthened in some or all of its stages by curtailing the rate of growth and development through food restriction. Slowing down the growth of beetle larvae extends their life from one to many years. In cockroaches, the optimal protein intake for longevity is about half that which produces the fastest development (8). McCay, Pope and Lunsford (9) showed that sexual maturation of rats could be delayed for periods up to 1000 days (longer than the normal life span) and that, after this period, survivors were capable of resuming growth and reproduction, thus considerably increasing their total life span; the gain in further expectation of life, however, was not equal to the period of underfeeding and was greater in males than in females. Carr, King and Visscher (10) have shown that life expectancy of the C3H strain of mice can be doubled by severe underfeeding during growth. Albino mice which were fasted two days out of seven had an increase in life span of more than 50 per cent (11). Similar experiments on other strains bear out the general conclusion that the beneficial effect on the total life span of retardation of growth and sexual maturation is much greater than what could be achieved with ad libitum feeding during growth followed by avoidance of obesity in adulthood.

It has been estimated that if our population were to avoid obesity through dietary control and exercise, the gain in life expectancy could be no more than four to five years. (Lest this be minimized, this increment is twice what the cure of cancer could bring.) Whether or not man, with his proportionately low growth rate and lengthy growth period, is similar to lower animals in being able to resume growth and sexual maturation after prolonged periods of consumption of a qualitatively complete but calorically inadequate diet, and whether or not such treatment would prolong life by decades, have never been tested. It is difficult to see how such an experiment could be conducted. Yet this fascinating possiblility may well offer the one way in which life expectancy could be spectacularly increased by nutritional means.

## OBESITY

There is little doubt that obesity is becoming more prevalent in this country (12) or that is is accompanied by increased mortality from a number of degenerative diseases (13). The relation between disease and mortality is certainly more complex than the simple causation often suggested (14), and it is likely that the relation between disease and obesity often is associative as well as causative. In the April 1959 issue of Postgraduate Medicine on page 471, a table was published showing the expected death rates from various causes among overweight men and women. While most correlations between causes of death and obesity are positive, at least two causes of death are negatively correlated with obesity, namely, suicide and tuberculosis. Moreover, the decreased association of obesity and tuberculosis is not simply a matter of reduced intake of food following infection; long-term studies show that there is a decreased probability of tuberculous infection among "overweight" persons (15).

The possible complexity of the interrelations of obesity and disease is exemplified by middle-age diabetes. This condition probably involves both associative factors (hyperphagia and diabetes being perhaps two facets of a common syndrome) and causative factors (the "lipoplethoric" state of adipose tissue contributing to the impairment of glucose tolerance, which can be improved by reduction of weight) (16).

It is also likely that the relation between obesity in the strict sense of the word (i.e. excess fat accumulation) and disease has been obscured by the fact that the insurance tables which provide the bulk of available data were established not in terms of individual fat content but in terms of weight. Selected "overweight" groups such as the California longshoremen studied by Buechley, Drake and Breslow (17) have a favorable health picture. Body build per se shows correlation with certain diseases (18). To my knowledge, somatotyping of aged patients has not been done on a large scale, so that we do not have a clear idea of the relation between body build and longevity or between body build and the incidence of degenerative disease, independent of the presence or absence of obesity. With these limitations, it is safe to say that the relation between obesity and degenerative disease is generally close enough to warrant consideration of prevention of obesity as the major nutritional measure to be taken in preparation for a successful old age.

While this association of obesity and degenerative disease is increasingly publicized, insufficient attention has perhaps been paid to the direct effect of obesity on functional disabilities. In the aged, obesity often prevents ambulation and self-care in hemiplegia, arthritis, and fractures of lower extremities. As Chinn (19) remarked, "It is difficult enough to train weakened muscle groups and damaged bones and joints to meet the disabilities of injury and disease without the considerable additional impediment of greater than normal extremity and total body weight."

Physicians often are reluctant to institute a program of weight reduction for a very old patient who has done well in spite of excessive weight. One can certainly sympathize with the desire not to upset a physiologic and psychologic balance which seems to have endured, but it must be realized that weight reduction is commonly accompanied by improved ease of movement in any present (or potential) locomotor disability. A reduction in weight of not more than 10 kg may be sufficient to increase appreciably the rate and extent of ambulation and thus enhance the patient's enjoyment of life. Even in the absence of visible improvement in muscular strength, such a reduction in weight also lessens the probability of further locomotor disabilities consequent to arthritis, cardiovascular disorders, or accidents. Weight reduction in the aged is admittedly difficult. Activity is restricted, and thus a decrease in caloric intake may be the only variable available to create a deficit in the energy balance.

Weight reduction in an aged patient may necessitate not only severe restriction of the diet but also a qualitative change to assure adequate intake of protein, vitamins and minerals. Formulation of a successful reducing diet may be complicated by resistance to changes in patterns of nutrition that have been followed for decades, by difficulties in mastication, and by economic factors. It may be advisable to enlist the services of an experienced dietitian to implement medical advice.

The always-undesirable practice of repeated "crash" programs of weight reduction may work an even greater stress on the elderly than it does on younger subjects. Follow-up observation is even more necessary for aging patients.

## UNDERNUTRITION

Because of the unfavorable relation between obesity and longevity, one would expect that undernutrition and resultant emaciation would be more common among persons who have reached old age, particularly among extremely old persons. There seems to be general agreement that among patients admitted to general hospitals with inanition or cachexia, old persons outnumber young and middle-aged ones. Specific or multiple deficiencies, although usually subclinical, also may be seen in this group, in addition to body wasting. Physiologic, psychologic and sociologic factors are involved, in various combinations. Structural disease of the esophagus or stomach may cause postprandial discomfort, and the patient therefore may not eat adequate meals. Senile or atheroselerotic psychosis and depression often have strong components related to food. Lack of teeth may make proper mastication difficult. (The fluoridation of water supplies, although its physiologic effect is in the young, may have its most beneficial nutritional effect in the aged, in that conservation of teeth permits continued proper mastication and thus greater choice of foods.)

Disinterest in eating because of loneliness is common, particularly among persons who live alone and are unable or unwilling to prepare meals. Economic factors are paramount in many cases. It has been estimated that 75 per cent of the people in the United States who are more than 65 years of age have a cash income of less than $1000 per year, and 15 per cent less that $500 per year. As Burton (20) has said, "Under the circumstances one is tempted to glibly generalize that the most important deficiency afflicting many of the aged is not the deficiency of vitamins or minerals, but of money."

Another important factor in the diets of many older patients is food faddism. In an era of rising educational standards, older persons often function at a lower level of information than young adults. Their often-incurable complaints cannot be eliminated by medical treatment, and in their search for relief they grasp at the irresponsible promises of wonder healers. Their isolation, sense of frustration, and distrust of novelty are exploited by food faddists: the field of arthritis, for example, is infested by these. The net effect is that a great deal of the propaganda for youth elixirs, nature foods, and fad diets is directed toward the aged. Expenditures for such items may work great hardship on limited budgets and may be made at the cost of variety in the diet and proper medical care.

Hospitalization, with particular attention to diet, often results in gains of 15 per cent of body weight or more in chronically emaciated persons. A number of ill-defined deficiency symptoms also disappear. Such treatment is by no means always or even generally successful, for irreversible physiologic and psychiatric factors and insurmountable social problems may continue to operate to restrict the intake of food. Nevertheless there is little doubt that partial anorexia is a frequent accident of the aged. By weakening the patient and making him feel sick, it may be self-perpetuating and even self-accelerating. Undernutrition not only decreases the older patient's enjoyment of life but may make him more difficult to care for and less likely to resist infectious or surgical trauma.

## NUTRITION AND HEART DISEASE

The possible relation between heart disease and dietary fat, obviously relevant to the problem of nutrition in aging, has been exhaustively reviewed by a number of writers (21) and will not be reexamined here. Suffice it to say that while there are widely divergent views on the relative importance of the proportion of monounsaturated and polyunsaturated fatty acids, on the specific role of linoleic acid, and on possible unknown factors in certain oils, there is almost general agreement that, by and large, saturated acids tend to elevate serum cholesterol. Incidentally, it may be useful to recall that a number of other factors, ranging from dietary cholesterol to purines and pyrimidines, to types of carbohydrates, fiber content, trace minerals and various vitamins, have also been found to have some effect on serum cholesterol. Recent studies emphasize the possible influence of exercise and the unfavorable effect of cigarette smoking in regard to heart disease. From a practical viewpoint it appears reasonable to suggest that aging persons (and probably all adults, men in particular) should consume a diet not too high in fats (saturated fats especially) and should adopt methods of food preparation that will minimize the total content of saturated fat.

The advisability of a drastic decrease in salt intake in many cardiovascular diseases is well documented. Available experimental data on rats (22) and data on man are at best suggestive that limitations of salt intake are useful in the prevention of hypertension and coronary accidents.

## CALCIUM

The possible increase in calcium requirements in old age, the relation of osteoporosis to calcium intake, and the possible effect of a high-calcium diet on osteoporosis, whether or not the latter is due to low calcium intake, are problems which evoke opinionated responses from experts but which have not yet been dealt with critically on a large scale. There is general agreement that individual calcium requirements may vary fairly widely. It has also been shown that the human body can adapt to restriction of calcium intake by lowering the urinary calcium content and possibly by improving the calcium absorption (23). Such findings, important though they are, have relatively little bearing on the problem of calcium requirements in old age. Malm's (24) observation that some persons remain in negative calcium balance for years is, again, not necessarily conclusive in regard to osteoporosis based on low calcium intake. Nordin (25), studying 81 consecutive cases of primary osteoporosis, found that 10 of 53 patients tested had steatorrhea and thus, conceivably, decreased absorption of calcium as well. The remaining 71 patients had intakes of calcium, vitamin D and protein significantly lower that those of persons of the same age and socioeconomic level who did not have osteoporosis; the greatest differences (30% to 40% involved calcium and vitamin D. Hayes, Bowser and Trulson (26), on the other hand, in a study of 47 elderly women with fractures of the hip or femur and suspected osteoporosis could not find differences in intakes of calcium between these patients and 47 control subjects. Nordin classified his cases of osteoporosis as spinal (involving the spine only), peripheral (involving cortical bone) and mixed; dietary intake of calcium appears to have been lowest in the third group, and it is not excluded that this may explain part of the difference between the findings in the two groups.

The fact that a number of physicians feel that increased intake of calcium has a beneficial effect on the evolution of osteoporosis does not necessarily prove that osteoporosis is due to lack of calcium any more than does the effectiveness of vitamin $B_{12}$ in pernicious anemia prove that the latter is a primary dietary deficiency. At best, we may conclude that there appears to be no decrease in calcium requirements in old age in comparison with requirements in youth or middle age (excluding pregnancy or lactation).

If one wants to speculate, it is intriguing to recall that there is some evidence that experimental animals, rats in particular, may be better able to retain calcium in old age if they are fed low-calcium diets during growth. This finding may be related to the observation that osteoporosis appears to be rarer in Japan than it is in Western countries where calcium intakes are high in youth. As is the case for calories, a low intake of calcium during the growth period may be beneficial in old age. Testing of this hypothesis is again likely to prove difficult.

## VITAMINS

Vitamin deficiencies are not common in aged persons in our population but are nevertheless seen not infrequently in oldsters who subsist on monotonous and nondiversified meals (this is usually due to replacement of normal foods by fad diets or alcohol). Jolliffe and colleagues (27) in New York described a condition exceptionally seen in the aged which they named nicotinic acid deficiency encephalopathy. The onset is insidious and the earliest sympoms are vague (fatigue, irritability, depression, nervousness). Later, impairment of intellectual function supervenes, followed by stupor and coma. Associated with the clouding of consciousness are certain other neurologic signs, rigidity of the limbs, grasping and sucking reflexes, extensor plantar responses, exaggerated tendon reflexes, and sometimes polyneuritis and spinal cord lesions. Signs of classic pellagra (scaling, erthematous skin rash, glossitis, diarrhea) may or may not be present.

Polyneuritis (in particular, alcoholic polyneuritis) is not an exceptional disease in the aged. Large doses of thiamine lead to early relief of pain and muscular tenderness, but further recovery often is extremely slow and it may not be accelerated by the use of such therapy.

Earl (28) believes that mild cases of nutritional neuropathy are frequently overlooked in the aged. Early symptoms may be fatigue, pain in the limbs, and mild paresthesias; slight muscular weakness is easily missed by physicians not used to testing critically the strength of muscular contractions. Polyneuritis, sometimes even of a mild degree, causes distress and may be enough to immobilize an already elderly and frail patient.

Wernicke's encephalopathy, while rare, is found in elderly persons who are alcoholics or who are suffering from malignant disease with repeated vomiting. It responds strikingly to parenterally administered thiamine as far as ocular movements are concerned, but the mental sympoms (in particular the mental confusion) are consequently much more resistant to treatment. Nutritional retrobulbar neuritis is also seen in elderly alcoholic patients and, if treated soon after the onset, sometimes responds quickly to B vitamins.

Glossitis has been emphasized by Vinther-Paulsen (29) as a symptom which often is correlated in the aged with a galaxy of other signs such as lack of appetite, lack of vitality, sideropenic anemia, and chelitis; spinal osteomalacia often is also present. In a hospital in Copenhagen, 16 women with glossitis were found to have been consuming diets providing fewer than 1300 calories, while 16 otherwise comparable patients with normal tongues all had received more than 1300 calories per day. There was a similar lack of overlap between intake of thiamine and of protein, 550 mcg and 40 gm representing the respective dividing points. Almost all the patients with glossitis had low serum protein values (less than 6.8 gm per 100 ml). Incidentally, in none of these cases was glossitis a sign of pernicious anemia. Intake of riboflavin was not particularly correlated with the presence or absence of glossitis.

Scurvy may not be as rare as is generally supposed. Woodford-Williams (30) noted that in one hospital in England three men and one woman with frank scurvy were admitted in a recent 12-month period. All the patients were more than 75 years of age, and the diagnosis had not been made prior to admission in any of the cases. Subclinical scurvy may be even more common and may be overlooked frequently because of the lack of quick routine tests for its detection.

Mild deficiency of vitamin A may be found in elderly persons subsisting on low-fat diets and may account in part for the excessive drying of the skin and mucosa as well as for the decreased secretion of mucus.

## CONCLUSION

The very apt comments of R. C. Garry, a distinguished Scottish physician and nutritionist, might well be quoted in conclusion. "Above all, we must see the elderly in continuity with youth and middle age. We accept that the child is father of the man. We could equally well say the elderly person is the child of his youth and years of maturity. The elderly do not form a special isolated section of the community: we must continually hark back to the earlier years." Nowhere is this more true than in the fields of nutrition and personal hygiene. Consumption of a varied diet, adapted in amount to individual needs; avoidance of dietary excesses, of an excessively fat diet; moderate salt intake; generous fluid intake, and sufficient exercise and rest are recommendations that are as valid for old age as they are for young and middle-aged adults.

## REFERENCES

1. Caloric Requirements, FAO Publication, Volume 5, Washington, D. C.,

1950. English, French and Spanish edition, with A. Keys and Calorie Committee.

2. Arimoto, K., Bergami, G., Dols, M. J. L., Garry, R. C., Hollingsworth, D. F., Karvonen, M. I., Keys, A., Mayer, J., Passmore, R., Pett, L. B., Tremolieres, J., Aykroyd, W. R., Rao, K. K. P. N., and Bengoa, J. M.: Calorie Requirements. Second Committee on Calorie Requirements Report. FAO, Rome. 1957.

3. Durnin, J. V. G. A.: Intake and expenditure of calories by the elderly. In Proceedings of the Nutrition Society. Cambridge, Cambridge University Press, 1960, vol. 19, no. 2, pp. 140-144.

4. Norris, A. H., Shock, N. W., and Yiengst, M. J.: Age differences in ventilatory and gas exchange responses to graded exercise in males. J. Gerontol., 10:145, 1955.

5. Brozek, J. and Keys, A.: Relative body weight, age and fatness. Geriatrics, 8:70-75, 1953.

6. Carlson, A. J., and Hoelzel, F.: Apparent prolongation of the life span of rats by intermittent fasting. J. Nutrition, 31:363, 1946.

7. McCay, C. M.: Diet and aging. J. Am. Dietet. A., 17:540, 1941.

8. Comfort, A.: Nutrition and longevity in animals. In Proceedings of the Nutrition Society, *ibid.*, (3) pp. 125-129.

9. McCay, C. M., Pope, F., and Lunsford, W.: Experimental prolongation of the life span. Bull. New York Acad. Med., 32:91, 1956.

10. Carr, C. J., King, J. T., and Visscher, M. B.: Delay of senescence infertility by dietary restriction. Fed. Proc., 8:22, 1949.

11. Robertson, F. B., Marston, H. R., and Walters, J. W.: The influence of intermittent starvation plus nucleic acid on the growth and longevity of the white mouse. Australian J. Exper. Biol. & M. Sc., 12:33, 1934.

12. Hundley, J. H.: In Weight Control. A collection of papers presented at the Weight Control Colloquium, Iowa State College. Ames, Iowa, Iowa State College Press, 1955, chap. 1, p. 1.

13. Dublin, L. I., and Marks H. H.: Mortality among insured overweights in recent years. Tr. A. Life Insur. M. Dir. America, 35:235, 1951.

14. Barr, D.: Obesity: Red light of health. In Overeating, Overweight and Obesity. Nutrition Symposium Series No. 6. New York, The National Vitamin Foundation, Inc., 1953, p. 90.

15. Berry, W. T. C., and Nash, F. A.: Studies in aetiology of pulmonary tuberculosis. Tubercle, 36:164, 1955.

16. Shull, K. H., and Mayer, J.: Hyperglycemic states not primarily due to lack of insulin. Vitamins & Hormones, 14:187, 1956.

17. Buechley, R. W., Drake, R. M., and Breslow, L.: Height, weight and mortality in a population of longshoremen. J. Chron. Dis., 7:363, 1958.

18. Kurlander, A. B., Abraham, S., and Rion, J. W.: Obesity and disease. Human Biol., 28:203, 1956.

19. Chinn, A. B.: Some problems of nutrition in the aged. J.A.M.A., 162:1511 (December 22) 1956.

20. Burton, B. T.: Nutrition in old age or nutritional requirements of the aged. Proceedings of the White House Conference on Aging. January 9-12, 1961, pp.66-72.
21. Mayer, J.: Nutrition and heart disease. Am. J. Pub. Health, 50:5 (March) 1960.
22. Meneely, G. R., Tucker, R. G., Darby, W. J., Ball, C. O. T., Kory, R. C., and Auerbach, S. H.: Electrocardiographic changes, disturbed lipid metabolism and decreased survival rates observed in rats chronically eating increased sodium chloride. Am. J. Med., 16:599, 1954.
23. Hegsted, D. M., Moscoso, I., and Collazos, C.: The study of minimum calcium requirements of adult men. J. Nutrition, 46:181, 1952.
24. Malm, O. J.: Calcium Requirement and Adaptation in Adult Men. Oslo, Norway, University Press, 1958.
25. Nordin, B. E. C.: Osteoporosis and caldium deficiency. In Proceedings of the Nutrition Society, *ibid.*, (3) pp. 129-137.
26. Hayes, O. B., Bowser, L. J., and Trulson, M. F.: Relation of dietary intake to bone fragility in the aged. J. Gerontol., 11:154 (April) 1956.
27. Jolliffe, N., Bowman, K. M., Rosenblum, L. A., and Fein, H. D.: Nicotinic acid deficiency encephalopathy. J.A.M.A. 114:307, 1940.
28. Earl, C. J.: Disorders of the nervous system in malnutrition. In Proceedings of the Nutrition Society, *ibid.*, (3) pp. 137-139.
29. Vinther-Paulsen, N.: Glossitis as indicator of nutritional deficiency in the aged. Rev. Med. Liege, 5:652, 1950.
30. Woodford-Williams, E.: The clinical medicine of old age. In Proceedings of the Nutrition Society, *ibid.*, (3) pp. 120-125.
31. Garry, R. C.: Nutrition and the elderly. In Proceedings of the Nutrition Society, *ibid.*, (3) pp. 107-108.

# PART IV
## Hunger and Obesity

*Chapter 29*

# THE VENTROMEDIAL GLUCOSTATIC MECHANISM AS A COMPONENT OF SATIETY

## ANATOMIC DATA

As early as 1912, postmortem examinations of very hyperphagic obese subjects suggested that lesions of the hypothalamus (rather than the pituitary) may be involved in disturbances of the regulation of food intake. Experimental work by investigators on both sides of the Atlantic in the 1930s and 1940s definitely dispelled the myth of the pituitary (Frohlich's) obesity syndrome. The work of Hetherington and Ranson and of Brobeck and co-workers demonstrated that bilateral destruction of the ventromedial nuclei causes hyperphagia in the rat. My co-workers and I subsequently demonstrated that unilateral destruction of the ventromedial nucleus in the rat may cause a slowly developing obesity. We also produced obesity in the mouse; in that species, bilateral lesions of the ventromedial area are necessary before obesity of even the slightest degree appears. Obesity follows bilateral destruction of the ventromedial area in a number of species. The possible relation of that area to other centers is illustrated by the fact that obesity is also seen following the production of lesions of the base of the anterior hypothalamus in the monkey and following the production of lesions caudal to the paraventricular nuclei in the dog. Bilateral damage to the ventromedial area of the thalamus, the rostral mesencephalic nuclei, the temporal area of the amygdala, or the hippocampus also causes hyperphagia in rats, as do separation of the frontal lobes from their thalamic connections in rats, frontal lobotomy in

Reprinted from *Postgraduate Medicine, 38* (No. 1), July, 1965.

man, and selective decortication in various animals.

Conversely, Anand and Brobeck found that bilateral destruction of more lateral parts of the hypothalamus in the rat is followed by complete cessation of eating. This observation was confirmed by Teitelbaum and Stellar, who found this inhibition to be temporary and the resumption of eating to be dependent on the nature and consistency of the food presented. Morrison and I, noting that lesions in the lateral hypothalamus at the same rostrocaudal level as the ventromedial nucleus caused both aphagia and adipsia, tried to find out whether these two responses were separate consequences of the lesions. Careful plotting of "aphagic" and adipsic" lesions and comparison of sham-operated animals deprived of food or water, or both, suggested that feeding and drinking were controlled by different centers. Morgane further analyzed the anatomy of the lateral area and concluded that lesions causing aphagia may interfere with at least two distinct systems of fibers of which the more important is lateral to the median forebrain bundle. Stimulation of various hypothalamic areas has given similar indications.

## BEHAVIORAL DATA

Use of the behavioral technics developed by B. F. Skinner and his associates has made possible a better definition of the role of the ventromedial hypothalamic area in the regulation of food intake. In an early application of these technics in mice trained to press on a lever to obtain food, Anliker and I demonstrated that bilateral destruction of the ventromedial area does not increase the rate of lever pressing, generally considered a reliable behavioral measure of hunger. What such lesions do is to eliminate, or at least shorten, the "satiety" periods during which no lever pressing takes place. This experiment confirmed pervious suggestions (in particular by Miller, Bailey and Stevenson) that the ventromedial area appears to act as a "satiety" brake inhibiting constantly activated lateral "feeding" areas. Bilateral destruction of the ventromedial area also prevents the expected increase in food intake following exercise and exposure to cold; in other words, metabolic requirements no longer exercise their normal influence on food intake.

This apparently simple picture, suggesting that the ventromedial area responds to metabolic requirements by inhibiting or releasing an inhibition on the lateral area, has been complicated recently by the results of behavioral experiments by Teitelbaum and Epstein. These workers have shown that there were taste concomitants of the destruction of the ventromedial area so that animals thus made hyperphagic responded more strongly than normal animals to consistencies or tastes that they did not like. The significance of these interesting observations is still difficult to assess. It may be that when one source of possible inhibition is removed, other sources are potentiated. It is also possible that the stereotaxic lesions produced in these animals also destroyed cells involved specifically in reactions to taste. The fact that animals can maintain their weight when feeding through a gastric fistula suggests that taste (if not exaggeratedly aversive) is not, in the long run, an essential component in the regulation of food intake.

The behavioral technics of Olds, who combined lever pressing for food in the rat with autoexcitation of a number of central nervous areas, together with the use of an electric grid permitting the examination of the circumstances under which the drive to eat is particularly intense, have allowed Morgane to explore the role of the ventromedial area, the pallidum, the median forebrain bundle and the lateral areas in the regulation of food intake. His experiments, performed in intact and in lesioned animals, suggest the presence in the lateral hypothalamus of two systems of fibers, one having to do with purely quantitative aspects of the regulation of food intake – and subject to ventromedial inhibition – and one having to do with more qualitative aspects of appetite; the relationship to the ventromedial area is still obscure.

## GLUCOSTATIC MECHANISM: EARLY WORK

My co-workers and I propounded the concept of the glucostatic mechanism of regulation of food intake in the early 1950s. It was proposed that in the ventromedial (satiety) hypothalamic centers (and possibly in other central and peripheral areas as well) there exist glucoreceptors sensitive to blood glucose in the measure that they utilize it. This concept was based on the facts that the central nervous system is dependent for its function on the availability of glucose; that carbohydrates are preferentially oxidized and are not stored in any appreciable amount, so that their depletion is rapid; and that in the intervals between meals there is an incomparably greater proportionate drop of carbohydrate than of protein and fat reserves, and only intake of food will replenish fully these depleted stores. Furthermore, carbohydrate metabolism is not only regulated by a complex edifice of endocrine inter-relationships but is in turn a regulator of fat oxidation and fat synthesis, of protein mobilization and breakdown, and of protein synthesis. Thus, a mechanism of regulation of food intake based on glucose utilization could and should be successfully integrated with energy metabolism and its components. Such a theory also permitted successful interpretation of the known effects of cold, exercise, diabetes mellitus, hyperthyroidism, hypothyroidism and other metabolic changes, provided that the additional postulate was made that carbohydrate metabolism in the ventromedial area differed from that in the brain in general. In particular it was postulated that the ventromedial area is highly glucoreceptive and that, unlike the rest of the brain, it would show considerably heightened utilization. Such a theory could also account for the self-perpetuating effect of hyperphagia, which of itself causes a more rapid utilization of glucose.

Early experimental work designed to test the theory has often been and apparently still is misinterpreted. Because of the (then) apparently insuperable difficulty in measuring glucose utilization in the ventromedial area and the postulate that, in general, ventromedial utilization must parellel peripheral utilization, Van Itallie and I attempted to correlate hunger feelings (and, later, Stunkard attempted to correlate gastric contractions) with diminished peripheral glucose utilization in an easily accessible area, the forearm. Utilization was measured by capillary-venous (of arteriovenous) differences (or $\Delta$-glucose); in patients at rest, variations of blood flow were not taken into effect. In general, there was a satisfactory degree of correlation between small $\Delta$-glucose and the appearance of hunger sensations and gastric contractions. (That the correlation is far from perfect, even when carotid-jugular vein determinations are made, is emphasized in recent work.) It was also shown, in particular by Stunkard and Wolff, that whenever glucose utilization is proceeding satisfactorily, a slow intravenous glucose infusion in hungry individuals eliminates both the feeling of hunger and gastric contractions. In diabetics, and in persons with hunger diabetes, glucose infusion does not affect hunger to a similar degree. While other authors at times have not observed the correlation between cessation of hunger and rises in the glucose utilization, they may have been operating under some of the conditions described by Van Itallie in which peripheral glucose arteriovenous differences are not reliable indexes of overall glucose utilization by the body, much less by the satiety mechanisms. Such conditions include changes in circulation dynamics because of increase in blood flow, rapid rises in blood glucose, certain effects of insulin, and the presence of overriding dominant conditioning. Again, the peripheral arteriovenous differences, although still associated in the thinking of many workers with the foundation of the glucostatic theory, have never really held any direct significance in it and were used in this early work "merely to obtain more reliable information about the changes which take place in carbohydrate supply than is available from arterial or venous glucose alone."

It is interesting to note that Van Itallie and Hashim have shown the reciprocal evolution of blood nonesterified fatty acid levels and arteriovenous glucose differences. While these authors point out that it is unlikely that nonesterified fatty acid levels per se act directly as a signal to the food-regulatory centers, their work provides yet another indirect way to evaluate patterns of metabolic utilization and their possible correlation with the hunger-satiety balance.

## RECENT DEVELOPMENTS

Major recent developments have entirely altered the status of our knowledge in this field by providing means whereby we can assess much more directly the hypothalamic events in the regulation of food intake without having to rely on mere statistical correlations. These include the effect of glucagon on hunger feelings and gastric contractions and the role of the ventromedial area in the regulation of gastric contractions, the elucidation of the mode of action of gold thioglucose, the demonstration of the special characteristics of metabolism of the ventromedial area of the hypothalamus and the determination of the electric activity of the ventromedial hypothalamic area under the influence of variations of blood metabolites, glucose in particular.

## ACTION OF GLUCAGON: HYPOTHALAMIC GLUCOSTATIC CONTROL OF GASTRIC HUNGER CONTRACTIONS

Stunkard, Van Itallie and Reiss made the interesting observation that the injection of 2 mg of glucagon reproducibly eliminates gastric contractions (and hunger sensations) in human subjects. They demonstrated that the elimination of gastric contractions lasts as long as glucose utilization proceeds actively and ceases when glucose utilization is reduced, even though the absolute level of blood glucose may still be well above the fasting level.

Stunkard also observed a patient who had lost practically all of his brain cortex in an accident and was incapable of feeding himself. After one week of fasting, the patient exhibited almost continuous gastric contractions. A variety of treatments, including the infusion of amino acids and induction of pyrexia (by rolling the patient in an electric blanket), did not inhibit gastric contractions. The only treatment (with the exception of food) which proved effective in inhibiting gastric contractions was the administration of glucagon.

My co-workers and I found that in rats, too, intravenous injections of glucagon inhibit gastric hunger contractions. The dose that was 100 per cent effective in a large series of animals was 75 mcg. The inhibition starts between 45 and 60 seconds after administration of glucagon. By the time inhibition takes place, the glucose in the blood has already risen considerably from the control fasting value and inorganic phosphorus has decreased, indicating active utilization. Blood glucose continues to increase as inorganic phosphorus returns to the fasting level and gastric hunger contractions appear.

Sudsaneh and I found that rats in which the ventromedial hypothalamic area has been destroyed show no significance in their pattern of fasting contractions as compared with normal animals. The inhibitory response to epinephrine and to norepinephrine is normal. On the other hand, the intravenous administration of 75 mcg of glucagon almost invariably fails to produce complete inhibition of hunger contractions in animals with lesions of the ventromedial nuclei whether they are allowed to become and remain obese or whether their weight is reduced to the preoperative level after demonstration of hyperphagia. Response of these animals to prolonged exposure to cold is delayed, on the average by 100 per cent. The lack of response to glucagon and the delay in response to prolonged exposure to cold are obviously not caused by refractoriness of gastric contractions as such. The finding may be interpreted as indicating that the ventromedial area does exercise a definite measure of control over gastric hunger contractions and does so in response to an increase in its glucose utilization. An anatomic basis for such a mechanism may be provided by the existence of the bundles of Schutz which seem to originate in the general area of the ventromedial hypothalamus and extend to the roots of the vagus.

## MODE OF ACTION OF GOLD THIOGLUCOSE

Brecher and Waxler in 1949 observed a syndrome of hyperphagia and obesity in mice after a single intraperitoneal or subcutaneous injection of gold thioglucose. Marshall, Barrnett and I confirmed the observation by demonstrating that gold thioglucose caused extensive damage to the ventromedial areas as well as damage of varying degree to the supraoptic nucleus, ventral part of the lateral hypothalamic area, arcuate nucleus, and median eminence. Marshall and I showed that there was minimum impairment of functions other than the regulation of food intake, in contrast to the effects of stereotaxic lesions. Gold-thioglucose-obese animals, unlike animals made obese by stereotaxic lesions, not infrequently will mate and rear their young. Like the animals with stereotaxic lesions, gold thioglucose-treated animals show impairment of satiety mechanisms as well as impaired reaction of the regulation of food intake to cold, exercise and caloric dilution. Marshall and I later showed that gold thiogalactose, gold thiosorbitol, gold thiomalate, gold thioglycerol, gold thiocaproate, gold thioglycoanilide and gold thiosulfate did not produce the brain damage which follows administration of gold thioglucose. Nor were hyperphagia and obesity seen following the administration of any of these compounds even though their toxicity is similar to that of gold thioglucose. It was also shown that gold thioglucose produced lesions in the rat similar to those observed in the mouse. The fact that simultaneous administration of sodium thioglucose protects animals against hypothalamic damage is probably traceable to competitive inhibition. On the basis of these observations, I suggested that the toxic gold moiety of accumulated gold thioglucose destroyed the ventromedial neurons specifically because of the affinity of these cells for the glucose component of the molecule, in accordance with the general proposal that glucose is a cardinal activator of the satiety center.

Recent work by Debons and associates, using radioautographic and neutron-activating analytic technics, confirms and considerably extends these conclusions. These Brookhaven workers determined the gold content of the rostral, middle and caudal portions of brains of control animals. They found that some gold accumulated in the brains of all gold-treated animals, but with notable differences in localization. Animals which received gold thioglucose but did not become obese had a lesser total gold content and a smaller amount localized in the medial sections than the animals in which the hyperphagic syndrome developed. In gold thioglucose-treated animals, radioautographic localization of gold activity was found consistently in four regions. The greatest concentration was in the hypothalamus, chiefly at the lateral angles and floor of the third ventricle. (Histologically this region consisted of collapsed glial scar tissue, and in some instances it showed cystic changes.) A second concentration of radioactivity was noted in the midline, dorsal and cephalad to the optic chiasm and immediately dorsal to the anterior commissure. A third was noted in the caudal portion of the septum and ventrohippocampal commissure, and a fourth in the hindbrain in the midline at about the level of the vestibular nuclei in the floor of the fourth ventricle. The fact that administration of gold thioglucose, but not of gold thiomalate, led to such localization even though gold diffused throughout the brain in each instance was taken to mean that the gold moiety probably is responsible for the focal accumulation of sufficient gold in the hypothalamus to produce a destructive lesion which can result in hyperphagia and obesity. Luse, Harris and Stohr, in electron microscopic studies of the early lesion, noted that gold thioglucose brought about initial changes in the hypo-thalamic oligodendroglial cells followed by focal neuronal degeneration. Luse and Harris suggested that the oligodendroglial cells, within certain areas of the central nervous system, share a high degree of specificity to glucose.

Debons and his colleagues point out that while it is true that the foci of gold accumulation in the hindbrain, in the hippocampal commissure, and above the optic chiasm are at sites where lesions have been reported by Perry and Liebelt, this by no means proves the suggestion of these authors that such extrahypothalamic lesions indicate that gold thioglucose passes through deficient areas in the blood-brain barrier and is not selectively accumulated at "glucoreceptor" sites. Indeed, they add, in view of the extreme chemical specificity demonstrated for the gold thioglucose molecule, consideration must be given to the possibility that the sites of extrahypothalamic gold accumulation may themselves be glucoreceptive sites.

That there are, incidentally, a number of physiologic functions distinct from the regulation of food intake which must be dependent on the existence of glucoreceptors is suggested by a number of facts, some of them known for a long time. One example is the classic absence of a secretory gastric (hydrochloric) response to insulin after total vagotomy. Another striking illustration is given by the famous experiment of Zunz and LaBarre, confirmed more recently by Duner, demonstrating that when the circulation of a dog's head was isolated from the rest of the body, with the nerve supply from head to body intact, hyperglycemia of the head resulted in hypoglycemia of the body. Edelman, on the basis of his analysis of the differential sensitivities of various area cells, has constructed an interesting theory of satiety, with various degrees of inhibition corresponding to greater and greater numbers of glucoreceptors of decreasing sensitivity being brought into action. When a relatively large amount of glucose is injected at the same time as gold thioglucose, more gold rather than less is taken up by the glucosensitive cells. This finding suggests that glucose itself may have a potentiating effect due perhaps to its role in dialating capillaries or increasing their permeability.

## SPECIAL METABOLIC CHARACTERISTICS
## OF THE VENTROMEDIAL AREA

A number of recent experiments have emphasized the metabolic heterogeneity of the hypothalamus and the very special metabolic characteristics of the ventromedial area. Forssberg and Larsson, seeking to test the glucostatic hypothesis, reasoned that the hunger state must be accompanied by changes in the concentration of those compounds through which brain tissue, which cannot burn or store fat, can nonetheless achieve some energy storage, i.e. phosphagens: creatine phosphate and adenosine triphosphate. Rates of incorporation of glucose and phosphorus would be expected to be particularly affected in the ventromedial area if it was designed to be sensitive to the rate of utilization of glucose. To this end, these workers studied the incoproation of $P^{32}$ and $C^{14}$ glucose in three areas, one including the "feeding" and satiety areas and two situated directly above the optic chiasm, the upper one cutting across the columna fornicis. In hungry rats, the sample which included the feeding area showed a preferential uptake of $P^{32}$, indicating an increase of physiology activity over in the fed state. In the fed state, by contrast, activity of the two control regions was enhanced while that of the feeding area was proportionally decreased. Experiments with $C^{14}$ glucose showed the same type of response. In hungry rats, the region including the feeding area had a greater uptake of glucose as compared with the control areas. While these studies demonstrated that various parts of the hypothalamus differ in their metabolic reactions, interpretation was difficult in that the experimental samples which were studied and compared with "control" areas included both the ventromedial and the lateral area as well as other structures presumably not directly concerned with the regulation of the intake of food.

Chain, Larsson and Pocchiari in a subsequent study confirmed differences in the fate of radioactive glucose in different parts of the rabbit brain, particularly the labeling of amino acids. Andersson, Larsson and Pocchiari extended the findings and mapped the incorporation of $C^{14}$ alanine, aspartic acid, glutamic acid, $\gamma$-aminobutyric acid, glutamine and arginine in the hypothalamus of the goat, again demonstrating differences between various parts. Interpretation of the results, beyond the demonstration of heterogeneity of the hypothalamus, is again difficult.

Anand, studying glucose and oxygen uptake of various parts of the hypothalamus in the monkey, arrived at clearer-cut results because of the better anatomic definition of his sample. He found that in the fed animals there is a relative increase in the oxygen and glucose per unit of nucleic acid activity by the satiety (ventromedial) region as compared with that of the feeding center. In the starved animal the uptake of oxygen and glucose is less than that of the feeding region. In this experiment the arteriovenous glucose difference was low in the starved animals and high in the ones which had been fed. Anand concluded that the results demonstrated an increase in activity of the satiety centers during fed states, which is accompanied by an increase in the uptake of glucose and is presumably determined by the changes in availability of glucose. " . . . the medial regions are activated as a result of changes in the levels of the blood sugar produced by food intake, which subsequently produces satiety and abolition of further eating by inhibiting the lateral mechanisms. The electroencephalographic recordings from feeding and satiety centers under conditions of hyperglycemia (mentioned previously) lend further support to this hypothesis, as changes in the activity of satiety centers are more pronounced than changes in the activity of feeding centers."

## ELECTROENCEPHALIC DETERMINATIONS

Anand and his co-workers have evaluated in rats and monkeys

the role played by changes in the blood levels of various nutrients on the electric reactions of various hypothalamic areas. Electrodes were bilaterally implanted in the lateral, ventromedial and various control areas of the hypothalamus. Still other electrodes were implanted in the cortex. Connections were brought through the skin at the back of the neck. Four to five days after the operation, hyperglycemia was produced by the intravenous injection of concentrated glucose solution. The consequent rise in blood glucose caused an increase in the frequency of encephalographic waves from the ventromedial (satiety) area (from six to seven per second to 9 to 10 per second). The glucose injection was followed by a drastic decrease in activity in the lateral (feeding) area, with reductions in potential by two-thirds or more being noted. Electric activity of control areas in other parts of the hypothalamus was not affected. Conversely, hypoglycemia (produced by intravenous injection of insulin) caused a reduction in frequency of ventro-medial waves (from six to seven per second to two to three). Activity in the feeding area was increased.

Changes in blood amino acid concentration and blood lipid concentration did not affect the electric activity of the satiety and feeding centers. Increase in glucose utilization following the consumption of a meal was similarly found to be associated with a doubling of the frequency of ventromedial pulsation and a decrease in the activity of the feeding centers.

In a series of recent experiments, these Indian workers obtained beautiful correlations between the electric activity of single ventromedial cells and carotid-jugular glucose differences. The activity of lateral area cells showed an inverse picture.

## CONCLUSION

The glucostatic mechanism appears to be one of the essential processes through which metabolic requirements influence the "feeding mechanism" and through which energetic homeostasis is maintained. There are, of course, many other factors which, at a given time, influence food intake. A thermostatic component, sensitive to elevations of body temperature, may act on a safety valve situated in another hypothalamic area to shut off feeding behavior. Other safety valves may be similarly sensitive to protein imbalance, to excessively high protein intakes, to gastric distention, and to dehydration. Metering of food intake by the mouth or the pharynx, taste, emotions and habits may, at a given moment, also influence intake. Long-term factors such as the state of the adipose tissue also appear to act to regulate food intake. (It may well be, however, that because of the relation of free fatty acid release to the size and metabolic state of fat cells and because of the mutual interrelationship of glucose and fatty acid availability, that particular factor is mediated through the glucostatic mechanism.)

The physician, daily confronted by obese patients, children who won't eat, and patients who respond to cortisone by becoming voracious, may well wonder at the significance for him of the detailed exposition of one component (even if it has special homeostatic significance) of the regulation of food intake. It is my hope, in discussing this factor at this particular point in a series devoted to recent work in obesity, to show both the considerable progress made in the analysis of appetite and satiety and the vast reaches of unknown territory that remain to be explored. In a more pragmatic vein, it is likely that the understanding of at least some of the biochemical phenomena which are involved in hunger and satiety can provide a basis for the systematic search for specific anorexigenic agents.

## REFERENCES

(References to work conducted prior to 1964 will be found in Mayer (1).)
1. Mayer, J.: Appetite and the many obesities. Aust. Ann. Med., 13:282, 1964.
2. Brecher, G., Laqueur, G. L., Cronkite, E. P., Edelman, P. M. and Schwartz, I. L.: The brain lesion of goldthioglucose obesity. J. Exp. Med., 121:395, 1965.
3. Edelman, P. M., Schwartz, I. L., Cronkite, E. P., Brecher, G. and Livingston, L.: The effect of hyperglycemia on hypothalamic gold uptake and hyperphagia in goldthioglucose-treated mice. J. Exp. Med., 121:403, 1965.
4. Anand, B. K., Chhina, G. S., Sharma, K. N., Dua, S. and Singh, B.: Activity of single neurons in the hypothalamic feeding centers: Effect of glucose. Amer. J. Physiol., 207:1146, 1964.

*Chapter 30*

# HUNGER AND SATIETY
# SENSATIONS IN MAN

Written in collaboration with
Lenore F. Monellow and Carl C. Seltzer

## INTRODUCTION

THIS chapter deals with one of the most basic aspects of the regulation of food intake, yet one which neither researchers nor clinicians had studied systematically until our laboratory started working on it a little over a year ago: the matter of hunger and satiety sensations which, in the last resort, determine eating behavior in most individuals. Extensive studies have been available of course, which deal with the physiologic or psychologic background underlying the sensations. A number of excellent physiologic studies have been performed on energy balance, gastric contractions, the effect of hypothalamic and frontal lobe damage, and various metabolic correlates of the nutritional state; psychologic studies have been conducted in large numbers (on experimental animals) on the characteristics of "food getting" under various conditions; psychiatric reports have dealt — not always under the best controlled conditions — with the emotional background in certain personality disturbances which have nutritional implications such as "psychogenic" obesity or anorexia nervosa; social and psychologic anthropology textbooks always contain sections dealing with the symbolic or the cultural significance of food. However, virtually the only descriptions of conscious sensations and feelings of hunger are to be found in the report of the Minnesota wartime study of semistarvation in human volunteers and in anecdotal reports of accidental and total

Reprinted from *Postgraduate Medicine, 37* (No. 6), June, 1965.

starvation. The sensations and moods associated with less extreme states of "everyday" hunger and satiety, the urge to eat, the preoccupations with thoughts of food in the course of the day in normal individuals, and the extent to which differences are encountered from one individual to another, and from one sex or one age group to another, and from obese to nonobese individuals are the objectives of this preliminary and summary report.

## METHODS OF STUDY

The data on which this study was based were accumulated through the use of a self-administered, highly structured questionnaire consisting of eight single and 70 multiple-choice (average of five or six) questions designed to help the subjects recollect their sensations or moods. The questionnaire was administered to five groups of subjects totaling approximately 800 persons. They were chosen to represent various ages in both sexes, subject to the limitation that their age, level of education, cooperation and verbal ability be sufficient to intelligently complete long and detailed questionnaires calling for the desired degree of competence in self-analysis and expression. The five groups, each comprising between 100 and 200 subjects, included two groups of adult college graduates, 20 to 67 years of age (the women were school teachers, the men, drug detail men); one group of adolescent boys; one group of adolescent girls; and one group of obese adolescent girls, 9 to 20 years of age, coming from middle to upper income families and attending summer camps.

A number of initial questions concerned age, height, weight, attitudes toward present and desired weight, schedules and size of meals and snacks and their relative importance (i.e. meal most anticipated, meal for which the individual is most hungry, skipping, dieting, etc). Subjects were then asked to describe their physical sensations and moods during extreme hunger (defined as "the hungriest you can remember being") two hours before a meal on a typical weekday, half an hour before this meal, sitting down to this meal, after a few bites of food, and at the end of this meal. Checklists of physical sensations were provided in the multiple-choice questionnaire for (1) gastric sensation (emptiness, rumbling, ache, pain, tenseness, nausea); (2) mouth and throat sensations (emptiness, dryness, salivation, pleasant or unpleasant taste or sensation); (3) cerebral sensations (headache, dizziness, etc.); (4) general overall sensations (weakness, fatigue, restlessness, coldness, warmth).

Moods categorized were (1) negative active mood (irritable, nervous, tense); (2) negative passive mood (depressed, apathetic); (3) positive passive mood (calm, relaxed, contented); (4) positive active mood (cheerful, excited).

Preoccupations with thoughts of food were graded as (1) not at all preoccupied (no thoughts of food); (2) mildly preoccupied (only occasional thoughts of food); (3) moderately preoccupied (many thoughts of food but can easily concentrate on other things); (4) quite preoccupied (most of thoughts are on food and it is difficult to concentrate on other subjects).

Satiety was studied during and after meals through questions dealing with sensations, moods, degree of urge to eat, pre-occupation with thoughts of food, quantity of food the subject felt he could still consume at the end of the meal, most important reason for stopping eating (no extra food readily available, feeling of satisfaction, desire to limit intake for the sake of figure control or health), and extent of willpower needed to stop eating (none – stopping is an abrupt process; none – stopping is a gradual process; some willpower required because some urge to eat is still felt; considerable willpower is required). Other questions dealt with sensations of discomfort felt at the end of the meal, if any; the description of such sensations (ranging from a "full" to a "distended" or "bloated" stomach, nausea) and their frequency (the extent to which subject continued to eat in the presence of such sensations); attitude toward plate-cleaning and its practice under a variety of circumstances. Additional comments were requested if subjects felt them appropriate. Results were categorized and significant differences established on the basis of sex, age and degree of obesity using an IBM 1620 computer to cope with the large amount of data obtained. Only some of the major findings will be described in general terms in this chapter. A more detailed although still preliminary report will be published later.

## EATING PATTERN

As expected, in spite of considerable variability among individuals within each group, there were significant responses common to each group which differed from those of the other groups. Adults, and adult men in particular, differ from adolescents in that an overwhelming majority are far hungrier for dinner than for any other meal. In contrast, a large proportion of boys are hungriest for breakfast or lunch and almost half of the girls for lunch. Similarly, an overwhelming proportion of adults "look forward" most to dinner (the largest meal of the day for all groups) while one-third of the adolescents look forward most to lunch.

Our data confirm the well-known prevalence of breakfast skipping. Forty per cent of adolescent girls admit it to be a frequent practice; other groups do so less frequently, with women doing it least (15%). Frequent skipping of lunch is highest in our group of men (46%) and lowest again in the women of our sample (14%). Virtually all the adolescents partake daily of between-meal snacks (boys: 3 on the average: girls: 2.3). Half of the men and one-fifth of the women do not; those who do average only 1.4 and 1.4 snacks per day. Only 4 per cent of the adults consume three or more snacks per day as compared with 46 per cent of adolescents.

## HUNGER

### Sensations

Over 90 per cent of each group of subjects record some specific gastric sensations when experiencing "extreme hunger," with approximately 60 per cent recording only one (tenseness, rumbling, feeling of emptiness, ache, pain or nausea) and 30 per cent experiencing two or more.

Approximately 50 per cent of all subjects note some gastric sensations two hours before the major meal; about half an hour before this meal, the proportion increases to 75 per cent of the adolescents, as compared to 83 per cent of adult men and 64 per cent of adult women. The proportion increases as deprivation is more prolonged.

The incidence of mouth sensations (salivation, tightness, dryness, emptiness, tenseness, unplesant taste) is higher at all degrees of hunger in males than in females, is higher in men than in boys, and increases as deprivation is more prolonged. Throat sensations (dryness, emptiness, tightness, tenseness, unpleasant feeling, nausea) have a similar distribution within groups and degree of hunger but are less frequent than mouth sensations. Head sensations (headache, dizziness, faintness, spots before the eyes, ringing in the ears) are rare except during extreme hunger, where they are seen more frequently among adults than among adolescents.

During extreme hunger, the great majority of subjects (80% of adults, 60% of adolescents) experience one or more general body sensations such as weakness, sleepiness, tiredness, restlessness, cold and muscular spasms. Suprisingly, close to one-third of all subjects experience several sensations half an hour before the main meal. Thus, in general, gastric sensations appear to be the most sensitive indicators of hunger, followed by general sensations, and by mouth, throat and head sensations.

## Moods, Urge to Eat, and Preoccupation with Food

Moods, like sensations, show considerable individual variability, but there are significant differences among groups. The triad of irritability, nervousness and tenseness ("negative active" mood) is much more frequent during the extreme hunger in adults (78% of the men, 66% of the women) than in adolescents (38% of the boys, 48% of the girls). Two hours before the main meal of the day, only half of the subjects describe themselves as calm, relaxed, contented (positive passive mood), a few as negative active, the rest equally divided between positive active and negative active. As deprivation is prolonged, more subjects switch to a negative active mood.

Under conditions of prolonged deprivation (extreme hunger) only a very small minority of subjects (2% of adults and 8% of adolescents) indicate that they feel no urge to eat, a percentage virtually identical to that seen half an hour before a major meal. In most individuals, however, the variation of the urge to eat evolves, as can be expected, as deprivation increases. Two hours before a meal, the urge to eat is absent in 20 to 30 per cent of the members of the various groups and mild in the others, particularly in adults. Half an hour before a meal, most adults described their urge to eat as mild rather than moderate, while adolescents tend to report it more frequently as moderate. During more prolonged deprivation, the frequency of "strong" urges increases in all groups.

Preoccupation with thoughts of food is reported as mild or absent in all groups two hours before the major meal, with women, however, reporting the greatest degree of preoccupation with thoughts of food. Approximately one-half hour before the major meal of the day, there is a sharp upsurge in the number of persons reporting a moderate degree of preoccupation with thoughts of food and, among adolescents, a strong degree of preoccupation. Conversely, the number of persons reporting no preoccupation with thoughts of food drops dramatically in all groups − particularly in adults − as one approaches the time of the major meal.

## Events During a Meal

Abrupt changes in sensations and moods, differing between the sexes, appear to take place after a few bites of food. Males experience an increase in mouth and throat hunger sensations while females experience a rapid drop in number and intensity of hunger sensations of all types. Both groups record a rapid drop in hunger sensations as the meal proceeds, with all hunger sensations ceasing completely, well before the meal is completed. Most subjects report a gradually relaxed stomach with pleasant "taste" or "feelings" in the mouth and throat; a few subjects report feelings of warmth. As they sit down to eat, all groups experience an abrupt change in mood from negative to positive (cheerful, excited). After a few mouthfuls, the mood starts shifting to positive passive (calm, contentment). The urge to eat is strong in most subjects as they sit down to eat, particularly adolescents. Adult males report a more frequent increase of their urge to eat after a few mouthfuls than adolescents. The urge to eat decreases in all groups as the meal progresses.

## SATIETY

The phenomenon of satiety, in striking contrast to hunger, appears to our subjects most difficult to describe. It is associated with far fewer sensations, and in many subjects, none at all. Unlike hunger which builds up slowly and brings in, one by one, sensations, moods and urges to eat which then increase in intensity, satiety occurs rapidly, in some cases in a matter of minutes or at most of a half hour. From a subjective standpoint changes in moods, more difficualt to describe than sensations, accompany cessation of the urge to eat. The phenomenon of satiety thus appears uniform and relatively simple in contrast to the complexity and diversity of descriptions of hunger. This is illustrated by some responses to the questionnaire. In response to the question, "What is the one most important reason you stop eating at the end of the major meal of the day", the great majority of subjects in all groups state that they eat until they are satisfied. A few subjects, particularly adolescents, state that they stop eating because no more food is readily available. A sizable minority, particularly females (18% of the men, 38% of the women, 10% of the boys, and 27% of the girls), stop eating voluntarily for reasons of health or figure control. Subjects thus "dieting" indicate that they need to apply varying degrees of self-control or "will power" ranging from mild to extreme. Most subjects who do not exercise self-restraint report that the end of all urge to continue eating is an abrupt process, with the abruptness more marked in adults than in adolescents. Adolescents report less plate-cleaning than adults.

Three-quarters of all adults report that they never (or almost never) feel uncomfortable after the major meal, as do half of the boys and two-thirds of the girls. By contrast, one-fifth of the men, one-fourth of the women and girls, and almost 40 per cent of the boys frequently or customarily report discomfort ranging from excessive stomach fullness to, in some cases (up to 8% in adolescents), nausea.

As the meal proceeds and ends, a mood of calm contentment often accompanied by warmth and sleepiness, particularly among adults, replaces the mood of cheerfulness and excitement which develops at the beginning of the meal. Adolescents tend to report more active positive moods than adults.

## SIGNIFICANCE OF FINDINGS

Should we want to speculate on the significance of these findings, it would appear that the multiplicity of hunger sensations hammering at the consciousness of man is probably necessary to prod him to hunt and to find or work for food and hence is essential to the survival of the species. However, satiety, which simply causes eating to cease, seems to occur unconsciously or subconsciously — perhaps at the hypothalamic level — as the meal has progressed to nutritional adequacy and some appreciable time after hunger sensations have disappeared.

The differences in satiety patterns between youngsters still growing and adults — in particular, the greater prevalence of gastric fullness in children and adolescents — may be related to the well-known phenomenon that the bilateral lesioning of the ventromedial hypothalamic "satiety" areas in experimental animals has little or no effect until growth has slowed down or stopped, indicating that some of the midbrain mechanisms which limit food intake are less important in the young.

## OBESE AND NONOBESE SUBJECTS

The analysis of our data on this aspect is still going on. We are attempting to correlate hunger and satiety characteristics not only with degree but also with the duration and types of obesity. At this point in our study we feel that we can make only the following statements.

Eating patterns of obese subjects differ from those of nonobese in a number of ways. A greater percentage of obese subjects skip breakfast, lunch or dinner than do nonobese; they eat sweet desserts less often, clear their plates more often, and tend to eat more snacks in the absence of hunger sensations but report that they eat fewer large meals.

In general, there appear to be no important differences between obese and nonobese subjects in sensations during extreme or moderate hunger except that there may be a somewhat greater number of obese individuals who report very few or no sensations after prolonged deprivation. Obese subjects report fewer sensations of gastric emptiness or rumble but more extreme pangs. Mouth, throat and head sensations are similar in obese and nonobese subjects; obese subjects report less frequent weakness and tiredness during hunger. Urges to eat are comparable in obese and nonobese subjects in extreme hunger and preoccupation with thoughts of food is somewhat greater in the absence of hunger.

It is at the end of meals that obese subjects differ most from nonobese. Obese subjects report they require more willpower to stop eating, even though they report more frequent sensations of discomfort (distention and nausea) at the end of meals. The obese are often preoccupied with thoughts of food half an hour after a meal, a phenomenon of exceptional occurrence in subjects who are nonobese.

## COMMENT

These preliminary observations suggest that abnormalities in satiety may be much more prevalent than abnormalities in hunger among obese subjects. It seems reasonable also to conclude that the physician or the dietitian dealing with a given obese patient should inquire in some detail as to his or her patterns of hunger and satiety. The spacing of the meals and, if indicated, the snacks which are components of the reducing diet best calculated to reduce hunger and promote a sufficient degree of satiety to make continued dieting tolerable depends on this knowledge. So does the choice of the proper dosage and timing of anoretic agents and the indications for their use.

## REFERENCE

1. Monello, L. F., Seltzer, C. C. and Mayer J.: Hunger and satiety sensations in men, women, boys and girls. A preliminary report. Bull. N. Y. Acad. Sci., 131:593, 1965.

*Chapter 31*

# GENETIC FACTORS IN
# HUMAN OBESITY*

## EXPERIMENTAL GENETIC OBESITY

IT is easy to demonstrate the importance of genetic factors in experimental obesity. In mice, for instance, the hereditary obese hyperglycemic syndrome — a recessive syndrome which has been extensively studied in our laboratory — is characterized *inter alia* by extreme adiposity, hypercholesteremia, a marked degree of hyperglycemia in spite of increased circulating insulin, marked hyperplasia of the islets of Langerhans with degranualtion, and a host of other metabolic and behavioral idiosyncrasies. The obese hyperglycemic syndrome is not only a clear example of genetically determined obesity but also a good example of pleitropism. The very large number of observable anatomic, metabolic and behavioral abnormalities (1) presumably all stem from one inborn error, which may be the presence of a glycerokinase in the adipose tissue of these animals.

The biochemical evidence leading to this conclusion has been reviewed in detail elsewhere (2). In terms of known genetic mechanisms, it could be further suggested that the inherited trait may be the absence of a represser. The genetic code for the production of glycerokinase is presumably present in all mammalian cells, but glycerokinase activity is normally absent in white adipose tissue. The observed increased concentration of glycerophosphate may be responsible for the hyperglycemia, which may in turn be responsible for the islet hypertrophy and hypersecretion of insulin, with the increased circulating insulin and hyperglycemia causing in turn the increased hepatic

---

*Adapted from an address presented at a symposium on fat metabolism and adiposity, New York Academy of Sciences, New York.
Reprinted from *Postgraduate Medicine, 37* (No. 4), April, 1965.

lipogenesis. Other observed metabolic abnormalities may be similarly derived, however remotely, from the same abnormality.

Yellow obesity, a dominant syndrome seen in mice heterozygous for this gene; New Zealand obesity, a recessive syndrome of obesity and diabetes quite different in many ways from the obese hyperglycemic syndrome (one difference being that the affected animals will mate; and a genetically controlled spontaneous degeneration of the ventromedial area of the hypothalamus are further examples of such hereditary obesity. Other examples of genetic obesity in various types of experimental and farm animals have been discussed in previous papers (3, 4).

## FAMILIAL OCCURRENCE IN MAN

The demonstration of the hereditary nature of familial obesity in man is much more difficult. That obesity does "run in families" is well established (5). In a series of over 1000 obese patients in Vienna, Bauer found that 73 per cent had one or both parents obese. This figure is close to the 69 per cent found by Rony for a series of 250 patients in Chicago. In his studies in Philadelphia, Angel found that half the offspring of an obese and an average parent were obese, as were two-thirds of the offspring of obese and obese matings. Eighty per cent of the obese children had at least one fat parent; the parents of 25 per cent of the obese children were both obese. Gurney in a previous survey of a similar population found that only 9 per cent of the children of average-weight parents were overweight. Fellows, studying the overweight fraction of a life insurance sample, found that 58 per cent of the mothers and 43 per cent of the fathers of these individuals were or had been overweight. Dunlop, studying a group of obese subjects in Edinburgh, found that 69 per cent had at least one overweight parent (39%, mothers only; 12%, fathers only; 18%, both parents).

Ellis and Tallerman, studying 50 very obese children, found that 60 per cent of them had a parent or a sibling similarly affected; in particular, 26 per cent had a grossly overweight mother, 12 per cent a grossly overweight father, 6 per cent both parents grossly overweight. Iversen, following 40 obese children, found that in 78 per cent (31 cases) one or both parents were obese. Only in 10 per cent (four cases) was there no obesity in parents or siblings. Our own studies in Boston also show a high degree of correlation between overweight in parents and in children.

## ETHNIC DIFFERENCES

Interpretation of these data is difficult, as cultural background interacts with genetics to determine the incidence of overweight (5). Angel (6) found that the large obese group which he studied showing a relative excess of first and second generation Americans; 42.7 per cent had American-born parents (more than half "old Americans") 8.7 per cent were American–born, with one foreign-born parent and one American-born parent; an unusual 35 per cent were American-born of foreign-born parents, and 13.6 per cent were foreign-born. On the other hand, while it has been claimed on the basis of small samples that children of South European and Jewish stock have an unusually high incidence of obesity, studies in Boston did not confirm this. Fry did not find any significant association between ethnic (white) origin and severity of obesity. Johnson, Burke and Mayer (7) did not find any significant differences between the incidence of obesity in two prosperous suburbs of Boston — Brookline (mostly Jewish) and Newton (mixed background). The fact that in the Southern United States overweight is more prevalent in white males than in white females but less prevalent in Negro males than in Negro females may be the result of a socioeconomic situation wherein the Negro men are still frequently employed in jobs entailing physical labor while Negro women no longer are so employed but are not yet subjected to social pressure for weight control. On the other hand, this difference between the white and the Negro population may be determined, at least in part, by genetic factors.

The possible interaction of environmental and genetic factors, the mixed genetic background of most human groups — particularly in Europe and North America — the fact that human genetics deals with generations whose life expectancy is similar to that of the geneticists, and the fact that some of the most useful tools of genetics (e.g. parent–offspring and brother-sister matings) are not applicable to human studies emphasize the significance of two tools which are applicable to problems such as that of genetic factors in human obesity, namely, the study of twins and the study of sex ratios.

## EVIDENCE FROM STUDIES OF TWINS

Much more cogent evidence of the importance of genetic factors in the cause of at least some forms of obesity other than the simple demonstrations of the frequent familial association is derived from Siemens' "Zwillings-Pathologie," the study of diseases in twins (5). The method is, briefly, as follows: Assuming that it is possible to diagnose with accuracy identical (monozygotic) and fraternal twins, it is then reasonable to say that if pathologic and other characteristics occur at all, they are always or nearly always present in both members of identical twin pairs, but rarely or never appear in both members of fraternal twin pairs, and that they are hereditary. (This statement does not imply the reverse, i.e. that the characteristics which are found in members of both types of pairs are not hereditary.) Newman, Freeman and Holzinger have applied the twin method to measurable characteristics such as height, weight and intelligence quotient. In this case, comparison of the variability of the quantity measured in identical twins and in fraternal twins permits a preliminary assessment of the role of heredity and of environmental factors. (A comparison of variability among siblings and individuals of the same age and sex shows far less clear-cut distinction between environmental and herediatary causes.)

Newman and associates' study bore on a large number of subjects, identical and fraternal twins, and siblings of like sex. Variability of weight was included among the many physical and mental characteristics compared. The correlation between identical twins for weight was found to be extremely high (0.973), exceeded only (and barely) by that for standing height (0.981), and higher than right and left finger ridges (0.919 and 0.931, respectively) and intelligence characteristics (Binet, 0.910, Woodward-Methews 0.562). The ratio of standard errors of estimated weight for fraternal twins to identical twins is 2.2

(22.96 lb for fraternal twin weights, compared to 10.33 lb for identical twin weights); this is of the same order as height and head length and superior to all such ratios for mental traits. When twins and siblings are paired, with the siblings being taken at comparable age, the mean pair difference in weight of siblings is 10.4 lb with 32.5 per cent differing by more than 12 lb; that of fraternal twins is 10.0 lb with 34.5 per cent differing by more than 12 lb; that of identical twins is 4.1 lb with only 2 per cent differing by more than 12 lb.

Von Verschuer, studying 57 pairs of identical twins aged 3 to 51 years, found weight somewhat more variable than other physical characteristics, but still very constant from twin to twin. Average percentage variation amounted to only 2.58 per cent. A separate calculation for those identical twins reared and living in identical environments and for those reared and living in dissimilar environments showed the average percentage variation in body weight for the first group to be 1.39 per cent and for the second group 3.6 per cent. These results would tend to demonstrate that while environmental factors play a role in the control of body weight, genetic factors are of paramount importance.

Suggestive of the importance of genetic factors in the cause of human obesity is the finding (6) that segregation can be shown to occur in the transmission of obesity. If the various types of matings — stout and stout, stout and nonstout and nonstout and nonstout — are considered, the variability of weight of the offspring is relatively small for the first type (most offspring stout, 73% in this study), least for the third type (almost none of the offspring stout, 9% in this study), and largest for the stout and nonstout matings (offspring almost evenly divided between obese, 41% and nonobese, 59%). Gurney has interpreted this as showing that stout individuals carry gametes for slenderness, while slender individuals rarely carry gametes for stoutness.

## EVIDENCE FROM SEX RATIOS OF CHILDREN

Perhaps the most striking indication of genetic determination in human obesity is Angel's (6) demonstration that the sex ratios of children in the various types of matings, as characterized by weight, are statistically different from that for the population as a whole. There are fewer males, and larger families, among the progeny of average and average matings and fat male and average female matings than among the offspring of fat and fat and average male and fat female unions. This is consistent with a hypothesis that one of the genes which in some cases helped to determine obesity is a sex-linked recessive lethal gene. Such sex-linked recessive lethals very probably occur in man. Such a gene might be expected to be more frequent among the females of the average and average matings with at least one obese daughter, where presumably the interactive nonrecessive genes mainly responsible for obesity would be less frequent, than in matings involving one or more fat parent, especially a fat father. On the other hand, the relatively larger family size of the average and average and fat female and average male matings may have purely psychologic or sociobiologic and not genetic determinants. Likewise, the relative excess of fat females aver fat males among the parents and siblings of the obese (about 60% of females are fat, as opposed to 40% of males) may express the effects of genetic sex limitation and social sex differences in activity as strongly as the effects of a hypothetical sexlinked recessive lethal factor which present data are inadequate to test. Here Angel noted that we are hampered by inability to record the potentially obese as well as the actually obese phenotypes.

## EVIDENCE FROM THE STUDY OF ADOPTED CHILDREN

Finally, in a recent study Withers (8) has attempted to differentiate genotype from phenotype in yet another way. He studied the possible correlation of overweight in adopted children and in their parents and compared it to the correlation observed between the weight of natural children and of their parents in a South London suburb. The weight picture in natural children was found to be correlated to the weights of the parents; that in the adopted children showed no correlation. I believe the evidence is convincing that in a society where food is abundant and hard physical labor unnecessary, genetic factors dictate predisposition and, to a significant extent, occurrence of overweight; but we still lack the data to permit elucidation of the mechanism of hereditary transmission.

## SOMATOTYPE, OBESITY AND GENETICS

Seltzer and Mayer (9), studying the somatotypes of obese adolescent girls, showed that these girls differed from the nonobese population in features other than differences in amount of fatty tissue. Obesity did not occur in all varieties of physical types. It occurred more frequently in some physical types than in others. The obese adolescent girls appeared to be more endomorphic, somewhat more mesomorphic, and considerably less ectomorphic than the nonobese girls of comparable age drawn from the general population. The obese series was somatotypically more homogeneous and less variable than the general population, as manifested by a lack of subjects low in endomorphy and high or even moderate in ectomorphy. In nonanthropologic language, the obese group was remarkable for large skeleton and muscle mass, which seems to be present in spite of the extreme inactivity of these obese adolescent girls (10), and by the absence of narrow, elongated extremities. Very few girls with long tapered fingers are obese. The authors caution that at present these findings are limited to adolescent females. In adults, in particular, the problem is more complex, since in that population group one must deal with those physical types which are prone to a relatively sudden blossoming into middle-age obesity, a group which to my knowledge has not yet been compared with the general population in regard to body build.

If there is a close correlation between obesity and body types in adolescents, this obviously further argues for the genetic determination of obesity, in that the hereditary character of the determination of body build has been repeatedly demonstrated. For example, Withers (8) has attempted to determine, in the working-class population of a South London suburb as well as in the sample from a boys' and a girls' school in a London borough, on whom he also reported in his study of overweight in adoptees, to what extent and in what manner endomorphy, mesomorphy and ectomorphy were transmitted from parents to children.

Several findings stood out when the results obtained in both studies were collated. The father definitely contributed meso-morphy to his sons, and the mother contributed endomorphy to her sons. The father may have also transmitted mesomorphy and ectomorphy to his daughters, and the mother endomorphy and ectomorphy to her daughters, although the size of the population studied was too small to establish these correlations definitely.

## CONCLUSION

Seltzer and Mayer's study on the association of certain somatotypes with obesity and Wither's study on the hereditary transmission of the various components of body build strongly indicate that overweight per se is probably an unsatisfactory phenotype in the study of the genetics of obesity. Lack of food and necessity for hard physical work in poor countries and extreme social pressure directed against obesity in Western countries (particularly the United States) may effectively prevent the phenotype from expressing genetic predisposition toward obesity. The complexity of the hereditary determination of body build is well known. For the present, it appears that the various approaches followed so far — studies of familial occurrence, sex ratios of offspring, twins, and adopted children; somatotyping of obese subjects; and studies of the inheritance of the various components of body build — will have to be pursued until specific inborn errors of the regulation of food intake or of fat metabolism are recognized and identified in man as they have been in experimental animals. In the long run, the examination of the mode of inheritance of such single, primary traits is likely to be easier and more fruitful.

## PRACTICAL CONSEQUENCES

From the viewpoint of the practicing physician, there was a time when the fact that a condition was genetically determined gave it a character of hopelessness. This is no longer true. In previous articles in this series, dietary treatments have been described for preventing the main pathologic consequences of phenylpyruvic oligophrenia, galactosomeia, disaccharidase deficiencies and pyridoxine dependency. Diabetes is an outstanding example of a condition which appears to be genetically determined and yet is the object of daily, and to a large extent successful, therapeutics. The same should be true of obesity, and its genetic aspects can actually be taken advantage of in at least three ways:

1. Detection of other obese patients. It is obvious from the preceding discussion that siblings and children of obese patients are much more prone to obesity than others.

2. Prevention. If there is one disease condition where an ounce of prevention is better than a pound of cure, it is obesity. It has been shown repeatedly that on a statistical basis treatment of obesity is not very successful. This may be in part because obesity sets up a psychologic chain of events which tends to make the condition self-perpetuating; i.e. obsessive concern with weight leads to passivity, expectation of rejection, greater inactivity, etc (11). Recent work from my laboratory also suggests that when a subject has once been obese some irreversible physiologic changes occur which may make the regaining of lost weight more "efficient" than the first weight gain. The realization of the susceptibility to obesity of obese patients' close relatives should provide the pediatrician or the school physician with a rationale for early institution of an adequate regimen of dietary instruction and exercise for likely candidates for overweight.

3. Pharmacologic treatment of specific syndromes. In the long run, if it is verified that certain obesity (or obesity and diabetes) syndromes in man are due to an inborn enzymatic abnormality, as the hereditary obese hyperglycemic syndrome in the mouse appears to be, it may become possible to find specific drug treatment for well-identified syndromes. While an increasing amount of research work is directed toward this end, practical measures are not yet in sight. For the time being diet, exercise and, in some cases, the judicious use of anorexigenic agents remain our only tools.

## REFERENCES

1. Mayer, J.: The obese hyperglycemic syndrome of mice as an example of "metabolic" obesity. Amer. J. Clin. Nutr., 8:712, 1960.
2. ——: Metabolism of the adipose tissue in the hereditary obese

hyperglycemic syndrome. In Rodah., K. and Issekutz, B., Jr. (Editors): Fat as a Tissue. New York, McGraw-Hill Book Company, Inc., 1964, chap. 16, p. 329.

3. ——: Genetic, traumatic and environmental factors in the etiology of obesity. Physiol. Rev., 33:472, 1953.

4. ——: Obesity. Ann Rev Med 14:111, 1963.

5. Bauer, J.: Constitution and Disease. New York, Grune & Stratton, Inc., 1945.

6. Angel, J. L.: Constitution in female obesity. Amer. J. Phys. Anthrop., 7:433, 1949.

7. Johnson, M. D., Burke, B. S. and Mayer, J.: Incidence and prevalence of obesity in a section of school children in the Boston area. Amer. J. Clin. Nutr., 4:231, 1956.

8. Withers, R. F. J.: Problems in the genetics of human obesity. Eugen. Rev., 56:81, 1964.

9. Seltzer, C. C. and Mayer, J.: Body build and obesity: Who are the obese? J.A.M.A., 189:677, 1964.

10. Bullen, B. A., Reed, R. B. and Mayer, J.: Physical activity of obese adolescent girls measured by motion-picture sampling. Amer. J. Clin. Nutr., 14:211, 1964.

11. Monello, L. F. and Mayer, J.: Obese adolescent girls: An unrecognized "minority" group? Amer. J. Clin. Nutr., 13:35, 1963.

## Chapter 32

# OBESITY: DIAGNOSIS

THE matter of caloric requirement is obviously fundamental to the analysis of the pathogenesis of disorders of energy metabolism. A caloric intake in excess of requirements eventually will cause obesity; a prolonged deficit will cause emaciation. The effect of the lack of physical activity on appetite, so often misunderstood and minimized, is probably the root of the slowly accumulating excess fat in many sedentary middle-aged persons who have no particular defect in the physiologic mechanism of the regulation of food intake and no psychogenic hyperphagia. Yet, these facts alone are quite insufficient to explain this most widespread condition. In fact, I am convinced that we can effectively treat obesity only when we recognize the extreme complexity of the problem. Hyperphagia and obesity may be common aspects of syndromes which have little in common otherwise. Before elaborating on a philosophy of treating the obesities, it may be pertinent to review recent investigations in the field of appetite and obesity, even though (as is true in the first stages of studying any disease or syndrome) most of the evidence is still largely experimental in nature.

## REASONS FOR DIAGNOSING AND IDENTIFYING OBESITY

It may be necessary to recall that obesity is a problem for the practitioner. Although this statement may appear self-evident, it must be recognized that the majority of obese subjects view their obesity first of all as an aesthetic problem and sometimes as a moral problem or, at least, a problem in human relations. Obesity has been so derided that obese patients feel unattractive, and they are afraid of being considered sensual and weak. Most persons are

Reprinted from *Postgraduate Medicine, 25* (No. 4), April, 1959.

motivated to place themselves on a diet or to ask for a reducing regimen because they are concerned with their appearance and with public opinion rather than with their health. If these were the only problems to be considered, one could well question whether it is the physician's function to devote time and effort to encourage and help weight reduction.

Actually, life insurance studies have clearly demonstrated that obesity is accompanied by increased mortality from a number of degenerative diseases. Dublin and Marks (1), of the Metropolitan Life Insurance Company, deserve particular credit for establishing incontrovertible evidence of the association of obesity and disease. They have shown statistically that obese persons who reduce and stay reduced may substantially increase their life expectancy. Yet, at the same time, it is highly probable that the link between obesity and disease is more complex than the simple cause-and-effect relationship often suggested. To be sure, the excess fat in some persons is obviously dangerous per se. It increases surgical risk by making administration of anesthesia more delicate and causing operations to be performed through layers of fat. It increases the probability of hepatic disease whenever it causes actual fatty infiltration of the liver. Increased mortality from accidents can be attributed to the fact that the obese person is a larger, clumsier and slower target as well as a poorer surgical risk after the accident.

On the other hand, it is likely that in many cases the relationship between obesity and disease is associative as well as causative. Table 32-1 indicates that while most correlations between causes of death and obesity are positive there are two causes of death which are negatively correlated with obesity: suicide and tuberculosis. In fact, it has been shown that the lesser mortality from tuberculosis in obese patients is not an artifact due to the decreased food intake of patients with a prolonged infection. Long-term studies (2) have shown that overweight persons are less prone to have tuberculosis. Incidentally, the decreased incidence of tuberculosis in overweight persons may explain why stoutness was so long equated with health in the Western world. (This is still the popular view in many underdeveloped countries.) Similarly, a causative relationship

TABLE 32-1

ACTUAL AND EXPECTED DEATHS OF OVERWEIGHT MEN AND WOMEN
BETWEEN 25 AND 74 YEARS OF AGE*

| Cause of Death | Men | | Women | |
|---|---|---|---|---|
| | Deaths | Expected deaths (per cent) | Deaths | Expected deaths (per cent) |
| Principal cardiovascular-renal diseases | 1,867 | *149* | 1,103 | *177* |
| Organic heart disease, diseases of the coronary arteries, and angina pectoris | 1,377 | *142* | 697 | *175* |
|    Organic heart disease | 748 | † | 515 | † |
|    Coronary disease and angina pectoris | 629 | † | 182 | † |
|    Cerebral hemorrhage | 247 | *159* | 226 | *162* |
|    Chronic nephritis | 243 | *191* | 180 | *212* |
| Cancer, all forms | 385 | 97 | 476 | 100 |
|    Stomach | 62 | 85 | 34 | 86 |
|    Liver and gallbladder | 33 | *168* | 46 | 211 |
|    Peritoneum, intestines and rectum | 103 | 115 | 93 | 104 |
|    Pancreas | 19 | 93 | 21 | 149 |
|    Respiratory organs | 39 | 78‡ | – | – |
|    Breast | – | – | 81 | *69* |
|    Genital organs | – | – | 132 | 107 |
|    Uterus | – | – | 103 | 121 |
|    Leukemia and Hodgkin's disease | 26 | 100 | 23 | 110 |
| Diabetes | 205 | *383* | 235 | *372* |
| Tuberculosis, all forms | 24 | *21* | 20 | *35* |
| Pneumonia, all forms | 98 | 102 | 78 | 129 |
| Cirrhosis of the liver | 96 | *249* | 32 | 147 |
| Appendicitis | 76 | *223* | 41 | *195* |
| Hernia and intestinal obstruction | 39 | *154*‡ | 31 | *141*‡ |
| Biliary calculi and other gallbladder diseases | 32 | 152‡ | 30 | *188*‡ |
|    Biliary calculi | 19 | *206* | 50 | *284* |
| Ulcer of stomach and duodenum | 30 | 67 | – | – |
| Puerperal conditions | – | – | 43 | *162* |
| Suicide | 63 | *78* | 23 | *73* |
| Accidents, total | 177 | 111 | 74 | *135* |
|    Automobile | 76 | *131* | 27 | 120 |
|    Falls | 32 | 131 | – | – |

*According to estimates of contemporary mortality experience on standard risks. From 1925 to 1934 issues of the *Statistical Bulletin, Metropolitan Life Insurance Company,* ordinary department; traced to policy anniversary in 1950. Numbers in italics indicate statistically significant deviations from experience on standard risks.

† Satisfactory basis for comparison not available.

‡ Based on mortality of standard risks from 1935 to 1939.

obviously is ruled out for the association of overwieght with a decreased mortality from suicide. Apparently, the physical and psychologic characteristics which favor the development of obesity do not favor the development of the suicidal state.

Nonketotic diabetes in middle-aged obese patients is an illustration of the complexity of the association of obesity and disease. This syndrome probably entails associative factors (both hyperphagia and diabetes may result from the basic impairment in metabolism of carbohydrate) as well as causative factors. The "lipoplethoric" state of adipose tissue undoubtedly contributes to the deterioration of the glucose tolerance, which is generally improved by weight reduction. The relationship of obesity to heart disease may well be even more complicated. By exerting pressure on the capillaries, excess fat may cause increased peripheral resistance to flow; it may impair the function of the heart, because the heart itself is infiltrated with fat; and it may increase the work of an inefficient cardiovascular system because of the extra weight to be moved. Obesity and deficient cardiovascular function both may result from a sedentary, sluggish mode of life and from excessive consumption of an atherogenic diet.

It also is likely that the relationship between obesity property, i.e. excessive adiposity, and disease has been obscured by the fact that the insurance tables which provide the bulk of available data were established in terms of body "weight," not body "fat." Selected "overweight" groups, such as the California longshoremen studied by Buechley, Drake and Breslow (3), have a favorable health picture. In spite of these complexities, it is reasonable to conclude that the relationship of obesity and disease is sufficiently close to allow obesity to be considered a serious menace to health. Within certain limits, which I shall try to define, the known facts justify vigorous efforts to try to bring most patients to a reasonable weight.

## DEFINITION OF OBESITY: LIMITATIONS
## OF HEIGHT-WEIGHT TABLES

It already has been implied that we are principally concerned with obesity, i.e. excess fat accumulation. Such a definition denotes a weight in excess of some norm for the height, ususally that established on the basis of the weight of insurance policy-holders less than 30 years of age. Tables of "normal," "standard," "ideal" and "desirable" weights are widely available. In theory they make the diagnosis of obesity easy. If a patient weighs in excess of the normal weight for his height, he is overweight; if he weighs less, he is underweight. Actually, there are a number of reasons why the thoughtful physician will not be satisfied to substitute a table for clinical judgment.

The first tables of normal or standard weights in general use in the United States were compiled by Charles B. Davenport for the Medico-Actuarial survey of 1912. Heights of subjects were recorded with their shoes on, weights with their clothes on (1885 to 1900 clothes at that). So many of the weights ended in 0 and 5 that some observers concluded that the weights were estimated, not measured. There is even greater uncertainty when the phrase "with shoes on" is applied to women. The weight of women's street clothes also must have varied more from year to year in that era, which saw rapid changes in women's fashion.

The basis of these older tables is also vitiated by the fact that at the end of the nineteenth century the practice of buying life insurance was not as widespread as it is now. It was confined to a relatively small group of prosperous persons. Thus, the normal weight for a given age was normal for only a wealthy and relatively inactive group. This limitation was only partly corrected by the later life insurance company tables, which are based on the following modifications of the 1912 figures. The weights for men are predicated on their standard weight at age 30. This is based on the generally justified assumption that any increase in weight from then on is essentially adipose tissue. It may have been that the 1912 figures represented the weight of subjects after several years of inactivity, which would have caused all weights to be higher than they would have been at, say, age 25.

Corrections were made in the 1912 tables, because it was felt that those figures tended to overestimate the correct body weight of tall subjects and to underestimate that of short persons. Further adjustments were made to correct the gradation of values at successive heights. Then, groups were set up on both sides of the figures thus obtained. The three columns thus arbitrarily achieved were designated as ideal or desirable weights for persons with small, medium or large frames.

It must be noted that the weights for the various frames were never based on actual measurements of persons classified by frame. No method was given to determine the size of the frame, nor, for that matter, was the term defined. To be sure, the experienced physician may have acquired an implicit concept of frame based on skeletal size, as estimated by the size of the wrist and the ankle, width of the shoulders, etc. This concept is difficult to apply and certainly open to differing interpretations. Patients tend to give themselves the benefit of the doubt by "adopting" a large frame.

Obviously, if fatness is the problem, a definition based on fatness is necessary. While tables based on height-weight ratios may be useful for actuarial predictions or for public health studies on populations, they do not give the information the clinician needs in order to work with individual patients.

## MEASUREMENT OF BODY FAT

About half the total body fat is deposited in the subcutaneous adipose tissue and is readily accessible for observation and measurement. Cursory visual examination of the naked subject generally will tell an experienced physician whether or not the patient is obese. The time-honored method of pinching the patient in appropriate places can settle doubt in many cases in which observation alone is inconclusive. While to date the caliper has been more an instrument of research than a tool of the general practitioner, its use is simple and permits actual measurement of subcutaneous fat thickness. Thus, the qualitative indication of manual pinching can be put on a systematic basis and validated by comparison with other methods. The true skin is only about 1 mm thick, so that most of the variation in thickness of skinfolds pinched up in different patients represents differences in subcutaneous fat. Thickness of fat layers at many points on the surface of the body has been found to be closely correlated to the total fat content. Two locations are particularly informative and easy to reach. The first is the area over the triceps muscle on the back of the upper arm, midway between the elbow and the tip of the shoulder. In adult men, the thickness of the skinfold at this point varies from about 4 to 50 mm or more. The next most useful site to test is over the tip of the scapula on the back. Other places for measurement include over the pectoral muscle on the chest, over the biceps, and various points on the abdomen.

As is well known, there are differences in localization of subcutaneous fat between children and adults. Small children have more fat on the arms than on the abdomen; adults show the opposite picture. There are classic differences in fat distribution between men and women. For instance, the thickness of fat layers on the calf of the leg is better correlated with total body fat in women than in men. Incidentally, this area is difficult to use for skinfold measurements, because the subcutaneous later tends to be more tightly adherent, and it may be difficult to obtain a real skinfold.

Data obtained with calipers* of standard dimensions, which exert standardized pressure (usually 10 gm per square millimeter of caliper jawface in contact with the skin), have been successfully compared with measurements obtained from roentgenograms of soft tissue. In turn, these determinations of subcutaneous fat have been correlated with calculations of total body fat obtained by densimetry. This method, based on weighing the subject first in air then under water (with elaborate corrections for the air in the lungs and respiratory passages at the moment of weighing), was pioneered by Behnke and further refined by Keys and Brozek (4). Total body fat can also be estimated from weight and total body water, which is obtained by heavy water dilution.

These methods have made it possible to demonstrate the differences in fat content between the sexes, between age groups, and between sedentary workers and those employed more strenuously, as well as to differentiate between overweight, and obesity. It has been shown, for example, that the total body fat content of 25-year-old women is at least 50 per cent greater than that of men of the same age. Thin, 40-year-old women may have

---

*Harpenden skinfold calipers are available from British Indicators, Ltd., Sutton Road, St. Albans, Herts, England.

up to twice as much fat as muscular men of the same age. A picturesque determination conducted by Welham and Behnke (5) exemplified the distinction between overweight and obesity. The average guard or tackle on a college or professional football team weighs 200 lb or more. Even in relation to his height and even when he is considered in the "large frame" class, the 6-foot, 200-lb lineman is at least 10 per cent overweight, according to the best-known table of ideal weights. Yet, when navy scientists examined 17 professional football players, several of whom were former All-Americans, they found them endowed with a greater than normal specific gravity, indicating an abnormally low fat content. These overweight men were underfat. Conversely, it has been repeatedly shown, particularly by Keys and Brozek, that sedentary men of normal weight may, in fact, be obese in terms of being excessively fat.

Aging in the adult is particularly interesting. The old tables of normal height and weight appeared to condone the progressive accumulation of weight during maturity. This adjustment for age is one criticizable feature which has been eliminated in more recent tables. Data obtained by calipers and by densimetry clearly show that weight which accumulates after completion of muscular and skeletal growth is useless or dangerous fat.

Even if the same weight is maintained throughout adult life, active tissue is progressively replaced by fat. Keys (6) compared 33 younger (age 22 to 29) men with 33 older (age 48 to 57) men of the same height and weight. The fat content of the older men was found to be 50 per cent greater than that of the younger men (38% at mean age 56, and 25% at mean age 24). Active persons who continue to exercise into middle age maintain a proportionately greater lean body mass than do sedentary people, but even in these subjects there is, if weight remains constant, a steady increase in total body fat. It would appear that the only way by which all patients (particularly highly muscular persons who stop intensive exercising) can prevent the progressive accumulation of fat is to stop gaining weight at the age of 25 and, over the later years, slowly to lose weight. In other words, patients should be encouraged to do what the French clinicians call *vieillir sec* − "to age dry."

The distinction between overweight and obesity and the variations in body composition with age pose some interesting problems of medical statistics. Is the 6-foot, 200-lb overweight athlete really in the same risk category as the sedentary overfat person of the same height and weight? Is it as bad from the viewpoint of prognosis to carry too much muscle as it is to carry too much fat? Or, if disease were correlated with fatness rather than with weight, would the correlation between obesity and increased morbidity and mortality be even more striking; Certainly, the improvement due to losing weight (in this case, weight must be synonymous with fat) would suggest that the latter hypothesis is the correct one; however, the final proof of this theory has yet to be given.

The way in which a patient is obese may be important. Certain European clinicians attach considerable importance to the distribution of excess fat. Android obesity (the "John Bull" type) is characterized by accumulation of excess visible fat in the upper half of the body, and gynecoid obesity affects the lower half. Vague and associates (7) distinguished five categories of obesity, from hyperandroid to hypergynecoid, and considered that hypertension and diabetes occur much more frequently in the android than in the gynecoid type. Whether or not statistical evidence confirms this finding, Vague's studies testify to an analytic view of the relationship of obesity to disease which is likely to be more fruitful in defining types of syndromes that is classifying of weight according to universal standards which are doubtful.

## PRACTICAL CRITERIA OF DIAGNOSIS AND FINAL TARGETS OF TREATMENT

A practical definition of obesity can be evolved from this general approach: A man may be described as definitely obese if his total fat content exceeds 25 to 30 per cent of total body weight; a woman, if her total fat content exceeds 30 to 35 per cent.

Obviously, no elaborate measurements are needed to diagnose obesity in a man of of ordinary height who weighs 250 lb or in a woman who weighs 200 lb. On the other hand, clinical observation

— looking at the nude body or pinching up skinfolds — is necessary to diagnose obesity in a patient who is 10 to 30 per cent overweight according to standard height-weight tables. The use of skinfold calipers, while not necessary for diagnosis, may allow obesity to be classified on a more quantitative basis. Obesity can thus be redefined on the basis of skinfold thickness. Obesity is present in men if the skinfold thickness of the triceps is greater than 15 mm. An exception may be made for very tall men (6 ft, 2 in or more), in whom 18 to 20 mm can be taken as the lower limit of obesity. Similarly, obesity is present in women if the skinfold thickness over the triceps is greater than 25 mm. As a practical guide for the patient, male patients may be told that they should be unable to pinch a skinfold mor than 1 inch thick on the abdomen under the navel; female patients should be unable to pinch more than 1.5 inches.

A patient's desirable weight should be determined by his physician, not from an automatic reading in a table. Such a judgment should be based on the patients appearance, his age, the natural history of his obesity, and information on his ancestry. It is often useful to know whether the obese patient resembles an obese parent or grandparent and to know the weight, duration of life, and cause of death of the latter. In a middle-aged man, the best target for weight reduction is often his weight at age 25; in a middle-aged woman, it is her weight at age 21 or 22. Weight accumulated after that time is excess fat, except, perhaps, in extraordinary cases in which muscle development has been pursued since that age. Setting these weights as goals avoids questions about body build and gives the patient a sense of identification with the aim of the reduction program.

The physician may want to keep a youngster's weight near constant and to let the patient grow to the height considered approximate for the weight. Indeed, the role of the physician may be to convince his young patients, particularly adolescent girls, that they should increase their weight to what he regards as reasonable. There is little doubt that a proportion of the anemias, amenorrheas, etc. seen in adolescent girls result from self-inflicted malnutrition based on a wish to be thinner than is desirable for their health and, more often than not, for their appearance. The use of high-protein, high-mineral, high-vitamin, calorically restricted diets may permit pregnant women not to reduce their weight as such, but to maintain a constant weight during pregnancy and let delivery and postpartum weight losses effect the desired weight. Again, this desired weight should be determined by the physician, not by a mechanically applied and easily misinterpreted table or by the dictates of fashion.

The use of anthropometric data — skinfold thickness, waist circumference, size of clothes, etc. — will bring home to the patient the point which she or, more particularly, he may not have been willing to face; namely, that he is not just "stout" or "heavy," but *fat*. The use of skinfold or body measurements may thus help to motivate the patient. Determination of body fat is particularly interesting in situations in which muscle development and resultant protein weight gain are desired at the same time as in loss of fat, such as in inactive adolescents who should be reduced, at least in part, by increase in physical exercise.

Finally, only the application of systematic observation will allow "typing" of obese patients, a prerequisite for describing the various syndromes entailing obesity and a help in organizing clinical data. More important, the anthropometric, metabolic and psychologic identification of such types is a necessary step if the chances of success and effectiveness of treatment are to improve.

## REFERENCES

1. Dublin, L. I. and Marks, H. H.: Mortality among insured overweights in recent years. Tr. A. Life Insur. M. Dir. America, 35:235, 1952.
2. Berry, W. T. C. and Nash, F. A.: Studies in the aetiology of pulmonary tuberculosis. Tubercle, 36:164, 1955.
3. Buechley, R. W., Drake, R. M. and Breslow, L.: Height, weight and mortality in a population of longshoremen. J. Chron. Dis., 7:363, 1956.
4. Keys, A. J. and Brozek, J.: Body fat in adult man. Physiol. Rev., 33:245, 1953.
5. Welham, W. C. and Behnke, A. R., Jr.: The specific gravity of healthy men; body weight ÷ volume and other physical characteristics of exceptional athletes and of naval personnel. J.A.M.A., 118:498, 1942.
6. Keys, A. J.: Weight changes and health of men. In Weight Control. A collection of papers presented at the Weight Control Colloquy. Ames, Iowa, The Iowa State College Press, 1955, p. 108.
7. Vague, J., Jouve, A., Delaage, M. and Teitelbaum, M.: Les relations de l'obesite et de l'ateriosclerose. Semaine hôp. Paris, 14:1 629 (September) 1957.

*Chapter 33*

# A SIMPLE CRITERION
# OF OBESITY*

*Written in collaboration with Carl C. Seltzer*

IN an article (1) published in 1959, one of us (J.M.) discussed existing definitions of overweight and obesity and pointed out that excessive adiposity, not simply a weight in excess of published averages, was the object of the clinician's concern. It was noted that while tables defining the normal limits of variations of weight for height were available and had been widely publicized, no such standards were available for obesity. It was suggested that of all exsisting methods for measuring body fat on which a definition of obesity might be based, caliper determination of skinfold thickness offered the greatest promise in terms of a basis for definition and of practical application.

Since that time several studies of body fat have been performed, some in our own laboratory, by a number of methods. Methods based on multiple anthropometric measurements (2) and on naturally occurring total body radiopotassium (3) have been described. Other studies have been based on measurements of total body water and body density and on indirect attempts at estimating fat by measuring skinfold thickness by means of radiography of soft tissues, krypton absorption, etc. Performance or observation of these studies has reinforced our belief that while methods other than skinfold determinations are important research tools, their execution is too difficult and time-consuming

*This publication is based on data obtained from studies supported in part by a grant-in-aid from the Bureau of State Services, Research and Development Division of Chronic Diseases (DC-00082-01), National Institutes of Health, United States Public Health Service, Bethesda (Department of Nutrition, Harvard University School of Public Health); from the Elsie T. Freedman Foundation (Adolescents' Unit, Children's Hospital); and from the Fund for Research and Teaching of the Department of Nutrition, Harvard University School of Public Health, Boston.
Reprinted from *Postgraduate Medicine, 38* (No. 2), August, 1965.

for the physician who wants to make a rapid diagnosis of obesity, obtain a reasonably accurate estimate of its extent, and follow its changes. We are convinced that the measurement of skinfold thickness and particularly of the most accessible, the triceps skinfold, permits a clear definition of obesity and a satisfactory assessment of its extent (4).

In this chapter we will review the basis on which the height-weight tables were established, point out their serious weaknesses and the difficulties inherent to their use, and suggest alternative criteria of obesity for males and females in the 5-to 50-year-age range based on the size of the triceps skinfold.

## HEIGHT-WEIGHT TABLES

The appearance of the naked patient is the usual basis for the diagnosis of obesity by the experienced clinician and, as a qualitative guide, is usually reliable. When a quantitative estimate is desired, the patient's weight is usually compared with the "standard" weight for his height as given by one of several tables. For children and adolescents, the standard is usually an average weight for height, age and sex. The variety of tables available included the Baldwin-Wood, Bayer and Bayley, Stuart, Hathaway, Falkner, etc. Some of these tables show percentiles as well as medians. The Wetzel grid defines channels expressing percentiles of weight for height, independent of age.

For adults, such standards are either average weight for height, age and sex or so-called ideal or desirable weight for height, age, sex and, in some cases, frame. For many decades the most commonly used were the life insurance standards based on the Medico-Actuarial investigations of insurance companies and published in 1912 (5). The two tables, one for each sex, listed the average weights for various heights and ages for men and women. These tables were based on measurements or, in some instances, estimates of the height (with shoes on) and weight (with clothes on) of life insurance policy holders who had bought their policies from 1885 to 1908. In 1929 a large sample of additional heights and weights collected from 1909 to 1927 was collated in connection with the "Medical Impairment Study" and found to be so similar to the 1912 averages that it was not considered worthwhile to prepare new tables.

In 1943 the Metropolitan Life Insurance Company actuarians introduced a new standard table based on the different principles. First they recognized the undesirability of continued increase in weight during adulthood past the termination of growth and, secondly, they realized, at least in theory, that people have different builds. Accordingly, the age scale was eliminated and the new table was based on averages obtained from younger age groups. Furthermore, the single average weight values were replaced by weight ranges corresponding to three classes of frame size — small, medium and large. As in the previous tables, the height measurements were made with shoes on and weight measurements with clothes on "as ordinarily dressed." Apparently the classification of a given individual's frame into one of the three categories was left to the subjective judgment of the examiner, as no specific definitions for the three frames were given.

The "Build and Blood Pressure Study, 1959" (6) of the Society of Actuaries provided the basis for the latest (and currently most used) "average" and "desirable" weight tables. The average weight tables are based on data obtained by 26 United States and Canadian life insurance companies on several million policyholders. Mortality of this population was followed for periods up to 20 years and analyzed for its relationship to body build (height and weight). The subjects' weight was recorded in ordinary indoor clothing and their height was measured with their shoes on. The authors of the study estimated that nude weights are 7 to 9 lb less than recorded weights for men and 4 to 6 lb less for women and that the height differential without shoes was 1 inch for men and 2 inches for women. Body frame was classified as small, medium or large on the basis of chest breadth and hip width; no data or description of method was given. Furthermore, the significance of these measures for proper body build assessment is extremely limited. In addition, the Metropolitan Life Insurance Company followed with a new table of desirable weights based on the pooled experience of greatest longevity.

## Limitations of Tables

It is obvious that if overweight (weight in excess of average) is very marked, obesity (excessive fatness) is present. For moderate degrees of overweight, however, obesity is by no means clear. College football linemen are generally not obese. Conversely, some extremely sedentary persons can be obese without being markedly overweight. Without a more direct measurement of adiposity, the diagnosis of obesity cannot be certain.

The standards derived from the "Build and Blood Pressure Study, 1959" have additional weaknesses. First, there is some question as to how representative the insurance data are for the general population of the United States. One of us (C.C.S.) has shown that average weights in the Metropolitan Life tables are 9 to 10 lb less for men and 3 to 4 lb less for women than the average values obtained in the National Health Examination Survey of the United States Public Health Service on a stratified, non-institutionalized random sample of men and women from all classes and areas of the country from 1960 through 1962 (7). Secondly, the Metropolitan Life Insurance Company tables give no definitions of frames, so that the user is unable to characterize his frame in the same way as the authors of the tables.

Recent epidemiologic data have shown that properly defined variations in body structure are important not only in terms of defining obesity, but also possible in terms of longevity. Our analysis of the data of the "Build and Blood Pressure Study, 1959" tends to suggest this. In general, for each broad height category, mortality increased as weight increased. These data have been interpreted to mean that increased overweight is responsible for increased mortality. However, since persons who have the lowest weight for height (referred to by the life insurance companies' acutarians as underweights) and who must be for the most part dominant ectomorphs (rather than emaciated meso-morphs and endomorphs) have the highest longevity, it appears that this body type is associated with a longer-than-average life expectancy. The significant association of obesity with bones and muscles larger than average, which we (8) have demonstrated in females, suggests that at least among females there may be an association between increased mortality and body type, irre-spective of adiposity. Gertler and White (9) and Spain, Bradess and Greenblatt (10) also have suggested the association of certain body types with specific diseases. The ultimate answer to the question of the relation of obesity to mortality may lie in treating each type of body build separately and in correlating the extent of adiposity of each category of body build with mortality and disease manifestations.

While it is not our intention to quarrel with the general concept that excessive weight gain after growth has ceased is bad for the patient, it appears questionable to base the diagnosis of obesity and the prescription of ideal weight for a given patient on height-weight tables, even those as seemingly sophisticated as the ones derived from the "Build and Blood Pressure Study, 1959." A knowledge of the patient's actual fatness is preferable not only from the viewpoint of diagnosing obesity, but also because it emphasizes that component of body weight which can, in fact, be modified.

## MEASUREMENT OF SKINFOLD THICKNESS

Measurement of skinfold thickness appears to be the simplest and most practical available method of determining the extent of obesity. These measurements, obtained by using a suitable caliper on selected sites, have been shown by comparison with results of other methods to give good indication not only of subcutaneous fat (about 50% of the total fat) but also of total body fat. The technic is simple, and the caliper relatively inexpensive.* With proper directions and a minimum of demonstration by an experienced person, the physician can obtain reproducible measurements with the skinfold caliper.

Standardization of skin-fold calipers has become a necessary requiremnt for universal comparability of fatfold measurements and conversion to total body fat. The accepted national recommendation is a caliper so designed as to exert a pressure on the caliper face of 10 gm per square millimeter and with a contact surface of 20 to 40 mm (2).†

The skinfold measurement to be obtained is the (doubled)

---

*Calipers usually range in price from $65 to $75.

†Skinfold calipers meeting these requirements include the Lange Skinfold Caliper manufactured by the Cambridge Scientific Industries Inc., Cambridge, Maryland, and the Harpenden Skinfold Caliper, Manufactured by British Indicators, Ltd., St. Albans, Hertsfordshire, England.

thickness of the pinched "folded" skin plus the attached sub-cutaneous adipose tissue. The person making the measurement pinches up a full fold of skin and subcutaneous tissue with the thumb and forefinger of his left hand at a distance about 1 cm from the site at which the calipers are to be placed, pulling the fold away from the underlying muscle. The fold is pinched up firmly and held while the measurement is being taken. The calipers are applied to the fold about 1 cm below the fingers, so that the pressure on the fold at the point measured is exerted by the faces of the caliper and not by the fingers. The handle of the caliper is released to permit the full force of the caliper arm pressure, and the dial is read to the nearest 0.5 mm. Caliper application should be made at least twice for stable readings. If the folds are extremely thick, dial readings should be made three seconds after applying the caliper pressure.

## Sites Measured for Skinfold Thickness

Various workers have used a number of sites, including the triceps, subscapular, abdominal, hip, pectoral and calf areas. For the general population, the Committee on Nutritional Anthropometry of the National Research Council has recommended the triceps and the subscapular skinfolds as good indexes of an individual's overall fatness (11).

## Triceps Skinfold

The triceps skinfold is located at the back of the right upper arm midway between the acromion and olecranon processes. The midpoint can be marked with the aid of a steel tape. The arm should hang freely during the skinfold measurement. Because of the gradation of subcutaneous fat thickness from shoulder to elbow, location of the midpoint is somewhat critical.

## Subscapular Skinfold

The subscapular skinfold is located just below the angle of the right scapula (shoulder and arm relaxed). The fold is picked up in a line slightly inclined in the natural clevage of the skin. Because the subcutaneous fat is fairly uniform in this region, precision of location is less critical.

Our work (4) as well as that of others leads us to believe that for obese individuals the triceps skinfold, which is the easiest to measure, is also the most representative of total body fatness. No special advantage is gained in utilizing any other skinfold in addition to the triceps skinfold.

## CRITERION FOR OBESITY

Extensive data on the distribution of triceps skinfold values, such as those obtained by Young and Blondin (12) and Novak (13), allow determination of the normal variation of such skinfolds in our population (at least for Caucasian subjects). The next step, setting up a cutoff point for obesity, is obviously arbitrary. Because of its association with certain body types, the distribution of fatness within the general population may not be strictly monomodal; it does, however, represent a continuum, and any cutoff point would be a practical rather than a theoretically based selection. Furthermore, while this selection may represent a common fat content, it may not represent a common risk, because the significance of a given body fat content may differ with body type. Finally, it must be noted that the relation of skinfold thickness to body fat content is virtually independent of height (4). This permits giving a single value for each sex and age as a cutoff point.

Based on these concentrations, we recommend that in the American population the qualification of obesity be reserved for those individuals less than 30 years old in whom the triceps skinfold is greater by more than one standard deviation than the mean.* Furthermore, the standard established for subjects 30 years old should be applied to men and women in the 30-to 50-year-age group. Table 33-1 shows the details of this definition in numerical terms; the minimal limits of our obesity criteria are shown graphically in Figure 33-1.

The very definition of standard deviation signifies that 16 per

---

*The triceps skinfold frequency distribution is typically skewed to the right. To normalize the distribution, the logarithmic mean rather than the arithmetic mean is determined before establishing the cutoff point. This prevents very obese members of the population from unduly influencing the determination of the mean.

## TABLE 33-1

### OBESITY STANDARDS IN CAUCASIAN AMERICANS

| Age (Years) | Minimum Triceps, Skin Fold Thickness Indicating Obesity (Millimeters) | |
|---|---|---|
| | Males | Females |
| 5 | 12 | 14 |
| 6 | 12 | 15 |
| 7 | 13 | 16 |
| 8 | 14 | 17 |
| 9 | 15 | 18 |
| 10 | 16 | 20 |
| 11 | 17 | 21 |
| 12 | 18 | 22 |
| 13 | 18 | 23 |
| 14 | 17 | 23 |
| 15 | 16 | 24 |
| 16 | 15 | 25 |
| 17 | 14 | 26 |
| 18 | 15 | 27 |
| 19 | 15 | 27 |
| 20 | 16 | 28 |
| 21 | 17 | 28 |
| 22 | 18 | 28 |
| 23 | 18 | 28 |
| 24 | 19 | 28 |
| 25 | 20 | 29 |
| 26 | 20 | 29 |
| 27 | 21 | 29 |
| 28 | 22 | 29 |
| 29 | 22 | 29 |
| 30-50 | 23 | 30 |

cent of the present American population less than 30 years of age are obese. Our experience with obesity in children, adolescents and young adults leads us to believe that experienced workers in the field, whatever the basis for their criteria, would recognize at least a similar proportion as obese.* For example, for 16-year-old girls the median skinfold thickness is 16 mm corresponding to

---

*This does not mean that a physician may not consider some patients whose skinfolds are slightly below our cutoff points to be too fat for their body builds. Our criteria defines frank obesity.

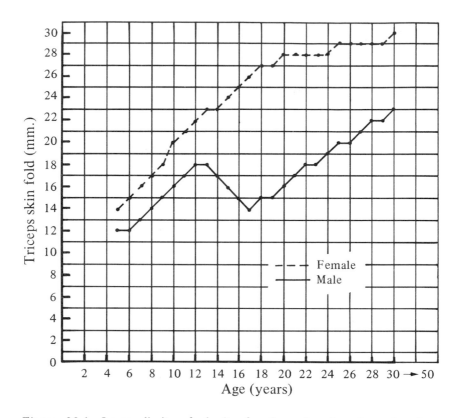

Figure 33-1. Lower limits of obesity for Caucasian Americans based on measurements of skinfold thickness.

about 23 per cent of the body as fat. The suggested criterion for obesity is 25 mm corresponding to 39 per cent of the body as fat. For persons more than 30 years old the proportion of obesity as defined by the criterion proposed here would increase far above 16 per cent in accordance with the general observation that middle-aged obesity is more prevalent than in the population at the younger ages.

## COMMENT

The interpretation of the proposed standards for determining obesity in terms of health awaits the results of research on the relation of mortality and morbidity to adiposity. Meanwhile, criteria of obesity actually based on a measurement of fatness seem superior to criteria based on inference of fatness.

## REFERENCES

1. Mayer, J.: Obesity: Diagnosis Postgrad. Med. 25:469 (April) 1959.
2. Behnke, A. R.: Anthropometric estimate of body size, shape and fat content. Postgrad. Med., 34:190 (August) 1963.
3. Christian, J. E., Combs, L. W. and Kessler, W. V.: Potassium 40 measurements of body composition. Postgrad. Med., 36:156 (August) 1964.
4. Seltzer, C. C., Goldman, R. F. and Mayer, J.: The triceps skinfold as a predictive measure of the body density and body fat in obese adolescent girls. Pediatrics. (In press.)
5. Medico-Actuarial Mortality Investigation. Trans. Ass. Life Insur. Med. Dir. Amer., 1912, vol. 1.
6. Build and Blood Pressure Study, 1959. Chicago, Society of Actuaries, 1959, vol. 1.
7. Seltzer, C. C.: Limitations of height-weight tables. New Eng. J. Med., 272:1132, 1965.
8. Seltzer, C. C. and Mayer, J.: Body build and obesity: Who are the obese? J.A.M.A., 189:677 (August 31) 1964.
9. Gertler, M. M. and White, P. D.: Coronary Disease in Young Adults. Cambridge, Massachusetts, Harvard University Press, 1954.
10. Spain, D. M., Bradess, V. A. and Greenblatt, I. J.: Post mortems on coronary atherosclerosis, beta-lipoprotein and somatotypes. Amer. J. Med. Sci., 229:294, 1955.
11. Brozek, J.: Body Measurements and Human Nutrition. Detroit, Wayne University Press, 1956, pp. 10-11.
12. Young, C. M. and Blondin, J.: Estimating body weight and fatness of young women. Use of "envelope" anthropometric measurements. J. Amer. Diet. Ass., 41:452 (November) 1962.
13. Novak, L. P.: Age and sex differences in body density and creatinine excretion of high school children. Ann. N.Y. Acad. Sci., 110:545 (September 26) 1963.

*Chapter 34*

# OBESITY:
# ETIOLOGY AND PATHOGENESIS

$O$NLY a few studies of weight reduction based on large groups of patients and pursued for a year or longer are available. In general, results are not encouraging. They show that it is relatively easy to obtain weight reduction in most patients for a short time, but that prolonged success is rare. This was demonstrated in Boston by a three-year study (1) of nearly 200 patients, of whom half received individual clinical instruction while the other half participated in group therapy. Three years after treatment was initiated, only three patients had reduced to or below their "ideal" weight. These patients initially were only 9, 10 and 13 per cent overweight, respectively, while the average figure for the group was 40 per cent overweight. (The limitations of gauging obesity by referring to tables have been discussed in the previous article (2) in this series.) Fifty per cent of the patients studied had lost some weight at the end of three years, but the remaining patients had maintained or increased their excess weight. Obviously, failure of this magnitude calls for reappraisal of the problem. Granting that obesity results from an intake of food in excess of the output of energy, these results indicate that we do not know how to control food intake.

Hilde Bruch a pioneer in the study of psychiatric aspects of obesity, has observed, "In this field we know all the answers; it is the questions we do not know." If we dig beneath the surface of easy generalization, we realize how little we understand of the mechanism of regulating food intake and, hence, of the etiology and pathogenisis of the obesities. As in any other disease condition, successful treatment of obesity must be based on proper diagnosis and identification and on understanding the

Reprinted from *Postgraduate Medicine, 25* (No. 5), May, 1959.

mechanism of development of the condition. While recent experimental work cannot yet fulfill these various criteria, it points toward future clinical advance and may thus be useful in considering the obesities.

## MECHANISM OF REGULATING FOOD INTAKE

### Gastric Factors

The earliest experimental approach to the problem of hunger was made by Cannon, who found that sensations of hunger appeared simultaneously with contractions of the stomach. In further investigations, Carlson (3) showed that in starvation the frequency and intensity of the empty stomach's contractions became progressively more pronounced — at least until the fourth day. Carlson actually based an entire theory of the control of hunger in health and disease on the appearance and inhibition of gastric hunger pangs. His ideas were widely accepted.

Doubt concerning the central role of the stomach in the mechanism regulating food intake arose not only from our increasing understanding of the role of hypothalamic structures but also from the work of Adolph, who showed that diluting the ration of experimental animals with inert material and thus increasing its "bulk" (the "stomach-filling" property of advertisements for methylcellulose) had only a very transient influence on food intake. Grossman and Stein (4) found that vagotomy and sympathectomy, which eliminate respectively the pattern of gastric contractions and the consciousness of gastric pangs, while eliminating the gastric components of hunger, do not affect the timing or the intensity of the extragastric components (feelings of weakness and emptiness associated with the desire for food).

Recent studies on experimental animals and on human subjects have reemphasized the excellent correlation between the presence of hunger contractions and the existence of the hunger state, hunger feelings and hunger behavior. Further investigation in this writer's laboratory has shown that damage to the ventromedial area of the hypothalamus impairs the response of gastric contractions to glucagon (see below). Gastric contractions thus appear to be one of the elements in the total awareness of hunger, and they can be integrated in a general scheme which includes also metabolic phenomena and at least two sets of centers in the hypothalamus (Figure 34-1).

## Central Nervous System

Pathologic studies of patients with hypothalamic obesity first established the importance of this general area in the control of food intake. Experimental work by investigators on both sides of the Atlantic clearly eliminated pituitary lesions from the possible causes of obesity. Identification of the areas in which lesions will cause obesity was advanced by surgical exploration and through the use of stereotaxic instruments. These devices make it possible to place electrodes in the brain of standard-sized animals in reproducible positions that are set in reference to a rigid set of rectangular or spherical coordinates.

Intensive studies of the rat, particularly by Brobeck, have

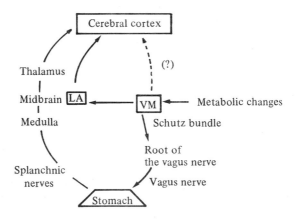

LA : lateral area of the hypothalamus
VM: ventromedial hypothalamic area

Figure 34-1. An integrated view of the mechanism of the regulation of food intake.

shown that bilateral destruction of the ventromedial nuclei was necessary for the rapid developement of obesity, although a slow increase in adiposity may follow unilateral lesions. This writer found that bilateral involvement of the ventromedial area also caused hyperphagia and obesity in mice. Others have demonstrated that obesity follows superficial lesions of the base of the anterior hypothalamus in the monkey, while lesions caudal to the paraventricular nuclei which intercept descending fibers leaving the ventromedial nuclei produce obesity in the dog. Damage to the ventromedial portion of the thalamus and rostral mesencephalic tegmentum also produces obesity in the monkey. Frontal lobotomy and selective decortication cause hyperphagia in rats and, frequently, in humans. Conversely, Anand and Brobeck (5) found that rats stopped eating entirely following bilateral destruction of the more lateral parts of the hypothalamus. The areas destroyed included the extreme parts of the lateral hypothalamic nucleaus at the same rostrocaudal level as the ventromedial nucleus. Morrison and Mayer further defined the anatomic localization of these lateral areas and showed that while these lesions cause adipsia as well as aphagia, the aphagia is not a result of the adipsia. Stimulation in the vicinity of the mammillothalamic tract produces morbid appetite for not only edible but also indigestible material. Temporary increases in food intake follow electric stimulation of the lateral hypothalamus at the level of the ventromedial nucleus.

In a particularly careful study involving sheep and goats, Larsson (6) found that electric stimulation of the hypothalamus just caudal to the optic chiasm, backward throughout the hypothalamus, and lateral to the sagittal level through the descending columns of the fornix and the mammillothalamic tracts results in hyperphagia. The most pronounced effect was obtained by stimulating the region of the lateral hypothalamic nucleus anterior to the descending columns of the fornix or at the same transverse level as this tract. It also has been shown that electric stimulation of different hypothalamic areas can produce inhibition or activation of the movements of the stomach and intestine.

We are thus led to the concept that a number of structures,

some peripheral in nature, are concerned with the mechanism of regulating food intake. Gastrointestinal structures are particularly involved. Although gastric contractions, in part controlled by hypothalamic centers (via the Schutz bundle and vagus nerves), cause consciousness of hunger (probably via the splanchnic nerves), they perhaps are not quantitative determinants. Oral structures undoubtedly are involved, as has been shown by a number of experiments demonstrating the influence of taste on intake; however, their role is of limited importance. Anliker and Morrison have shown that rats will regulate their food intake even when the mouth is bypassed by feeding through the gastric fistula. The most important regulating structures are a system of central areas, some cortical and some situated at intermediary points between the hypo-thalamus and the cortex. Various types of stimuli will influence these structures at various levels (Figure 34-1). It is very interesting to note that recently developed behavioral technics have partially elucidated the role of some of these structures, especially that of the ventromedial nuclei.

## Adjustment of Food Intake to Metabolic Need

Legitimate preoccupation with obesity as a widespread fundamental fact that the majority of mammalians, including most humans, do regulate their food intake; i.e. they adjust their caloric intake to their caloric requirements. Until a few years ago, studies of the regulation of food intake were hampered by lack of recording technics. Food intake for large animals and man was determined on a daily basis or, at best, on a meal basis. New technics permit the recording of every mouthful of food and every tongueful of water taken by experimental animals. The animals studied may be normal or they may have lesions in various areas of the central nervous system. It thus becomes possible to relate behavior to the corresponding structures. For example, during the course of the day, normal animals exhibit a period of rapid eating followed by a period of satiety. Animals with ventromedial hypothalamic lesions do not show any increase of the rate of ingestion (which constitutes a behavioral measure of hunger) over the maximal rate of ingestion of normal animals. But the satiety plateau has disappeared. This finding and related results confirm that the role of the ventromedial area is to brake a constantly activated feeding area. Lesions of the ventromedial area also eliminate the increase in food intake which normally follows exposure to cold or prolonged exercise. It thus seems probable that the metabolic state intervenes to regulate food intake by modulating the inhibition exerted by the ventromedial area on a constantly activated feeding mechanism originating in part in the lateral area. Of course, many other regulations, such as that of circulation, are affected by modulating inhibitions.

The nature of the mechanism by which metabolic events influence the ventromedial area is especially interesting. Brobeck (7) proposed a theory in which variations of heat production, particularly those associated with specific dynamic action of food, directly regulated food intake. While it is doubtful that heat production as such does, in fact, play a direct role in the quantitative adjustment of intake to requirements, a degree of facilitation or inhibition attributable to small temperature variations in the hypothalamus remains an interesting probability. Soulairac (8) suggested a limited but intriguing theory which primarily emphasized the rate of absorption of carbohydrate through the gastrointestinal tract. However, while it has been confirmed that prolonged overconsumption of a high-carbohydrate diet increases the rate of intestinal absorption of glucose, this is a secondary phenomenon which may help to perpetuate the hyperphagia but does not appear to be of etiologic significance.

The glucostatic hypothesis, which the author and his associates (particularly Van Itallie) proposed and which Stunkard and co-workers supported, postulates that the influence of the metabolic state on feeding behavior and its role in regulating food intake are mediated through the rate of passage of glucose or of ions associated with the passage of glucose, e.g. glucose phosphate and potassium, into the cells of the ventromedial hypothalamic area. When first proposed, the theory seemed difficult to test directly because of the apparent inaccessibility of the hypothalamus. For this reason, initial efforts were concentrated on correlating feelings of hunger, gastric hunger contractions, and hunger behavior with the peripheral measurements of the utilization of glucose by the critical midbrain area. It has since been shown that the metabolism of carbohydrates in the ventromedial hypothalamic area does, in fact, present certain idiosyncrasies which make it much more representative of metabolic events in the body as a whole rather than in the central nervous system. It was shown that the presence or absence of hunger sensations in normal persons in various states of nutrition and in diabetic patients correlated well with respectively small and large arteriovenous or capillary-venous glucose differences ("Δ-glucose"). Stunkard and Wolff have confirmed this correlation. In addition, they have shown that the presence of gastric hunger contractions correlates well with the absence of hunger feelings and large Δ-glucose values.

Bernstein and Grossman (9) interpreted the fact that glucose infusions do not invariably eliminate hunger as an insuperable objection to the glucostatic theory. The question was successfully reexamined by Stunkard and Wolff (10), who infused 50 ml of 50 per cent solution of glucose in 40 normal and diabetic subjects. Gastric hunger contractions were eliminated in 19 persons. Ten and 20 minutes after the infusion, arteriovenous differences were significantly higher in the persons in whom gastric contractions were eliminated, indicating a more active utilization of carbohydrates. In 14 of the 19 persons, contractions resumed after a lapse lasting an average of 47 mintes. In the other five persons, arteriovenous differences (Δ-glucose) remained elevated.

Administering glucagon, the pancreatic glycogenolytic factor which apparently acts through activation of hepatic phosphorylase, is a more reproducible method of increasing the availability of carbohydrates to nonhepatic tissues. Glucose thus released is well utilized, and both the blood glucose level and Δ-glucose are invariably increased when this hormone is administered. Over 50 experiments on humans have been conducted since the first report on the effect of glucagon on gastric contractions (10). In all cases gastric contractions and hunger sensations were immediately and strikingly eliminated by administration of glucagon. At the same time, Δ-glucose values were drastically increased, As these waned (after variable intervals), hunger sensations and gastric contractions reappeared, even at absolute levels of blood glucose, which continued to be higher than the fasting values. Particularly striking was Stunkard's (11) observation on a decorticate starved patient in whom continuous gastric hunger contractions were eliminated by administration of glucagon when attempts to eliminate contractions by other methods (excluding ingestion of food) had failed. Glucagon also eliminates gastric contractions in rats, in which intragastric balloons can also be inserted. In these animals, it is possible to correlate the presence or absence of gastric contractions with behavior through the use of operative conditioning technics.

An even more cogent indication in favor of using a glucostatic component in the regulation of food intake is that gold thiogulcose, but not other gold thio compounds of similar toxicity, produces destructive lesions in the ventromedial hypothalamic area. These lesions are most severe in the ventromedial nuclei, but they also involve the ventral part of the lateral hypothalamic area, the arcuate nucleus, and the median eminence. Gold thiosorbitol does not cause such lesions or produce obesity, in spite of the structural similarity between glucose and sorbitol. Similarly, compounds in which gold is linked by a sulfur bridge to normal metabolites other than glucose, such as malic acid, caproic acid or glycerol, do not induce hypothalamic lesions or obesity. Gold-thioglucose-hypothalamic lesions can be induced in rats as well as in mice. It thus appears that gold destroys the ventromedial hypothalamic cells because of the peculiar affinity for glucose displayed by these cells. Forssberg and Larsson (12) have shown that this particular hypothalamic area exhibits an atypical glucose and phosphate metabolism.

While it thus appears probably that the regulating mechanism is in part glucostatic, its quantitative operation is still not understood. Some indications of the overall characteristics are available. The intake in adult animals is in constant ratio to the output. A. Mayer and co-workers further showed that the precision of regulation in caged animals was better when the energy output was increased by exposure to cold. Recent studies have demonstrated that the precision of the regulation is better when animals and men have to perform moderate exercise than when they are inactive. In rapidly growing animals (rats, chickens, pigs) on good diets, food intake seems to be so determined that the thermo-chemical efficiency of growth, i.e. the ratio of calories depositied to calories ingested, is constant from weaning to puberty. No data of this type have been established for children. It is also possible that in addition to the short-term mechanism which operates to adjust intake to output, another mechanism — slower, somewhat sluggish and perhaps based on the state of fat depots — intervenes to correct imprecisions of the short-term mechanism on a long-term basis and permit greater constancy of adult size and growth rate.

## MULTIPLE ETIOLOGY OF OBESITY

The development of obesity can be considered from the viewpoint of either etiology or pathogenesis. The various etiologies are perhaps best considered by the classic epidemiological approach, dividing causative factors into those pertaining to the host, the agent and the environment and thus considering genetic , traumatic and environmental elements (Figure 34-2 and Table 34-1). Although such a distinction is useful, it obviously entails a certain degree of oversimplification. For obesity to develop, there must be a permissive interaction of genetic and environmental factors or of traumatic factors with genetic and environmental background. However, this very simplification permits a useful classification through simply singling out the characteristic element in the etiology.

Genetic factors in obesity are easily demonstrated in experi-mental animals. For example, a yellow dominant form of obesity in the mouse has been recognized for some time. The obesity is associated with a yellow color of its coat, unless this coloration is superseded by the albino gene. The homozygous combination of genes is lethal. Female mice are hypercholesteremic and are fatter than male mice.

A recessive form of obesity, the hereditary obese-hyperglycemic syndrome, has been studied more extensively in this writer's laboratory and will be considered in greater detail below (as the example of metabolic obesity in Table 34-2). Animals with this syndrome do not mate; the condition is perpetuated by mating nonobese carriers of the obese gene. The NZO syndrome also is recessive but differs from the obese-hyperglycemic syndrome in spite of certain resemblances. Mice with the NZO syndrome mate and produce offspring; they also present abnormalities of metabolism of carbohydrate which are different from those exhibited by mice with the obese-hyperglycemic syndrome. Many other forms of genetically transmitted obesities have appeared

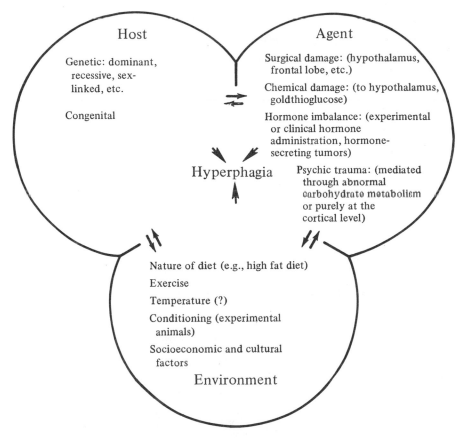

Figure 34-2. A schematic view of constitutional (genetic and congenital), traumatic and environmental factors in the etiology of obesity.

TABLE 34-1

TYPES OF OBESITY

**In Mice**

Genetic: Yellow obesity, associated with coat color: heterozygous, dominant character, normal mating. Hereditary obese hyperglycemic syndrome: homozygous, recessive character, absence of mating. NZO obesity: homozygous, recessive character, normal mating

Of hypothalamic origin: Spontaneous; surgically induced; induced by gold thioglucose

Of endocrine origin: Caused by injection of pituitary tumors secreting adrenocorticotropic hormone

Otherwise induced: By high fat diet

**In Rats**

Genetic: Associated with diabetes

Of hypothalamic origin: Induced by bilateral or unilateral lesions

Of other central nervous system origin: From frontal lobe damage

Of endocrine origin: From hypertrophy of adrenocortical tissue; prolonged treatment with protamine zinc insulin or insulin with forced feeding; after thyroidectomy with hypothalamic lesions or with forced feeding

Otherwise induced: By immobilization; high-fat diet; conditioning

**In Dogs**

Genetic: In the Shetland sheep dog, recessive character

Of hypothalamic origin: Spontaneous; surgically induced; paraventricular degeneration caused by corticotropin or cortisone

Otherwise induced: By immobilization

**In Monkeys**

Of hypothalamic origin: Surgically induced

Of other central nervous system origin: Surgically induced by lesions of the thalamus

**In Farm Animals**

Genetic: In strains selectively bred for fat, particularly in pigs

Of endocrine origin: Induced by castration and by estrogens in fowl; by castration and implants of estrogens in male cattle

Otherwise induced: By immobilization in pigs, cattle and geese; by forced feeding in geese for production of *foie gras*

**In Man**

Genetic: In congenital adipose macrosomia; in monstrous infantile obesity; associated with Laurence-Moon-Biedl syndrome; associated with hyperostosis frontalis interna; associated with von Gierke's disease; in familial hypoglycemosis (congenital lack of alpha cells); in genes predisposing to obesity

Of hypothalamic origin: In adiposogenital dystrophy, with discrete or diffuse hypothalamic injury; occasionally with panhypopituitarism and narcolepsy; Kleine-Levin syndrome

Of other central nervous system origin: After frontal lobotomy; in association with cortical lesions, particularly, bilateral frontal lesions

Of endocrine origin: With insulin-producing adenoma of the islets of Langerhans, with diffuse hyperplasia of the islets, and in association with diabetes; with chromophobe adenoma of the pituitary without hypothalamic injury; in Cushing's syndrome (hyperglycocorticoidism); from treatment with cortisone or adrenocorticotropic hormone; in the Bongiovanni-Eisenmenger syndrome; in disorders of the reproductive system including gynandrism and gynism, aspermatogenic gynecomastia without aleydigism, male hypogonadism (sometimes with bulimia), postpuberal castration, menopause, ovarian disorder, paradoxical (Gilbert-Dreyfus) disorder

Otherwise induced: By immobilization in adults and children; psychic disturbance; social and cultural pressure

TABLE 34-2

COMPARISON BETWEEN REGULATORY AND METABOLIC OBESITIES: TWO ILLUSTRATIONS WHICH
HAVE BEEN OBTAINED IN LITTERMATES: GOLD THIOGLUCOSE OBESITY AND
OBESE-HYPERGLYCEMIC SYNDROME IN MICE

| Object of Comparison | Obese-Hyperglycemic Syndrome | Gold Thioglucose-induced Obesity |
|---|---|---|
| Etiology | Mendelian recessive | 1 mg gold thioglucose per gram of body weight |
| Pathology and mechanism | Pancreatic dysfunction; hyperplasia of islets of Langerhans; increased insulin and glycagon secretion | Hypothalamic lesions (destruction of cells regulating intake in ventro-medial area) |
| Energy balance | Positive through moderate hyper-phagia; moderate or small increase in oxygen consumption; drastically de-creased activity | Positive through considerable hyper-phagia |
| Effect of diet | Maximal weight gain on high-carbo-hydrate, less on protein, less or de-creased on high-fat | Maximal weight gain on high-fat, less on carbohydrate, decreased on high-fat |
| Effect of weight reduction | Composition remains obese; i.e. ani-mal loses nitrogen as well as fat and is still obese when weight is normal or below normal | Brings body composition back to normal |
| Resistance to cold | Drastically reduced | Normal |
| Blood glucose levels | Generally hyperglycemic; further in-creased by growth hormone, etc. | Normal |
| Total blood lipids | Elevated | Elevated |
| Blood cholesterol levels | Elevated; further elevated by growth hormone, etc. | Normal |
| Effect of hormones | Abnormal sensitivity to hypergly-cemic effects of growth hormone, glucagon, etc.: increased resistance to insulin | Normal |
| Mating behavior | Absence of mating | Less frequently than normal; normal pregnancies and lactations |
| Lipogenesis | Increased with hyperphagia; in-creased in fasting | Increased with hyperphagia; normal when fasting |
| Cholesterogenesis | Increased in fasting | Normal when fasting |
| Acetate pool and turnover | Increased pool; greatly increased turnover | Normal |
| Liver glycogen turnover | Greatly increased | |
| Enzymatic activities | Increased liver phosphorylase | Normal phosphorylase |
| Intestinal absorption | Increased in proportion to hyper-phagia | Increased in proportion to hyper-phagia |
| Body composition; size of organs | High body fat; decreased protein; cholesterol content increased with weight; enlarged liver, heart, pan-creas, thymus, adrenals; decreased uterus, ovaries, brain | High body fat; slightly increased pro-tein; cholesterol content normal; en-larged liver, kidneys, ovaries and uterus |
| Retention of steroid hormones | Increased in proportion to body fat | Increased in proportion to body fat |
| Ketone levels during normal eating | Slightly increased | Slightly increased |
| Ketone levels during fasting | Decreased | Normally elevated |

from time to time in mice colonies; a hereditary tendency to spontaneous degeneration of ventromedial nuclei with resultant hypothalamic obesity has been particularly noted. Genetic obesity also has been observed in rats, dogs and chickens. In animal husbandry, obese animals, especially pigs, formerly were selected for breeding in order to produce animal fats. The current trend is to breed nonobese animals in this species, since lard is no longer in much demand and lean meat is desired.

Genetically determined accumulations of lipids other than triglycerides have been demonstrated in man in the Niemann-Pick and Tay-Sachs diseases (phospholipids), in Gaucher's disease (cerebrosides), and in the Schuller-Christian disease (cholesterol and its esters). A clear-cut but isolated association of obesity and genetic lesions can be demonstrated in the frequent occurrence of general or localized obesity in Von Gierke's disease, in the macrosomnia adiposa congenita syndrome and some other rare diseases (Table 34-1), and in the sex-limited steatopygia of Bushmen and Hottentot women.

More cogent evidence is derived from studies of twins. As in other genetic conditions, pathologic or other characteristics which are always or nearly always present in both identical twins, but rarely or never present in both fraternal twins, are hereditary. This statement does not imply the reverse, i.e. that characteristics which are found in each member of both types of twins are not hereditary. Newman and Von Verchuer have shown that identical twins have much more similar weights than have fraternal twins; when identical twins are reared in different environments, differences in weight increased. This demonstrates that while the genetic factors play a paramount role in determining body weight, the environmental factors also are important.

In the light of such definite demonstrations of the influence of genetic factors on normal weight, studies of the familial incidence of obesity assume additional significance from the viewpoint of hereditary determination. In 73 per cent of a series of over 1000 obese patients in Vienna, Bauer found that either one or both parents were obese. This figure agrees with that determined by Rony in Chicago, who found parental obesity in 69 per cent of obese patients studied. In his studies in Philadelphia, Angel found that half of the offspring of one obese and one average parent were obese, as were two-thirds of the offspring of parents who were both obese. Eighty per cent of the obese children had at least one obese parent; both parents of 25 per cent were obese. Similar proportions were found in a number of separate studies conducted in Boston.

While there is evidence to support the idea that there are genes which predispose to obesity, the mechanism of transmission is still obscure. Because both environmental and hereditary factors are involved and because many types of obesity are probably considered simultaneously, the incidence of obesity, the sex ratios, etc. in children of obese and nonobese parents do not fit any simple pattern. It has been stated that there are fewer male offspring and larger families among the progeny from marriages of men of average weight to women who are either average weight or obese than among the offspring of either an obese man and an average woman or an obese man and an obese woman. This would suggest that one of the genes predisposing to obesity is a recessive sex-linked lethal gene, but data are as yet inadequate to confirm this hypothesis. To the hereditary factors predisposing to obesity through physiologic factors may be added hereditary psychologic characteristics. The part played by hereditary factors in determining obesity actually can be a useful tool in the detection and early prevention of this condition.

## TRAUMATIC FACTORS

A number of physiologic as well as psychologic factors may lead to obesity. As previously mentioned, lesions have been produced in experimental animals by stereotaxic technics and by introducing gold thioglucose into the hypothalamus and other parts of the central nervous system. While hypothalamic events appear to dominate the subcortical picture and hypothalamic hyperphagia may be a sequela of encephalitis as well as of increased pressure due to pituitary tumors, lesions of the frontal lobe may be of greater interest in interpreting psychogenic obesity. Cobb (13) reported that 70 of 74 patients subjected to frontal lobotomy had an increase in appetite. The associated symptoms were lack of initiative in 73 patients (30 persistent), procrastination in 56 patients (29 persistent), and laziness in 52 patients (22 persistent). Similar results have been confirmed by other authors.

Endocrine factors in obesity have been the object of extremes in fashion. In the early part of the century, haziness about the distinction between myxedema and obesity and the mistaken belief that Fröhlich's syndrome was of pituitary origin led enthusiasts to expect an early solution of the problem of obesity along purely endocrine lines. In a second period of investigation, the possibility that endocrine factors may directly or indirectly cause the hyperphagia leading to obesity or may orient metabolism toward a greater rate of lipogenesis was discounted in all save rare and exceptional cases. It may be more realistic to remember that while it is true that hypopituitarism or hypothyroidism as such does not cause obesity, it is known that a number of hormones influence food intake and fat metabolism. In view of their close relationship, it is not surprising that an endocrine disturbance which affects metabolism of carbohydrate usually also affects regulation of food intake. Obesity can be induced in experimental animals by prolonged treatment with long-lasting insulin. Combination of thyroidectomy or propylthiouracil treatment with insulin leads to rapid development of obesity. The obese-hyperglycemic syndrome in mice, in many ways similar to maturity-onset diabetes in man and which is generally associated with obesity, appears to be due to a hyperplasia of the islets of Langerhans, increased insulin secretion, and probably increased glucagon secretion as well. The yellow obese mice and NZO obese mice also show disturbances of carbohydrate metabolism which are probably of endocrine origin. Grafting of ACTH-secreting pituitary tumors in mice of the $LAF_1$ strain also has been used to produce obesity, a syndrome which is in some respects similar to Cushing's syndrome in man.

In man, the response of body weight to sex hormones administered under various conditions is not well known. The response of experimental animals to both sex hormones and gonadectomy varies with the species and conditions. Similarly, it has been stated that castration after puberty in men seems to promote obesity; castration before puberty prolongs growth. Of perhaps greater relevance to the possibly endocrine etiology of some cases of obesity in man are the frequent deviations of glucose tolerance from both sides of the normal in obese patients. In addition, Stunkard and others observed that episodes of particularly acute hyperphagia in obese patients, including those brought about by psychogenic factors, often are preceded or accompanied by marked disturbances of carbohydrate metabolism. It appears therefore reasonable to conclude that endocrine factors, particularly those centered in the pancreas and perhaps also in the adrenals, may play a more significant role in human obesity than has been heretofore suspected.

Finally, there is little doubt that psychologic trauma may lead to the development of hyperphagia in certain persons, as it does in experimental animals. While in animals the technics used are simple conditioning methods (the animals are punished if they do not overeat), the sequence of events is obviously more complex and not well understood in man. The fact that the same psychologic trauma may cause hyperphagia in some persons and partial anorexia in others may provide an example of the interaction of physiologic and psychologic factors.

## ENVIRONMENTAL FACTORS

A number of environmental factors, such as diet, exercise, temperature, culture, etc., are important in determining obesity. The availability of enough food to permit an intake in excess of expenditure is obviously a necessary prerequisite. The nature of the diet also may be of importance. It has been shown that certain strains of rats and mice become spontaneously obese on high-fat diets. Their regulatory mechanism, adequate to cope with diets lower in fat, seems unable to adjust when the diet contains a very high (60% or more) proportion of calories as fat. Hypothalamic hyperphagic rats and mice become fatter quicker on a high-fat diet. By contrast, obese-hyperglycemic mice become obese quicker on high-carbohydrate diets. These obeservations indicate that the influence of diet composition varies according to different constitutional factors.

While it has been well established that obesity in man follows the habitual ingestion of a caloric intake in excess of energy expenditure, until recently there has been little reliable information comparing the selection of nutrients or the meal patterns of obese persons with those of similar groups of nonobese persons. It has often been stated that obese persons eat more frequently, often eat enormous amounts of food at one sitting, derive a larger proportion of their caloric intake from evening meals and snacks, or consume most of their food in one meal. However, many such statements have been made without confirmatory evidence.

In a study conducted in Boston, Dr. Beaudoin and this writer found that the average caloric intake of a group of obese women was derived from the same proportion of calories from fat (37%) and carbohydrate (49%) as that of a comparable group of women of normal weight (control group). The women in both groups ate substantial snacks. The center of gravity of caloric consumption appeared to be shifted to the later hours of the day in the obese as compared with the control group. These observations, particularly the high caloric intake during the evening meal and evening snacks, have been confirmed by others. Stunkard coined the apt designation of the "night eating syndrome" for this phenomenon. Of course, it is possible that when we know better how to type obesities we will be able to associate certain types of cravings for food with certain types of obesities, but the statistical foundation for indicting certain foods is lacking at this point. The importance of considering the intake of excess calories in the evening in the treatment of obesity will be explained in the next chapter.

The influence of the level of activity, all too often minimized, was discussed at length in a preceding chapter. Little is known at this time about the influence of environmental temperature on obesity. Exposure to moderately cold temperatures tends to produce an appreciable increase in stores of fat and an elevation of the iodine number in the fat depots in animals. An experiment on army personnel showed that shifts from a hot to a cold environment tended to lead to an increase of a few pounds in body weight. Increase in weight was more marked in persons who had short daily exposure to cold than in persons who had markedly increased caloric expenditure because of prolonged exposure to cold.

It is obvious that familial, socioeconomic and cultural factors also are important in the development of obesity. Familial and social environments help to determine eating patterns. Parental preoccupation with the health of children often results in directive overfeeding, which eventually may be metabolically and psychologically self-perpetuating. In many societies, the value of food as a symbol of economic security and as a token of good will leads families and groups of friends to congregate at frequent intervals around excessive amounts of appetizing foods and "fermented" beverages. Significant events of human life, from christening to burial, and commercial transactions thus may be marked by almost compulsive, self-inflicted forced feeding.

## DUAL PATHOGENESIS OF OBESITY: REGULATORY AND METABOLIC FORMS OF OBESITY

This writer and his associates have been led to introduce a general distinction between regulatory obesities, in which the primary impairment is in the central mechanism regulating food intake, and metabolic obesities, in which the primary lesion is an inborn or acquired error in the metabolism of tissues other than the regulating centers. In regulatory obesities, habitual hyperphagia may lead to secondary metabolic abnormalities. In metabolic obesities, peripheral metabolic dysfunction may in turn interfere with the proper function of the central nervous system. This difference has been illustrated in the laboratory by comparing different types of obesity in mice. Results of this study are presented in Table 34-2. Points of comparison other than those presented in the table have been drawn, but the latter suffice to establish the fact that certain characteristics are nonspecific consequences of hyperphagia and obesity and are found in both regulatory and metabolic obesities. Examples of such characteristics are increases in fat content, intestinal absorption, total blood lipids or lipogenesis under adlibitum feeding. Characteristics such as increased lipogenesis and cholesterogenesis under fasting conditions, maintenance of a high-fat content even when weight is reduced to normal or below normal levels, and failure of blood ketones to rise normally when the animal is fasted are found in metabolic obesities, not in regulatory obesities. In addition, certain characteristics are specific for one or another metabolic obesity not in regulatory obesities, for example, liver phosphorylase activity is elevated in the obese-hyperglycemic syndrome, while phosphorylase activity is normal but hepatic glucose 6-phosphatase is increased in the obesity induced by ACTH-secreting tumors.

At this time, similar documented distinctions cannot be applied to various classes of obesity in man. However, research is actively proceeding in this field; the study of the reaction of blood ketones to fasting is particularly promising. It is hoped that before too long it will become possible by simple clinical tests to determine whether a case of obesity is regulatory (psychogenic or neurologic) or metabolic (endocrine or due to an enzymatic abnormality). While this is obviously only an initial step in diagnosis, it should help to place the problem of obesity in man on a more rational basis.

## REFERENCES

1. Bowser, L. J., Trulson, M. F., Bowling, R. C. and Stare, F. J.: Methods of reducing: Group therapy vs. individual clinic interview. J. Amer. Dietet. A., 29:1193, 1953.
2. Mayer, J.: Obesity: Diagnosis. Postgrad. Med., 25:469-475 (April) 1959.
3. Carlson, A. J.: The Control of Hunger in Health and Disease. Chicago, University of Chicago Press, 1914.
4. Grossman, M. I. and Stein, I. F.: Vagotomy and the hunger-producing action of insulin in man. J. App. Physiol., 1:263, 1949.
5. Anand, B. K. and Brobeck, J. R.: Localization of a "feeding center" in the hypothalamus of the rat. Proc. Soc. Exper. Biol. & Med., 77:323, 1951.
6. Larsson, S.: On the hypothalamic organization of the nervous mechanism regulating food intake: I. Hyperphagia from stimulation of the hypothalamus and medulla in sheep, goats. Acta physiol. scandinav. (supp. 115), 32:1, 1954.

7. Brobeck, J. R.: Neural factors in obesity. Bull. New York Acad. Med., 33:762, 1957.
8. Soulairac, A.: Les regulations psycho-physiologiques de la faim. J. physiol., Paris, 50:663, 1958.
9. Bernstein, L. M. and Grossman, M. I.: An experimental test of the glucostatic theory of regulation of food intake. J. Clin. Invest., 33:627, 1956.
10. Stunkard, A. J. and Woff, H. G.: Studies on the physiology of hunger. I. The effect of intraveneous administration of glucose on gastric hunger contractions in man. J. Clin. Invest., 35:954, 1956.
11. Stunkard, A. J.: Studies on the physiology of hunger. II. The effect of intravenous administration of various nutrients on the gastric hunger contractions of a man with severe brain damage. Am. J. Clin. Nutrition, 5:203, 1957.
12. Forssberg, A. and Larsson, S.: On the hypothalamic organization of the nervous mechanism regulating food intake: II. Studies of isotope distribution and chemical composition in the hypothalamic region of hungry and fed rats. Acta physiol. scandinav. (supp. 115), 32:41, 1954.
13. Cobb, S.: Technic of interviewing a patient with psychosomatic disorder. M. Clin. North America, 28:1210 (September), 1944.

## Chapter 35

# OBESITY: PSYCHOLOGIC
# ASPECTS AND THERAPY

I N the previous chapter we reviewed a number of recently described etiologies of obesity in experimental animals. We showed that genetic, traumatic and environmental factors all could contribute to a positive energy balance leading to obesity. From the standpoint of mechanism, we saw that obesities could be classified in two general types: (1) metabolic obesities, in which an error in metabolism causes increased synthesis of fat even when hyperphagia is eliminated, and (2) regulatory obesities, in which a lesion in the central nervous mechanism regulating food intake directly leads to overeating. Among the examples of the latter type is conditioned obesity, which can be induced in experimental animals by punishing them unless they overeat. We are not at present in a position to point to a strict correspondence between models studied in rats, mice, etc. and types of obesity in men, but we are in a position to assume that the diversity of origins of hyperphagia and obesity found in animals is also present in man. Furthermore, because the central nervous system, the intellectual and emotional activities and the sociocultural environment are so much more complex in man than in lower animals, it is reasonable to assume that phychogenic obesity is much more widespread in humans. In fact, this assumption has received such overwhelming acceptance that it has tended to obscure in the mind of many clinicians the fact that there are probably a number of cases of obesity which are not due to psychologic causes alone. A striking example of such cases, the obesity due to inactivity, has been examined in some detail previously by the author. While in some patients [well studied by Bruch (2) and by Stunkard and Dorris (3)], inactivity may be due to acute psychologic disturbances,

Reprinted from *Postgraduate Medicine, 25* (No. 6), June, 1959.

inactivity is in general the result of social and economic conditions which have eliminated the need for physical work without creating the leisure, the means or the incentive for voluntary physical exercise.

Other forms of nonpsychogenic obesity in man have been listed in the previous chapter. Once these forms of obesity have been ruled out, it remains true that an important although undetermined fraction of obesities in man is probably due to psychologic disturbances.

In addition to psychogenic obesity, the fact of being obese for whatever cause, particularly in a society which has been conditioned to view obesity as a sign of gluttony, self-indulgence and lack of will power, does in itself bring about important psychologic consequences. Finally, cutting down food intake to bring about weight loss also has important psychologic implications, because of both the resulting hunger and the weight loss itself. Failure to reduce in spite of repeated attempts also has psychologic connotations.

In the first part of this chapter we shall attempt to summarize what is known of these psychologic aspects of obesity: psychologic factors in etiology, psychologic aspects of being obese, and psychologic aspects of reducing. In the second part we shall try to derive from the evidence presented in previous chapters (devoted to caloric requirements, effects of exercise, diagnosis of obesity, and etiology of obesity) and from the first part some simple rules which may be useful to the practitioner in treating obesity.

## PSYCHOLOGIC FACTORS IN THE ETIOLOGY OF OBESITY

One of the ablest psychologists in the field of obesity, Hilde Bruch (2,4,5), has classified the possibilities of associating body weight and adjustment in the following fashion: (1) slenderness with good adjustment: (2) slenderness with poor emotional adjustment; (3) continued obesity, usually of a moderate degree, with good adjustment; and (4) continued obesity with maladjustment.

In her thinking, continued obesity with good adjustment

represents a "constitutional" obesity compatible with an otherwise normal personality. She assumes the obesity in this case to be due essentially to physiologic factors. Patients of this type are usually obese from childhood and stay continuously heavy, with their height and weight moving steadily in the overweight area of the growth diagram. They function adequately with this degree of obesity. Bruch believes that in such patients psychologic difficulties are likely to arise or to become serious only if they are forcibly reduced.

The situation is quite different in what Bruch terms "reactive" obesity and in "developmental" obesity of nonconstitutional origin. She believes that in reactive obesity, overeating is a response to and a compensation for tension and frustration. In many patients, as Stunkard and Dorris (3) also emphasized, the situations leading to overeating also provoke a drastic decrease in activity. Both these factors are synergistic in causing markedly positive caloric balance. Episodes of grief or of severe depression thus coincide with drastic elevations of weight. As this type of obese patient does, in fact, tend to become depressed easily, a considerable degree of obesity can develop in a few years. Bruch considers this reactive obesity the characteristic form of psychologic obesity in adulthood and middle age. She has observed few instances of reactive obesity in childhood. Stunkard, Grace and Wolff (6) emphasized that among such potentially depressed, reactive obese patients they frequently found a distinctive eating pattern which they called the "night eating syndrome." In a study conducted a few years ago in Boston, Dr. Beaudoin and this writer (7) observed that an unselected group of obese women tended to distribute their calories so that they consumed more in proportion during the later hours of the day. Stunkard showed that this effect was particularly marked in obesity associated with frequent bouts of depression. In many such patients, the acutal bulk of the daily calories may be consumed in the evening hours and at night, which are also the periods of the day when depression is most severe. Stunkard and Wolff (8) showed that, in addition to this characteristic eating pattern and the decreased activity during periods of intense depression, this type of obese patient exhibits in many instances drastic changes in carbohydrate metabolism, particularly abnormally increased glucose tolerance, which coincide with the episodes of drastic weight gain. It is thus possible that physiologic changes mediate in many of these patients the psychologic trauma which indirectly leads to over-eating. Interaction between psychologic and endocrine factors may explain why certain patients will tend to accumulate considerable excess weight during a period of grief while others faced with the same trauma may lose weight.

Developmental obesity is described by Bruch as a common form of obesity during childhood. She believes that in many obese children in whom the obesity is not due to purely physiologic factors the emotional development centers around eating as much as they want, avoiding physical activity and social contacts, and being fat. Usually, such children are growing in a family setting in which they are used by one or the other parent (sometimes by both) as an object fulfilling his needs and compensating for failure and frustration in his own life. The child is fussed over excessivly, overprotected and overfed. Generally, the mother plays the dominant role in the emotional life of such families; she indulges the obese child and keeps him close to her by constant and excessive demands. Thus, the problems of children of this type are not unlike those seen in the premorbid stage of schizophrenia. The combination of this environment and of being obese tends to promote a sense of helplessness and inadequacy which causes flight into fancy and sometimes hostility and sadism.

## PSYCHOLOGIC ASPECTS OF BEING OBESE

Hyperphagia and obesity, due either to physiologic lesions or to psychologic factors of various types, have in themselves physiologic and psychologic consequences. The nonspecific "physiologic consequences" of obesity have been mentioned in previous articles by the author (1, 9). Examples are hypertrophy of certain organs such as the gastrointestinal tract, liver, kidney, etc.; increased rate of intestinal absorption; and, generally, some degree of decrease in spontaneous activity, even in the cases in which inactivity was not the origin of the obesity.

Obesity also has "psychologic consequences." The manner in which these manifest themselves depends on the cultural environment of the obese persons. In certain societies or at certain periods, fat men and women have been described as jovial, cheerful and easygoing. In our society there has been a tendency to describe obese persons al lethargic, lazy and weak-willed, so that obesity becomes an object of ridicule and humiliation. Obese persons not only feel excluded, but in a number of social situations and job competitions they are discriminated against. This hostile attitude is likely to have profound influence on obese persons, particularly on the young. The fact that siblings, parents, teachers and physicians all tend to reproach the obese child for his bulk and appetite may have a destructive effect on his personality. It often makes the obesity self-perpetuating. Obese young people may be so embarrassed by the persons in their immediate enviornment that they become more and more withdrawn and avoid sports and physical activities done in public, thus placing themselves in the very conditions most likely to perpetuate a constant imbalance between food intake and energy expenditure.

## PSYCHOLOGIC ASPECTS OF REDUCING

The all too widespread belief that a fat patient will not be hungry while on a reducing diet is at the root of many failures in therapy. Actually, when we place an obese patient on a reducing diet, we add to the physiologic or psychologic difficulty he had to start with, that of being hungry a large part of the time. The work of Keys and co-workers (10) illustrated the psychologic reactions of normal-weight persons placed on a prolonged negative caloric balance. Their volunteers showed an extreme narrowing of interest. They became continuously preoccupied with food. The experiment had to be discontinued in several patients because of increasingly serious emotional disturbances. It is true that obese persons do have large stores of fat which should decrease the physiologic diffuculties associated with losing weight. It must be recalled, however, that patients with certain types of experimental obesities — the metabolic types — go into very negative nitrogen balance when fasted (1,9). Animals with these forms of obesity can be brought down to normal-weight or even to underweight levels by prolonged undernutrition; yet, even at these weight levels, they are obese in terms of composition. Their normal or subnormal weight still contains a much larger proportion of fat than that of normal animals. While they have lost fat they also have lost considerable protein. It may well be that there is a substantial proportion of human subjects with metabolic obesity in whom the effect of underfeeding is similar. Ohlson and co-workers (11) demonstrated that even when large amounts of protein are included in reducing diets some subjects are constantly in markedly negative nitrogen balance. It is thus not surprising that these persons experience the greatest discomfort during reduction and most quickly regain the lost weight at the end of the experimental reducing period. Even in those persons in whom metabolic factors are not primary in the etiology of obesity, burning of body fat does not fulfill satiety requirements to the same extent as does food. This may explain why so many fat patients react to dieting as though they were starving. They show an acute craving for all sorts of food, even some which they do not usually like. They are constantly in a state of extreme tension; they feel dizzy and are sleepless at night, and in some extreme cases they may show an almost complete disintegration of their personality. Bruch (5) warned against the danger of precipitating acute nervous disorders and even psychoses in emotionally unstable patients who are reduced too vigorously. In a study at a New York hospital, Stunkard (12) observed untoward responses to weight reduction in an alarmingly high proportion (50%) of a group of unselected female obese patients. Of 25 patients who were studied in detail, nine had severe emotional disorders connected with dieting. Stunkard also found that the incidence of severe illness was statistically higher during the period of reducing than in other periods in the patients' lives. The excessive food intake and underactivity may be protective factors in the emotional health of these obese patients.

It must be recognized that the obese population of a nutrition outpatient department or of a psychotherapy clinic is probably not a cross section of the obese population at large. There are many persons who can quite successfully cope with their own weight problem without requiring professional help. Those persons who do seek medical help or are directed to do so probably already have had excessive difficulty in coping with this problem. They may thus represent the most refractory part of the population. "Paradoxical as it may sound, " Bruch said, "weight loss and food restriction are not rational and causal treatments of obesity." This striking statement must be taken (fortunately) with some reservation, but it probably best applies when the obesity is of psychogenic origin.

## PRACTICAL SUGGESTIONS

### General Attitude of the Therapist

Obesity is not a moral issue. It is a complex medical problem. It cannot be cured by blaming the patient and shifting the entire responsibility for the treatment onto him. In many cases, a censorious or punitive attitude is likely to do more harm than good. The patient may be afraid to come back to his physician if blame is going to be incurred. The time-honored aim of medicine also applies to the treatment of obesity: "To cure sometimes, to alleviate pain whenever possible, to comfort always."

### Diagnosis of Obesity

The mechanical application of "standard," "ideal" or "desirable" height-weight tables is not a proper diagnostic procedure. There are obvious weaknesses inherent in the construction of these tables. They are based on highly approximate heights ("with shoes on") and weights ("with ordinary clothing on") of a biased sample of people (insurance policyholders of a generation or two ago, when such policies were much less widespread than they are now). The reworking of the data rightly eliminated from calculations of averages those persons more than 30 years of age. It also introduced the concept of "frame," but did not give any definition of frames of various sizes. In practice, immediate diagnosis of obesity or emaciation without any need for tables is easy when the weight deviates widely from the average. Smaller deviations from tabulated standards cannot be interpreted without physical examiniation of the patient for skeletal size and muscular development. Since approximately half of the excess fat is deposited directly under the skin, the old-fashioned office or clinic technic of pinching (with or without calipers) is a cheap and simple substitute for underwater weighing, measurement of thiocyanate or deuterium space, etc.

## Inducement to the Patient and Limitation of Potential Success

There is enough evidence to advocate weight reduction on the basis of health as well as aesthetics. On the other hand, there are dangers in too much emphasis on the threat of obesity to health; there are also dangers in excessive promises of reward if reducing succeeds. This is particularly important for obese children and adolescents who may have organized their mental balance around unrealizable fantasies dealing with the improvement of their fate after they reduce; disappointment may be severe if weight reduction succeeds. In addition, present-day methods are often ineffective, and the patient may need considerable support if intense hunger is a corollary of weight loss. In some cases, weight reduction may be undesirable. A target based on the constitution of the patient (e.g. weight at age 25) should be selected but not dangled before the patient prematurely.

## Informing the Patient

The importance of informing patients about probable daily energy expenditure and about the caloric value of foods cannot be overemphasized. Most patients have very inaccurate concepts of the caloric content of the usual foods. They pay more attention to the type of food consumed than to the amount, and they have been filled with misinformation on the whole area of energy expenditure. Sound knowledge of the caloric value of foods not only will guide the patient during treatment but also will protect him against the dishonest claims of manufacturers of "miracle" foods (such as "low-calorie" bread, "nonfilling" beer, etc.).

## Use of Dietitians and of Nutrition Clinics

The practicing physician does not have the time to spend the hours required to correct misinformation about the caloric value of foods, to give advice on menus, to recommend certain methods of food preparation, etc. Such a job is best handled by a competent dietitian or by the dietetic service of an outpatient department. There is every advantage in directing the patient or his parents to make use of such services.

## Psychotherapy

Psychotherapists have not, in the past, been successful in reducing many patients. However, psychotherapy is indicated for the obese patient if he clearly has emotional and psychologic difficulties; it also will help him adjust to the difficulties entailed by his obesity if it is refractory to treatment. In the opinion of this writer, if an obese patient needs psychotherapy, he needs "individual" attention. Group psychotherapy, supervised reducing groups, etc. have proved notoriously unsuccessful in dealing with obesity on a long-term basis.

## Use of Hereditary Data

It has been shown repeatedly that obesity runs in families. Genetic as well as environmental factors are involved. Studies in the United States have shown that less than 10 per cent of the children of normal-weight parents are obese, but that the proportion rises to 40 or 50 per cent if one parent is obese and to 80 per cent if both parents are obese. Comparative lifetime studies of identical and fraternal twins have shown that food habits are not the only or even the main factor. Instead of denying the facts of heredity, it is more effective to use them (as done with diabetes) to track down obese relatives and, more important, to try to prevent the development of obesity in those subjects in whom this condition is most likely to develop. Obesity is most malignant when the onset is early. Sound dietary exercising habits should be developed as soon as possible in susceptible children.

## Exercise

The mechanism of regulating food intake is apparently not adapted to function well at very low levels of activity. In order to keep obesity from developing under modern living conditions, many of us either will have to work consciously at stepping up our activity above the level required in daily life or we will have to endure mild or acute hunger all our life. The first alternative is difficult, especially in the United States and Canada, where the cities offer little inducement to walking and often are poorly provided with facilities for adult exercise. Lack of easily accessible facilities for sports and lack of parental or medical encouragement further decrease activity in the young, thus accentuating the tendency toward inactivity of many obese youngsters (13). Even among the young, highly competitive team sports for the few are often emphasized at the expense of individual sports which all could learn and continue to enjoy after school and college years are over. If the first alternative — stepping up activity — is difficult, it is well to remember that the second alternative — lifetime hunger — is so much more difficult that to rely on it for weight control in cases of sedentary overweight can only continue to produce the fiascoes of the past. Strenuous exercise on an irregular basis in untrained persons already obese is obviously not what is advocated here. But a reorganization of one's life to include regular exercise adapted to one's physical capacity is a sound preventive measure and a justified return to the wisdom of the ages. When practicable, moderate exercise during weight reduction also helps in promoting positive nitrogen balance and muscle tone.

## Drugs

As our knowledge of the mechanism of regulation of food intake increases, it will perhaps become possible to devise drugs which will act specifically on structures (e.g. the ventromedial areas of the hypothalamus) concerned with the hunger process. So far, such drugs are not available. As a result, compounds which have been used in the past have tended either to have dangerous side effects, as has dinitrophenol, or to become rapidly ineffective, as does amphetamine. Among pharmacologic methods for the treatment of obesity, thyroxin has been too often used and abused. There is no possible justification for prescribing thyroxin to nonhypothyroid patients. Side effects such as increased nervousness, irritability, lack of ability to concentrate, etc. are undesirable; if there is any risk of heart involvement, use of thyroxin may be disastrous.

Hypothyroidism is not to be diagnosed lightly in the obese person. To do it on the basis of the basal metabolic rate (B.M.R.) alone is an error, especially if the decrease of the B.M.R. is not marked. The ratio of oxygen consumption to body surface may be sufficiently abnormal in a markedly obese patient to lead to an apparent decrease in the B.M.R. which is not confirmed by determinations of protein-bound iodine or radioiodine uptake by the thyroid. An apparently moderate decrease in the B.M.R. not confirmed by such determinations does not constitute an indication for thyroid treatment.

With no specific drugs available, we might as well recognize that the presently available pharmaceutical preparations provide at most a temporary crutch. Van Itallie (14), studying a large group of obese patients under reducing treatment, some of whom received amphetamine, found a statistically significant but clinically negligible difference in weight loss in favor of the patients receiving amphetamine during the first six weeks of treatment. After that, even this small difference vanished. The patient should not be led to expect or desire too rapid a rate of weight loss. He should be made to understand that reducing is going to take a long time, that the course of weight loss is easily reversed (it could be quipped that the price of reducing is eternal vigilance), and that the use of drugs for a few days or even a few weeks is not going to be a lasting help and thus might as well be eschewed altogether

## Low-salt Diets

A number of physicians, particularly in Europe, routinely put reducing obese patients on low-salt regimens. There are three possible justifications for this measure.

1. Salt depletion makes less likely the water retention which often takes place as the patient loses weight. This water retention tends to obscure for a while the fact that fat has been lost. Weight tends to decrease only after a certain delay, and the weight loss curve corresponding to a constant daily caloric deficit tends to look more like the steps of a flight of stairs than like a descending straight line. Such delays in weight loss may have adverse effects on the morale of the reducing patient.

2. Lack of salt in the diet also makes food less palatable and therefore decreases the temptation to overeat. In a way, such a prescription is thus a special case of the facetious advice on reducing: "Eat all you want of the foods you most dislike."

3. Finally, it is argued that inasmuch as obese persons are more prone to heart disease, a low-salt diet is a useful preventive measure from a cardiologic viewpoint.

None of these arguments appear convincing to this writer. Again, a better course is to tell the patient that weight loss is not likely to proceed along a perfectly smooth course, even if a constant caloric deficit is maintained. The facts about water retention should be explained. Patients — particularly women in whom periodic variations in water retention occur as part of the menstrual cycle — should be cautioned against weighing themselves too frequently; once a week or once a fortnight is enough.

A "salt-free" diet is notoriously difficult to adhere to, even for patients to whom a heart attack has already given warning. In cardiologically normal persons it is unlikely to be maintained for long. Again, it is at best only a temporary measure and therefore not a part of the long-term education of the patient. It is a crutch no more to be relied on for the long pull than are "bulk" pills, present-day reducing drugs, etc. Finally, the association between obesity and heart attacks is not so marked that any nonsick obese patient should receive other than preventive treatment (by reducing the excess weight) for diseases he has no evidence of having. Of course, avoiding excessive use of salt (like avoiding an excessive proportion of saturated fat in the diet, selection of a balanced diet, etc.) is sound practice for any patient, obese or nonobese.

## Diets

The essential principle to follow in devising reducing diets is that a good reducing diet is one on which the patient does not feel too hungry. The diversity of probable etiologies makes it likely that different patients will feel more comfortable on different types of diet. In practice, the choice of foods and the feeding patterns of obese persons are as diverse as those of normal subjects. It has been repeatedly found that most obese patients tend to do their overeating late in the day and at night, which indicates that evening eating should be controlled with particular care.

Diet prescription should be an individual operation, adapted to the patient's rate of energy expenditure and desired rate of weight loss. It should furnish an opportunity for education in the caloric value of foods. It also should permit nutrition education in general. Finally, it should be experimental; trial and error will permit the finding of the most effective diet as well as the most suitable schedule of exercise. "Fad" diets may have a short-term value, but they have no lasting educational or practical worth. If, as some have claimed, it is possible to "shrink" the stomach or "retrain the appetite," special diets might perhaps be used for that purpose before a change is made to a more normal diet. The evidence offered in favor of this process is, however, very scant. In some cases, better success is obtained with smaller and more frequent meals. The practice of eating slowly seems desirable on physiologic grounds, since satiety mechanisms are likely to need time to take effect. It is also desirable on psychologic grounds.

## Desirable Rate of Weight Loss

Too rapid a rate of weight loss is unnecessary and undesirable. Excess weight has been accumulated over the years. The patient should get used to the idea that weight loss also is going to be a progressive process and that it is infinitely more important to maintain a reduced weight than to achieve a dramatic but transient result. Too great a rate of weight loss will invariably go with fatigue, nervousness and inability to concentrate, and it may have untoward somatic and psychologic effects. At best, such a drastic regimen has no educational value. The diet is so extreme that it will have to be considerably augmented eventually, and this creates the obvious danger of falling back into the old errors. In fact, those patients who are proudest of their success in losing weight quickly are often those who have had to lose weight often. There are indications that repeated weight gains and weight losses may be a greater stress on the organism than is static obesity. In fact, a loss of 2 lb per week (corresponding roughly to a deficit of 1000 calories per day) seems to be reasonable for most adult patients; a loss of 1 lb a week (corresponding to a deficit of 500 calories per day) would still lead to a weight loss of 50 lb in a year. Such moderated deficits still permit the establishment of diets centered around three adequate meals a day and can be used as a basis for the education of the patient.

It goes without saying that the desired rate of weight loss in turn determines the caloric content of the reducing diet. It is necessary to establish the proper "deficit." To put all patients to be reduced — truck drivers, small elderly ladies and even children — on a "standard" reducing diet, e.g. a 100 calorie diet, is absurd.

## Obesity in Childhood and Pregnancy

It seems undesirable as a rule to attempt to reduce weight by diet restriction in children or pregnant women. In a child, a better solution consists of manipulating the diet and the schedule of exercise in order to keep the child's weight at its existing value and to let the child "grow up" to the weight. Similarly, in pregnant women, postpartum weight loss can be used to achieve at least part of the desired result. When dealing with obesity in childhood, it is important to remember that inactivity may be the major factor in the caloric imbalance, and that it may be easier and more effective to step up activity than to reduce food intake. Care must be exercised, particularly with children who have been obese since early childhood, not to do more harm than good. With present methods, the prognosis for such subjects is generally poor, and the psychologic trauma of persistent and tactless attempts at reduction may be considerable. Another old medical adage, *"Nil nocere"* (Do no harm), also applies to the therapy of obesity.

## REFERENCES

1. Mayer, J.: Exercise and weight control. Postgrad. Med., 25:325 (March) 1959.
2. Bruch, H.: Psychopathology of hunger and appetite in Changing Concepts of Psychoanalytic Medicine. New York, Grune & Stratton, Inc. 1956.
3. Stunkard, A. J. and Dorris, R. J.: Physical activity: Performance and attitude of a group of obese women. Am. J. M. Sc., 233:622, 1957.
4. Bruch, H.: Fat children grown-up. The Johns Hopkins Medical and Surgical Association, Baltimore, February 25, 1955.
5. ——: The Importance of Overweight. New York, W. W. Norton & Co., 1957.
6. Stunkard, A. J., Grace, W. J. and Wolff, H. G.: The night eating syndrome; pattern of food intake among certain obese persons. Am. J. Med., 19:78, 1955.
7. Beaudoin, R. and Mayer, J.: Food intakes of obese and nonobese women. J. Am. Dietet. A., 29:29, 1953.
8. Stunkard, A. J. and Wolff, H. G.: Pathogenesis in human obesity. Psychosom. Med., 20:17, 1958.
9. Mayer, J.: The physiologic basis of obesity and leanness. Nutrition Abstr. & Rev. Part I, 25:597, Part II, 25:871, 1955.
10. Keys, A. et al.: The Biology of Human Starvation Minneapolis, University of Minnesota Press, 1950.
11. Ohlson, J. et al.: Weight control through nutritionally adequate diets. In Weight Control: A Collection of Papers. Ames, Iowa, Iowa State College Press, 1955.
12. Stunkard, A. J.: The dieting depression: Untoward responses to weight reduction among certain obese persons. Am. J. Med., 23:77, 1957.
13. Mayer, J.: A physiologist examines some psychiatric assumptions concerning obesity. Internat. Rec. Med., 171:13, 1958.
14. Van Itallie, T. B.: Combined staff clinic: Obesity, Am. J. Med., 19:111, 1955.

*Chapter 36*

# REDUCING BY TOTAL FASTING

$T$HE very multiplicity in dietary fads and clinical fashions in the treatment of obesity testifies to our continued ignorance of the deeper causes of the many syndromes entailing prolonged positive energy balance and hence, of their rational treatment. The latest popular method of dealing with intractable obese patients (those in whom "self-control," bolstered by the doctor's most persuasive manner, has failed) is total, prolonged fasting. Recently advocated by Duncan and his co-workers (1), this method has been tried in hospitals all over the United States with, many clinicians feel, some measure of success. Whether it will remain permanently an important part of the medical armamentarium used against obesity in more than a few special cases is perhaps doubtful.

In a comprehensive article, Duncan, Jenson, Cristofori and Schless (2) have presented the responses of 107 obese patients to restricted intake and intermittent or prolonged fasting. By and large, these individuals had abandoned all hope of weight reduction by "dieting."

Each patient was hospitalized for intitial observation and careful examination of his metabolic behavior during the first fasting period. Infection, diabetes, liver diseases, recent myocardial infarction, peptic ulcer, uncontrolled diabetes, and pregnancy were causes for exclusion. Glucose tolerance tests were performed in all patients and cholecystography in some. Patients less than 18 years old fasted for no more than one week. Other patients fasted from 5 to 14 days. In most instances, diets providing 900 to 1500 calories were resumed abruptly following the fast; these apparently exceeded the patient's appetite for several days following the fast. Eventually patients were allowed to consume

Reprinted from *Postgraduate Medicine*, *35* (No. 3), March, 1964.

"more liberal diets than formerly," e.g. 1300 to 1900 calories, but, to compensate for the fact that on such caloric intakes patients did not lose and sometimes gained weight, this procedure was "overcorrected" by one or two day fast periods at appropriate intervals. After a few weeks of "adaptation," the patient may be readmitted for a repetition of the "long fast."

Duncan and his colleagues feel that this method of weight control presents great advantages: loss of weight varying from 1.5 to as much as 4 lb a day (average loss between 2 and 2.7 lb a day); sense of well-being and cheerfulness; anorexia, "notably after the first day," with a close relationship between hyperketonemia and loss of appetite; and lowering of blood pressure during the fast in cases of hypertension. Follow-up, covering 1 to 32 months (no breakdown of this information was given, which makes interpretation impossible), showed that while 40 per cent of the patients regained or exceeded their former weights, 43 per cent maintained their reduced state and 17 per cent continued to lose. Drawbacks observed in this series included "mild degrees of weakness" (especially in fairly active subjects), headaches and lightheadedness in a few instances, transient waves of nausea (usually mild) in one-third of the cases, and a prompt, moderate gain in weight ("attributed to fluid retention") when food intake was resumed.

Reports from other institutions suggest additional drawbacks, not observed in the series reported by Duncan and his associates: The disappearance of hunger does not appear to be as universal as stated by the Philadelphia authors. After a fast of a few days, some patients exhibit hyperuricemia (3). In a small series in one hospital (4), at least one case of previously unapparent or nonexistent ulcerative colitis and one case of severe and unanticipated depression occurred after fasts of 8 to 10 days.

From a practical viewpoint, it is difficult in the absence of a longer follow-up and a more detailed presentation of Duncan's results to evaluate whether this new therapeutic method has substantial merits. From a theoretical viewpoint, there are a number of obvious points which need to be clarified before reduction by total fasting can be considered a rational (as opposed to an empirical) procedure. First is the matter of weight loss.

While it is true that daily weight losses in cases of total starvation are much greater than those seen in patients on restricted but appreciable diets, this does not mean that total fasting causes much greater losses in body fat, which is, after all, the object of "weight" reduction. First, the fact that the central nervous system requires glucose as its exclusive fuel forces the fasting organism to provide glucose by glyconeogenesis, i.e. the breakdown of protein for the purpose of providing carbohydrate. Inasmuch as 1 gm of adipose tissue is probably equivalent to eight caloreis, while protein yields only four calories per gram and each gram is accompanied in tissue by 3 gm of water, the breakdown of "protein tissue" will cause a weight loss many times — perhaps as much as eight times — greater than the loss of adipose tissue.

In animals, the size of the liver, salivary glands, pancreas and eventually the muscles and other organs is markedly reduced by prolonged inanition. In man, the older but very well-controlled studies of Benedict (5) on a fasting subject showed that during a two week fast (during which basal metabolism dropped 31%), protein catabolism rose from 42.6 gm per day the first day to 71.2 gm the fourth day, and then dropped slowly to 46.4 gm at the end of two weeks. By this time the protein catabolism still contributed 20 per cent of the calories consumed and, one surmises, at least half of the weight loss. The ketosis itself, of course, leads to weight loss; the excessive loss of sodium chloride in the urine, by reducing the size of the extracellular fluid compartment, magnifies the loss of weight to a much greater value than would correspond to loss of fat alone. After all, even if a caloric deficit of 3500 calories could be achieved in hospitalized patients (less than half that amount may be realistic), the maximum weight loss which could be achieved by atrophy of the adipose tissue alone is 1 lb a day instead of the average of 2.5 lb a day ovserved by Duncan and his colleagues. Even this could be achieved in patients formidably larger or obese enough at the start to have a maintenance requirement of 3500 calories. The weight loss of 4 lb a day reported by Duncan, if it was actually sustained over the whole duration of the fast, must represent a tremendous — and to this worker, an alarming — degree of dehydration. In fact, the excessive weight loss not due to fat is a measure of the extraordinary stress under which the organism of the patients is placed.

In one study Duncan and his colleagues called obese subjects "adults with uncomplicated exogenous obesity." I take this simply to mean that by existing tests no abnormality could be detected. Work in experimental animals suggests, however, that obesity may be the end product of a number of syndromes, several with metabolic components, which would not be detected by clinical tests such as those described by Duncan and associates. This makes it all the more important to try to use reaction to total fasting as one of the possible methods for differentiating various forms of obesity; a more careful analysis of which patient reacted to fasting by very marked hyperketonemia, for example, would be important.

The rise in blood ketones in obese subjects is often lower than would be seen in nonobese individuals. Kekwick, Pawan and Chalmers (6) have suggested a difference in susceptibility to ketosis of obese and of lean patients on low-calorie, low-carbohydrate diets. More relevant is the study of fasting ketosis conducted by Bloom (7) on six obese men and seven obese women with limited and comparable activity. Bloom reported that on the average his subjects showed a lower rise in blood ketones than individuals of normal weight. Furthermore, the female susceptibility to ketosis seems to disappear in obesity. (Incidentally, I am struck by the fact that Bloom's patients did not present a homogeneous picture but that some of them showed an extreme resistance to rise in blood ketones with fasting while others did not, finding in agreement with his experience in adult men and in adolescents. The fact that blood ketones similarly fail to rise in certain forms of metabolic obesity in animals may be significant.) Folin and Dennis (8) and McKay and Sherril (9) have similarly observed marked differences in evolution of blood ketones among obese individuals, with some showing a normal or severe rise with prolonged fasting and a minority showing very little rise. Whether the disappearance of acute hunger pangs after one or two days of fasting observed in many but not all individuals is in fact correlated with hyperketonemia does not appear to have been studied on an individual basis.

Similarly, data on nitrogen balance would be essential, not only for an appraisal of how much of the weight loss is really fat loss but also because this might again allow differentiation between patients in whom fat reserves are relatively freely available, as is the case in regulatory obesities, and those in whom a metabolic hindrance to fat mobilization, such as has been described in the obese hyperglycemic syndrome in animals (10), may exist. In such a syndrome, much more marked depletion of body protein reserves takes place under fasting condition than is seen in regulatory obesities.

Many other questions are still unanswered. What is the effect of prolonged fasting on patients who are still growing? What types of personality may react to total fasting with serious psychiatric or psychosomatic disturbances? What is the composition of the tissue which is regained rapidly after fasting? Are there any pathologic consequences of hyperketonemia and dehydration? What are the long-term effects on the liver and other organs of alternating total fasting and refeeding? And many others.

From a public health viewpoint, certain dangers should be kept in mind. First, as a result of the newspaper and magazine publicity given this procedure, a number of obese subjects will try — some are trying already — total fast as a method of weight reduction without hospitalization and, in fact, without consulting their physicians and without changing their modes of life. The prospect of fasting obese teen-agers attempting to study or of fasting subjects driving automobiles is not a happy one. Secondly, unless careful instruction, supervision and follow-up are available, the publicity given this procedure once again is leading to a widespread feeling the weight control can be an on-and-off business and that knowledge of the caloric content of foods and establishment of proper dietary and exercise regimens, which alone can be effective over long periods, can be evaded. Total fasting is an interesting tool of clinical research, if properly conducted and evaluated, particularly with respect to the types of obese patients in which it is tried. It is to be hoped that the interesting observations of Duncan and his colleagues are not going to be a pretext for yet one more — and a particularly dangerous — wave of faddism in dealing with the important health problems constituted by obesity.

# REFERENCES

1. Duncan, G. G., Jenson, W. K., Fraser, R. I. and Cristofori, F. C.: Correction and control of intractable obesity. J.A.M.A., 181:309, 1962.
2. Duncan, G. G., Jenson, W. K., Cristofori, F. C. and Schless, G. L.: Intermittent fasts in the correction and control of intractable obesity. Am. J. M. Sc., 245:515, 1963.
3. Emerson, K., Jr.: Personal communication.
4. Van Itallie, T. B.: Personal communication.
5. Benedict, F. G.: A Study of Prolonged Fasting. Wahsington, D. C., Carnegie Instituition, 1915, No. 203.
6. Kekwick, A., Pawan, G. L. S. and Chalmers, T. M.: Resistance to ketosis in obese subjects. Lancet, 2:1157, 1959.
7. Bloom, W. L.: Fasting ketosis in obese men and women. J. Lab. & Clin. Med., 59:605, 1962.
8. Folin, O. and Dennis, W.: On starvation and obesity, with special reference to acidosis. J. Biol. Chem., 21:183, 1915.
9. McKay, E. M. and Sherril, J. W.: A comparison of ketosis developed during fasting by obese patients and normal subjects. Endocrinology, 21:677, 1937.
10. Mayer, J.: Obesity. Ann. Rev. Med., 14:111-132, 1963.

*Chapter 37*

# UNDERSTANDING PORTION SIZES

Written in collaboration with Johanna Dwyer

$A$ BUSY medical practitioner confronted with a patient who should lose weight has only enough time to advise him that he needs to reduce and to hand him a low-calorie diet to follow. Often when the patient returns for a follow-up visit, he has lost much less weight than predicted from the caloric deficit imposed although he insists he has religiously followed the diet. If the patient has not knowingly concealed deviations from his diet, something must have been lacking in the instructions he received. The critical element in many cases is that portion size of foods is not stressed sufficiently when the diet is prescribed. The patient has a good notion of "what" to eat, but he often has no idea of exactly "how much" he should eat. Many patients do not understand that quantity is more important than the nature of foods in a reducing diet.

Obviously, obese persons trying to lose weight should eat smaller portions than the nonobese. If they are to reduce, they must have a good idea of the size of servings prescribed. This information is essential not only for the success of the weight reduction program but for maintaining the weight loss after satisfactory conclusion of the reduction phase.

Many people assume that an "average" portion is that which they normally eat, regardless of how large or small it may be. Ideas of the size of an "average potato" or an "average serving of meat" vary greatly among different people. Portion sizes specified in diets are often smaller than those which patients consider to be average. Prescribing a diet which has portions of TV dinner size is useless if the patient pictures the larger-sized portions he usually

Reprinted from *Postgraduate Medicine, 44* (No. 3), September, 1968.© McGraw-Hill, Inc.

takes at home.

Minor errors in estimating portion size easily add up to enough calories per day to greatly inhibit weight loss. For example, if the patient eats his customary half-pound of roast beef or his usual large serving of mashed potatoes rather than the smaller servings specified in his diet, he will add an extra 500 calories to his reducing diet without being aware that he is overeating. Five hundred calories per day is the caloric equivalent of 1 lb of body fat per week. Excesses of this type can sabotage dieting efforts.

It is difficult to judge portion sizes accurately without instruction. Anyone who has tried to determine if a piece of pizza is equivalent to the 3-inch section of a 14-inch pie listed as an average serving in calorie tables recognizes how easily one can become exasperated with the whole procedure. If portion sizes are not judged accurately, the caloric values assigned to them are worthless. The patient must be shown the exact sizes of portions he is to eat so that he will have an image of the proper portions fixed firmly in his mind.

Ease of measurement differs with various foods. Foods which are reported on an item or count basis or measured in cups or tablespoons are most accurately measured. Foods measured in other units, such as ounces or inches, are less accurately measured. Yet often the latter foods (meat is an important example) are major sources of calories in the reducing diet. Patients tend to consistently underestimate the size of servings of foods measured in ounces as the actual size increases; the size of servings measured in cups or tablespoons is often overestimated. It is relatively easy to judge amounts of foods when the portion size is discrete as for fruits and cookies. The task is much more difficult when one must judge the size and caloric content of a portion of steak or roast beef. The sizes of servings of these foods are on a continuum. Geometric problems also interfere with estimating caloric content of foods like these because the way the meat is cut or the potato served may vary greatly and make portions appear to be more or less than they actually are.

## WHAT SHOULD THE PATIENT KNOW?

What then is the best way to treat those who want to reduce?

First, both the physician and the patient must realize that obesity is not an acute condition which can be quickly treated and cured. Obesity is a chronic disease which requires lifelong therapy and attention. The goal of any reducing program is not merely to lose weight but to keep it off. For this reason, adapting a diet to the patient's long term food habits is extremely important. No one particular diet is appropriate for everybody. The diet should be planned specifically to fit the individual patient's style of living.

The downward caloric adjustment of existing food habits by reducing portion size (if food habits already provide an adequate amount of basic nutrients) is an easy way to place the patient on a diet acceptable to him in terms of economics and style of eating. This method of formulating a diet has additional merit in that it will not introduce revolutionary changes in the cooking practices of the household. Furthermore, once the patient attains the required weight, portions can be adjusted to provide a proper maintenance diet in the future.

Models of food are practically indispensable in helping the patient comprehend the size of portions prescribed in the diet. The person instructing the patient should use models or in some cases actual foods to illustrate a portion of a given size. Without such models, instruction is often meaningless. The obese patient should visualize and memorize portion sizes and their corresponding caloric content. He also needs thorough training in appraising the size of servings of various foods.

Many people have only the vaguest idea of what a calorie is. Some believe that calories are substances in foods which cause fat to accumulate. Few people realize that protein, carbohydrates and fat are all sources of calories in the diet. The patient on a diet may be counting arbitrary units which he does not understand if he is not given some instruction in basic nutrition. Much folk knowledge regarding weight control is also inacurate and often patently false. For example, the belief that carbohydrates and starchy foods calorically surpass meats is common. Another widely held falsehood is that only solid foods contain calories. Dietary instruction should correct any misconceptions the patient may have.

The patient needs to know how much less of each food he must consume, the amounts of the particular foods he must eat, and the particular foods he must avoid because they contribute too many calories and too few essentials nutrients to his diet. If the formulation of a diet adapted to the patient's needs, the dietary instruction, and the follow-up visits take more time than the physician can give, a referral to a dietitian or nutritionist is in order.

## SUMMARY

Understanding what calories are, knowing portion size, and memorizing enough representative caloric values of common foods are essential components of basic nutrition education for the dieting patient. Physicians have given too little attention to instructing their obese patients on proper portion sizes of the foods in their diets. Weight reduction programs will be more effective when physicians eschew generalities in explaining a diet and when they spend enough time with each patient really to teach him what he needs to know.

## Chapter 38

# TREATMENT OF OBESITY IN ADULTS

## MEDICAL HISTORY AND BASIC DATA

IT is essential that in the medical history particular attention be given to the age of onset of obesity and its past course: The psychologic aspects and prognosis are quite different in persons who become obese in their adult years and in persons who were obese as children and as adolescents. Persons who were obese as youngsters are much more likely to be obsessively concerned with self-image and to view their obesity as a badge of shame rather than as a medical problem which can be attacked by rather simple means; they are more likly to have failed repeatedly to control their weight in the past, they are more likely to be victims of as yet little understood physiologic or psychologic abnormalities. While the classic "endocrine" abnormalities are rare, the possibility of hypothyroidism, hyperadrenocorticism and, the male, hypogonadism should be ruled out. The possible occurrence of abnormal fluid retention should be ruled out. Dietary habits should be investigated thoroughly together with the familial, psychologic and economic background. Patterns of hunger and satiety should be understood and their modification when the patient is on a reducing diet followed, as they form the basis of decisions on the division of the calories allotted to the reducing diets among the proper number of meals and snacks and of decisions on the eventual use of anorexigenic agents, their dosage, and timing of administration. The actual time spent in activities not involving sitting or lying down and some idea of the vigor with which these activities are pursued should be known; these elements, together with the sex of the patient and his or her size and age, form the basis of the estimate of the daily caloric

---

Reprinted from *Postgraduate Medicine, 38* (No. 3), September, 1965.

requirements for energy balance. An oral glucose tolerance curve is a useful element of information. (The presence of a marked secondary hypoglycemia may be an indication to attempt a low-carbohydrate diet.) Availability of serum iron data as well as hemoglobin, etc. may be useful as possible indications of a tendency toward iron deficiency, a condition which seems much more prevalent among obese subjects than among the general population (1).

As regards psychologic data, it is important, before searching for possible psychogenic factors, to evaluate as carefully as possible the psychologic effects of obesity on the patient. The psychologic impact on the patient of newly discovered pathologic conditions (e.g. diabetes, hypertension) ought also to be appraised in terms of their possible effect on motivation.

## INDICATIONS FOR WEIGHT REDUCTION

Outside of some (rare) situations involving either somatic or psychiatric problems, weight reduction is desirable in all obese individuals. The attitude that in the absence of any clear reason for reducing the patient he or she should be left alone is a counsel of laziness. Should one wait for hypertension or diabetes or immobilization consequent to the superimposition of excess weight on arthritis to do something about the problem? Furthermore, the patient's general fitness is visibly improved; his employability is increased in both government and industry; and, in a society which, for better or for worse, puts a great deal of emphasis on appearance, his social acceptability — and in some cases, his happiness — is improved.

In some serious conditions indications for weight reduction are particularly pressing:

1. Respiratory difficulties — The work of breathing is increased if considerable additional weight is carried on the chest wall. Excessive adipose tissue also increases the complexity of the problem of keeping the whole body oxygenated. Obese people consequently have a diminished exercise tolerance and may show greater difficulty in normal breathing, particularly in the presence

of any — even mild — respiratory infection. At the extreme, very marked obesity may lead to the Pickwickian syndrome where, through decreased ventilation, accumulation of carbon dioxide in blood leads to lethargy and somnolence. Lowered oxygenation of arterial blood may also lead to reactive polycythemia, which may compound the possiblility of thrombosis and abnormal blood clotting. Cardiac enlargement and congestive heart failure may also result from pulmonary difficulties due to extreme obesity. The removal of obesity is essential to the treatment of the Pickwickian syndrome. It can aid greatly the treatment of congestive heart failure

2. Hypertension — While it is true that in some early reports the correlation between obesity and hypertension was exaggerated by the use of pressure cuffs of ordinary size, which excessively compressed the tissues in the upper arm, even when a cuff of proper size is used, a significant association between obesity and hypertension is seen. In general, it can be said that hypertension is more prevalent among obese than among nonobese persons and that obese hypertensives show a greater morbidity and mortality rate and, in particular, a greater risk of coronary heart disease than nonobese hypertensives (or than obese nonhypertensives).

The results of weight reduction on hypertension are by no means universally present, but when there is a change, it tends to be favorable, with the drop in blood pressure a function of the drop in body weight. Recent experience shows that in large groups of hypertensives, at least half — and in some instances as many as 75 per cent — of the patients experience significant decreases in blood pressure (20 mm systolic or 15 mm diastolic) if they lose at least 15 lb. While certain authors have claimed that the most important effect of weight reduction regimens is the curtailment in sodium chloride which accompanies the caloric restriction, it appears that this is only one of the variables involved. There is no doubt that, whatever the mechanisms involved, hypertension in an obese patient is a compelling indication for weight reduction. The favorable effect of weight reduction on the survival of post-coronary patients is well documented. While improvement in angina pectoris is always difficult to measure, there is little doubt that weight reduction is also a favorable factor in this condition.

3. Endocrine and metabolic disturbances — Hirsutism and menstrual irregularities, much more freqent among obese women than among nonobese, can often be mitigated after sufficient weight loss. There are somewhat conflicting reports on the association of obesity with high cholesterol levels, triglycerides and fatty acids. It is probable that such conflicts are due to a lack of differentiation of the phase of obesity (active weight gain, static obesity) and to our inability at present to differentiate among various forms of obesity. It can be stated in general that while abnormal plasma lipid levels frequently fail to respond to weight reduction, any response which takes place, particularly in blood cholesterol level, tends to be favorable; i.e. the abnormally high lipid level is decreased temporarily or permanently.

There is a high prevalence among obese subjects of impaired glucose tolerance and, in many cases, of hyperglycemia. This type of maturity-onset "diabetes," which often responds dramatically to weight reduction, may be less likely to lead to vascular degeneration than juvenile, "nonobese" types of diabetes. Nevertheless, avoiding the need for insulin, preventing skin and other infections related to hyperglycemia, and avoiding the risk of acidosis provide strong indications for immediate institution of weight reduction in such patients. After suitable weight reduction, insulin can very frequently be replaced by oral hypoglycemic agents. In many cases, the need for pharmacologic agents to control blood sugar may be eliminated altogether. For example, in a large series of obese diabetics, glucose levels returned to normal in nearly 75 per cent of those achieving the desired weight reduction. Glucose tolerances were improved in about half of the remainder.

4. Other pathologic conditions — Serious difficulties in reproduction associated with obesity can often be diminished or eliminated by weight reduction. The risk of toxemia and delivery problems can be decreased if the woman's weight is controlled, preferably by reduction before the beginning of pregnancy, but at least by cutting down on the weight gain during pregnancy. Infertility in obese men may be the result of excessively high temperature of the scrotum if it is surrounded by folds of adipose tissue.

While there is a significant association between obesity and gallbladder disease, there is yet no documented evidence that once the disease is present, it is ameliorated by weight reduction.

Certain skin problems may similarly be mitigated or eliminated by weight reduction. Obesity, because it restricts normal heat loss by the body, tends to promote excessive perspiration. Contact or friction between moist skin areas in adjacent folds often leads to rashes, inflammation and furuncles. While obesity per se probably does not cause varicose veins, weight reduction considerably lessens the risk of ulcers and other skin complications in women who have varicose veins.

A number of bone and joint diseases are greatly benefited by weight reduction, which decreases the pressure on the damaged structure and facilitates mobility. Rupture of intravertebral disks, osteoarthritis and intermittent claudication are examples in point.

In spite of steady advances in anesthesiologic and surgical technics, obese patients still have an increased risk in operations and, if possible, should be reduced before elective procedures.

Finally, especially in adolescents but also in many obese adults, particularly in women, the adverse psychologic effects of obesity — "losings one's looks," anxiety about its effects on marital relationships, etc. — may by themselves constitute a pressing medical indication for weight reduction.

## CONTRAINDICATIONS TO WEIGHT REDUCTION

Certain diseases, in particular tuberculosis, gout and diverticulitis, are often quoted as examples of conditions in which weight reduction is contraindicated. Actually, weight reduction, if needed, can be accomplished safely in these diseases if done very gradually with a sensible dietary regimen. Weight reduction is contraindicated in Addison's disease, regional ileitis and ulcerative colitis; it is, however, rarely associated with these diseases.

Cases in which rapid weight loss was associated with profound depression or acute psychosis have received wide attention and have frequently been cited as illustrating the dangers attendant on weight reduction. While such cases are indeed documented, the following points must be made: (1) The occurrence of depression or psychosis during weight reduction is very rare; (2) the patients had manifestly unstable personalities before the reduction therapy; (3) treatment was usually aimed at a rapid rate of weight loss and was based on a drastic curtailment of food intake rather than aimed at a slow rate of weight loss with the combination of increased exercise and a moderate diet to create the caloric deficit necessary for weight loss. Previous instances of successful weight loss, even though the lower weight was not maintained, can be taken as a sign that the patient can probably tolerate a course of weight reduction. Certainly, in the enormous majority of cases, the physician need not fear such drastic psychologic complications of the treatment, although regular checks of the patient's outlook, a careful examination of the degree of hunger and fatigue experienced by the patient, and proper remedial measures if both appear excessive are essential parts of the sound therapy of obesity.

## METHODS OF WEIGHT REDUCTION

It cannot be emphasized enough that the various methods which we are about to examine are not alternative methods. Diet and exercise are complementary measures in establishing the caloric deficit. The manipulation of the dietary schedule and the use of artificial sweeteners, formula diets and anorexigenic agents are all directed at making the limitation in caloric intake more acceptable. Salt restriction may help to provide a more even rate of weight reduction by avoiding excessive fluid retention. Psychologic support is always an essential element of any long-term therapy.

### Dietary Regimen

A proper diet must provide all necessary nutrients other than calories in sufficient amounts, be palatable, easily available from the viewpoints of economics and convenience, and be limited in calories so as to permit the desired caloric deficit. Ideally, the diet must be such as to help in the reeducation of the patient so that by increasing somewhat the size of the portions, it will provide a proper maintenance diet when the desired weight has been obtained.

The determination of the desired deficit is based on the fact that a pound of body fat is the caloric equivalent of 3500 calories. This, in turn, means that a daily deficit of 500 calories will lead, over a long enough period to an average rate of loss of 1 lb a week, a deficit of 1000 calories, to an average rate of loss of 2 lb a week. This rate of 2 lb a week is, incidentally, as much as should be lost by a patient not under close, frequent medical supervision; if patients are very obese and are followed very carefully both metabolically and psychologically, greater rates of weight loss can be obtained safely, at least at the beginning of the reduction regimen, but indications for such a rapid rate must be pressing (e.g. impending surgery).

It is generally true that in ambulatory, busy patients, a caloric intake of less than 1500 calories for men and 1000 for women is poorly tolerated over long periods. An increased rate of energy expenditure through stepped up physical activity makes it possible to obtain a caloric deficit of 500 or 1000 calories per day without having to cut food intake below these (low) limits.

Once the rate of weight loss has been decided (e.g. 2 lb per week, tantamount to a deficit of 1000 calories per day), a guess is made as to the requirements to maintain the patient, given his or her size and pattern of activity. Let us assume that the best guess is of the order of 2200 calories. Adding an hour of walking to the usual activity pattern will bring it to 2500 calories; the diet should be geared then to provide 1500 calories, with the intake adjusted as the results of the trial become available over, say, a two-week period.

Determining the caloric content of the diet is but one aspect of dietary prescription. Knowledge of the patient's familial and economic status, his usual eating pattern, his tastes, and the capabilities of the person who does the marketing and cooking are necessary before the choice of foods to be included in the diet can be made (always remembering that the more varied a diet, the greater the chances that it will be nutritionally adequate, thus eliminating the need for nutritional supplements such as vitamin pills).

Education of the patient as regards the caloric content of the various foods in various-sized portions is essential not only to the success of the weight reduction program but also of the subsequent maintenance program. Models are a necessary tool in demonstrating the size of portions. Such expressions as an "average" potato or an "average" serving of lean meat are understood to mean widely different sizes by various individuals.

The distribution of the food in a number of meals and snacks is a matter for individual prescription and experimentation: A "good" reducing diet is one on which the patient does not become too hungry. Knowing the normal pattern of hunger and satiety of the patient, a guess can be made as to the number of meals and snacks which will prevent the development of excessive hunger. If this does develop once caloric restriction is instituted, further fragmentation of the daily food allowance may help to mitigate the problem. If this is still unsuccessful, a clear indication for the use of anorexigenic agents exists.

There is at present no evidence available which would support the idea that some of the more extreme diets recently popularized have any advantage over a calorically restricted, balanced, "normal" diet. A low-protein, low-fat, "rice" type diet was popular a few years ago. It was followed by a very low-protein diet, dubbed the "Rockefeller" diet by its promoters. The very high-protein, moderate-carbohydrate diet has been recommended by a number of groups, in part on the basis of a misconception of the order of mangnitude of the specific dynamic action of proteins in a mixed diet. The high-fat, low-carbohydrate (or carbohydrate-free) diet reappears every now and they under a variety of names, most recently the 'DuPont" or "Pennington" or "Mayo" diet. With alcohol added, it has become the "drinking man's diet." Again, advocates of these diets who are sincere are apparently misguided on a number of counts. While it is true that a high-fat diet depresses fat synthesis, it by no means prevents fat deposition when the fat is copiously available in the diet. Fat does have "satiety" value, but so do other foods. A carbohydrate-free, high-fat diet does cause an immediate weight loss (over and above the steady decrease due to caloric deficit), but this is due to partial dehydration and is of no lasting significance in a program designed to reduce adiposity, not simply to decrease weight per se over the short term. A diet high in fat, where calories and alcohol can be consumed ad libitum, not only tends to make your patients fat (and inebriated) but also may be highly atherogenic.

A balanced diet, containing no less than 12 to 14 per cent of protein, no more than 30 per cent of fat (with saturated fats cut down), and the rest carbohydrates (with sucrose cut down to a very low level), provided by foods of sufficient variety is infinitely preferable to the fad diets mentioned (and their congeners, the grapefruit diet, the banana diet, the hard boiled egg diet, etc.).

Formula diets have become very popular in the past 10 or so years. Whether purchased in liquid form or as powders to be suspended in water, their main advantage is that they provide strictly established amounts of food (three times 300 calories or four times 225 calories per day in general) and thus provide a simple, rigid regimen which does not need to be based on any knowledge of foods and food values. While this is often an advantage at the beginning of the reducing period (two to four weeks), it should not retard the dietary education which sooner or later is absolutely necessary to carry the patient over a prolonged weight reduction period and through the maintenance, lifelong phase. The enormous majority of patients do not in fact stay exclusively on such formula diets, and as the formula diet is supplemented by other foods, its intrinsic value is lost. Formula diets may, nevertheless, be found useful during maintenance as the exclusive replacement of one meal a day.

Bulk-producing agents (such as methyl cellulose) have not been shown to have any special merit. Apples, celery, raw carrots or salads are more palatable, more likely to become parts of lifelong dietary pattern and thus are superior on all counts to artificial bulk-producing agents. Work done in our laboratory suggests that bulky foods may be particularly valuable as satiety adjuncts not so much because of their stomach-filling role as because they slow down the course of the meal and provide time for satiety phenomena to supervene. Artificial bulk-producing agents do not make a similar contribution to satiety.

The use of artificial sweeteners can be a useful adjunct to reducing diets. Certainly there is little to say for the extensive consumption of sucrose, an "empty" source of calories which in large amounts may excessively stimulate insulin production. A small amount of sucrose (e.g. one sourball once or twice a day at the end of a meal as "dessert" or as a snack if a meal is excessively delayed) is useful with some patients, but the use of sugar in the numerous cups of tea and coffee often consumed by reducing patients and the use of sugar-containing soft drinks should be strictly eliminated. If reducing patients have to drink a number of cups of black coffee a day (a questionable practice for some patients on other grounds) and if the coffee has to be sweetened, the use of saccharine and other artificial sweeteners should be encouraged.

Strict restriction of salt is a therapeutic procedure which should be prescribed only if the clinical picture warrants it. On the other hand, cutting down on the salt intake decreases the tendency to excessive fluid retention seen in many reducing obese subjects particularly middle-aged and older women and sedentary individuals. It may also have some effectiveness in the prevention of hypertension. Salt restriction is a much sounder and sager measure to prevent excessive water retention during weight reduction than the use of diuretics which, if prolonged, may cause renal damage. It is unfortunate that certain "reducing" pills containing diuretics (ammonium chloride) are still available for over-the-counter sale. Patients ought to be warned against such preparations.

## Anorexigenic Agents

The current anorexigenic agents are sympathomimetic amines, amphetamines and related compounds. It is generally agreed that they act chiefly by stimulating the ventromedial (satiety hypothalamic centers, but they may have other accessory actions, including some stimulation of spontaneous activity and of free fatty acid release by the adipose tissue. The dosages used vary from patient to patient (from 5 to 20 mg per day for the amphetamines). They are most usefully employed after the hunger-satiety pattern on the desired reducing diet has been determined and whatever adjustment could be made by shifting snacks has been effected, so that the physician knows that the critical periods of extreme hunger are in fact covered. There is little point in giving a small or moderate dose early in the morning, so that the effect has worn off by the end of the afternoon if one is dealing with a patient who is hungry, eats and overeats only in the evening. A frequently successful practice is to give a long-acting amphetamine preparation in the morning with a booster in the late afternoon.

In general, the effective duration of amphetamine treatment is of the order of a month to six weeks; amphetamines are most useful at the onset of treatment and with the patients who have become obese relatively recently. Unfortunately, in many, if not most patients, some side effects are observed: dry mouth, restlessness, irritability, insomnia and sometimes constipation. Cardiac patients are not good candidates for amphetamine therapy because of the adrenergic effects of such agents on the heart (increase in heart rate, potentiation of cardiac arrhythmias); in cases of moderate hypertension, the favorable effect of steady weight loss on blood pressure often outweighs the slight risk of increase due to the amphetamine. The superiority of modifications of the amphetamines (such as phenmetrazine, phentermine, chlorphentermine and benzphetamine) both in terms of effectiveness and avoidance of side effects is not yet convincing to this observer. Supplementation of amphetamine therapy with sedatives or tranquilizers can be useful in certain cases.

It cannot be emphasized enough that the use of such agents by a physician does not in any way decrease the importance of dietary prescription and dietary instruction as previously described. It goes without saying that patients should also be warned against increasing the dose of the prescribed agent on their own or supplementing it with over-the-counter medications (most of which are worthless and some of which are dangerous).

## Exercise

The value of exercise in the prevention of obesity and the treatment of moderately obese persons in otherwise good health has been discussed at length in an article by the author (2). Its value in the prevention of heart disease has also been discussed (3). Let it be recalled simply that: (1) Exercise is the great variable in energy expenditure. Caloric equivalent of exercise of various types has been given (2). The caloric expenditure due to exercise is proportional to the duration of exercise; it is also proportional to the weight of the subject, so that an obese person will use up proportionately more calories to perform the same task than a thin subject. The caloric expenditure increases rapidly with the intensity with which the exercise is performed. (2) Exercise does not increase voluntary food intake in inactive subjects until it has reached a certain critical duration and intensity, depending on the individual.

While obviously a very obese subject, even in good cardio-vascular state, should not be put suddenly to exercise, it is a good idea to start him to walk every day and to increase the duration and eventually the intensity of the exercise as his weight reduction progresses. An understanding of the schedule and of the mode of life of the patient is neccessary if exercise is going to be built into his daily life. Advantage of every opportunity for walking, stair climbing, etc. can be taken so as to restore mobility in patients used to the constant use of automobiles and elevators.

The physician must remind the patient that the insulation provided by the excessive adiposity will restrict his rate of heat loss on hot days so that particular caution must be exercised in the summer to interrupt the exercise with sufficient rest periods and keep hydrated (preferably with water!)

## Thyroid Preparations

There is still too much thyroid hormone prescribed to obese patients (usually in the form of desiccated thyroid preparation) without any clear indication that the patient is in a hypothyroid state. Such medication is based on the misconception that most obese patients are hypometabolic, an old idea originating from relating basal oxygen consumption to body weight. At present, sophisticated methods ($I^{131}$ uptake, PBI determinations, etc.) should be used before a diagnosis of hypothyroidism is arrived at and acted on. The administration of thyroid hormone is in part self-defeating anyway as it depresses endogenous thyroid secretion, the depression being very slow to reverse. If higher doses are given, tachycardia, palpitation, nervousness and insominia appear, creating an unpleasant and potentially dangerous situation.

Triiodothyronine has been advocated by some as a useful aid to dietary restriction. It enhances in vitro the lipolytic effect of epinephrine and is said not to depress thyroid action to the extent shown by throid preparations and not to cause thyrotoxicosis. The evidence to support the claim of usefulness in reducing treatment is not sufficient to recommend its general use.

## Other Methods

A number of "heroic" measures have recently been advocated. One, total fasting, has been discussed at some length in Chapter 36. I was unimpressed with total fasting as a therapeutic measure (as distinct from a research procedure). Reports published since, including reports of accidents during total fasting, do not impel me to look at this method more favorably, although there may be situations, such as impending surgery, where the risk of total fasting for a hospitalized patient under close laboratory and psychologic supervision may be less than that of continued extreme obesity. If surgery is contemplated, it is important that the patient have a week of moderate feeding at the end of the fasting period and immediately before the operation. Patients ought to be strongly warned against self-administered total fasting because of its dangers to themselves (as well as to others if they drive a car!).

Surgical procedures which permit temporary bypass of part of the small intestine have been used in "intractable" obesity. In patients in whom adequate follow-ups are available, the experience has been miserable. Not only did the patients exhibit serious difficulties while the shunt lasted (including some cases of uncontrollable hypocalcema) but the weight was generally recovered rapidly after the shunt was discontinued.

## PSYCHOLOGIC SUPPORT

The physician should be concerned with certain psychologic aspects of the therapy of obesity. In order of increasing diagnostic and therapeutic difficulty, these are:

1. The psychology of weight reduction. He should ease the

discomforts attending the continued sensations associated with a prolonged period of caloric deficit, such as mitigating hunger and fatigue by appropriate measures and counseling, and fix realistic short-term and long-term targets, arriving at the latter by his clinical judgment and based on the actual body structure of the patient and his mode of life and capabilities.

2. The psychology of being obese. Particularly in patients who were obese in adolescence, when the body image appears to be developed, there is a galaxy of psychologic traits which appear to be due to the obesity-obsessive concern with self-image, passivity, expectation of rejection, and progressive withdrawal, which must be coped with if the patient is to be a happy, well-adjusted person (4). Many of these psychologic effects of obesity may tend to make the obesity self-perpetuating.

3. Psychologic factors leading to obesity. These are the least known and thus this area is particularly difficult to deal with adequately. Anxieties and stresses which burden an obese patient may be instrumental, if the patient is otherwise predisposed to obesity by genetics and by constitution (5), in causing overeating and immobilization and, hence, weight accumulation. The development of new interests can be useful, particularly in middle-aged women with little to do outside of the home, too much time on their hands, and a tendency to view their interpersonal relationships in terms of sitting down together at meals.

## REFERENCES

1. Seltzer, C. C. and Mayer, J.: Serum iron and iron-binding capacity in adolescents. II. Comparison of obese and nonobese subjects. Amer. J. Clin. Nutr., 13:354, 1963.
2. Mayer, J.: Exercise and weight control. Postgrad. Med., 25:325 (March) 1959.
3. ——: Exercise and prevention of heart disease. Postgrad. Med., 34:601 (December) 1963.
4. Monello, L. F. and Mayer, J.: Obese adolescent girls, an unrecognized "minority" group? Amer. J. Clin. Nutr., 13:35, 1963.
5. Seltzer, C. C. and Mayer, J.: Body build and obesity — who are the obese? J.A.M.A., 189:677 (August 31) 1964.

*Chapter 39*

# WEIGHT CONTROL IN
# PUBLIC SCHOOL CHILDREN

 $S$ TATISTICS from weight control programs in adults usually are not encouraging. The only basis for human variability is a change in either heredity or environment. In adults, with the genotype established and the mode of life difficult to modify, particularly food and exercise habits, there is little likelihood of permanently altering the phenotype. The situation is more hopeful in children. The whole process of education is a continuing effort to change values, knowledge and habits, and this should pertain to the body as well as to the mind. Furthermore, many educational processes take place outside the home in day schools, boarding schools, camps, etc., where the possibility of modifying food and exercise habits obviously is enhanced. Finally, there is a major (and favorable) difference between the comparative caloric balances of obese and nonobese adults and those of children.

In adults obesity generally is associated with a food intake that is greater than normal. In our urbanized, mechanized society the energy expenditure due to exercise, including walking, is very low in nonobese as well as in obese subjects. In children obesity generally is associated with food intake in the normal or low range and with extremely low expenditure of energy. Our studies have shown repeatedly that in both sexes and at various ages obese children eat no more, and generally eat less, than nonobese children. However, they spend far less time (about one-third as much time) in activities in which they are on their feet — walking, exercising, playing competitive athletic games, etc. Furthermore, we have found that when obese youngsters exercise, they spend far less energy and much less time in actual motion than do

Reprinted from *Postgraduate Medicine, 45* (No. 6), June, 1969.© McGraw-Hill, Inc.

nonobese youngsters. The excess calories available for fat deposition thus come actually from "underexercising" rather than from "overeating." This is not to say that the food habits (as distinguished the food intake) of obese youngsters are in any way superior to those of the nonobese, although our studies have shown that in the older groups obese girls know more about nutrition than thinner girls.

Conversely, we have shown in limited, controlled situations that while increasing the energy expenditure of normally active youngsters increases their food intake so that their weight is maintained, a moderate increase in the activity of fat, inactive children is followed not by an increase in food intake but by a loss of adiposity. This fact is the basis of the program of at least one medically supervised commercial summer camp for obese youngsters. While the results obtained by this camp over the course of the summer usually have been gratifying, they have rarely been permanent. Furthermore, our work showed that summer is not the critical period for obese children in New England. At this time of year their weight is usually plateaued. Fall and winter usually are the periods of weight gain. Finally, the very high cost of summer camps means that only the wealthy can take advantage of this method of weight control.

For these reasons we concluded that the obvious site for a weight control program is the school, where it will reach all children, regardless of economic status, for nine months that include the critical period. Although obesity is fraught with medical consequences, its prevention is best organized within an educational context because it requires reeducation of the individual with regard to food habits, exercise habits, and the whole mode of life. Since we had found previously that from 12 to 20 per cent of the public school students in the Boston area are obese, it seemed that on a national basis only a program carried out in the public schools would suit the size of the problem.

## FEATURES OF THE PILOT PROGRAM

From 1964 through 1967, my associates (Dr. C.C. Seltzer, physical anthropologist; Dr. H. E. Rose, pediatrician; Miss J. A.

Schoonmaker, physical educator and field director; Mrs. J. Goodman, dietitian), their assistants and I carried out a program of weight control for obese youngsters in elementary and junior high grades of the public schools in Newton, Massachusetts, a large suburb of Boston. The program provided increased daily physical education, nutrition education and psychologic support for 350 obese children and adolescents, with other obese youngsters serving as untreated or partly treated controls. Participation was entirely voluntary. The school committee authorized the program and it was organized in cooperation with the regular staff, in particular the superintendent, Dr. Charles Brown, and the director of physical education, Miss Helene Breivogel.

We weighed and measured all participating children and determined their triceps skinfold, a measure of fatness that best correlates with overall adiposity. Subjects were selected on the basis of criteria Dr. Seltzer and I developed for determining adiposity by measuring the triceps skinfold. Medical records, psychologic evaluation, achievement, and record of cooperation between school and parents were also obtained on each child. Parental permission was sought for all children invited to participate and obtained for all who joined, but in the younger age group, participation in the program was based on parental decision only; in the junior high school grades the youngsters made their own decision.

Although we wondered if identification with the "fat" group would present an insuperable barrier, we found that small children were indifferent to the label and older children and adolescents were so anxious to improve their appearance, which caused them increased misery as they became older, that they were delighted to join a daily program that functioned as an integral part of the curriculum and offered them help with a hitherto intractable problem. Nor did we experience the difficulties that we had expected to have with the mothers. In a weight-conscious middle-class community, mothers are anxious that their children, particularly their daughters, receive help with their weight problem. Quite unexpectedly, however, we had difficulty with some of the fathers, who vigorously protested any aspersion on the physique of their sons. Children are realistic about their appearance, and in the case of teen-age girls may even tend to exaggerate any figure problem. Mothers are reasonable in the matter, but we found that it was not always easy to convince a father that his son's adiposity was well outside the limits of normal variability and that a problem existed that should be corrected before the child was enmeshed in the self-perpetuating physiologic and psychologic implications of obesity.

The youngsters in the program took part in special physical activity classes on days alternating with the regular school physical education classes, thereby increasing physical activity sessions from two to five a week. Each session lasted 45 minutes and was conducted by an experienced physical education teacher who was indoctrinated in the physiologic, psychologic and nutritional problems involved, acquainted with the practices and regulations of the Newton school system, and thoroughly appraised of the results of similar pilot programs in physical education conducted on smaller groups of obese youngsters during 1963 and 1964. The teachers were free to plan their own activities within the framework of the program. Classes, consisting of about 15 pupils each, were large enough for group activities yet small enough to permit careful supervision of individual activities.

Vigorous exercise of sufficient duration was the target of the physical education program. Emphasis was on team sports like soccer and volleyball, games, and individual races against the clock, stressing self-improvement rather than competition. Games such as dodge ball, "shipwrecked," chase and relays were chosen because they involved everyone and keep as many people as possible in motion at one time. Instructors encouraged the obese youngsters to remain active during weekends and vacation by pursuing sports or exercises that they liked.

We did not attempt to place most of the obese children on low-calorie diets since we were dealing essentially with growing children on moderate food intake and with low energy expenditure. Under these conditions, restriction of calories results in a slowdown or cessation of growth. Instead we concentrated on improving the youngsters' food habits. The project nutritionist held a series of six classes in nutrition for each age group, followed by individual conferences with the junior high children and conferences with both students and parents at the elementary school level. Instructors used visual aids — wax models to illustrate size of food portions, films and printed material.

All members of the special staff, and eventually those of the regular staff, gave the youngsters constant psychologic support. Their chief aim was to break up the vicious circle — obesity leading to (1) censorious attitudes of peers and elders, leading to (2) obsession with self-image, passivity and expectation of rejection, leading to (3) awkwardness, social isolation, actual rejection, decreased opportunity for exercise outside the home, and increased exposure to food, leading to (4) greater obesity (1).

## RESULTS AND CONCLUSIONS

The effectiveness of such a program is best assessed by comparing changes in the skinfold thickness of subjects and controls; comparison of weight changes in the two groups does not take into account the replacement of fat by muscle in those youngsters exercised most successfully. By all criteria the program was very successful. In boys in the elementary schools, changes in stature were similar in exercised and control groups; the average weight increase and percentage of skinfold increase were more than twice as great in the control group as in the exercised group; the differences for girls were similar but smaller. In the junior high school participants, triceps skinfolds increased in the control goups but decreased in the exercised group. The average weight increase was over 50 per cent greater in the controls than in the exercised youngsters. Analysis on the basis of linearity (height/$\sqrt[3]{\text{weight}}$), which paralleled our visual impression of the youngsters, was equally encouraging. We will publish full data elsewhere (2).

We are now convinced that an effective voluntary weight control program consisting of increased physical exercise, dietary education and psychologic support can be successfully incorporated in public school systems. Success of the program depends on the availability of facilities and the degree of cooperation from the community, school board and school staff. Individual success, of course, depends on the persistence of the child, the extent of his participation in classes, and the family's cooperation in helping him to improve his food habits. Essentially, our experiment showed that most youngsters will benefit from such a program.

A similar program could and probably should become an integral part of all public school systems at all levels. Our pilot study showed that the earlier the age at which the weight control program is started, the better it is for the obese child. At present, our school physical education programs are geared primarily to the physically fit, not to the handicapped students such as the obese. Only pressure and cooperation from the school physician and community practitioners, particularly pediatricians, can effect the necessary broadening of physical education programs to make them valuable agents in preventitive medicine.

## REFERENCES

1. Mayer, J.: Overweight; Causes, Cost, and Control. Englewood Cliffs, New Jersey, Spectrum Books, Prentice-Hall, Inc., 1968.
2. Seltzer, C. C. and Mayer, J.: An effective weight-control program in a public school system. Amer. J. Public Health, 60:679, 1970.

*Chapter 40*

# ANOREXIA NERVOSA

$A$NOREXIA nervosa is probably the only kind of malnutrition which still kills young people in the United States. As such it deserves more attention on the part of clinical nutritionists than it has received. It is this writer's experience that the syndrome can be defined clearly, and that the essential aims of therapy are logical corollaries of its definition.

## A TRIAD OF DENIALS

A number of authors have unnecessarily confused the definition of anorexia nervosa by terming it the particular component of any psychiatric condition associated with a refusal to eat sufficient food to maintain caloric balance. Such a broad definition would include anorexias associated with hysteria, compulsion neurosis, schizophrenia and borderline states of diverse origins (1). By this broad concept, the anorexia exhibited by the paranoic who fears his food is being poisoned could be classified as anorexia nervosa. Such a general definition loses any usefulness. Attempts such as those of Eissler (2) and of other workers, among them Rose and Falstein, to relate the defensive structure of the ego to all such anorexias lead to inconclusiveness. Anorexia occurs both in patients with strong egos and in those with weak egos. Other authors, in attempting to see what such anorexias had in common by delving into the patients' fantasies, have uncovered a great variety of such associations. Lorand (3) had described guilt associated with the combination of the patient's subconscious wish to be impregnated through the mouth and the presence of fat on the abdomen, such guilt being responsible for nausea and vomiting. Waller, Kaufman and Deutsch (4) have described similar

Reprinted from *Postgraduate Medicine, 34* (No. 5), November, 1963.

fantasies of oral impregnation and constipation representing pregnancy. Rose (5) and other authors, Cobb for one, who also studied fantasies or oral impregnation in adolescent girls, noted that such fantasies are far more common than anorexia nervosa. Similarly, the observation by Masserman (6) and other researchers, including Leonard, of an association of eating disturbances with orally destructive incorporative wishes (e.g. patients who, in an "inverted oedipal attachment," wish to incorporate the father's penis in order to become masculine and please the mother) is by no means specific for anorexia nervosa.

Actually, it appears that if one does not insist on indiscriminately naming all severe anorexias associated with psychiatric disorders anorexia nervosa, it becomes possible to reserve this name for the severe anorectic condition, usually found in young women and adolescent girls and exceptionally in adolescent males,* characterized by the following traits: (1) In spite of extreme emaciation, the patient has such a disturbance of body image that she denies being excessively thin. (2) In spite of prolonged inanition, the patient denies ever being hungry. (3) In spite of frantic and usually ritualized exercise done in a state of chronic underfeeding, the patient denies ever being tired.

## Denial of Excessive Thinness

This writer agrees with Bruch (7) that one cannot over-emphasize that disturbance of body image is an essential and diagnostic aspect of anorexia nervosa. This is one of the characteristics which usually differentiate this condition from the malnutritional states generally observed in other psychiatric syndromes. The patient so dreads obesity that she not only is unconcerned with her emaciation but is actually pleased with it as a step toward avoiding fatness. The picture is thus quite different from that seen in hysterical patients who refuse to eat but often complain about becoming too thin, or in schizophrenics who often show some disturbances of body image but are not specifically

---

*Anorexias seen in younger children are usually quite different in character. This important subject will be the topic of later review; in this article, only patients no younger than adolescence will be considered.

delusional about their weight or appearance. In contrast, the patient with anorexia nervosa, while obsessed with the importance of her appearance, will deny vehemently that excessive thinness detracts in any way from her looks.

Monello and Mayer (8) have described the obsessive concern with obesity shown by obese adolescent girls. Bruch (9) has described a similar compulsive preoccupation in "thin fat people." In young women with anorexia nervosa we see the acme of such obsessive concern to the extent of denying not only that all danger of obesity has been eliminated but also that the opposite danger has in fact been reached. Not infrequently, a patient goes from obesity to anorexia nervosa; such a sequence is particularly difficult to manage, as the patient clearly sees the anorexia nervosa as a victory over a great handicap of long standing.

## Denial of Hunger

Almost as striking as the denial of excessive thinness is the denial of hunger. This is clearly either an inability or an unwillingness to recognize hunger and not simply the lack of appetite which follows prolonged starvation and is a component of the terminal phase of starvation. The patient claims that she never feels hungry, not even when only enough food is consumed daily to avoid ketosis, and she complains bitterly of extreme fullness after she has been induced to consume ridiculously small amounts of food. Moreover this denial of hunger is strikingly similar to that which Stunkard (10) noted in many obese patients. Again the fact that anorexia nervosa is frequently noted in patients who have been obese, including patients who go through eating binges, illustrates that some of the psychosomatic background of anorexia nervosa and certain types of obesity may be similar. It is also possible that both the obsessive concern with fat and the denial of hunger are induced in susceptible individuals by society's punitive attitude toward obesity and by the frequent equating of obesity with gluttony (8).

## Denial of Fatigue

Analytically oriented psychiatrists have ignored the activity component of anorexia nervosa just as they have ignored the inactivity component of the obesity of many if not most obese adolescents (11). Bruch (7), ever a keen observer, has noted that "overactivity" is present with great regularity and that the drive for activity continues until emaciation is far advanced, with a subjective feeling of alertness and "wanting to do things." I have been struck with the extreme and usually highly ritualized rate of activity exhibited by adolescent girls and young women with anorexia nervosa. The patients are usually intelligent and have a clear, although not always precise, idea of the caloric cost of exercise. They are determined not to allow themselves to eat certain amounts of particular foods unless and until they "deserve" them by accomplishing certain tasks: walking at a set speed to a specific point and back, running so many blocks, playing tennis, hitting tennis balls against a board for so long, etc. Unlike the other two characteristics, this ritualized activity is particularly extreme in persons who have never been obese. All such patients deny fatigue generally, sometimes vehemently, even though it appears highly probable that keeping up such effort in their debilitated state cannot be comfortable. In fact, this writer feels that for most such patients this very need to ritualize activity is an attempt to make sure it is going to be done, however exhausted they may really feel and however weakened they may be.

## OTHER BEHAVIORAL AND PERCEPTUAL TRAITS

In an effort to reduce further the number of calories they consume, many patients of anorexia nervosa use laxatives, enemas and self-induced vomiting. Such behavior is not infrequently seen in obese subjects and even in "thin fat people." Amenorrhea, as will be discussed later, is probably the result of endocrine changes consequent to starvation, although there may be a psychologic component in its genesis. Bruch has emphasized that many patients with anorexia nervosa exhibit passivity and a sense of helplessness.

Passivity is a trait also seen in many obese patients, which may be a result of social pressures rather than being of primary etiologic significance. Bruch (9) goes so far as to believe that a sense of profound ineffectiveness is characteristic of the patient with anorexia nervosa. This writer has not received this impression from the patients he has seen. One common characteristic among these patients which this writer has not seen pointed out elsewhere, is their tremendous sensitivity to criticism of their appearance by one key male member of their environment, such as the father, a guardian uncle, a boy friend, or even, as in the case of a hitherto highly successful female athlete, a coach. After recovery starts, the patient almost invariably admits that the syndrome was precipitated as indicating that the key male figure involved considered her to be fat.

## TREATMENT

Examination of the literature reveals a baffling diversity of therapeutic approaches, all of which are claimed to have restored the disire to eat in at least one patient. A favored form of treatment has been hormonal; estrogens, thyroid, insulin, desoxy-corticosteroid, pituitary extracts, ACTH and cortisone have all been used in treatments associated with remission and sometimes cure. Forcing fluids by mouth, intravenously administered fluids, isolation, prolonged hospitalization with the round-the-clock nursing care, intragastric tube feeding or the threat of it, and the doctor's insistence that the patient eat, as well as massage, rest, hydrotherapy and electric stimulation were frequently advocated treatments in the pre-World War II period. Since then, variously structured psychotherapy, ranging from informal discussions to psychoanalysis, existential analysis, narcoanalysis and hypnosis, have been used "successfully." Other physicians have even used lobotomy, electroshock and insulin coma (1).

The combination of insulin and chlorpromazine or reserpine has been particularly favored lately for emergency treatment of anorexia nervosa. The most successful method appears to be that of Dally and Sargant (12). Large doses of chlorpromazine (150 mg a day initially, increased by 75 mg a day to the limit of tolerance — as much as 1 gm a day has been used in difficult patients) are combined with insulin (5 units initially and progressively increasing the dose until the patient perspires and becomes drowsy). A large meal interrupts the treatment. The British authors use a morning dose of insulin which varies from 40 to 80 units. Precautions are taken to avoid late hypoglycemia. Small doses of benzhexol also can be used if signs of parkinsonism increase as the dosage of chlorpromazine is increased. The dosage of the drug is reduced after the food intake has been maintained at 4000 calories (starting at 1500) long enough to bring the weight back to an approximately normal level. While reassurance and attempts to gain the patients confidence are essential throughout the treatment, it appears unwise and unprofitable to uncover and handle the psychologic problems until use of the drugs is discontinued or until only chlorpromazine is used in a maintenance dosage.

Actually, it would appear that the first determination should be whether malnutrition — specifically electrolyte imbalance, degree of emaciation, and present rate of weight loss — is so severe as to endanger the patient's life. The risks of emaciation are not simply proportional to the total weight loss; obviously a patient who is obese to start with can withstand a much greater weight loss than a normal or thin individual. Rapid losses, even in smaller amounts, may constitute a great threat to life, because their very speed indicated that protein tissue rather than fat is being lost. A deficit of 1000 calories will correspond to a loss smaller than one-third of a pound if adipose tissue is being consumed, a pound or more if protein tissue is jettisoned. Certainly, in an adolescent girl or young woman any drop in weight to less than 70 lb or any loss of 40 per cent of the ideal weight calls for emergency action if the patient still is not eating or is not retaining adequate calories. At that point emergency refeeding must be started as a last resort.

The problems of and procedures for refeeding are similar to those encountered in refeeding victims of concentration camps or famine. It is perhaps useful to recall that World War II experiences showed that victims of even extreme starvation usually could swallow and digest "normal" simple foods. Intravenous feeding, predigested foods and protein hydrolysates generally were not found to be superior to skim milk powder and water administered orally or by gastric tube followed by other such readily available foodstuffs.

## ENDOCRINE, METABOLIC AND
## ELECTROLYTE DISTURBANCES

Among the effects of the severe self-inflicted malnutrition of anorexia nervosa are a number of disturbances of the endocrine system. Almost invariably seen are low levels of urinary gonadotropins and of 17-ketosteriods, 17-ketosteroid oligomenorrhea and generally amenorrhea — a situation stimulating panhypopituitarism. However, actual panhypopituitarism is contradicted by the usually normal thyroid function and levels of protein-bound and butanol-extractable iodine. This endocrine picture, the result of inanition, does not per se justify hormonal treatment (insulin-chlorpromazine treatment specifically directed at the appetite mechanism falls in a different category). Vitamin therapy sometimes advocated, generally appears unnecessary, although contraindications are missing.

In contrast, one of the most frequent complications of anorexia nervosa and one which poses an urgent therapeutic problem is electrolyte deficiency. Sunderman and Rose (13) described the first case, a patient with hypokalemic alkalosis. Since then, Wigley (14) has reviewed 17 more cases of electrolyte disorders secondary to anorexia nervosa and has added three cases of his own. Most of the patients had alkalosis; some had hyponatremia and eight showed evidence of renal dysfunction, probably due in turn to potassium depletion. In some cases, habitual purgation probably contributed to the potassium deficiency. The patient described by Siebenmann (15) showed. vacuolation of the renal tubules and fragmentation of heart muscle at post mortem. Wigley's three patients showed tubular vacuolation, hypokalemic paralysis, and transient renal involvement, respectively. From a therapeutic viewpoint, conventional treatment in such cases should correct the deficit, but oral or intravenous administration of potassium chloride may be necessary.

## ANALYSIS OF WEIGHT GAIN

Russell and Mezey (16) have analyzed the weight gain of patients with anorexia nervosa who were successfully refed. Four female patients, 18, 18, 22, and 22 years old, respectively, whose weight ranged from 30.3 to 44.1 kg were given a high-calorie diet and induced to gain 5.6 to 11.8 kg in five to six weeks. During this period, the patients were investigated in a metabolic unit; the caloric expenditure was determined by indirect calorimetry and the nitrogen balance was measured. From these data, the composition of tissue deposited was calculated; it consisted of 77 per cent fat, 7 per cent protein, and 16 per cent water. The high rate of fat deposition was confirmed by measurements of skinfold thickness and, in a more quantitative way, by determinations of respiratory quotients. In contrast with reports in the literature on undernourished male patients, in particular the painstaking study of Widdowson and McCance (17), there was a relatively low rate of protein synthesis, which suggests that these patients were not too markedly depleted of protein at the start of the refeeding. In fact, the composition of the weight gained was more similar to that observed by Keys, Anderson and Brozek (18) and by Passmore and his co-workers (19) in males in a state of good nutrition experimentally given excess food to study deposition of obese tissue. Quite reasonably, Russell and Mezey considered this finding to be due to the normally larger fraction of body weight represented by fat in females than in males rather than to a hitherto unrevealed primary metabolic peculiarity of patients with anorexia nervosa.

## SPECIFIC PSYCHOTHERAPEUTIC ASPECTS

When the patient's weight has not reached dangerously low levels, the choice by refeeding is best left to the individual physician's judgment. Some have advocated an easygoing approach to avoid re-creating the type of conflict which the patient usually has experienced with her relatives. Others have emphasized the frequent success of more authoritarian frontal attacks on anorexia. It is argued that the mixture of authority and dispassionate kindness displayed by a physician who spends enough time with his patient, particularly at mealtimes, is quite different from the tangled emotional approach typical of relatives who alternately plead, vacillate and accuse.

Whatever the physician's technic, certainly in the long run

psychotherapy should take into account and eventually correct not only whatever neuroses or psychoses may be associated with anorexia nervosa but first and foremost the triad of denials which are characteristic of the disease:

1. The patient must be reeducated to see herself as others see her, as an abnormally and unaesthetically thin individual. Patients with anorexia nervosa are often quite aware that their arms are too thin. This is frequently a useful point of departure to make them see that the rest of their body is too thin. Careful examination of her body in a mirror, often deferred, not infrequently comes as a shock to the patient and may be the first step in overcoming the dread of being monstrously fat. Bruch has rightly emphasized that the patient will be subjected indefinitely to new episodes of anorexia nervosa as long as the disturbance of body image is not corrected.

2. The patient must be reeducated to feel hungry. Denial of hunger, as we have seen, is a universal trait of patients with anorexia nervosa; it is a common trait in obese patients. In both cases, this nullifies the elaborate machinery which normally adjusts energy intake to energy expenditure (20). One may wonder to what extent schedule-feeding in infancy and a program of feeding which gratifies the mother's needs rather than the child's have been instrumental in weakening or confusing the recognition of hunger signals. At any rate, it is essential that just as the denial of thinness be overcome, that of hunger also be corrected.

3. The patient must be reeducated to feel fatigue. Frantic or ritualized exercise has to be stopped or at least minimized if emaciation is to be overcome. In this writer's experience, patients with anorexia nervosa, although usually intelligent and articulate, have a background of food faddism or at least are ingnorant of the caloric and nutritional value of foods. The physiologic significance of the balance between sensible exercise and rest usually is equally shrouded in ignorance and superstition. In many patients with anorexia nervosa obsessive preoccupation with apearance is present, with good health a secondary concern. This pre-occupation with appearance can be used, as it can in cases of obesity, to lead the patient to a better understanding of true fitness.

# REFERENCES

1. Bliss, E. and Branch, C. H.: Anorexia Nervosa. New York, Harper & Brothers, 1961.
2. Eissler, K. R.: Psychiatric aspects of anorexia nervosa demonstrated by case report. Psychoanalyt. Rev., 30:121, 1943.
3. Lorand S.: Anorexia nervosa; report of a case. Psychosom. Med., 5:282, 1943.
4. Waller, J. V., Kaufman, M. R. and Deutsch, F.: Anorexia nervosa; a psychosomatic entity. Psychosom. Med., 2:3, 1940.
5. Rose, J. A.: Eating inhibitions in children in relation to anorexia nervosa. *Ibid.*,[3] p. 117.
6. Masserman, J. H.: Psychodynamisms in anorexia nervosa and neurotic vomiting. Psychoanalyt. Quart., 10:211, 1941.
7. Bruch, H.: Psychopathology of hunger and appetite. In Rado, S. and Daniels, E. G. (Editors): Changing Concepts of Psychoanalytic Medicine. New York, Grune & Stratton, Inc., 1956.
8. Monello, L. F. and Mayer, J.: Obese adolescent girls: An unrecognized minority group? Am. J. Clin. Nutrition, 13:35, 1963.
9. Bruch, H.: Perceptual and conceptual disturbances in anorexia nervosa. Psychosom. Med., 24:187, 1962.
10. Stunkard, A.: Obesity and the denial of hunger. Psychosom. Med., 21:281, 1959.
11. Mayer, J.: A physiologist examines some psychiatric assumptions concerning obesity. Internat. Rec. Med., 171:13, 1958.
12. Dally, P. J. and Sargant, W.: A new treatment of anorexia nervosa. Brit. M. J., 5188:1770, 1960.
13. Sunderman, F. W. and Rose, E.: Studies in serum electrolytes. XVI. Changes in the serum and body fluids in anorexia nervosa. J. Clin. Endocrinol., 8:209, 1948.
14. Wigley, R. D.: Potassium deficiency in anorexia nervosa, with reference to renal tabular vacuolation. Brit. M. J., 5192:110, 1960.
15. Siebenmann, R. E.: Zur pathogischen Anatomie der Anorexia nervosa. Schweiz. med. Wchnschr., 85:530, 1955.
16. Russell, G. F. M. and Mezey, A. G.: An analysis of weight gain in patients with anorexia nervosa treated with high calorie diets. Clin. Sc., 23:449, 1962.
17. Widdowson, E. M. and McCance, R. A.: The Effect of Undernutrition and of Posture on the Volume and the Composititon of Body Fluids. Studies of Undernutrition. Special Rep. Series No. 275. London, His Majesty's Stationery Office, 1951.
18. Keys, A., Anderson, J. T. and Brozek, J.: Weight gain from simple overeating. Metabolism, 4:427, 1955.
19. Passmore, R., Meiklejohn, A. P., Dewar, A. D. and Thow, R. K.: An analysis of the gain in weight of overfed thin young men. Brit. J. Nutrition, 9:27, 1955.
20. Mayer, J.: Obesity. Ann. Rev. Med., 14:111, 1962.

# PART V

# Inborn Errors of
# Metabolism and Nutrition

*Chapter 41*

# PHENYLKETONURIA AND NUTRITION

IN his 1908 Croonian Lectures to the Royal College of Physicians, Sir Archibald Garrod (1) suggested that four metabolic disorders — albinism, alkaptonuria, cystinuria and pentosuria — were "inborn errors of metabolism." These diseases had at least four features in common: (1) Onset was early and could, in fact, be traced to the first days or weeks of life; (2) at least one other case could usually be found among the patient's relatives; (3) the conditions were relatively benign and compatible with prolonged survival if not normal life expectancy; and (4) cases frequently occurred among offspring of consanguineous marriages. This article deals with one of the most interesting of such conditions, phenylketonuria, a disease which, through its proper treatment, illustrates how much medicine can make the phenotype differ — for the better — from the genotype.

## DISCOVERY OF PHENYLPYRUVIC IMBECILITY

The story of phenylketonuria is relatively short. Unknown at the time of Garrod, the disease was not identified until the early 1930s. From then on, our understanding of it progressed rapidly, and now stands as the prime example of a disease which is clearly genetically determined and yet generally preventable — in this case through nutritional technics.

The story started in Norway, where the mother of two retarded children, bothered by the peculiar odor which further stigmatized her youngsters, pursuaded a distant relative, the biochemist Asbjorn Folling, to examine them. He observed that when ferric chloride was added to their urine a green color developed, and he identified phenylpyruvic acid as the component responsible for this

Reprinted from *Postgraduate Medicine, 35* (No. 5), May, 1964.

abnormal color reaction. Folling went on to discover eight additional cases within a few months; he described a number of their characteristics and in 1934 published the fundamental paper, in which he named the disease imbecillitas phenylpyruvica. He has continued to study the syndrome ever since (2).

Folling's findings elicited great interest in a number of countries. Phenylketonuria was found in a substantial number of institutionalized mentally defective patients — as many as one in 200. Both sexes were equally affected. Although statistics are imperfect, it appears that the disease may be more common in the white race than in Negroes or Chinese. It also appears that within the white race the disease is more common among persons of Anglo-Saxon and Nordic descent than among those of Jewish ancestry. The disease was discovered to be familial, with approximately one-fourth of the children in the involved families affected. This is consistent with autosomal recessive transmission, with both parents carriers of the gene and the disease manifest in the homozygous offspring, who carry two such recessive genes. Inasmuch as the disease occurs in about every 20,000 live births, it is possible to calculate that one of 70 individuals is a carrier of the gene (3).

## DESCRIPTION OF THE DISEASE

Although phenylketonuric children appear normal at birth and seem normal during their first weeks of development, following objects with their eyes and smiling at one month of age, they progressively deteriorate mentally and rarely reach an intelligence quotient (IQ) over 50. (A very few patients with higher IQ's have been reported.) Most of them are in the imbecile-idiot range. The average age at which they start sitting alone is more than one year; they are at least two when they walk (if they ever do), and those who learn to talk are more than three before they start (4). They are frequently hyperactive. Unlike mongoloic children, they have unpleasant and schizoidlike personalities. Eighty per cent have electroencephalographic abnormalities. Convulsions are common. These children often have eczematoid rashes and most of them also exhibit the characteristic odor noted by Folling, which has been described variously as a horsy, barnlike or musty. Phenyl-pyruvic imbeciles are usually blonder and have lighter irises than their parents and normal siblings. These observations are consistent with the nature of the metabolic block, inasmuch as it appears that phenylalanine competes with tyrosine for the enzymes which produce pigments from tyrosine, particularly tyrosinase (5).

## BIOCHEMICAL DEFECT

The fundamental defect in phenylketonuria is the absence of the parahydroxylase which normally oxidizes the amino acid phenylalanine to tyrosine in the liver. Tyrosine is in turn metabolized through various pathways. One of them, through 3,4-dihydroxyphenylalanine and various quinones, eventually leads to melanin formation, a fact which may also explain the greater degree of blondness of patients with deficient tyrosine formation. The absence of a functioning phenylalanine parahydro-xylase leads to an elevated phenylalanine level in blood and to spillage of phenylpyruvic acid in the urine. Normal levels of phenylalanine are between 1 and 3 mg per 100 ml; those of phenylpyruvic oligophrenics are usually in the 15 to 60 mg range (6). It must be noted that at birth phenylalanine levels in the cord blood are normal; as the child begins to take breast or cow's milk, the blood phenylalanine level rises. Phenylpyruvic acid appears in the urine when the blood phenylalanine level reaches 12 to 15 mg per 100 ml. Incidentally, the characteristic diaper odor seems to be due to phenylacetic acid, resulting from the oxidative decarboxylation of phenylpyruvic acid. Phenylpyruvic acid causes the green color reaction the the presence of ferric chloride.

The exact mechanism of the mental retardation, while related to the accumulation of phenylalanine and some of its derivatives in blood and cerebrospinal fluid, is not known. Various authors have suspected phenylalanine, phenylpuruvic acid, phenylacetic acid and various indole derivatives. (In fact, indicanuria has been suggested as a substitute determination to check the dietary control of the condition.) It has also been suggested that at least two factors are responsible for the clinical picture, one which damages the central nervous system in early infancy (when the brain may be functionally more sensitive or when rapid growth may make it more vulnerable) and one (or the same) factor responsible for the day-to-day status of the patient. Phenylacetaldehyde may be one such factor (7).

## DETECTION OF CARRIERS

It is of interest to note that the heterozygous carriers, although immune from any pathologic effect, can actually be identified through a number of biochemical means. Carriers have significantly higher fasting plasma phenylalanine levels than noncarriers, although they overlap with noncarriers (8). If a load of 200 mg of L-phenylalanine per kilogram of body weight is given by mouth and phenylalanine levels are determined after one, two and four hours, plasma levels are twice as high in carriers, with the difference highly significant. A third, and better, method is based on the phenylalanine-tyrosine ratio in plasma after a load test. The measurement of tyrosine after a phenylacetic load test is equally indicative (9). While it is true that orthohydroxyphenylaceitc acid is present in the urine of heterozygotes but not of noncarrier controls after a phenylalnine load test, this substance also appears in the urine of normal individuals given enough phenlalanine to raise the plasma level to the heterozygote value. Because plasma levels of phenylanine are not as specific as those of tyrosine or the phenylalanine-tyrosine ratio, this urinary test is perhaps not as good a method for genetic investigation. Phenylalanine levels may go up in carriers during pregnancy; this does not seem to have deleterious effects.

## SCREENING

It is obvious that if the physician waits until the first symptoms of phenylketonuria appear in a patient, it is likely that irreversible changes leading to at least some degree of mental retardation will have occurred. Checking on the siblings of a retarded phenylpyruvic child is obviously essential; however, it does mean that one child has already contracted what could have been a preventable disease. There is only one way to deal satisfactorily with the problem, namely, to test routinely all well babies. Such a practice is already in effect in a number of situations and is expanding rapidly. For instance, when the urinary test was still the only available method of detection, the department of pediatrics of the College of Medical Evangelists, Loma Linda, California, under the impulsion of Dr. W. R. Centerwall (6) and with the cooperation of a large number of the health departments of the state of California and their well-baby clinics, launched a large testing program (10). They used a test consisting of placing a drop of a clear 10 per cent aqueous solution of ferric chloride on the infant's wet diaper. A blue-green color fading within a minute was indicative of phenylpyruvic acid. (In case the child did not wet at the clinic, the mother was asked to bring the latest wet diaper.) The test, ususally started at three weeks of age, had to be repeated at least three times during subsequent visits in case the condition had been slow to develop. Positive or doubtful reactions can be checked by observing the characteristic turbidity appearing within a minute when equal volumes of urine and acid solution of 2,4-dinitrophenylhydrazine are mixed and, of course, by plasma phenylalanine determination. Commercially prepared papers can be used to replace the diaper test *

The greatest step in screening was accomplished when Guthrie (11) developed a serum phenylalanine test which was sensitive enough to detect high concentrations of phenylalanine in blood before babies are discharged from the hospital (thus obviating the problem of getting them back, sometimes repeatedly, for testing). Urine methods, as previously mentioned, do not work before plasma levels reach a figure of 20 mg phenylalanine per 100 ml. Guthrie observed that inhibition of *Bacillus subtilis* ATCC 6051 by $\beta$-2-thienylalanine was specifically prevented by addition of proline, phenylalanine, phenylpyruvic acid or atrolactinic acid. This finding permitted the development of a convenient agar diffusion microbial assay employing small filter paper disks impregnated with serum on the agar surface. Specifically, blood from a skin puncture is spotted on a piece of Whatman No. 3 filter

*Research Test Paper (RT974), Eli Lilly and Company, Indianapolis; Phenistix Reagent strips, Ames Company, Inc., Elkhart, Indiana.

paper, dried and mailed to a laboratory where a single technician can test up to 200 of these paper specimens daily. The papers are steamed to coagulate blood protein, after which a disk is punched our from each blood spot with an ordinary paper punch. These disks are marked and placed in rows on the surface of large agar dishes. Control disks are prepared from normal blood to which has been added 2, 4, 8, 12, 20 mg L-phenylalanine per 100 ml. After overnight incubation, barely normal rings of turbid growth are observed around the disks corresponding to normal blood. A response similar to that of the 12 or 20 mg per 100 ml disks is considered positive and leads to confirmation by quantitative blood assay. The method has been successfully used in many laboratories. The Children's Bureau of the Public Health Service has sponsored a nationwide screening program, ascribing a quota of tests to each state. The Massachusetts Department of Public Health decided to go far beyond its assigned quota and since mid-July 1962 has offered the program to all maternity hospitals, including the military hospitals with obstetric services. Three cases were identified within the first three months. By July 1963 nine cases had been found. All patients were placed immediately on a low-phenylalanine diet (12).

## PREVENTION AND TREATMENT

The first effective treatment of phenylketonuria dates back to 1953, when Bickel, Gerrard and Hickmans (13), followed in 1955 by Woolf, Griffiths and Moncrieff, prepared protein hydrolysates low in phenylalanine. Administration of diets based on these preparations as protein sources caused the plasma phenylalanine to drop and pheylpyruvic acid to disappear from the urine. Similar experiences with phenylpyruvic infants and children of various ages led to the conclusion that children raised on such diets since early infancy usually develop normally; the diet has little or no effect on retarded phenylketonuric children three years of age or older. (There is one reported case of a six-year-old phenyl-ketonuric child who had a normal IQ at the age of six but was definitely retarded two years later and who probably should have been given a low-phenylalanine diet (14). Most children started on started on such a diet between the ages of a few months and three years benefit to a variable extent (including the development of normal or near normal intelligence); however, some may be permanently retarded. Obviously these results emphasize the crucial importance of very early detection.

It must be noted that practically all food proteins contain 4 to 6 per cent of phenylalanine. No amount of manipulation of natural foods is therefore likely to produce a diet low in phenylalanine and yet high enough in protein generally — particularly in essential amino acids — to permit adequate growth (15). Requirements for phenylalanine are of the order of less than 1 gm per day for an adult, but 60 to 90 mg per kilogram of body weight per day for a newborn infant. Requirements decrease with age and may be of the order of 25 mg per kilogram per day at six months and 10 to 15 mg per kilogram daily at 15 years of age. Some authors have recommended daily intakes of 15 to 50 mg of phenylalanine per kilogram of body weight for infants. Again 25 mg per kilogram daily seems a reasonable, conservative figure. While phenylalanine is itself an essential amino acid for man, the requirement can be in part (up to 70 per cent) fulfilled by tyrosine, ingestion of which does not have undesirable effects in the phenylketonuric child. The special diets must be therefore based on amino acid mixtures or on hydrolysates.

### Special Preparations

To my knowledge, there are at present two such preparations on the market. Ketonil®* is a powder made from casein hydrolysate from which most of the phenylalanine has been removed and amino acids, mineral salts and choline chloride added. The powder is mixed at home with vegetable oil or shortening, sugar and water to make a paste like peanut butter or a liquid formula (which may have to be supplemented with vitamins and iron). Lofenalac®† is also based on a protein hydrolysate from which most of the phenylalanine has been removed and to which methionine, tyrosine and tryptophan have been added.

*Merck Sharp & Dohme, Division of Merck & Co., Inc., West Point, Pennsylvania.
†Mead Johnson Laboratories, Evansville, Indiana.

Lofenalac also contains vegetable fat, Dextri-Maltose®, minerals and vitamins to make a complete food. It can be used as a powder mixed with low-protein foods or as a formula when mixed with water. Both preparations have given satisfactory results.

It seems essential to restrict phenylalanine intake particularly drastically at the beginning of treatment in order to bring phenylalanine levels back to normal. The diet should therefore consist exclusively of either formula given in lieu of milk. It is perhaps helpful in this respect that Lofenalac looks like milk. As the child grows and becomes older, natural foods low in phenylalanine will be added, but plasma levels should be maintained between 2 and 6 mg per 100 ml. Abnormally low levels are signs of phenylalanine deficiency, which slows down and stops growth and may result in paradoxical secondary elevation of plasma phenylalanine levels due to the breakdown of tissue protein.

## Use of Natural Foods

Lyman and Lyman (14) and Acosta and Centerwall (16) particularly have studied supplementation of diet by natural foods. Both of these authors' excellent publications have attempted to place the formulation of low-phenylalanine diets on the basis of exchange lists based on equivalents corresponding to 15 mg phenylalanine. For example, Acosta and Centerwall divided foods into eight lists. List 1 is Lofenalac, of which 4 tablespoonfuls correspond to 2 equivalents (or 30 mg phenylalanine). List 2 vegetables, gives the portions of green and strained beans, beets, cabbage, carrots, celery, cucumbers, lettuce, spinach, squash and tomatoes corresponding to 1 equivalent. List 3, fruits, gives similar equivalent portions for bananas, dates, fruit cocktail, grapefruit, oranges, grape juice, lemon juice, peaches, pears, pineapples, plums, prunes, raisins, tangerines and watermelons. List 4 gives 2 equivalent portions of raw and cooked cereals, Irish potatoes and sweet potatoes, and certain wafers and crackers. List 5 gives one-third equivalent (5 mg phenylalanine) portions of butter, cream, margarine and mayonnaise. List 6 is desserts (1 equivalent), **rice flour, cornstarch, cookies and ice creams** and puddings made by certain recipes given in another part of the article. List 6 is the free foods, containing little or no phenylalanine — candy, honey, jams, jellies, molasses, oils, syrups and tapioca. List 8 is the foods which should be avoided because of their very high phenylalanine content such as most breads, all cheeses, eggs, dried legumes, meat, poultry, fish, nuts and nut butters. It is readily seen that there is considerable diversity in taste left, particularly if advantage is taken of the seven low-phenylalanine pudding and four low-phenylalanine ice cream recipes. Acosta and Centerwall also give a number of additional low-phenylalanine recipes for cookies, biscuits and blancmange. Knowing the caloric and other nutrient contents of the foods from the usual food composition tables and using the phenylalanine equivalents given by such a list, it becomes possible to prescribe diets of sufficient versatility in protein and energy content to adjust to the need of the growing phenylketonuric patient. This is all the more important since, although it is recognized that the patient will have to be maintained on the low-phenylalanine diet a number of years, it is not known at present how long this means in practice; however, there are indications that the need may decrease by school age.

## CONCLUSION

The determination of the mechanism of phenylketonuria and the elaboration of a successful dietary method of treatment put an onus on all of us to make sure that this disease or, at least, its pathologic results are eliminated in the United States. This will require vigilance on the part of all physicians in charge of caring for newborns. Testing is cheap — a matter of pennies — and should be done on absolutely all infants. Practicing physicians all over the nation should press their hospital and their state health departments to make the Guthrie test universally available. Treatment may be relatively expensive, but is worth it to mobilize the resources of the community — dietitians, health educators and visiting nurses, plus whatever source of funds may be needed — to do a thorough job of treatment. After all, the cost to the community of lifelong full-time care of a phenylketonuric imbecile would be \$100,000 to \$200,000. The cost in suffering to the patient and his parents would be, of course, incalculable.

## REFERENCES

1. Garrod, A. E.: Inborn Errors of Metabolism. Ed. 2. London, Hodder & Stoughton, 1923.
2. Folling, A., Mohr, O. L. and Ruud, L.: Oligophrenia Phenylpyruvica. A Recessive Syndrome in Man. Oslo, Dybwad, 1945.
3. Hsia, D. Y. Y.: Medical genetics. New England J. Med., 262:1172, 1222, 1273, 1318, 1960.
4. Knox, W. E. and Hsia, D. Y. Y.: Pathogenetic problems in phenylketonuria. Am. J. Med., 22:687, 1957.
5. McKusick, V. A.: Medical genetics 1959. J. Chron. Dis., 12:70 1960.
6. Centerwall, W. R.: Phenylketonuria. J. Am. Dietet. A., 36:201, 1960.
7. Seidenberg, M., Martinez, R. J. and Guthrie, R.: Phenylalanine metabolism: The production of phenylacetaldehyde by a *Proteus* species. Arch. Biochem., 97:470, 1962.
8. Knox, W. E. and Messinger, E. C.: The detection in the heterozygote of the metabolic effect of the recessive gene for phenylketonuria. Am. J. Human Genet., 10:53, 1958.
9. Jervis, G. A.: Detection of heterozygotes for phenylaketonuria. Clin. chim. acta, 5:471, 1960.
10. Woolf, L. I., Griffiths, R., Moncrieff, A., Coates, S. and Dillistone, F.: The dietary treatment of phenylketonuria. A.M.A. Arch. Dis. Child., 33:31. 1958.
11. Guthrie, R.: Blood screening for phenylketonuria. J.A.M.A., 178:863, 1961.
12. MacCready, R. A. and Guthrie, R.: Phenylketonuria screening programs. New England J. Med., 269:52-53 (July 4) 1963.
13. Bickel, M., Gerrard, J. and Hickmans, E. M.: Influence of phenylalanine intake on phenylketonuria. Lancet, 2:812, 1953.
14. Lyman, F. L. and Lyman, J. K.: Dietary management of phenylketonuria with Lofenalac. Arch. Pediat., 77:212, 1960.
15. Mayer, J.: Amino acid requirements of man. Postgrad. Med., 26:252, 1959.
16. Acosta, P. B. and Centerwall, W. R.: Phenylketonuria: Dietary management. *Ibid.*, (6) p. 206.

## Chapter 42

# GALACTOSEMIA AND NUTRITION

$G$ALACTOSEMIA was first described by von Reuss (1) in 1908. He reported the case of a four-month-old infant with malnutrition, hepatomegaly and melituria. The melituria ceased when the infant was placed on a milk-free diet, but the patient died anyway. Liver cirrhosis was found at autopsy. The disease was reported only occasionally between 1908 and 1945. Since then, the condition has attracted considerable interest, especially since it was recognized that, like phenylketonuria, it rapidly led to irreversible mental disease, the development of which can be prevented through nutritional technics. As in the case of phenylketonuria, it is essential that physicians caring for infants be alert to the possibility of galactosemia in one of their patients, particularly if he or she is related to an individual with galactosemia; they should be aware of the very simple and effective method of treating this condition.

## GENETIC CONSIDERATIONS

The disease is inherited but the precise mode of transmission is not known. Most genetic studies have been based on galactose tolerance tests, a method which, as will be seen when metabolism of galactose is examined, is not entirely specific. Galactosemia is the result of the deficiency of one enzyme closing one pathway may be available and may become more so as the individual matures. Be that as it may, the fact that in galactosemia one is dealing with an inborn error of metabolism is plain enough: for example, in four families of galactosemic patients carefully studied by Holzel, Komrower and Schwarz (2) in England, at least one parent had decreased tolerance for galactose and in one family

Reprinted from *Postgraduate Medicine, 35* (No. 6), June, 1964.

both parents did. In one family in which the parents were first cousins, two children died in infancy and two living children had decreased tolerance for galactose. Clinical reports and autopsy findings both indicated that the deaths were due to galactosemia. There was a high incidence of decreased galactose tolerance without clinical signs of galactose tolerance without clinical signs of galactosemia among the members of these four families. Hsia, Inouye and Walker (3) have reviewed their experience with galactosemia in 27 North American families containing 45 homozygous galactosemic patients. In spite of the fact that all these showed total absence of galactose-1-phosphate uridyl transferase in their red blood cells, marked differences were observed in tolerance to milk. In children with some tolerance to milk, incidentally, significant amounts of galactose-6-phosphate and galactose-1-phosphate were formed when their erythrocytes were incubated with galactose. One-third of the homozygotes were mentally retarded, and 14 out of 22 showed galactose in the urine. A 63-year-old man, although clearly homozygous by chemical tests, appeared to have been essentially free of symptoms all his life.

The most likely interpretation is that galactosemia is inherited as a heterozygous character with the disease becoming overt in subjects homozygous for the same gene. Other genes in the background may then influence the relative severity of the condition. While it has not been possible to show abnormal tolerance in both parents in all cases, as already suggested, this is probably because of the lack of specificity of the tolerance test. At present, it would seem that the only way to "clinch" the mode of genetic transmission would be through enzymatic studies, ideally in liver biopsies of healthy parents. To my knowledge, this method has not been carried out on a large scale. What data there are in this area do support the recessive hypothesis.

## CLINICAL PICTURE

Galactosemia is associated with the following symptoms: anorexia, growth failure, vomiting, diarrhea, jaundice, a considerable degree of hepatomegaly, albuminuria and melituria. Cataracts, splenomegaly and mental retardation are frequent consequences.

Holzel, Komrower and Schwarz (2) have distinguished three degrees of the disease. In severe cases, signs usually appear during the first two weeks of life. Vomiting is usually the first indication, followed by jaundice and weight loss. The liver enlarges steadily and may descend below the umbilicus; ascites may develop, and spenomegaly may occur. Anorexia and lethargy, hypotonia, failure to thrive, and diarrhea are seen at this stage. Cataracts are seen in more than half the cases, often as early as the third week. Gangrene has been observed in a number of infants.

In less severe cases, the signs and symptoms develop more slowly; the child may thus not be seen until several months have elapsed since birth. The child usually is brought to a physician because of feeding difficulties, occasional vomiting and retarded development. Hepatomegaly and cataracts are then often noted. Hsia and Walker (4) have described a striking example of such mild galactosemia: A business executive in his 60's had long been thought to be diabetic until the reducing sugar was shown to be galactose. His intelligence was above average, but he had a cataract and an enlarged liver. Determination of enzyme levels showed him to be homozygous for the galactosemic gene. Incidentally, his daughter married a carrier of galactosemia and had two galacto-semic children.

Finally, mild cases are usually found by chance because a sibling is galactosemic. Such children have never liked milk and are happier when milk is omitted; they show an abnormal level of galactose tolerance but no apparent liver damage. The first two groups show amino-aciduria and proteinuria, as well as grossly abnormal galactose tolerance tests, with 50 per cent of the ingested galactose recovered in the urine. (In such cases, the carrying out of the test involves a degree of risk, as it may cause acute hypoglycemia; in the third or mild group, the risk is much less, and the test is actually more necessary to confirm the diagnosis.) Disturbances of liver function are seen in untreated infants with the more severe cases.

## METABOLISM OF GALACTOSE IN MAN
## AND BLOCK IN GALACTOSEMIA

The early work of Leloir, followed by that of Kalckar and his associates, has permitted the elucidation of the general lines of conversion of galactose to glucose. Galactose is phosphorylated (in the presence of galactokinase and adenosine triphosphate) to galactose-1-phosphate in order to be absorbed. Galactose-1-phosphate can then be transformed into glucose-1-phosphate, essentially in the liver, in order to be utilized. The reaction involves uridine diphosphate glucose (UDPG) and the enzyme galactose-1-phosphate uridyl transferase and yeilds glucose-1-phosphate and uridine diphosphate galactose (UDP Gal). UDP Gal, under the influence of the enzyme uridine diphosphate galactose-4-epimerase, is then transformed into uridine diphosphate glucose. Finally, the last compound in the presence of a source of pyrophosphate is transformed into uridine triphosphate and glucose-1-phosphate, the reaction being catalyzed by the enzyme uridine diphosphate glucose pyrophosphorylase. Kalckar, Anderson and Isselbacher (5, 6,) have demonstrated that in galactosemia the body's inability to utilize galactose efficiently is caused by a deficiency of the enzyme galactose-1-phosphate uridyl transferase. The result is an accumulation of galactose-1-phosphate primarily in the liver, where conversion to glucose phosphate would normally take place.

Actually, later work by Isselbacher (7) has shown that mammalian tissues have two pathways for converting galactose-1-phosphate to uridine diphosphate galactose. One of these is that described previously, which is interrupted in galactosemia by the absence of galactose-1-phosphate uridyl transferase. The other concerns catalysis by another enzyme, uridine diphosphate galactose pyrophosphorylase, which directly forms uridine diphosphate galactose from uridine triphosphate and galactose-1-phosphate. Isselbacher finds both enzymes present in low concentration in fetal and neofetal liver tissue. The concentrations increase with age. This phenomenon makes it likely that the symptoms of galactosemia are particularly severe in infants because of the absence of one pathway and the low activity of the other. Galactosemic subjects can utilize some galactose (8), and their tolerance of galactose appears to increase with age (9). This improvement could be the result of increase in the activity of the uridine diphosphate galactose pyrophosphorylase-catalyzed alternate pathway. Specific determinations of galactose-1-phosphate uridyl transferase are therefore a much better genetic tool in confirming the recessive transmission than methods based on galactose utilization.

The risk of hypoglycemia may be due to the fact that galactose, like glucose, may stimulate insulin production. Insulin, however, does not decrease the galactose level; galactose may thus continue to stimulate insulin to the point of hypoglycemia, in spite of — or because of — a high total plasma hexose level.

Cataracts may be due to the accumulation of galactose-1-phosphate in lens cells characterized by a deficiency of galactose-1-phosphate uridyl transferase. Lens cells are essentially dependent on glucose for energy, and galactose phosphate specifically inhibits glucose-6-phosphate dehydrogenase.

## CHEMICAL DIAGNOSIS

From a clinical viewpoint, the main problem is early detection of the disease, inasmuch as the removal of galactose — in effect, of milk — within a few days following birth prevents the symptoms from appearing. A high level of blood sugar consisting in part of nonfermentable sugar, a positive reaction to Tollens' test and the mucic acid test, and a high galactose level make the diagnosis of galactosemia likely. Unfortunately, most of the more specific tests are complicated, although new findings give encouragement and may permit the development of a simple paper test. Galactose tolerance tests are not entirely specific; there is also the possiblity that they might harm the patient. Other methods used have been determination of galactose-1-phosphate uridyl transferase in the erythrocytes, for example, by incubating cord red blood cells with galactose. Some authors (10) have used a manometric determination of ozygen uptake, others (11) the production of carbon dioxide from galactose-1-carbon 14 through the hexose monophosphate pathway. (It has already been pointed out that at least some of the heterozygous carriers are detected through such enzyme determinations.) Such procedures are well worth performing in suspected cases or in relatives of galactosemic patients. They are too cumbersome to lend themselves to the routine screening of galactosemic cases in the newborn population.

Rorem and Lewis (12) have recently reported the preparation of a test paper sensitive to and specific for very small amounts of galactose and galactose-containing sugars. While the prime object of the development of the test paper was the determination of galactose-containing material in plants, it appears possible to adapt it to the detection of galactose in blood or urine. The critical ingredient is galactose oxidase extracted from cultures of the fungus *Polyporus circinatus* F 2 by freeze-drying of the filtered and dialyzed culture medium. In the presence of oxygen, the enzyme catalyzed the oxidation at the carbon 6 position of the primary alcohol group to an aldehyde group with the formation of hydrogen peroxide. The test papers are made from filter paper treated with *o*-tolidine. One end of the paper is dipped into the enzyme solution and Carbowax® 6000 in phthalate buffer. The papers are dried in the dark. The working end has a light-tan color and turns deep blue-green in 10 minutes when dipped into a solution that contains as little as one part in 10,000 galactose at 25° C. Complex carbohydrates containing galactose such as lactose and raffinose react at much higher concentrations. Interfering substances such as fluoride and chloride ions and ascorbic acid can be removed from unknown solutions by de-ionizing with Amberlite® ion-exchange resins, which must be freed from hydrogen peroxide by washing with a catalase solution; the catalase is then inactivated by heating on a steam bath. The authors suggest that the test can be made semiquantitative by standardization with solutions of known galactose concentration. It is obvious that the adaptation of such a test paper to the routine detection of galactosemia would be of inestimable value.

## TREATMENT: THE GALACTOSE-FREE DIET

The treatment of galactosemia consists of the complete exclusion of milk, lactose or galactose-containing foodstuffs, following whatever immediate correction of dehydration and acidosis is necessary. It is important to realize that many processed foods contain small amounts of lactose; some of the soybean milks, although free of lactose, containing some polymers of galactose. Two "galactose-free" preparations commercially available in this country are Sobee®, a soybean milk which is diluted 1:1 and contains 3.2 per cent soybean protein, 2.6 per cent soybean oil and coconut oil, 7.7 per cent Dextri-Maltose and sucrose, and 0.5 per cent minerals; and Nutramigen®, which is diluted 1:7 and contains 2.2 per cent hydrolyzed casein, 2.6 per cent corn oil, 8.5 per cent Dextri-Maltose and arrowroot starch and 0.6 per cent minerals. Holzel, Komrower and Schwarz (13) in Great Britain feel, however, that preparations such as Nutramigen are not really free of galactose, and they fear the repeated assault of even small quantities of the sugar. They have devised a formula consisting of egg, sugar, margarine and rice flour which they supplement with fruit juices. They start with dilute feeds to avoid gastrointestinal disturbances — even at the risk of slowing down weight gain — and progressively increase concentrations. Whatever the initial galactose-free formula, it is supplemented as the infant grows with vegetables, fruit, meat (excluding brain, which is high in galactose) and eggs. Butter should be excluded.

Unlike the many theoretical and practical problems arising in the development of diets for phenylketonuric patients, the difficulties involved in the dietary prescription for galactosemia are thus few and relatively easy to solve. (One point to remember is that a number of drugs and even some vitamin preparations are prepared in pills containing lactose.) It is generally agreed that this rigid exclusion of all lactose-containing foods — including butter — should be maintained for at least three years and that the longer this exclusion is maintained beyond that point the better. Milk should be excluded forever (14). Even clinically normal adults with abnormal galactose tolerance who can tolerate small amounts of milk without apparent harm feel better when milk and milk products are totally removed from the diet.

## PROGNOSIS

Early diagnosis and adequate nutritional treatment lessen

mortality and reduce the risk of irreversible liver and lenticular damage. Cataracts frequently disappear and liver function generally returns to normal following introduction of the galactose-free diet, although cirrhosis may be too advanced by then to be reversible. The evidence also favors Holzel's (2) view that the mental retardation seen in the untreated disorder is not a genetic error independent of the metabolic disorder, as suggested by Clay and Potter (15), but is a consequence of the enzyme deficiency, whether or not mediated through hypoglycemia. Whether all persistent pathologic symptoms could be eliminated if the diagnosis could be made at birth and susceptible infants completely shielded from any trace of galactose from the very first is for the future to show.

## REFERENCES

1. Von Reuss, A.: Zuckerausscheidung im Sauglingsalter. Wien. med. Wchnschr., 58:799, 1908.
2. Holzel, A., Komrower, G. M. and Schwarz, V.: Galactosemia. Am. J. Med., 22:703, 1957.
3. Hsia, D. Y., Inouye, T. and Walker, F. A.: Galactosemia: Clinical, genetic, and biochemical study. J.A.M.A., 178:944, 1961.
4. Hsia, D. Y. and Walker, F. A.: Variability in the clinical manifestations of galactosemia. J. Pediat., 59:872, 1961.
5. Kalckar, H. M., Anderson, E. P. and Isselbacher, K. J.: Galactosemia, a congenital defect in a nucleotide transferase. Biochim. et biophys. acta, 20:262, 1956.
6. Anderson, E. P., Kalckar, H. M. and Isselbacher, K. J.: Defect in uptake of galactose-1-phosphate into liver nucleotides in congenital galacto-semia. Science, 125:113, 1957.
7. Isselbacher, K. J.: Evidence for an accessory pathway of galactose metabolism in mammalian liver. Science, 126:652, 1957.
8. Eisenberg, F., Jr., Isselbacher, K. J. and Kalckar, H. M.: Studies on the metabolism of carbon[14]-labeled galactose in a galactosemic individual. *Ibid.,*[6] p. 116.
9. Townsend, E. H., Jr., Mason, H. M. and Strong, P. S.: Galactosemia and its relation to Laennec's cirrhosis; review of literature and presentation of six additional cases. Pediatrics, 7:760, 1951.
10. Schwarz, V., Wells, A. R., Holzel, A. and Komrower, G. M.: A study of the genetics of galactosemia. Ann. Human Genet., 25:179, 1961.
11. Weinberg, A. M.: Detection of congenital galactosemia and the carrier state using galactose C[14] and blood cells. Metabolism, 10:728, 1961.
12. Rorem, E. S. and Lewis, J. C.: A test paper for the detection of galactose

and certain galactose-containing sugars. Anal. Biochem., 3:230, 1962.

13. Holzel, A., Komrower, G. M. and Schwarz, V.: Low-lactose milk for congenital galactosemia. Lancet, 269:92, 1955.
14. Zellweger, H. V.: Enzyme deficiency diseases. 1. Galactosemia. J. Am. Dietet. A., 34:1041, 1958.
15. Clay, P. R. and Potter, C. T.: A case of galactosemia with special referance to mental development. Arch. Dis. Childhood, 30:147, 1955.

*Chapter 43*

# DISACCHARIDASE DEFICIENCIES
# AND THEIR NUTRITIONAL SIGNIFICANCE

## NORMAL DIGESTION AND
## ABSORPTION OF DISACCHARIDES

THE finding that certain subjects exhibit serious intestinal disturbances and other symptoms as a result of deficiencies of intestinal disaccharide-splitting enzymes has revived interest in the normal digestion and absorption of these sugars in humans. It had been recognized for some time that while the lumen content of disaccharide hydrolases in low, digestion and absorption of such sugars as lactose are normally rapid and efficient, a finding which suggested that these enzymes reside and act in the mucous membrane of the intestine.

Dahlqvist and Borgstrom (1), to whom we owe much of our knowledge of the physiologic and pathologic aspects of digestion of disaccharides, used intubation of the small intestine in young male volunteers after ingestion of standard formula meals containing known amounts of fat, protein, sucrose, maltose and lactose or starch as a means of obtaining samples from chosen sites. They were able to demonstrate that following such 400 gm, 550 calorie meals, about three hours were required for complete stomach emptying, with the nature of the carbohydrate exerting apparently no effect on this phenomenon. The upper part of the intestine diluted the meal two to five times; the chyme was again concentrated in the lower part. The bulk of the meal was in the proximal part of the ileum in about four hours. Sucrose was found to be absorbed in part in the jejunum and in greater part in the

Reprinted from *Postgraduate Medicine, 36* (No. 3), September, 1964.

ileum. No absorption occurred in the duodenum. Invertase activity of jejunal samples was low; no more than 10 per cent of the sucrose was hydrolyzed in the lumen. Maltose, like sucrose, was not absorbed in the duodenum. Unlike sucrose, however, most of it was absorbed in the jejunum. Maltase activity in that area was again low, with no more than 10 per cent hydrolyzed. Maltase activity was high in the ileum, with half of the remaining maltose hyrolyzed in the lumen of the ileum. Results suggested that most of the maltose was absorbed in the disaccharide form, since it would have taken too long (upward of 10 hours) for the maltase to hydrolyze all the ingested maltose to glucose. This conclusion holds true for lactose as well; absorption of lactose starts in the duodenum and is completed in the jejunum. The low activity of the lumen lactase would suggest that no less than 100 hours would be required for its absorption. Starch, by contrast, is rapidly hydrolyzed in the lumen, with perhaps as much as 90 per cent reduced to disaccharide form. No more than 10 per cent, however, goes on to glucose.

It seems logical to conclude from these studies, as Dahlqvist and Borgstrom have done, that most of the disaccharides are hydrolyzed within the cells of the intestinal mucous membranes, with the monosaccharides excreted into the portal blood. This conclusion is consistent with the normally high content of disaccharide hydrolases in these cells. It is, incidentally, interesting to note that these processes occur at least in part in different sites, with lactose being essentially absorbed in the duodenum and proximal jejunum, maltose in the jejunum and proximal ileum, and sucrose in the distal jejunum and ileum.

With this background of normal physiology, let us turn now to the curious diseases increasingly recognized in children and in adults which appear to be caused by deficiencies of these intestinal mucosal disaccharide hydrolases.

## DEFICIENCIES IN DISACCHARIDASE

The first significant observation in this field was that of Weijers and associates (2), who remarked that some children with chronic fermentative diarrhea were apparently intolerant of sucrose. (We also are indebted to this group for their superb studies of celiac disease.) Furthermore, such patients appeared to lack invertase in their intestinal mucosa. The addition of invertase to a sucrose meal produced a normal rise in blood glucose which otherwise was not observed.

Weijers and co-workers (3) also observed other infants in whom chronic diarrhea which began during first year of life appeared to be the result of intolerance to maltose; in these infants the addition of maltase alleviated the condition. While maltose or starch administration gave rise to a flat glucose tolerance curve, the addition of maltase caused a near normal rise in blood sugar. Sucrose and maltose-intolerant infants all showed watery, voluminous, frothy and malodorous stools, high in mucus and acid in reaction. The infants showed moderate growth failure, with muscle hypotonia, pallor and irritability.

In a subsequent publication the Dutch authors (4) elaborated on their initial findings as well as on those of a number of other authors (5, 6) and further defined the concept of chronic fermentative diarrheas due to total deficiency of disaccharidase, to their "overloading," or to a decrease in their capacity caused by various factors such as a suboptimum pH. Such deficiencies in invertase, maltase, isomaltase or lactase would permit the growth of an intestinal flora which in turn would cause, among other effects, a marked production of lactic acid. This explains the fact that while nonabsorbed disaccharides can still be demonstrated in the stools after the first 24 to 48 hours following the addition of disaccharide to the diet, the nonabsorbed part of the sugar has been completely fermented to organic acids after a maximum of 48 hours. By then, the disaccharides can no longer be demonstrated in the feces.

## PRIMARY DEFICIENCIES

Weijers and van de Kamer (4) distinguished between primary and secondary deficiencies in sugar-splitting enzymes. Primary deficiencies are probably inborn errors, genetically determined, although single cases without known family histories of the disease have been described. For example, lactase deficiencies have been described in a father and son, with the disease likely to have been present in a grandfather; this disorder also has been observed in two brothers. Invertase deficiency has been described in two sisters. Often in similar cases, the apparent deficiency may be much more marked in one patient than in the other, with the fermentative chronic diarrhea a function of the deficiency.

As can be expected, lactase deficiency is likely to be seen in the earliest months of life, particularly if the infant is breast-fed, because of the high lactose content of the mother's milk. Weijers and van de Kamer reasonably speculated on the possibility that many infants who do not thrive on mother's milk, supposedly because of difficulty in coping with a milk of that general composition, are in point of fact partly deficient in lactase. It may be added that lactase deficiency is a particularly vicious syndrome, manifested by especially frothy stools with a high lactic acid content and usually accompanied by severe malnutrition, particularly in the young infant. The symptoms respond dramatically to the exclusion of lactose from the diet.

Invertase and maltase deficiencies obviously will not become manifest until sucrose or dextrin is added to the diet. The Dutch authors believe that an absolute deficiency is essentially incurable, with elimination of the chronic diarrhea essentially depending on the elimination of the corresponding disaccharide from the diet. A relative deficiency or partial deficiency may, by contrast, be overcome as the organism grows, as food intake decreases in proportion to body size, and as the diet gains in variety.

The work of Auricchio and his group (7) would suggest that sucrose and isomaltose intolerance disappears gradually with maturity. By contrast, a recent study by Dahlqvist and his colleagues (8) demonstrates that at least in some adults, lactase deficiency and its nutritional consequences are permanent. Four adult males, 39 to 54 years old, complained of diarrhea, intestinal distention and cramps after ingestion of milk. Intolerance to milk had developed in one patient four years previously and the other three had a history of milk intolerance dating back to childhood. These patients were subjected to oral lactose tolerance tests and to multiple duodenal biopsy. The biopsy specimens were used for histologic examination and for determination of disaccaridase activity. Similar studies were run on controls. The patients with a long history of milk intolerance had flat blood glucose after ingestion. They also showed the expected distress and diarrhea and, incidentally, a sharp increase in blood glucose after ingestion of a mixture of glucose and galactose. The mucosal biopsy specimens of these subjects showed the normal sucrase. maltase and invertase activity, but a drastically decreased lactase activity; the highest value was only 6 per cent of the lactase activity of the controls. The fourth patient showed a normal rise in blood glucose following lactose ingestion, no distress or diarrhea, and normal mucosal lactase activity. His acquired intolerance obviously must depend on some other mechanism.

## SPECIFICITY OF PRIMARY DEFICIENCIES

Dahlqvist and his collaborators (9) have recently made a curious observation which may be of eventual significance not only clinically but also for our understanding of the mode of transmission of inborn errors of metabolism. In such diseases, as we now understand them, a single enzyme is missing. The European workers, first having observed that a certain intolerance for starch and maltose-dextrin was present in several patients with sucrose intolerance, have gone on to show that such patients show an intolerance for isomaltose and isomaltulose, a sugar with a close structural resemblance to isomaltose. To ascertain that separate enzyme deficiencies were in fact involved, Dahlqvist and co-workers checked the specificity of human small-intestine iso-maltase and invertase and showed by a variety of methods, particularly heat inactivation and mixed-substrate incubation, that these were indeed separate enzymes. Isomaltase was shown to be responsible not only for the hydrolysis of isomaltose but also for that of isomaltulose and 1,6-*a*-oligosaccharides. This reduces the number of enzymes involved in these multiple intolerances to two, invertase and isomaltase, but the frequent and perhaps constant association between hereditary intolerance for sucrose and isomaltose remains mysterious, Are the two activities controlled by two enzymes which are structurally very similar and whose formation is in turn partly controlled by a single gene? Are they controlled by a single protein with two different enzymatically active centers which respond differently to heat? It is to be hoped that further work will bring an answer to these interesting questions.

## SECONDARY DEFICIENCIES

Weijers and van de Kamer (4) have introduced the concept of secondary deficiency of disaccharidases. This concept has proved useful. They considered that inasmuch as the sugar-splitting enzymes are formed chiefly within the intestinal wall and develop their activity mainly in these cells, "each process by which the cells of the intestinal wall are damaged either anatomically or functionally may cause a decrease of the enzymatic function." Diarrhea would follow the development of such a secondary deficiency.

One likely cause of such damage would be the diffuse enteritis which often follows an enteral infection. Obviously, if such an enteritis is accompanied by considerable mucus production, the sugars may not reach the wall, and fermentative diarrhea will occur. But fermentative diarrhea may also occur as a result of decreased intracellular concentration of disaccharidases, even if the absence of excessive mucus allows the sugars to reach the mucosal cells. Children with dystrophy may also be expected to have all sorts of enzyme deficiencies.

Finally, the reduction of the absorbing surface of the intestine by resection may exert a very specific effect on the absorption of a given disaccharide if the area resected was that of maximum hydrolase concentration for that sugar. Weijers and van de Kamer cited only the case of a generalized decrease of absorption of sugar in a small boy (one and one-half years old) in whom about two-thirds of the small intestine had been resected and whose stools showed lactic acid with even a slight overloading. However, their conception of more specific secondary inhibitions of absorption seems logical.

A recent example of lactose intolerance with steatorrhea secondary to ideal resection and jejunocolostomy, described by

Kern, Struthers and Attwood (10), is related to this concept. In this case, a primary genetic deficiency, relatively benign, was made acute by the elimination of part of the intestine; this superimposed on the primary deficiency a secondary decrease as well. The patient they described, a 22-year-old woman, was admitted to Colorado General Hospital with a chief complaint of diarrhea of five months' duration. Signs of intestional obstruction had led, five months previously, to hospitalization in another institution where laparotomy and resection of the entire ileum and a portion of ascending colon had been performed to correct what was thought to be an internal hernia. The portions of intestine removed were histologically normal. Postoperatively the patient had done well, but as soon as oral feeding was begun, she had diarrhea, with four to six bulky, malodorous and frothy bowel movements a day. She had lost 20 lb before her weight stabilized. Further history revealed that the patient had had a long history of milk intolerance, with cramps, nausea and diarrhea, which antedated the operation but which had become much worse since the surgical procedure. Two brothers, aged seven and 19, had similar histories of milk intolerance; the younger brother was small and underdeveloped. The patient was shown to be unable to absorb orally or intraduodenally administered lactose even though glucose, D-xylose and disaccharides other than lactose were absorbed normally. Lactose administered with the enzyme lactase was absorbed normally. Assay of the jejunal mucosa for lactose activity indicated a partial deficiency of this enzyme. The steatorrhea following lactose or milk ingestion was ascribed to the bacterial decomposition of lactose in the small intestine.

From a nutritional standpoint, it is obvious that at present treatment of these disorders can consist only of the omission from the diet of the sugar which the organism is unable to absorb. It must be further noted that our increased understanding of such inborn or secondary biochemical errors of metabolism is growing. There is little doubt that besides taxing the ingenuity of the physicians and the dietitians, this development will put an evergrowing stress on the versatility of hospital laboratories.

# REFERENCES

1. Dahlqvist, A. and Borgstrom, B.: Digestion and absorption of disaccharides in man. Biochem. J., 81:411, 1961.
2. Weijers, H. A., van de Kamer, J. H., Mossel, D. A. A. and Dicke, W. K.: Diarrhoea caused by deficiency of sugar-splitting enzymes. Lancet, 2:296, 1960.
3. Weijers, H. A., van de Kamer, J. H., Dicke, W. K. and Ijselling, J.: Diarrhoea caused by deficiency of sugar-splitting enzymes. I. Acta paediat., 50:555, 1961.
4. Weijers, H. A. and van de Kamer, J. H.: Diarrhoea caused by deficiency of sugar-splitting enzymes. II. Acta paediat., 51:371, 1962.
5. Holzel, A., Schwarz, V. and Sutcliffe, K. W.: Defective lactose absorption causing malnutrition in infancy. Lancet, 1:1126, 1959.
6. Auricchio, S., Prader, A., Muerset, G. and Witt, G.: Saccharoseintoleranz. Helvet. paediat. acta, 16:483, 1961.
7. Auricchio, S., Dahlqvist, A., Murset, G. and Prader, A.: Isomaltose intolerance causing decreased ability to utilize dietary starch. J. Pediat., 62:165, 1963.
8. Dahlqvist, A., Hammond, J. B., Crane, R. K., Dunphy, J. W. and Littman, A.: Intestinal lactase deficiency and lactose intolerance in adults. Gastroenterology, 45:488, 1963.
9. Dahlqvist, A., Auricchio, S., Semenza, G. and Prader, A.: Human intestinal disaccharidases and hereditary disaccharide intolerance. The hydrolysis of sucrose, isomaltose, palatinose (isomaltulose) and a 1,6-*u*-oligosaccharide (isomalto-oligosaccharide) preparation. J. Clin. Invest., 42:556, 1963.
10. Kern, F., Jr., Struthers, J. E., Jr. and Attwood, W. L.: Lactose intolerance as a cause of steatorrhea in an adult. *Ibid.*,[8] p. 477.

*Chapter 44*

# NUTRITION AND GOUT

W E have records of dietary likes and dislikes of more famous patients with gout than with most other diseases. Louis XIV, Milton, Newton, Dr. Johnson, Franklin, the Pitts, Gibbon and Darwin all had gout. (Perhaps a consolation for hyperuricemic patients is the long-believed association of a high blood uric acid level and genius.) Syndenham wrote his famous 1683 description of the disease in part from his experinece as a gouty patient.

The views of famous as well as obscure patients toward the disease have varied both with the opinions of the period and with their own personal temperament. Viewed with fatalism during the seventeenth and eighteenth centuries as a disease of the wellborn, gout acquired a **hereditary** character during the nineteenth century. Because Lamarckism — belief in the inheritance of acquired characteristics — dominated thinking before Darwin and Mendel, gout often was thought to result from centuries of familial addiction to venison and port rather than simply from personal excess. The fact that 90 per cent of the victims were men led to special attention to the eating habits of male ancestors.

A more rational view of the dietary aspects of the disease was slow to develop. For at least half the period since Sir Alfred B. Garrod demonstrated (in 1848) that gout is characterized by an increase in uric acid in the blood, it was believed that the excess uric acid was derived directly and totally from the diet and that both prevention and treatment of the disease should be based on eliminating dietary nucleoproteins or, in practice, meat.

We understand now that dietary nucleoproteins contribute, at the very most, half the uric acid found in normal persons' blood and cannot in themselves be responsible for the high levels found

Reprinted from *Postgraduate Medicine, 45* (No. 5), May, 1969.   McGraw-Hill, Inc.

in the blood of patients with gout. On the other hand, acute attacks of gout often follow bouts of heavy eating and drinking. Medical lore in Britain purports that heavy wines such as port and Madeira are more likely to cause an attack than light wines such as Rhine wine or white Bordeaux. The fact that champagne (a white wine low in alcohol) is often incriminated, too, makes me doubt the validity of this British generalization. It is difficult to interpret our British friends' idea that "poor man's gout" is seen more often in beer drinkers than in those who partake of spirits. It seems more reasonable to assume that in a situation where purine metabolism is in a state of unstable equilibrium, the metabolic storm which may follow an excessive consumption of any form of alcohol may cause increased endogenous purine synthesis and precipitation of urate.

Similarly, at one time it was fashionable to think that food allergies were particularly important in precipitating a gouty episode. While this theory cannot be categorically ruled out, it seems more likely that dietary excesses (with or without alcoholic excess) may again start a storm in the metabolism of purines with gouty crisis as the result.

Better understanding of the pathogenesis of the disease and availability of extremely effective drugs have transformed the clinical picture of the disease in the treated patient, but going from extreme dietary caution to complete disregard of diet does not seem reasonable. The fear that attention to diet will lead the patient to omit his medication, or to be casual about the intervals between pills is not founded on extensive observation or confirmed by careful internists. The following dietary advice can and should be given in addition to pharmacologic prescription:

1. Weight control. The generalization that an unusually high proportion of patients in whom gout develops in middle age are obese appears to be valid. Obesity seems to be associated with gout at least to the same extent that it is associated with maturity-onset diabetes. Weight reduction seems an effective method of preventing attacks of gout in obese patients. The reduction in weight should be gradual; fasting or drastic dieting will increase blood uric acid. With the last provision in mind, I think it is fair to say that the effect of weight reduction alone in decreasing attacks

tends to be forgotten under the impact of the present-day pharmacology. The excessive preoccupation with the nature of the diet and the lack of attention paid to the quantity of food is in part responsible for many physicians' skepticism regarding the value of dietotherapy in gout.

2. Fat content of the diet. It has been repeatedly observed that a high-fat diet decreases urinary excretion of urates. This is a good reason to reduce the gouty patient's fat intake. Inasmuch as he is usually male, middle-aged, overweight and, hence, particularly susceptible to atherosclerosis, he already has good reason to decrease the fat content of his diet and to reduce the proportion of saturated fat within the fat intake.

3. Purines. The obsessive attention to the purine content of the diet and the drastic decrease in the meat and fish content of the diet, popular before the biochemical basis for uric acid synthesis was at all understood, are no longer justified. We now know that dietary purines are only partially responsible for the hyper-uricemia of gouty patients. On the other hand, patients with either acute or chronic gout should avoid the additional metabolic stress of consuming large amounts of meat, poultry or fish, and should particularly ˆavoid those foods which are excessively high in purines — fish roe, sardines, smelts, herring, sweetbreads (pancreas or thymus), liver, kidney and heart.

4. Alcohol. There is no reason to ban alcohol altogether from the regimen of the gouty patient. However, moderation appears to be essential. Excessive alcohol consumption, like exposure to cold, undue fatigue, and various traumas, tends to precipitate attacks.

5. Coffee and tea. The fact that caffeine is a methyl purine used to be considered as prima facie evidence that coffee and tea precipitated gouty attacks. However, it has been shown that caffeine is not converted into uric acid in the body, and there is no reason to ban them any longer. Of course, moderation in their use, particularly in the consumption of strong coffee, is advisable on other grounds (possible association with cardiovascular disease and perhaps diabetogenicity in susceptible individuals).

During an acute attack, the patient's appetite is usually depressed. Vague abdominal complaints are often present. Inasmuch as the acute attack is of short duration, there is no point in devising any special diet. Foods low in purines (milk, milk products, eggs and more particularly cereals, vegetables and fruit) are preferred to meat, poultry or fish. The consumption of whole milk and eggs should be moderate, not only on general principles of avoiding atherogenic diets but more specifically because fat tends to decrease the excretion of nucleic acid. The patient should drink as much fluid (water, fruit juices, soft drinks, etc.) as possible, and alcoholic beverages should be eliminated during this period. Sodium bicarbonate given in water between meals relieves gastric discomfort and promotes uric acid solution by alkalizing the urine; this decreases the likelihood of uric acid calculi formation.

To summarize, specific pharmacotherapy is undoubtedly the keystone of modern treatment of gout. While compulsive attention to dietary minutia is absurd and many past beliefs on the relationship of gout and diet have been disproved, there is no more reason to neglect the patient's diet than to ignore other aspects of his general hygiene. Weight control, avoiding excessively high intakes of purines, moderation in using alcohol, regular eating habits, and a balanced diet are important aspects of controlling this ancient but rarely ennobling disease.

*Chapter 45*

# NUTRITION AND CELIAC DISEASE

C ELIAC disease was for a long time a source of utter frustration for the pathologist and the biochemist, as well as for the pediatrician treating the disease. In recent years, largely through the efforts of a distinguished group of Dutch clinical investigators, the disease has lost some of its mystery and, thanks to nutritional management, much of its threat.

The entire group of diseases of intestinal absorption which Thaysen (1) called "idiopathic steatorrheas" was for a long time associated with no consistent histologic finding which could explain the defect in intestinal absorption that so often caused emaciation and death. This was true in particular of the celiac syndrome, a disease which ordinarily manifests itself between the first and fifth years of life, generally develops gradually, and, when fully developed, is characterized by marked emaciation of the trunk and extremities, distended abdomen, seborrheic dermatitis of the scalp, anorexia, depression and irritability. The feces are voluminous, fatty and generally foul-smelling. Although the duodenal juice contains normal amounts of bile acids and pancreatic enzymes, the children absorb fat and carbohydrates poorly. Oral blood glucose tolerance curves are low, as are rises in blood vitamin A in tolerance tests. Not infrequently, this condition, if untreated, leads to secondary nutritional deficiencies, and the lack of both calories and certain vitamins leads to marked retardation of growth as well as physical development.

Celiac disease has a variety of degrees; the symptomatology has been classified by Sheldon (2). First are the nutritional symptoms: diarrhea, abdominal distention, weight loss and, frequently, anemia. Second are the psychologic manifestations: depression, contrariness and, eventually, anorexia. These can be seen in the

---

Reprinted from *Postgraduate Medicine, 33* (No. 6), June, 1963.

absence of major intestinal pathologic findings, as described in particular in a classic article by Daynes (3). The third group of symptoms concerns growth failure, which is also compatible with an absence of severe intestinal dysfunction (4). This absence of obvious severe intestinal disturbance makes it likely that diagnosis is missed in a number of cases.

## ROLE OF WHEAT GLUTEN

Various diets were used before part of the mechanism of the celiac syndrome was elucidated. Because of the steatorrhea, low-fat or fat-free diets were tried; these were discarded when they did not markedly relieve the condition. In fact, it was found that even when fat was rigidly excluded from the diet, patients continued to excrete fat in the feces (5). The banana diet of Haas (6) and the vegetable-fruit diet of Fanconi (7) became well known, if not reproducibly successful. A considerable step was taken in 1950 when Dicke (8) observed that patients with the celiac syndrome react particularly unfavorably to wheat and rye. Van de Kamer and Weijers (9), following up on this initial observation, systematically examined the effect of inclusion of wheat flour in the diet of celiac patients. The results, soon confirmed by others (10, 11), were striking. Whenever the diet contained even small amounts of wheat flour, the patient became pale and showed increased steatorrhea and diarrhea. Removal of the wheat flour led to immediate improvement: this improvement persisted even if wheat starch was then given. It appeared, therefore, that the gluten of wheat flour might be responsible for the exacerbation of the condition. In subsequent studies the Dutch authors (12, 13) showed that the gliadin fraction of wheat gluten was the noxious part of gluten in this syndrome, with the steatorrhea a secondary consequence of the faulty metabolism of this protein. Gliadin is an unusual protein. It is insoluble in water, but soluble in 70 to 80 per cent ethyl alcohol. More significantly, it has a very unbalanced composition, characterized by small proportions of such essential amino acids as lysine, methionine and threonine and a very large proportion (43%) of glutamine, the mono-amide of glutamic acid. Van de Kamer and Weijers therefore investigated the effect of glutamine supplements (2 to 4 gm daily, equivalent to the glutamine content of 125 to 250 gm of wheat flour). No untoward symptom was elicited. The Dutch workers concluded that free glutamine was not the responsible agent in celiac disease.

## ROLE OF PROTEIN-BOUND GLUTAMINE

The next step in this analysis consisted in keeping gliadin substantially intact while decomposing glutamine by deamidization (induced by boiling gliadin with 1-N-hydrochloric acid for 45 minutes). This procedure is too mild to hydrolyze peptide bonds in the gliadin molecule to a substantial degree, but it causes 90 per cent of the glutamine to dissociate into glutamic acid and ammonia. Supplements of such treated gliadin caused no symptoms and the patients improved rapidly during the period of administration.

Van de Kamer and Weijers tentatively concluded that the noxious element was glutamine bound to gliadin. This hypothesis was supported by determining the ratio of amide nitrogen to nonamide nitrogen in various foods and correlating this ratio to tolerance of these foods by celiac patients. Specifically, the ammonia liberated by boiling for four hours with 1-N-hydrochloric acid is related to total ammonia set free by Kjeldahl's method (entailing prolonged boiling with concentrated sulfuric acid in the presence of a catalyst) according to the formula

$$\frac{\text{amide nitrogen}}{\text{total nitrogen} - \text{amide nitrogen}} \times 100.$$

Foods well tolerated by patients with celiac disease such as meat (including beefsteak), whole egg, fish (cod), soybean oil meal, green peas, and potato were found to have ratios of 11 or less. By contrast, foods leading to exacerbation of symptoms such as wheat flour, barley and rye, as well as such noxious fractions as glutenin, gluten and gliadin, all have ratios of more than 11, with gliadin of the order of 30.

Using the method of Prescott and Waelsch (14) to determine

blood glutamine, Van de Kamer and Weijers (13) developed a gliadin tolerance test to determine sensitivity to wheat. The fasting patient is given per os in 15 to 20 ml of buttermilk 350 mg of gliadin per kilogram of body weight. Plasma glutamine is determined at administration and at one, two, three, four and five hour (s) afterward. Under such conditions the rise in blood glutamine does not exceed 40 per cent in normal children. Celiac patients on diets including wheat show rises between 55 and 200 per cent, with a mean of 100 per cent. Patients on wheat-free diets show intermediate results. Van de Kamer and Weijers consider that a rise of 50 per cent is indicative of wheat sensitivity; the method seems preferable both from the viewpoint of simplicity and rapidity and from that of objectivity to the study of steatorrheic responses to wheat supplement.

The nature of the enzymatic error or errors in this impairment of the metabolism of bound glutamine is still obscure. Sakula and Shiner (15) have described a flattening of the lining membrane of the duodenum, with partial disappearance of the villi, a finding similar to that seen in adult idiopathic steatorrhea, which may be the same disease (2). Van de Kamer and Weijers (13) assume that the enzymatic error is in the intestinal mucosa and that the peptide-bound glutamine is responsible directly (rather than through allergic processes) for the manifestation of the disease. That this abnormality is in part at least controlled genetically is suggested by the finding of Boyer and Andersen (16) that there is a significantly higher incidence of celiac disease, recurrent diarrhea of unknown origin, and intolerance to fats and various other foods in the families of children with celiac disease than in control families, an observation confirmed by Sheldon (2).

## INFLUENCE OF FATTY ACID COMPOSITION AND MAGNESIUM DEFICIENCY

Fernandes, Van de Kamer and Weijers (17) studied the influence of molecular weight of fatty acids on their absorption in celiac patients (as well as in patinets with cystic fibrosis and ileectomy). They found that when butterfat was fed to children with celiac disease, the coefficient of excretion (100 x fatty acid excreted: fatty acid fed) of the saturated fatty acids rose with the molecular weight; the same was true of monounsaturated fatty acids. By contrast, polyunsaturated fatty acids were completely absorbed, irrespective of chain length. In addition, they found that the overall composition of the lipid fraction of the diet influenced the absorption of individual fatty acids. When oleic acid was fed as part of an oil high in linoleic and linolenic acid, it was absorbed in much greater proportion than when it was fed as part of a fat high in saturated long-chain fatty acids. The conclusion of the study was that patients with steatorrhea should be fed unsaturated fats rather than "hard" fats poor in unsaturated and polyunsaturated fatty acids.

The detailed study of a case of magnesium deficiency associated with celiac disease described by Goldman, Van Fossan and Baird (18) is a warning of a possible dangerous complication of this syndrome. The patient, a 16-year-old girl, had had the disease for no less than one and one-half years and probably much longer. Besides growth failure, abdominal distention and steatorrhea, she exhibited lethargy, carpopedal spasm and generalized convulsions; Trousseau's and Chvostek's signs were present. Serum magnesium was low (0.3 mEq per liter instead of the normal 2.5). Serum calcium was also depressed. Tetany was relieved by intra-muscularly administered sulfate; calcium administration had no effect on a gluten-free diet. The patient gained and grew rapidly (16 kg and 5 cm respectively, in six months). Serum magnesium rose to 1.2 mEq per liter and serum calcium to normal. Metabolic balances indicated that clinical improvement was accompanied by a decreased loss of magnesium (as magnesium soaps) in the feces.

Iron-deficiency anemia, low-calcium tetany, and even occurrence of megaloblastic anemia cured by folic acid have also been reported to be complications of celiac disease which are seen occasionally.

## PROGNOSIS

Sheldon (2) presented in the 1959 Kenneth D. Blackfan Memorial Lecture the results obtained at the Hospital for sick Children, Great Ormond Street, London, in 1958. Ninety-five children attending the clinic, all of whom had been for one to three years on a gluten-free diet, were restored to a normal diet. Forty-four continued to grow satisfactorily; 28 others, although persistenly more than one standard deviation below the average, were considered to be growing normally since their parents were of small stature. The remaining 23 underwent a relapse; in 11 all the typical symptoms returned and the other 12 showed a rapid decline in growth rate. All 23 children quickly improved when gluten was eliminated from their diet. When a year later gluten was put back in the diet, only seven continued to do unequivocally well. It thus appears that after a period of treatment three of four children tolerate gluten satisfactorily and grow at a normal rate. It is equally obvious that the child's progress must be carefully watched for several years after restoration of a normal diet. In particular, careful plotting of height and weight on a growth chart may give the only indication that intolerance is returning.

## DIETARY MANAGEMENT

The principles of dietary management of celiac disease are immediate consequences of the findings previously summarized. The diet should be free of gluten (no wheat, rye, oats or barley), high in other proteins, and moderately low in fat, particularly saturated fats. Administration of 5000 to 10,000 units of vitamin A daily is made necessary by the fat restriction and the impairment in absorption and administration of a liberal supplement of B vitamins is reasonable. If anemia is present, 10 mg of iron should be given and if prolonged prothrombin time is observed, particularly in babies, vitamin K should be given intravenously. Roughage should be avoided; pureeing the foods is useful. Allergies are common, with fish, particularly shellfish, often responsible. The use of such foods should be carefully supervised and, if necessary, restricted or avoided. In general, when any new food is introduced, the patient should be carefully observed for one week or longer, as the intolerance may take time to develop. At the same time, it must be remembered that the patient is an underfed child who has been deficient for some time. Even during the acute phase, the ill child requires frequent feeding, as often as every two or three hours. Caloric requirements are high if past deficiency is going to be remidied. Protein intake can be high; as much as 6 to 8 gm per kilogram of body weight has been used successfully, but such high levels should not be maintained long, and other sources of calories are indispensable. During the acute phase, simple carbohydrates are best tolerated, although ripe banana has classically also been successfully used. While visible fat should be avoided during the acute phase, the fat of egg yolk and lean meat is usually tolerated; skim milk rather than whole milk should be used. As the acute phase recedes, unsaturated fats (corn, cottonseed, olive and sesame oils) can be added to the diet, with progression to other fats as the disease recedes. There is no special indication for salt restriction. Mike (19) published a valuable list of low-gluten or gluten-free foods for patients with celiac disease, as well as a list of foods usually well tolerated and foods best avoided by such patients. She also cited examples of successful menus.

It would be presumptuous to say that celiac disease can now be "cured." But the combination of careful diagnosis, detailed prescription and conscientious and prolonged follow-up has eliminated the threat to life and much of the threat to growth and health that made the disease a malignant pediatric entity.

## REFERENCES

1. Thaysen, T. E. H.: Ten cases of idiopathic steatorrhea. Quart. J. Med., 4:359, 1935.
2. Sheldon, W.: Celiac disease. Pediatrics, 23:132, 1959.
3. Daynes, G.: Bread and tears — naughtiness, depression and fits due to wheat sensitivity. Proc. Roy. Soc. Med., 49:391, 1956.
4. Frazer, A. C.: Discussion of some problems of steatorrhea and reduced stature. *Ibid.*, p. 1009.
5. Weijers, H. A. and Van De Kamer, J. H.: Centraal Inst. v. voedingsonderzoek T.N.O. Publication No. 113. Utrecht, Netherlands, 1950.
6. Haas, S. V.: The value of the banana in the treatment of celiac disease. Am. J. Dis. Child., 28:421, 1924.
7. Fanconi, G.: Der intestinale Infantilisme und ahnliche Foremen det chronischen Verdauungfstörung. Abhand. aus d. Kinderh. Heft 16-21, No. 21, 1927-1928.
8. Dicke, W. K.: Coeliake. (Thesis.) Utrecht, Netherlands, 1950.
9. Van de Kamer, J. H. and Weijers, H. A.: The diet in celiac disease. Voeding, 14:37, 1953.

10. Anderson, C. M., French, J. M., Sammons, H. G., Frazer, A. C., Gerrard, J. W. and Smellie, J. M.: Coeliac disease: Gastrointestinal studies and the effect of dietary wheat flour. Lancet, 1:836, 1952.

11. Sheldon, W. and Lawson, D.: The management of celiac disease. Lancet, 2:902, 1952.

12. Van de Kamer, J. H. and Weijers, H. A.: Celiac disease: Some experiments on the cause of the harmful effect of wheat gliadin. Acta paediat., 44:465, 1955.

13. —: Celiac Disease: A rapid method to test wheat sensitivity. *Ibid.*, p. 536.

14. Prescott, B. A. and Waelsch, H.: A microdetermination of glutamic acid and its application to protein analysis. J. Biol. Chem., 164:331-334 (July) 1946.

15. Sakula, J. and Shiner, M.: Coeliac disease with atrophy of the small intestine mucosa. Lancet, 2:876, 1957.

16. Boyer, P. H. and Andersen, D. H.: A genetic study of celiac disease: Incidence of ceilac disease, gastrointestinal disorders, and diabetes in pedigrees of children with celiac disease. A.M.A. J. Dis. Child., 91:131, 1956.

17. Fernandes, J., Van de Kamer, J. H. and Weijers, H. A.: Differences in absorption of the various fatty acids studied in children with steatorrhea. J. Clin. Invest., 41:488, 1962.

18. Goldman, A. S., Van Fossan, D. D. and Baird, E. E.: Magnesium deficiency in celiac disease. Pediatrics, 29:948, 1962.

19. Mike, E. M.: Practical dietary management of patients with celiac syndrome. Am. J. Clin. Nutrition, 7:463, 1959.

# PART VI
## Nutrition and Disease

*Chapter 46*

# NUTRITION AND THE
# RHEUMATIC DISEASES

N O attempt will be made in this chapter to redefine and classify rheumatic diseases, because this is both outside the limits of competence of this writer and largely unnecessary for the purposes of this study. We shall consider the nutritional aspects of treating the following conditions: nonarticular rheumatism osteo-arthritis, gout, arthritis due to infections, rheumatoid arthritis, rheumatic fever, systemic lupus erythematosus, progressive systemic sclerosis (scleroderma), and polyarteritis nodosa. In general, in the present state of our knowledge, it can be said that nutrition has little or no specific relationship to the cause or treatment of these conditions, with the possible exception of gout. On the other hand, patients with these chronic diseases are exposed to many nutritional hazards; failure to inquire into their food habits and to follow their nutritional state may seriously jeopardize their well-being. Thus, while there is no specific diet for arthritis, it is essential to make certain that the patient with arthritis is on a balanced, palatable diet calorically adequate but consistent with the avoidance of obesity.

## NONARTICULAR RHEUMATISM

There is little evidence that nutrition has any part in the cause or the specific treatment of nonarticular rheumatism. In the 1930's it was fashionable to believe, on the basis of the most questionable and scanty evidence that certain food allergies might cause fibrositis. This condition can appear so suddenly and be elicited by such uncontrollable factors as exposure to draft or chilling of a particular area of the body and, conversely, the

Reprinted from *Postgraduate Medicine, 38* (No. 4), October, 1965.

spontaneous remission of attacks is so frequent that it is easy for a patient to mistake the coincidental ingestion of a certain food as a causal factor. It has also been suggested that in patients with psychogenic rheumatism, self-prescription of an unusual diet can be a substitute means of expressing their anxiety; the diet then "works" in terms of decreasing the frequency or severity of fibrositis.

The calcium deposits visible on x-ray examination in the painful shoulder syndrome occurring in the aged and in young patients such as violinists or baseball pitchers, who use the shoulder with unusual frequency or violence, do not indicate a generalized disturbance of calcium metabolism or a drastic cut in the patient's calcium intake.

## OSTEOARTHRITIS

As with most rheumatic disease, the cause of this most common of all forms of arthritis is essentially unknown, and there is no rational basis for any specific dietotherapy. Obesity, however, can be considered a serious complication of osteoarthritis. The strain of carrying an amount of weight considerably above that for which the joints were designed makes the symptoms of the disease more acute, accelerates its course, and, by making it difficult for the patient to move, complicates the treatment of both the obesity and the osteoarthritis.

Patients with osteoarthritis are often overweight, unlike patients with rheumatoid arthritis, who are typically thin, asthenic and visceroptotic. Institution of a reducing regimen, plus whatever exercise is possible and advisible, is obviously an important part of the therapy. As in nonarticular rheumatism, many patients believe that "excessive" calcium intake is in some way responsible for the bony malformations of osteoarthritis. As a result, they tend to eliminate calcium sources from the diet, so that osteoporosis of essentially dietary origin is frequently associated with osteoarthritis, particularly in older women.

## GOUT

Few patients realize that the urates which accumulate in the body in gout arise from two sources — exogenous urates for the utilization of food proteins and endogenous urates from tissue catabolism. Furthermore, patients are not aware that the endogenous sources of uric acid are by far the most abundant and that this endogenous production of uric acid is amenable to little if any dietary control such simple and ubiquitous compounds as glycine are precursors of uric acid. Patients must be impressed with the concept that although eliminating from their diet foods high in preformed purines is a reasonable measure, it is far less important than taking the colchicine or probenicid (Benemid®) and phenylbutazone prescribed.

Since stress of any type may precipitate acute attacks of gouty arthritis it should be avoided. This is just as true of dietary excesses as it is of stress from surgery, trauma, emotional disturbances and certain drugs. Certain dietary precautions must be observed. Excessive ingestion of alcohol also may precipitate an attack, perhaps because the resultant increase of lactic acid in the blood may suppress the excretion of uric acid. It is important to put the patient on an even keel nutritionally and to help him develop sensible food habits from which he will not suddenly depart. High-fat diets have been shown to cause an increased incidence of acute attacks, again possibly because of the resultant acidosis. Fasting, either because of illness or because of voluntary drastic reduction of calories, is equivalent to the feeding of a high-fat diet and will cause an elevation of blood uric acid and precipitate acute attacks. A marked and sometimes dangerously high increase in serum uric acid is often observed in nongouty patients subjected to weight reduction by total fasting, a practice which is obviously a fortiori contraindicated in patients with gout. If weight reduction is indicated, and it frequently is, it must be very gradual. I would suggest that a deficit of 500 calories a day is the most that should be attempted; this would correspond to a weight loss of no more than a pound a week, actually a very sizable rate if it can be maintained. In general, keeping the intake of fat relatively low and that of carbohydrate correspondingly higher seems a desirable practice in managing gout. A high fluid intake helps to prevent the deposition of urates in the urinary tract and thus helps to retard or prevent renal involvement.

Contrary to ancient and general opinion, severe restriction of purine, protein or alcohol does not help to control gout. It is reasonable, however, to avoid such high-purine foods as liver, kidney, brain, sweetbreads, meat extracts, anchovies, sardines and condiments, including pepper, as well as any particular food which seems to provoke an attack. While small amounts of alcohol apparently do not present a risk, the physician may feel it safer to recommend total abstinence if this seems the only way to prevent alcoholic excesses. Only in managing patients with severe chronic tophaceous gout, in the initial phase of uricosuric therapy, is there a rationale for some restriction of protein. Dietary protein can then be limited to thatfrom vegetable sources, supplemented by 1 pt to 1 qt of milk daily. A pleasant and safe dietary pattern for most patients provides one serving a day of moderate amounts of meat, fish or seafood (other than those previously mentioned as excessively high in purines); one serving of peas, lentils, asparagus, cauliflower, spinich or mushrooms; and unlimited amounts (restricted only as caloric intake requires) of other vegetables, fruit, milk, cheese, eggs and cereals other than whole grain. There is no general rationale for forbidding tea, coffee or cocoa in gout. The methyl xanthines (caffeine, theophylline and theobromine) of coffee, tea and cocoa are metabolized to methylurates and are not deposited in the tophus. Risk of gastric irritation due to phenylbutazone is minimized if the drug is taken with meals or at least a glass of milk.

## ARTHRITIS DUE TO INFECTION

Again, there is little specific nutritional advice that can be given with regard to treating arthritis due to infection, whether the infectious agent is introduced directly by way of a wound (e.g. staphylococcal infection) or through the bloodstream (e.g. tuberculosis, syphilis, gonococcal infection). As with all infectious diseases, a diet sufficient in amount as well as in quality is as much a part of the treatment as specific antimicrobial agents, rest or indicated surgical drainage.

## RHEUMATOID ARTHRITIS

By this time many of the old ideas on the supposedly specific merits of vitamins C, D and E in the treatment of rheumatoid arthritis have been repeatedly disproved. Abundant evidence is also available that rheumatoid arthritis does not increase the requirements for other vitamins over the amounts required by normal healthy individuals. Such bizarre regimens as the cod liver oil and orange juice treatment; the cherry, raw food and "natural" food fads; and the administration of molasses, honey or "sulfur-containing" foods have no justificiation whatsoever. The supposed intolerance to dietary carbohydrates at one time ascribed to the patient with severe rheumatoid arthritis was based on a misunderstanding. Although many patients exhibit a decreased "glucose tolerance" when subjected to the classic tests, this is probably a consequence of their chronic inflammatory state and in no way suggests that they are unable to assimilate dietary carbohydrates. The dispelling of such errors and hoaxes does not, however, in any way eliminate the need for careful dietotherapy.

Rheumatoid arthritis, a generalized systemic disease which can be very severe, is often accompanied by anorexia and critical weight loss, which may aggravate the muscular atrophy due to local disease and to the disuse caused by joint disability. In addition to the anorexia caused by general sickness, pain and fatigue, it has been estimated that about 5 per cent of patients with rheumatoid arthritis have involvement of the temporomandibular joints, which restricts, sometimes markedly, the ability to open the mouth and to chew. Restriction of movements of the joints of the hand and arms makes it difficult for many patients to feed themselves. Restriction of motion of the upper and lower limbs may make it more difficult for the homemaker to prepare food. Finally, in Sjogren's syndrome (also called the sicca syndrome), a complication of rheumatoid arthritis, the lacrimal and salivary glands become atrophied. The resultant dryness in the mouth and pharynx causes difficulty in mastication and swallowing.

The solutions of these problems are easy to state but often difficult to put into practice. Anorectic patients must be coaxed back to appropriate intake, an undertaking often representing a formidable challenge to the physician, dietitian and cook as well as to the patient himself. Whether this increase in intake is best accomplished through an increase in the size of the main meals or through the additon of supplementary snacks is very much an individual matter. The problem is particularly difficult to solve in the case of the severely handicapped patient living alone who not only has a very poor appetite but also has great difficulty in preparing his food. If institutionalization is impossible or undesirable, the delivery of at least one meal a day by a community program is helpful.

Patients with chewing difficulty should be instructed in the use of a semiliquid diet. The use of liquid formula diets for some of the snacks is often helpful and nutritionally sound. Self-help devices often can improve the self-sufficiency of patients with restricted use of the hands. A great many such devices have been developed and many were described in articles published in *Postgraduate Medicine* from April 1959 to November 1964. A booklet also describing them may be obtained from the Institute of Physical Medicine and Rehabilitation.* Occupational therapy departments of large hospitals are helpful sources of information on available devices designed both for self-help and for assisting the handicapped homemaker.

Finally, it is essential to recognize Sjögren's syndrome and, if it is present, to instruct and encourage the patient to drink enough liquid with his food to mitigate the otherwise unpleasant sensation of dryness which makes the ingestion of food difficult.

## RHEUMATIC FEVER

There is little doubt that improvement in nutrition, as well as in housing and in antistreptococcal prophylactic measures, is responsible for the decreasing incidence of this dreaded condition. While there is no specific nutritional measure in its treatment, it is important to maintain sound nutrition in the patients, many of whom are growing individuals (peak age of onset is between six and nine years). At the same time, many are victims of an infection and are receiving a number of powerful pharmacologic agents — such antibiotics as penicillin, salicylates, corticosteroids and sulfadiazine. If cardiac failure is present, a low-sodium diet

---

*Institute of Physical Medicine and Rehabilitation, New York University Medical Center, 400 East 34th Street, New York 10016.

must be given with enough care and culinary imagination to maintain sufficient caloric intake.

## SYSTEMIC LUPUS ERYTHEMATOSUS

It is impossible to suggest any specific dietotherapy for this chronic, dangerous and polymorphic disease. Such possible complications such as cardiac or renal involvement and such symptoms as nausea, anorexia and abdominal pain create nutritional problems which must be solved on an *ad hoc* basis such as a low-sodium or a low-protein diet for certain cardiac or renal complications, respectively. Patients who not only are victims of the disease but also are subjected to prolonged pharmacologic treatment, including salicylates and large doses of corticosteroids and antimalarials, must be maintained in as satisfactory a nutritional state as is feasible. Prolonged use of large doses of corticosteroids and the higher age of the patients seem to predispose them to a higher incidence of gastric ulcers and osteoporosis. The former must be dealt with by appropriate medical measures and, at least during the acute phase, by an ulcer regimen; the latter can be minimized by high calcium intake.

## PROGRESSIVE SYSTEMIC SCLEROSIS

There are serious difficulties in nutritional management of this condition whenever the mouth or the esophagus is affected. Patients experience difficulty in swallowing and may be able to take only a few mouthfuls of food at a time, particularly if the esophagogastric junction is involved. The patient may be unable to swallow when lying down. He may also have difficulty opening his mouth sufficiently due to tight atrophic facial skin.

The patient must be studied carefully and an estimate made of the relationship of the continuation of apprehension, pain and structural hindrance to the decreased ingestion of food. The use of concentrated liquid formula diets may ease some of the practical problems in feeding such patients, but if calcium deposits are forming in subcutaneous tissues, it may be best to restrict markedly the intake of calcium and phosphorus, which precludes use of the usual commercial formula diets.

## POLYARTERITIS NODOSA

Symptoms of this disease are extraordinarily varied; they may include fever, abdominal complaints, renal, pulmonary and cardiac diseases, peripheral neuritis, and skin, muscle and joint involvement. The disease can be acute or chronic and can have a prognosis which extends from recovery to death.

There is no specific diet for polyarteritis nodosa. Proper nutritional maintenance of the patient is necessary, with specific complications, such as cardiac or renal complications, or by certain treatment such as large doses of corticosteroids.

## CONCLUSION

Precisely because so little is known about the cause of the rheumatoid diseases, sound nutrition is of particular importance. If little can be done at present to "cure" the disease, it is particularly important to take care of the patient during the long course. The chronic character of the rheumatic conditions, their capricious onset and exacerbations, and their unpredictable remissions make it easy for patients to convince themselves or be convinced by food faddists and quacks — particularly numerous in the field of arthritis — that all sorts of weird and unbalanced regimens are beneficial. Nutritional quackery endangers such patients not only because it entails risks of deficiencies and unnecessary financial burdens but also because it thrives on distrust of medicine and can lead to even more dangerous forms of quack "therapy."

*Chapter 47*

# DIETOTHERAPY OF PEPTIC ULCER

$T$HE objective of treatment of an active peptic ulcer is to rest the stomach. Dietotherapy is generally considered an important part of such treatment, which also includes the use of antacids, anticholinergics and sedatives, and the avoidance of mucosal irritants in foods, condiments, alcohol and coffee. This discussion will be restricted to the dietotherapeutic aspects of the treatment.

## OBJECT OF DIETOTHERAPY OF PEPTIC ULCER

Dietary measures in the treatment of gastroduodenal ulcer (as is true of other therapeutic measures) have a threefold purpose: (1) reduction of free gastric acidity, (2) reduction of pyloroduodenal motility, and (3) enhancement of mucosal resistance.

The first aim, reduction of free gastric acidity, cannot be obtained adequately through dietotherapy. Food and alkalizing agents are used as anacids but are not very efficient. It is more effective to reduce gastric antacids but are not very efficient. It is more effective to reduce gastric most important of which is protein. Fat, in a concentration of 10 per cent or more, depresses secretion of acid by stimulating the release of enterogastrone. One basic nutritional problem in the management of peptic ulcer is the desirability of avoiding protein, because its role as a secretagogue coexists with the need for abundant protein to repair the gastric or duodenal mucosa, a dilemma which has to be solved by compromise. If the ulcer is open and active, avoiding the stimulation of acid and, above all, resting the stomach become paramount considerations. In the initial days of illness a regimen of rigid stomach rest, frequent small (less than 150 cc) feedings of milk

Reprinted from *Postgraduate Medicine, 40* (No. 3), September, 1966.

from 7 A.M. to 10 P.M. (and at night if distress is present) alternating every half-hour with anacid, and ingestion of an anticholinergic drug every four hours usually relieves the patient of symptoms in 12 to 18 hours and permits the ulcer to start healing.

If circumstances make it convenient, hourly milk feedings can be replaced by hourly feedings selected alternately from milk, cream soups, vegetable juices, farina, oatmeal, Jell-O®, pudding or custard, although milk alone usually serves well. Skim milk is often as effective as whole milk and has the advantage of contributing fewer calories (obesity) and less saturated fat (atherosclerosis). If delay in gastric emptying is desired because pain returns, milk can be fortified with cream to delay gastric emptying. If the patient is in a poor nutritional state and needs additional protein, protein concentrates or skim milk powder may be added (50 to 100 gm per quart of milk) (1).

After maintaining the rigid "stomach rest" diet for 10 to 14 days, a graduated advance is usually carried out, extending six to eight weeks. The first change is to supplement the hourly milk feeding by a breakfast of cooked cereal and prune juice, cream soup or vegetable juice at lunch, and Jell-O, Junket®, custard or pudding at dinner. After three or four days, soft-boiled eggs and bland cheese can be added to the meals and the between-meal milk feedings are reduced to six a day.

During the next few weeks, baked potatoes, rice, macaroni and other vegetable juices are added (as intermeal milk feedings are reduced to three a day), followed by white meat of chicken, fish, and finally tender red meats (six to nine weeks after the beginning of the treatment) (2). The diet to be followed then is summarized in Table 47-1.

Any recurrence of ulcer pain as the diet becomes more complex is a sign to return to the previous diet and to advance more slowly. The following conditions are also indications for a very slow progression from the hourly schedule: old age, persistence of night distress, gastritis, tension or epigastric tenderness, location of the ulcer in the antrum and cardia, long duration of ulcer attacks before treatment is instituted, and various complications such as penetration with adhesion of the ulcer bed or confined perforation (3).

## TABLE 47-1

### THREE-FEEDING GASTRIC SOFT DIET

Morning      1 small glass diluted strained fruit or tomato juice (to be consumed at the end of the breakfast if necessary).

Cereal with cream and sugar—Cream of Wheat , farina, cornmeal, oatmeal, boiled rice, puffed rice, Rice Krispies®, rice flakes, or cornflakes.

Egg—any way except fried.

1 slice bread—white, plain or toasted with butter. Finely ground wheat or rye bread allowed without crust.

10 A.M.      Milk or buttermilk—1 glass

Noon      Meat—scraped beef, minced chicken, flaked fish broiled, baked or creamed.

Potato—baked (do not eat skin), boiled, mashed or creamed. May substitute macaroni, noodles, spaghetti or rice with butter or cream sauce.

1 small glass tomato or fruit juice.

1 slice white bread with butter. Finely ground wheat or rye bread allowed without crust.

Dessert—Junket, custard, gelatin desserts without fruit or nuts, vanilla ice cream, bread, tapioca, cornstarch and rice pudding, plain cookies, unfrosted angel food or sponge cake.

Milk—1 glass.

3 P.M.      Milk or buttermilk—1 glass.

Night      Strained cream soup and crackers, chicken broth, strained vegetable soup.

Meat (see list above) or egg, cottage cheese, cream cheese.

Potato or substitute.

1 slice white bread with butter. Finely ground wheat or rye bread allowed without crust.

Dessert.

Milk—1 glass.

8 P.M.      Milk beverage or eggnog—1 glass.

Omit the following foods from diet: chocolate; stimulating, alcoholic or carbonated beverages; highly seasoned foods; smoked, dried, pickled or salted meats or fish; pork; shellfish; black pepper, chili, cloves, mustard seeds; fried foods; fruits and vegetables except as allowed; nuts, tea, coffee, cocoa; rich gravies and sauces. Eat slowly and at regular times.

## MAINTENANCE DIET

While there is no evidence that rigid adherence to dietary restrictions after apparent complete "cure" will prevent recurrence, most physicians will try to encourage regularity in eating habits and moderation in the use of spices, condiments, caffeine and alcohol. They will discourage eating occasional very large meals, advise against long intervals between meals, and advocate small snacks at midmorning, midafternoon and in the evening. In general they will try strenuously to discourage smoking and will advise that no more than one cup of coffee whould be consumed at breakfast. They will aslo try to discourage the patient from consuming strong alcoholic drinks, and they will certainly strongly recommend against the consumption of more than one or two dilute drinks. The use of aspirin will be forbidden.

## A DIFFERENT VIEW: IS DIETOTHERAPY SOUNDLY BASED?

It must be recognized, however, that a small number of gastroenterologists, Ingelfinger (4) foremost among them, are extremely skeptical of the benefits of the more rigorous dietary treatment of peptic ulcer after the early phase has elapsed. Their point of departure is our "gross ignorance" of the effects of individual foods on gastrointestinal structure and function and the little real knowledge about foods which enhance and foods which diminish gastric secretion, or foods which increase and foods which decrease the resistance of the mucosa.

In considering our ignorance, this school contends that it is better to avoid detailed dietary prescriptions which may not be effective and of which some components may even in the long run be harmful. Ingelfinger recognized that alcohol, caffeine, meat extracts, and probably all foods containing a very high proportion of proteins do increase gastric secretory activity over and above normal rates of secreting; but he has pointed out that, on the other hand, proteins – whether meat, fish, fowl, or cheese – tend to neutralize acid-peptic activity immediately upon their ingestion (by their buffer activity), even though the end products of their activity are active secretagogues. He has also questioned whether fat taken by mouth in a mixed meal under clinical conditions does in fact depress gastric acidity or whether it actually exercises a late secretory activity, at least if taken in large amounts.

As regards the rest of the diet, Ingelfinger stresses the "nebulous" character of the quality of blandness, although he recognizes that coarse, sharp particles may exercise a noxious mechanical action in an ulcer close to the esophagus or in the pyloroduodenal area where the strong milling effect may grind those rough particles into an open wound. He is more puzzled by what he calls "dietotherapy by analogy," best illustrated by the so-called white diet (white supposedly being tantamount to pure: breast of chicken, potato, rice, milk and cottage cheese), his point being that no evidence exists that white meats or that they stimulate gastric secretion less. He can see no rationale for preferring dairy or vegetable fat to meat fat and believes that, again, dietotherapy proceeds by analogy when forbidding spices which "burn" the taste papillae of the tongue and the mouth on the ground that they must similarly burn the gastroduodenal mucosa. He finds no justification for thinking that pork is more irritating than veal.

Deprivation of fruits and fresh vegetables, he feels, frequently induces in ulcer patients borderline ascorbic acid deficiencies. Even more serious, a diet as rich in fat as often been prescribed may be athermatous; and the very high calcium intake of an abundant consumption of milk and cheese by a patient who previously may have been on a relatively low calcium diet may seriously complicate any preexisting unsuspected renal disorder.

The orders and prohibitions with which an ulcer patient is faced — a specific diet at specified intervals, eating slowly and in peace, eliminating alcohol, tobacco and coffee, new rest habits, avoiding certain tasks or stress — all this Ingelfinger feels may lessen the patient's clear understanding of the first priorities, i.e. the regular and frequent intake of food and of antacids and anticholinergics.

## CONCLUSION

It must be first of all noted that there is no justification for not continuing to use a very restricted diet during the early phase of ulcer management. It would appear that in the present state of our knowledge it is reasonable to continue to instruct the patient in the principles of classic ulcer dietotherapy during the later phase of ulcer management, and to maintain the taboos on coffee, alcohol, strong condiments and coarse foods. Only the unjustifiable extremes of ulcer therapy should obviously be left out. While it is true that some of the theoretical basis for the components of the ulcer diet is still missing, the diet has been found to work as well as or better than others in actual treatment. In many cases, the prescription of a diet and a routine has by itself a therapeutic effect. Of course, care should be taken to make sure that the diet is nutritionally balanced (if necessary, it should be supplemented with vitamins). Care also should be taken to avoid too high an intake of saturated fat by avoiding an exaggerated emphasis on cream or butterfat. Finally, careful attention should be paid to the sensations experienced by the patient both in terms of schedules of meals and in the introduction of new foods. The ulcer diet is not terribly exacting; the patient can stay on it while the doctor uses the experimental method and introduces each new food under controlled conditions.

## REFERENCES

1. Friedman, G. and Janowitz, H. D.: Nutrition in diseases of the stomach. In Wohl, M. G. and Goodhart, R. S. (Editors): Modern Nutrition in Health and Disease. Philadelphia, Lea & Febiger, 1964, p. 713.
2. Krause, M. V.: Diet in gastric diseases. In Food, Nutrition and Diet Therapy. Ed. 4. Philadelphia, W. B. Saunders Company, 1966, p. 233
3. Roth, J. L. A.: The ulcer patient should watch his diet. In Ingelfinger, F. J., Relman, A. S. and Finland, M. (Editors): Controversy in Internal Medicine. Philadelphia, W. B. Saunders Company, 1966, p. 161.
4. Ingelfinger, F. J.: Let the ulcer patient enjoy his food. *Ibid.*, p. 171.

*Chapter 48*

# DIETARY TREATMENT OF
# CORONARY PATIENTS

E VER since the association of a high serum cholesterol concentration with a high-fat diet and with an increase in mortality from coronary heart disease (CHD) became apparent (1), clinicians have tried to control the serum cholesterol of survivors of myocardial infarction. Studies based on the use of estrogens showed that estrogen treatments which lowered cholesterol did exert a favorable effect (2), although responses in some series were ambiguous. Dietary trials seems to have been more numerous. Lyon and associates (3) and other investigators working with large numbers of patients showed a highly favorable effect of a low-fat, low-cholesterol diet. A few studies attempted to take advantage of the influence of the "nature" of the fat on serum cholesterol, as first demonstrated by Kinsell and by Groen and confirmed by recent work (4, 5). Indications were highly favorable (6).

Because the results of these studies were difficult to interpret, they did not inspire internists to strongly recommend plasma cholesterol-lowering diets for survivors of myocardial infarction. The studies have to last long enough. They have to be conducted with extraordinary care. The groups of patients must be large enough. Excellent matching of groups at the start is indispensable. Dropouts have to be avoided. Adherence to the diet has to be verified. Relatively few studies meet all these criteria.

It remained for Leren (7), a cardiologist in Oslo, Norway, to clinch the evidence in a carefully planned and beautifully executed demonstration of the use of diets high in polyunsaturated fats in treating male survivors of myocardial infarction.

Leren's five-year trial was conducted on 412 men 30 to 64 years

Reprinted from *Postgraduate Medicine, 44* (No. 1), July, 1968.   McGraw-Hill, Inc.

of age who were discharged from Oslo hospitals during the years 1956 and 1958 with a first diagnosis of myocardial infarction. One to two years after infarction, the patients were randomly placed in an "experimental" ("diet") group and a control group. Comparability of the two groups of 206 patients was thoroughly studied. They were comparable in every respect except for a slightly larger number of hypertensive patients in the diet group. Criteria for diagnosis of reinfarction were established, and this decision was left to a diagnostic board which did not know to which group the patient belonged. The study was intensive throughout the five years and included clinical examinations, dietary interviews, serum cholesterol determinations, electrocardiography, and review of hospital records.

The only difference in the treatment of the two groups was dietary. The dietetic instructions were given to the patients orally and were relatively simple. They were to eat as little meat as possible and to remove all visible fat from the meat. When boiled meat was eaten, the fat which formed on the broth when it cooled was to be removed. Beef, mutton and pork were to be replaced as much as possible by poultry and whale meat (a food that would be hard to procure in the United States; it might be useful here to emphasize the desirability of lean veal). Fish and shellfish were recommended.

Whole milk and cream were virtually eliminated (no more than 3 oz once a week) and replaced by skim milk. Butter, margarine, lard, shortenings and olive oil were not to be used. Fat cheeses were to be replaced by low-fat cheese such as cottage cheese. Eggs were limited to one a week. Breads eaten were to contain no fat. Breakfast cereals were permitted if consumed with skim milk. "Pure sugar should not be used abundantly." Vegetables, fruits and fruit juices, marmalades and jams were recommended.

Vegetable oils rich in linoleic acid were to be used abundantly. Soybean oil was the only such oil readily available in Oslo at the start of the trial. The desirable amount was set at half a liter (about a pint) a week. If it proved impossible to use that much in cooking, baking and salads, up to an ounce a day was to be taken as "medicine." Appreciable time was spent in giving instructions in the use of soybean oil in preparing foods.

Alcoholic beverages and soft drinks were allowed. A daily vitamin pill was prescribed (for patients in both groups). Twice a week the "dieters" received considerable quantities of Norwegian sardines canned in cod liver oil (one "animal" fat which is high in polyunsaturated fatty acids), which proved to be popular as a bread spread.

Continuous supervision and instruction of the dieters were emphasized. Dietitians visited the homes of dieters often and kept in touch by letter and telephone. Instructions were repeated at each clinical or laboratory examination. Adherence to the diet was tested by questionnaires issued six times. About 62 per cent of the dieters had a score of "excellent" (and a mean reduction of cholesterol of 22%), 22 per cent had a score of "good" (and a 12% reduction of cholesterol), and 10 per cent had a score of "fair" (and a 7% reduction of cholesterol). The remainder scored poorly and had little or no reduction of cholesterol.

Only three dieters had to reduce oil consumption because of diarrhea, and six because of short periods of nausea.

Analysis of the diets yielded an average of 39 per cent fat. Soybean oil represented 72 per cent of the fat ingested. Total caloric consumption was of the order of 2400 calories. Weight changes were similar in the two groups. In overall composition the diet was far from extreme, providing 92 gm of protein, 104 gm of fat, and 269 gm of carbohydrate. The average cholesterol content was low, 264 mg.

Striking differences between the dieters and the control group were observed. They were based on counting only one CHD relapse in each patient, the order of priority being myocardial infarction, new cases of angina pectoris, and sudden death. Sixty-four myocardial infarctions, 23 of them fatal, occurred in 54 patients in the control group; 43 infarctions, 10 of they fatal, occurred in 34 patients in the diet group. (The difference became significant after the third year of the trial.) Among subjects who did not have angina pectoris at the start of the trial, this condition developed in 29 of 79 control subjects and only 10 of the 75 dieters. (Even when nine control subjects and two dieters who also had reinfarction are excluded, this difference is significant.) The number of sudden deaths was 27 in each group. This is not surprising. Sudden death is considered to be caused in most instances by ischemia which induces ventricular fibrillation or cardiac arrest. Leren considers, it would appear reasonably, that sudden death in survivors of myocardial infarction, who presumably have rather advanced atherosclerosis, is related less to the degree of atherosclerosis than to other factors such as location of lesions in more dangerous areas.

The total number of CHD relapses, including sudden deaths, was 120 in the control group as compared with 80 in the diet group. A significant difference became apparent as early as the second year of the trial. When the patients were divided into age groups it was found that the difference was significant only in those less than 60 years of age. Among those over 60 there was no association between serum cholesterol levels and CHD relapses (nor was there at any age an association between serum cholesterol level and sudden death). Another interesting finding is that in the diet group there was no influence of blood pressure on CHD relapse, while in the control group there was the expected trend of higher CHD relapse rate in hypertensive subjects. The patients in whom the diet was most successful were those who had overcome myocardial infarction with no obvious signs and symptoms of heart disease (no angina pectoris, normal heart volume and blood pressure).

It seems unlikely that the small decreases in body weight and in sugar consumption in these patients were more than slight contributory factors in the improvement observed in the diet group. This leaves as the overwhelming factor the marked decrease in serum cholesterol. That this improvement was seen in the patients under 60 (in whom presumably the atherosclerotic process has not reached the point of no return), does not cover sudden death (which, on an atherosclerotic background, is likely to be triggered by other events), and takes more than a year to manifest itself actually strongly confirms the beneficial effect of dietary control, acting through modification of cholesterol level. I believe the case for dietary control of serum cholesterol through drastic reduction of saturated fats and drastic increase of polyunsaturated fats in the treatment of survivors of myocardial infarction is strongly supported by Leren's study, coming as it does in the wake of massive experimental, epidemiologic and clinical indications. Is it unreasonable to think that what is necessary for treatment is also useful for prevention?

## REFERENCES

1. Keys, A.: Atherosclerosis: A problem in newer public health. J. Mount Sinai Hosp. N.Y., 20:118, 1953.
2. Stamler, J., Pick, R., Katz, L. N., Pick, A., Kaplan, B. M., Berkson, D. M. and Century, D.: Effectiveness of estrogens for therapy of myocardial infarction in middle-aged men. J.A.M.A., 183:632, 1963.
3. Lyon, T. P., Yankley, A., Gofman, J. W. and Strisower, B.: Lipoproteins and diet in coronary heart disease. Calif. Med., 84:325, 1956.
4. Keys, A., Anderson, J. T. and Grande, F.: Serum cholesterol response to changes in the diet. Metabolism, 14:747, 1965.
5. Hegsted, D. M., McGandy, R. B., Myers, M. L. and Stare, F. J.: Quantitative effects of dietary fat on serum cholesterol in man. Amer. J. Clin. Nutr., 17:281, 1965.
6. Bierenbaum, M. L., Green, D. P., Florin, A., Fleischchman, A. I. and Caldwell, A. B.: Modified fat dietary management of the young coronary male. A five-year controlled study. Circulation, 31-32, Suppl. II:3, 1965.
7. Leren, P.: The effect of plasma cholesterol lowering diet in male survivors of myocardial infarction. Norwegian Monographs on Medical Science. Oslo, Norway, Universitetsforlaget, 1966, 92 pp. (Also published as Acta Med. Scand. Suppl., 466:1, 1966.)

*Chapter 49*

# HYPERLIPOPROTEINEMIAS AND
# DIETARY TREATMENT

$A$BNORMALLY increased concentrations of plasma cholesterol or triglycerides, or both, are commonly seen in clinical practice. These hyperlipidemias are classified as primary when not due to obvious disease and secondary when due to disease such as hypothyroidism, obstructive liver disorder, nephritis, or diabetes mellitus.

In secondary hyperlipidemias, treatment is directed toward the disease rather than the blood lipid levels per se. In primary hyperlipidemias, however, treatment is directed toward lowering the plasma lipids since the pathogenesis is essentially unknown. Certain types of primary hyperlipidemia are obviously inherited. Lowering plasma lipids diminishes the risk of early athersclerosis and premature death, prevents or reverses xanthoma, and in severe cases relieves recurrent abdominal pain and reduces the risk of acute pancreatitis.

Definitions of hyperlipidemias vary; the commonly accepted upper limits of normal levels of plasma cholesterol and triglycerides are given in Table 49-1. It should be emphasized, however, that while these values represent statistical normality in terms of being within 2 SD of the mean and clinical normality in terms of being below values associated with acute symptoms, they are well above the desirable values in terms of minimizing atherosclerosis and maximizing life expectancy. Thus, patients with plasma levels above values in Table 49-1 should receive the physician's urgent attention.

Because triglycerides and cholesterol circulate in the plasma in piggyback combinations with various types of four major groups of lipoproteins, the hypertriglyceridemias and hypercholester-

Reprinted from *Postgraduate Medicine, 48* (No. 6), December, 1970© McGraw-Hill, Inc.

TABLE 49-1. UPPER LIMITS OF NORMAL* LEVELS
FOR PLASMA CHOLESTEROL AND TRIGLYCERIDES

| Patient's Age (Years) | Cholesterol | Triglycerides |
|---|---|---|
| | (mg per 100 ml) | |
| 1-19 | 230 | 140 |
| 20-29 | 240 | 140 |
| 30-39 | 270 | 150 |
| 40-49 | 310 | 160 |
| 50 and over | 330 | 190 |

*The term "normal" as used in this table permits the definition of upper limits beyond which various types of hyperlipidemias can be characterized. It is obviously desirable to maintain the plasma cholesterol and triglyceride levels well below the upper limit.

olemias have been separated into a number of hyperlipoproteinemias. A diet for each type of hyperlipoproteinemia often permits closer control than a general diet for all types.*

Since the actions of drugs for treating this disorder are not well known and could interfere eventually with basic physiologic processes, these agents should be used only to supplement inadequate dietary therapy.

Biochemical classification of five main types of hyperlipoproteinemia is based on the appearance of a sample of plasma from blood that has been collected after a 12 to 14 hour fast, centrifuged, and stored overnight at 4° C. Before fasting, the patient should have maintained his usual weight on a normal diet for at least two weeks. The degree of turbidity of the infranatant fluid shown by the presence or absence of a creamy layer on top determines whether or not beta lipoproteins or prebeta lipoproteins are present.

Cholesterol and triglycerides are elevated in all five types of hyperlipoproteinemia. However, in type IV the cholesterol level may be almost normal, and in type II the triglyceride value may be close to normal range. Three determinations of these two lipid

*Diet menus for each type of hyperlipoproteinemia are given in "Dietary Management of Hyperlipoproteinemia: A Handbook for Physicians," and in separate booklets under the general title "Dietary management of Hyperlipoproteinemia" with a specific subtitle giving the type. These booklets were prepared by the National Heart and Lung Institute, National Institute of Health, Bethesda.

fractions at least one week apart are necessary to establish a solid base line before therapy.

## TYPE I

After centrifugation and overnight storage at 4° C, the plasma sample in type I hyperlipoproteinemia has a creamy layer on top and a clear infranatant layer. The cholesterol and triglyceride levels are elevated, with the latter often over 5000 mg per 100 ml. The chylomicrons are greatly increased, and the beta lipoproteins and prebeta lipoproteins are normal or decreased.

Type I is almost always familial and is probably associated with lipoprotein lipase deficiency. The patients usually are young and may have lipemia retinalis, hepatosplenomegaly, eruptive xanthoma, and abdominal pain. A low-fat diet drastically decreases plasma triglycerides and relieves abdominal pain.

This type of hyperlipoproteinemia does not respond to existing antilipemic drugs. The therapeutic diet is low in ordinary fats and possibly supplemented by triglycerides of medium chain length that are absorbed directly into the portal vein without forming chylomicrons. Fat intake should be less than 30 gm per day, and alcohol should be avoided. The ratio of polyunsaturated fat to saturated fat is unimportant, cholesterol intake is immaterial, and protein and carbohydrate intake is unrestricted.

## TYPE II

In type II hyperlipoproteinemia the processed plasma is usually clear but sometimes may be slightly turbid. Usually cholesterol levels are 300 to 600 mg per 100 ml, triglyceride levels are slightly elevated or near normal, beta lipoproteins are markedly increased, and prebeta liproteins are moderately increased or normal. Type II can be hereditary, affecting both sexes equally, or secondary to disorders such as myxeedema, nephrosis, and liver disease. The inherited type is detectable before the age of one year and, particularly if homozygous, is accompanied by xanthoma that often appears before age 10.

Therapy is based on lowering the cholesterol intake to less than

300 mg per day and on raising the polyunsaturated-saturated fat ratio by increasing the intake of polyunsaturates and decreasing the intake of saturates. In adults with familial type II, the dietary regimen is usually supplemented with a cholesterol-reducing drug. Cholesterol levels may be allowed to reach normal range except in homozygous familial cases.

The dietary polyunsaturated-saturated fat ratio should be between 1.8 and 2.8. Safflower oil, corn oil, and soft safflower margarine should be used to the exclusion of butter, lard, hydrogenated shortenings, and coconut oil. Cholesterol intake should be limited to 3 oz portions of cooked lean meat or fish (no shellfish or organ meats). Carbohydrates and proteins are unrestricted; limited alcohol is allowed.

## TYPE III

The processed plasma sample in type III hyperlipoproteinemia is usually turbid, with a faint chylomicron layer. The cholesterol and triglyceride levels range from 350 to 800 mg per 100 ml, and the plasma contains large amounts of beta lipoproteins with abnormally low flotation rates. Type III is relatively uncommon and is clinically characterized sometimes by tendon xanthoma but more often by tuberous eruptive lesions over elbows, knees and buttocks. These lesions are often associated with orange-streaked palmar xanthoma. The incidence of coronary and peripheral diseases at an early age is increased in these patients.

Therapy consists of reducing body weight to ideal standards, followed by a maintenance diet low in cholesterol.

## TYPE IV

The processed plasma sample in type IV hyperlipoproteinemia is usually turbid and does not have a creamy layer. The degree of turbidity depends on the degree of increase in endogenous triglyceride. Unless the triglycerides are greatly elevated, the cholesterol levels are normal. The plasma contains high levels of pre beta lipoproteins or lipoproreins of very low density. The disorder is usually asympomatic, but with very high levels of triglycerides, xanthoma and hepatosplenomegaly may be present.

Type IV is quite common and usually exacerbated by obesity. It is often seen in conjunction with hereditary metabolic diseases such as diabetes mellitus. About 50 per cent of patients have abnormal glucose tolerance, and a high proportion also have hyperuricemia.

Therapy is based on reducing body weight to ideal standards, which also reduces triglyceride levels. The maintenance diet is low in carbohydrates and alcohol.

## TYPE V

In type V hyperlipoproteinemia, the processed plasma sample has a creamy layer on top and a turbid infranatant layer. When diet is unrestricted, plasma triglycerides may range from 1000 to 6000 mg per 100 ml; cholesterol is much lower. The plasma contains large amounts of chylomicrons and prebeta lipoproteins.

Type V may be secondary to acute metabolic disorders such as diabetic acidosis, pancratitis, nephrosis and alcoholism, or it may be familial with symptoms often present by age 20. Patients with the familial type have creamy plasma, hepatosplenomegaly, attacks of abdominal pain and, in more acute cases, pancreatitis. They may also show varying degrees of fat intolerance.

Therapy consists of reducing body weight to ideal standards. This often will reduce plasma lipid concentrations to normal and increase tolerance to minor excesses of fat and carbohydrates. The ideal weight is maintained by a diet limited in carbohydrates and fats.

## ACKNOWLEDGMENT

The author gladly acknowledges his debt to the extremely useful series of booklets produced by the National Heart and Lung Institute, National Institutes of Health, Bethesda, under the direction of Drs. D. S. Fredrickson and R. I. Levy, with E. Jones, M. Bonnell and N. Ernst.

## Chapter 50

# HYPERTENSION AND OBESITY

W E may have considerably underestimated the importance of obesity as a risk factor in cardiovascular diseases, especially when it is relatively moderate ("overweight" is the term used then). Recent studies, the Framingham Heart Study in particular, ascribe only a small influence to obesity uncomplicated by the presence of hypercholesterolemia, hypertension, or other known risks. These studies imply that hypercholesterolemia and hypertension develop independently of obesity and then interact with this condition; the simultaneous presence of obesity then considerably increases the risk due to hypertension and hyper-cholesterolemia. It has become clear that, in fact, the association of obesity and hypertension in many patients is not fortuitous and that obesity actually may cause certain forms of hypertensive disease.

Let us lay to rest the old idea that the relationship between obesity and hypertension is an artifact caused by the increased circumference of the arm around which the blood pressure cuff is wrapped. Comparisons of direct intra-arterial measurements with stethoscopic determinations have shown that the supposed differences between the two methods were inconsistent and statistically negligible.

The prevalence of obesity, of course, depends on the criteria used. I have repeatedly advocated on definition of obesity based on measurements of actual fat by densitometry or the use of calipers, and data on the prevalence of obesity in children and adolescents based on these criteria are beginning to appear. They make somber reading, with a prevalence over 20 per cent, at least in the East. Data in adults are essentially based on deviation of body weight from insurance or other collective standards. The

Reprinted from *Postgraduate Medicine, 46* (No. 5), November, 1969.© McGraw-Hill, Inc.

481

Metropolitan Life Insurance Company considers 29 per cent of 40-to 49-year-old men to be 10 to 19 per cent above ideal weight and 32 per cent to be 20 per cent or more overweight. For women in the same age groups, the figures are 19 and 40 per cent, respectively. The incidence of overweight in persons 50 to 59 years old is even higher. These numbers indicate that the majority of middle-aged Americans are obese.

The prevalence of hypertension also depends on the arbitrary cutoff points used. If one considers the comprehensive study made in Tecumseh, Michigan, in a "typical" American population, 27 per cent of the men and 37 per cent of the women have hypertensive disease. Clearly, both obesity and hypertension affect tens of millions of Americans.

In the United Staes the correlation between overweight and hypertension is quite significant in the 30-to 59-year-age group but decreases for older persons. Available international data suggest that the correlation is higher in countries where obesity is common and that the increase in blood pressure with age is greater in denser populations. In populations living in subarctic regions and characterized by substantial seasonal variations in skinfold thickness, corresponding variations in blood pressure are seen.

Blood pressure and body weight correlate better in women than in men. The correlation is higher in patients with a family history of both hypertension and obesity, in very obese patients, and in patients in the younger age groups. The correlation between systolic pressure and weight is better than that between diastolic pressure and weight. Studies have shown that weight and blood pressure correlate more closely than skinfold thickness and blood pressure, suggesting that both body type and weight are factors to consider.

The general correlations described differ somewhat in various populations. The Charleston Heart Study and a study in Evans County, Georgia, showed differences between Negro and white populations. Negroes have a high incidence of hypertension, but the correlation between overweight and hypertension is weaker in Negroes than in whites, particularly in males. Yet, in the United States in general, the assocation is such that we can reasonably assert that one-fifth to one-third of all hypertensive adults are also markedly overweight or obese.

A study involving 22,000 U.S. Army officers showed that the prevalence of hypertension occurring after age 45 was 2.5 times higher among overweight subjects than among their lighter counterparts. The data obtained by Stamler in his study of 746 male workers of a large Chicago utility company are even more convincing. Among individuals followed over a 20-year period, men whose weight was markedly above the desirable level when they were young adults and who continued to gain during the observation period showed an incidence of hypertension four to five times that of thinner subjects.

In the Framingham Study, over a span of 12 years the risk of hypertension was eight times greater in those men and women who were 20 per cent overweight than in those who were 10 per cent underweight. The incidence of hypertension was five times higher in men who reported having significant weight gain in the 20 years preceeding examination than in those whose weight had remained normal, particularly if the weight was gained after age 25.

There are indications that weight reduction often will favorably influence hypertension, but the favorable effect is not by any means universal. Besides the well-known general favorable effect on mortality and morbidity reported by life insurance companies, several other studies may be cited. In a group of 37 middle-aged obese patients with weight ranging from 212 to 218 lb, 19 of whom were hypertensive and 18 normotensive, an average loss of 42 lb caused no change in systolic and diastolic levels in 12 hypertensive patients. Weight loss lowered the systolic pressure in five and both systolic and diastolic pressures in two. In normotensives similar effects were seen in three subjects and one subject, respectively.

Studies of large groups give similarly convincing indications that blood pressure falls substantially with weight loss. In a group of 194 obese patients who lost more than 10 lb, the average blood pressure fell from 154/96 to 133/86. Among a group of 62 patients with a systolic pressure of 200 mm Hg or more, blood pressure in 22 patients who had a substantial weight loss fell from

219/129 to 176/108. In a group of 100 consecutive cases of obesity, systolic blood pressure was elevated above 140 mm Hg in 61 cases. Weight reduction brought sysolic pressure down below 135 mm Hg for 75 per cent of the patients whose systolic level ranged between 140 and 180 mm Hg but had no effect on obese individuals with a higher level of hypertension. Examples could be multiplied, and all illustrate the wisdom of weight-reducing therapy in the obese hypertensive but caution against expecting a universally favorable effect.

The mechanism of the association between obesity and hypertension is not known. Obesity alone can increase oxygen consumption at rest, increase work when moving, and thus increase cardiac output and peripheral resistance. This forces greater left ventricular work. Hypertension has different effects on the cardiovascular system, but the increase in pressure and peripheral resistance also causes an increased left ventricular work load. This synergistic increase of the work of the heart is obviously dangerous and explains why the combined risk of the two conditions present simultaneously may be greater than the sum of the risks due to each condition.

Obesity has been suggested as a causal factor in hypertension in some patients. These patients may be unable to respond to the increased cardiac output demanded by obesity without increasing their blood pressure. The importance of weight reduction in this type of patient is obviously even greater than in other hypertensive subjects.

## REFERENCE

1. Mayer, J.: Overweight: Causes, Costs and Control. Englewood Cliffs, N.J, Prentice-Hall, 1968.

*Chapter 51*

# MEASLES AND THE STATE OF NUTRITION

I N many ways underdeveloped countries give us an opportunity to witness our own history. This is particularly true in medicine. Not so long ago — in fact as late as the nineteenth century — the mortality of children age one to four in Western countries equaled or exceeded the mortality of infants from birth to one year. And there was a time when in Europe and the United States measles was a highly dangerous disease, with a mortality over 10 per cent. As late as 1900 the mortality from measles in Britain was 32 per 100,000, compared with 0.2 per 100,000 today. In the United States the mortality was still as high as 10 per 100,000 in 1925, compared with a present mortality rate equal to the current British figure. In many parts of the world, high mortality from measles persists. In Africa, for example, mortality may be as high as 20 per cent or more, and in some villages well-authenticated records show a rate above 50 per cent.

As there appears to be no difference in the viruses seen in Africa and the United States and as Americans of African descent show a very low mortality from measles, the condition of the host, particularly his nutritional state, probably plays a paramount role in determining whether measles is the generally mild children's disease with which we are familiar or a dreaded scourge operating on a catastrophic scale. It also determines many of the signs of the disease. One can see in Africa the form of measles that old textbooks described as typical but that is rarely seen in America today.

A recent report on measles in Senegal is of interest not only historically and geographically but because it indicates how measles and other infectious diseases affect children in an environment where they are poorly fed. We do have poor and

Reprinted from *Postgraduate Medicine,* 45 (No. 2), February, 1969.© McGraw-Hill, Inc.

malnourished children in the United States — on Indian reservations (average life expectancy 42), in the migrant streams (mostly Negroes and Puerto Ricans in the East and mostly Mexicans in the West), in big city slums, and in the rural South. We also have patients who have chronic secondary malnutrition because of lifelong malabsorption diseases or metabolic abnormalities. In such patients, measles and other infectious diseases may be expected to follow a different course from that observed in healthy, well-fed persons.

Senegal is far from being the poorest of the African countries that have achieved their independence since World War II. Colonized very early by the French, it has a better economy and higher literacy than most African countries. This country, with a population of less than four million people, also has one of the best medical schools in Africa. What can be learned of the relation of poverty to infectious diseases in this area is all the more interesting because the conclusions were not evolved within the context of an extreme situation.

The authors of the Senegal study, Drs. André Deboise, Ismaila Sy and Pierre Satgé, are members of the pediatric staff of a well-known general hospital in the capital city Dakar. They studied six villages situated near a small town that has a hospital. In these villages, as elsewhere in Africa, measles is well known and very much feared, so that when a child shows signs and symptoms of the disease, quarantine is instituted. Unfortunately, mothers do not understand that children are contagious at the end of the incubation period, and the communal wells, where all mothers and their small children congregate every day, are sites of contagion for infectious illnesses other than the water-borne diseases. In general, epidemics are limited to the area served by a well because of the tendency of Africans to live in close communities within each village. The density of the child population within these areas determines the rate at which the epidemic grows. In a big city like Dakar most of the children have had measles by the time they are three, and practically all children in the villages studied had not had the disease by the latter age.

The cutaneous signs of the disease in Senegales children are similar to those observed in children of temperate countries. Skin desquamation, however, is much more marked than in present-day American or European children; the sign appears to have been characteristic of the nineteenth-century measles in these areas. Respiratory complications are also much more frequent and generally much more serious in African countries. Besides the rhinobronchial signs that are expected in "uncomplicated" measles, the investigators saw serious respiratory complications in over one-quarter of the cases studied. Almost all of these were pulmonary, but treatment kept mortality down to only a few patients.

Another facet of the disease is even more surprising for the physician used to "temperate area" measles. The most deadly and most widespread complication in Africa is diarrhea. This complication occurred in almost all of the several hundred patients examined. In 90 per cent of the cases, it set in at the very beginning of the cases, it set in at the very beginning of illness. The stools were liquid, sometimes with undigested solid material, and in some cases bloody. In a few cases shigellosis or salmonellosis was present but, in general, patients with diarrhea did not have the characteristic pathogens in their stools. Since the intestinal epithelium basically suffers from the same pathologic disorder as the epidermis, it, like the skin, is apparently hit much harder in the malnourished child.

The mortality of the various epidemic waves in the villages varied from 2.5 to 33 per cent; the overall mortality was 13 per cent. It is difficult to evaluate what part diarrhea plays in the mortality, but even more alarming is the fact that once initiated by measles, the diarrhea can go one for weeks and often for months. Over one-third of the children studied had a weight loss of 10 per cent. These children were followed carefully because the diarrhea often seems to trigger kwashiorkor or marasmus, both syndromes of protein-calorie malnutrition. Even with continued treatment some children had not regained their pre-illness weight five months after the "end" of their measles.

As I pointed out, the frightful picture described by Deboise and his colleagues is not an extreme. Moreover, the report does raise all sorts of questions for American pediatricians and general practitioners even if the disease observed here is generally so much milder.

We know that in the United States the nutrition of thousands, and perhaps millions, of children is far from optimal, even though in the great majority of cases it is better than that of the Senegalese children studied. While among very poor American children the mortality from measles and similar children's diseases is obviously much lower than that of African children, is it as low as that of well-fed American children?

How prevalent are the permanent complications (deafness, etc.) in these children? Medical examinations of children participating in Project Headstart have shown an unexpectedly high prevalence of auditory and other pathologic conditions. Could these be, in part, sequelae of infectious diseases acting on a terrain of less than adequate nutrition? In view of the lasting effect of measles on the gastrointestinal tract of African children, should children in poor families who have measles or other infectious diseases be followed for a longer period? Certainly present evidence suggests that near-adequacy is just not good enough when applied to the diet of children, exposed as they all are to a series of infectious assults throughout their years of growth.

## REFERENCE

1. Scrimshaw, N. S., Taylor, C. E. and Gordon, J. E.: Interactions of Nutrition and Infection. WHO Monograph Series Number 57. Geneva, World Health Organization, 1968.

*Chapter 52*

# NUTRITION AND TUBERCULOSIS

## DIET-AND SUSCEPTIBILITY TO TUBERCULOSIS

THE mechanism of nutrition-related susceptibility to tuberculosis is not completely understood. Studies indicate that kwashiorkor impairs formation of antibodies. Skin reaction to tuberculin also may be depressed, and response to immunization may be diminished. Severe malnutrition, which depletes body protein, also eventually inhibits phagocyte formation. Deficiencies of vitamin A and ascorbic acid reportedly have inhibited macrophage activity.

### Specific Deficiencies

*Protein*

There is a good deal of indirect evidence in man and direct evidence in laboratory animals that lack of dietary protein strongly increases susceptibility to infectious diseases and that adequate intake has a definite protective effect. For example, Leton's study in 1941 of Russian and British prisoners of war in Germany indicated that when the prison diet of the British was supplemented with 30 gm of protein and 1000 extra calories per day, the rate of tuberculosis was 1.2 per cent, compared with a rate of 15 to 19 per cent in the Russians.

*Vitamins*

Vitamin A deficiency has been proved to be related to infection, while vitamins D and E apparently have no significant influence. The contribution of vitamin A deficiency to tuberculosis has been documented in several species by laboratory studies, and a statistically significant relationship between tuberculosis and diets that are low in vitamin A has been demonstrated in a large series of human subjects.

Vitamin C deficiency shows an equally great correlation with tuberculosis. The variety of species tested is not large, since only guinea pigs and primates require dietary vitamin C, but the results

are consistent. Scorbutic guinea pigs show a heightened susceptibility to tuberculosis and a less marked skin reaction to tuberculin
than normal animals. Again, the same appears to be true in man; the
incidence of tuberculosis was greater in the series of human subjects
who lacked dietary vitamin A when dietary intake of ascorbic acid
also was low.

Of the B vitamins, only pyridoxine has exhibited an effect on
development of tuberculosis, and interestingly enough, a deficiency
of pyridoxine in the diet may have a protective effect. Guinea pigs
made pyridoxine-deficient and then inoculated with tuberculosis
have shown a depressed skin reaction to tuberculin but fewer and
less severe gross lesions than the control animals.

## Minerals

Apparently, mineral deficiencies alone have no effect on
susceptibility to tuberculosis infection.

## EFFECTS OF TUBERCULOSIS ON METABOLISM

What is the effect of tuberculosis and its treatment on the
patient's metabolic state? While it is certainly untrue to state that an
unbalanced diet, general undernutrition, or frank malnutrition is the
major precipitating cause of tuberculosis infection, faulty nutrition
obviously can be a contributing factor. Good nutrition also is an
important part of the treatment and cure of tuberculosis,
particularly in preventing reinfection. In frankly malnourished
patients, the disease is more virulent, spreads faster, and reinfects
more readily.

Unlike many other infectious diseases, tuberculosis does not
necessarily increase the metabolic rate or raise the temperature
much above normal. Other metabolic alterations are more typical. In
clinical experiments with various bacterial infections, a rise in the
level of amino acids in the blood has been noted as one of the first
responses to infection, sometimes occurring before any other
symptoms.

### Protein

A marked increase in nitrogen excretion was one of the first
observed consequences of active tuberculosis. Urinary excretion can
show a threefold increase; the ratio of urinary sulfur to nitrogen has
been seen to change from 1:7 to 10:7. Serum albumin levels are low
compared with those seen in other illnesses. Up to 1.7 gm of nitrogen
per day can be excreted in the sputum of healthy persons; the loss

may be much greater in active tuberculosis. Protein content of the liver has been shown to be depressed in infected experimental animals. In humans, liver tuberculosis causes amyloidosis and faulty metabolism of endogenous protein; thus, a high-protein diet is especially important for such patients.

## Vitamin A

Tuberculosis can precipitate serious avitaminosis A, but this is not often seen now in developed countries. Early in this century in the United States and western Europe, children with chronic tuberculosis (or other infections) also commonly had xerophthalmia or keratomalacia; both are still serious problems in the Far East and in other developing areas, where marginal deficiency in young children is still common.

## Ascorbic Acid

Tissue saturation of ascorbic acid decreases as severity of tuberculosis increases, and serum ascorbic acid values may be relatively low compared with intake. It has been estimated that patients with tuberculosis metabolize up to 150 extra milligrams of vitamin C each day.

## B Vitamins

As with the inhibitive effect of pyridoxine deficiency, the situation with the B vitamins in active tuberculosis is somewhat paradoxical. Pellagra, often seen in conjunction with tuberculosis that interferes with absorption or assimilation of nutrients, is seldom seen with pulmonary tuberculosis. High levels of niacin-amide appear in the tissues of such patients, and it has been noted that M. tuberculosis is capable of synthesizing niacin. Tryptophan, a niacin precursor, has been shown in guinea pigs to be an inhibitor of human strains of tuberculosis. It would appear that in this instance the microorganism itself generates an antagonistic effect.

## Minerals

Iron deficiency may occur as a result of hemorrhage in pulmonary tuberculosis or because of ulcerative lesions of the alimentary tract. The so-called anemia of infection does not appear to result from lack of dietary iron, but rather from decreased iron retention due to reduced iron-binding capacity, which in turn results from decreased erythropoiesis in the bone marrow.

One study has shown large increases of serum copper in

tuberculosis patients, but the reason for this increase and its significance are not yet apparent.

Blood calcium and phosphorus are markedly reduced in experimental animals with tuberculosis. In humans with active disease, a negative calcium balance is common, but can be corrected by increased intake over a number of months.

### Other Metabolic Disturbances

Other metabolic complications occur when pulmonary tuberculosis spreads to other sites. Malabsorption may be caused by ulcers or hypertrophy of the alimentary tract. Osteoporosis appears in tuberculosis of the bones. Tuberculous lesions in the genitourinary tract may precipitate renal disease. Amyloidosis of the liver and spleen results in faulty protein metabolism.

Moreover, drug administration may cause complications, such as folate deficiency and myeloblastic anemia during isoniazid therapy, thiamine deficiency after prolonged treatment with phthivazide, nephrotoxicity caused by streptomycin, and diarrhea and vomiting following use of aminosalicylic acid.

## DIETARY RECOMMENDATIONS

Individual diets must be planned with the various possible complications in mind. However, the following general dietary recommendations can be made.

While there is some evidence of increased susceptibility to tuberculosis in underweight patients (if the lack of weight is caused by undernutrition), there is no indication that marked overweight protects against infection. There is no evidence that a balanced weight reduction diet is harmful to tuberculosis patients.

As noted, basal metabolism is increased much less in tuberculosis than in most infections. However, in this infection as well as others, appetite is reduced and fever, however low, increases caloric needs. Therefore, the diet should have sufficient calories for the patient to attain his optimal weight, whether by loss or gain, and to maintain it at that level. The diet should include enough protein to counter nitrogen loss and to promote healing. A protein intake of approximately 75 to 100 gm per day should be sufficient for adults.

Particular attention must be given to the vitamin and mineral content of the food, especially in insuring adequate intake of calcium, vitamin D, ascorbic acid, and vitamin A. Iron supplements should be prescribed if bleeding occurs and B vitamins given to counteract depletion by drugs as well as to prevent additional anorexigenic effects.

*Chapter 53*

# HOOKWORM AND NUTRITION

*NECATOR AMERICANUS,* the American hook-worm, is unfortunately still very much with us. A large-scale survey conducted by the health department laboratories of nine southern states in 1955 gave the following incidences: Alabama 11 per cent positive, Louisiana 4.0 per cent, Florida 18.9 per cent, Georgia 7.1 per cent, Kentucky 3.8 per cent, Mississippi 6.3 per cent, North Carolina 12.3 per cent, South Carolina 8.0 per cent, and Tennessee 2.0 per cent. At the same time Puerto Rico showed a general prevalence of about 25.0 per cent. While improvement in sanitation and in living standards has reduced the scope of infestation, hookworm is still a major health hazard in the South and Southwest.

A distinction has often been drawn between hookworm infection and hookworm disease. The method for routine stool examination merely shows the presence of the parasite; it does not give exact evidence of the magnitude of the hookworm burden. Other methods involving egg count technics give data on the intensity of the infection, thus furnishing a basis for estimating an individual's worm burden. Hookworm "carriers" have few worms and no clinical evidence of hookworm disease; patients who have clinical disease carry many worms, and other things being equal, the severity of the disease depends on the number of parasites.

Adequate direct evidence that a firm immunity to hookworm infection can develop in man is lacking. In the United States the highest incidence of hookworm infection occurs among teen-agers with fewer and less severe infections in Negroes than in whites.

## PATHOLOGIC AND CLINICAL CHARACTERISTICS

The area of penetration into the skin by the filariform larvae of

---

Reprinted from *Postgraduate Medicine, 46* (No. 1), July, 1969.© McGraw-Hill, Inc.

*N. americanus* is often marked  by a local dermatitis with edema, erythema and an eruption which subsides in about two weeks unless a secondary bacterial infection arises. As the larvae leave the lung capilaries and penetrate the alveoli, small hemorrhagic lesions develop. In less severe infections the pulmonary reaction is mild.

From the nutritional viewpoint, the important pathologic finding is the intestinal picture. Adult hookworms inhabit the upper part of the intestine, where they attach themselves and suck blood. Mechanical and lytic destruction of cells at the point of attachment damages the mucosa. The resultant anemia is the chief pathologic condition. A single hookworm may remove as much as 0.1 ml of blood per day; the rate of removal per worm depends on the density of infestation. Hookworms digest only part of the blood they ingest. Previous points of attachment bleed for some time after the worm moves to a new location because the worm secretes an anticoagulant. Folic acid deficiency, apparently due to the combination of blood loss and intestinal damage, has been reported to occur in hookworm infection.

The clinical picture reflects the interaction between the severity of the infection and the patient's diet. Common symptoms are weakness, fatigue, dyspnea on exertion, cardiac palpitation, pallor and epigastric discomfort. A severe infection starting in early childhood also causes physical and mental retardation. Severely infected children often have a potbelly, and pica, geophagia, and other aberrations of appetite are not uncommon. In very severe cases, the extreme anemia and hypoproteinemia may cause extensive edema and cardiac damage.

## HOOKWORM AND ANEMIA

The anemia of hookworm infection is usually microcytic and hypochromic. It can be extremely severe, with hemoglobin values under 15 per cent and the erthrocyte counts below 1 million per cubic millimeter. When the disease is complicated by malnutrition (primary and consequent to intestinal damage) the anemia may be macrocytic or normocytic. The mechanism of the anemia has been the object of recent intensive research. Several studies in which the intestinal blood loss in chronic hookworm infection has been measured have generally confirmed the correlation between worm load and blood loss but have shown that other factors are also of importance.

In 1961, P. W. G. Tasker did a basic study using blood cells tagged with radioactive chromium to measure daily blood loss in patients with hookworm infection. After drawing some blood, the cells were were tagged and then reinjected into the patient. A daily (complete) stool collection was made, and the blood samples were obtained every other day. The amount of radioactivity in the stools gave a measure of the blood loss in the intestine; the loss of radioactivity in the blood provided a check. After two weeks, the patients were given tetrachloroethylene (the preferred vermifuge for *N. americanus)* and a purgative. Then radioactive chromium was determined again both in the feces and in the blood to gauge the effect of deworming. A secondary deworming treatment was used as a check on the effectiveness of the first treatment. Tasker checked the method itself by determining the amount of chromium reabsorbed – less than 15 per cent – by introducing chromium-tagged cells into the gastrointestinal system through a stomach tube.

The results of this careful study showed that the daily blood loss into the intestine varied from 2 ml per day for patients with mild infections (100 worms) to close to 100 ml per day for patients with severe infections (1500 worms). The amount of blood lost per worm decreased from 0.1 m. for mildly infected patients to 0.02 ml for severely infected patients. Tasker pointed out that at a hemoglobin level of 14 gm per 100 ml, 8 ml of blood represents 14 mg of iron per day, a considerable loss when one considers that this is approximately the daily iron intake, of which only 5 to 10 per cent is absorbed! The role of hookworm infection in causing anemia even in adequately fed subjects is thus fairly obvious.

## EFFECT OF IRON THERAPY

Since Tasker's initial work, a number of studies have increased our knowledge of the dynamics of anemia associated with hookworm infection. The work of M. Roche and co-workers

(1967) is particularly noteworthy. They showed that contrary to previous belief, blood loss does not decrease in the presence of a low hemoglobin level. In fact, red blood cell survival is abnormally low when the hemoglobin level is low, a phenomenon which clearly points to the dangerous instability of the situation. The same group also showed an excellent correlation between the number of eggs in the feces, the number of parasites, intestinal blood loss, and the anemia.

These authors studied a small group of patients in particular detail to discover the effect of iron therapy. All these patients carried heavy parasite loads and had a low hemoglobin (less than 8.9 gm per 100 ml). Twelve day test periods, during which fecal blood loss, hookworm egg counts, and red blood cell survival (radioactive chromium was used as tag) were determined, alternated with one month periods when the patients were left untreated or were given intravenous therapy. The patients were completely dewormed at the end of the study.

The patients showed the expected heavy fecal blood loss, with no decrease as hemoglobin decreased. In all patients the life-span of red blood cells was greatly decreased. In almost all cases, red blood cell survival time returned to normal when iron therapy normalized the hemoglobin level, even though the high parasite load was not reduced. It appears that the toxin of *N. americanus* does not interfere directly with the life-span of the erythrocyte.

By contrast, deworming without iron therapy did not correct the reduction in survival time of red blood cells in hookworm anemic patients. Tagged erythrocytes from anemic patients infected with hookworms showed a short survival time when injected into normal recipients.

## THERAPEUTIC CONSIDERATIONS

From an epidemiologic viewpoint, the various correlations thus demonstrated permit a general prediction that in a population not particularly malnourished, anemia due to hookworm is found in men when the fecal egg counts reach 5000 per gram and in menstruating women and in children when counts reach 2000 per gram. For example, an adult male with 15 gm hemoglobin per 100 ml of blood and 5000 eggs per gram of feces has a daily intestinal blood loss which contains 5 mg of iron. Even if 40 per cent of the iron that is discharged into the intestine is reabsorbed, about 3 mg of iron is lost every day, about twice the amount expected to be absorbed from food. If the diet is poor, as is often the case in hookworm-infected populations, lower levels of infection will cause or exaggerate anemia.

Hookworm infection in young women is particularly grave. Women of childbearing age lose iron through menstruation (45 mg per month and often considerably more, particularly in anemic women), through lactation (about 1.0 mg per day), and during childbirth (variable but large amounts). Pregnancy increases the iron requirement through the increase in blood volume of the mother-placenta-fetus system. Under these conditions even a light parasite load may precipitate anemia — with resultant threat to the health of the pregnant mother, increase in pregnancy risks, and through prematurity, increased threat to the physical and mental health of the offspring.

The work presented here suggest that *iron therapy is indispensable whether or not the population is dewormed.* In cases in which control of infection is difficult, it is particularly important to provide iron for the children and other members of the population, and of paramount importance to provide it for pregnant and lactating women. To suggest, as some have, that there is little point in doing anything about the nutritional problems of groups infected with hookworm until sanitation can be improved and deworming practices is to misunderstand the nature of the problem.

## Chapter 54

# NUTRITION AND RENAL CALCULI

RENAL calculi were well known to Hippocrates, and paleopathologic studies show that they have plagued the human race for thousands of years. Contemporary studies of 25,000 autopsies at the University of Minnesota Hospitals showed an incidence of stones in 1.12 per cent of cases, with 0.38 per cent of the deaths related to the presence of calculi. Another recent study estimated that each year one person per thousand in the United States is admitted to a general hospital for treatment of urinary stones. In the "stone belt," an area extending from Southeast Asia to the Middle East, the disease can reach epidemic proportions, notably in Thailand, where it is undergoing intensive investigation. In these areas, about 80 per cent of the stones are vesical, and about 50 per cent are found in children ages 1 to 10, with the male to female ratio about 8:1. The Western world has known similar epidemics. The records of the Norfolk and Norwich Hospital in England show that between 1772 and 1816, about 3 per cent of patients admitted had a bladder stone.

In the absence of the intensive investigation carried out in other widely prevalent chronic diseases, the likely elements of the pathogenesis of nephrolithiasis remain those considered by Hippocrates: soil, climate, water, and food habits.

Therapeutic diets are used less often now in treating renal calculi, but dietary modification continues to be a sound preventive measure against recurrence of stones, particularly after surgical removal. In patients with chronic production of stones, prevention is of paramount importance.

## ETIOLOGY

The first step in the care of a patient with a stone is to

---

Reprinted from *Postgraduate Medicine, 46* (No. 2), August, 1969.© McGraw-Hill, Inc.

determine the stone's composition. Usually this means the crystalloid component rather than the organic matrix. Sometimes, crystal content indicates the pathogenesis: A cystine stone reveals cystinuria; an ammoniomagnesium phosphate stone indicates urinary tract infection. In mixed stones, topographic analysis of radial structure can be translated into time sequences.

Stone pathogenesis can be conveniently considered under two general headings: (1) urinary changes that increase the concentration of constituent crystalloids, such as reduced volume of urine or increased excretion of calcium, oxalate, cystine, uric acid, xanthine, ammonia or phosphate, and (2) urinary changes that lead to formation of stones even though the concentration of the precipitating crystalloids is within normal limits, such as altered pH, presence of stone matrix or foreign bodies, stasis, and presence or absence of protective substances such as magnesium ion, pyrophosphate, citrate, inhibitor peptides, and other normal constituents. We know more about the first category than the second although the latter is probably at least as important in many cases.

Statistics vary on the relative importance of the types of stones. Usually, however, in 90 per cent of cases, the chief cation of the crystals is calcium. In more than half the cases, stones are mixtures of calcium, ammonium and magnesium phosphates and carbonates; oxalate is also an important anion. Most statistics indicate that uric acid stones represent about 4 per cent and cystine stones less than 1 per cent of the total incidence, although some authors think these figures are too low.

Hypercalciuria is the most frequent metabolic abnormality found in nephrolithiasis. The study of renal excretion of calcium is a complex problem and involves consideration of protein binding, ion associations, chelation, hormonal control, and the relationship of the clearance of calcium to the clearance of other electrolytes. Smith (1) has stated that idiopathic hypercalciuria remains "a baffling and important disorder or group of disorders, clearly separable from primary hyperparathyroidism." The availability of orthophosphates and specific diuretics has simplified management of renal stones, but dietary measures are helpful.

Oxalate is present in about two-thirds of the stones, but hyperoxaluria is rare in the United States. Genetically, the condition is of at least two types, related to specific enzymatic defects. Gershoff's vitamin $B_6$ and magnesium oxide therapy has been helpful in these patients.

Cystinuria, one of Garrod's original four inborn metabolic errors, has been studied extensively for many years. Penicillamine offers some hope of control, a finding all the more important since the dietary approach has had very limited success.

Uric acid stones result directly from the insolubility of uric acid, particularly in acidic urine. There is a rationale for modifying the diet to prevent chronic stone formation.

## DIETARY THERAPY: GENERAL PRINCIPLES

I must emphasize that nephrolithiasis is a chronic condition and that in most cases, the patient may have recurrences throughout his life. Thus in all types of dietary therapy, long-term dietary adequacy should not be sacrificed to theoretical short-term advantages. Since partial magnesium deficiency, low-phosphorous diets, and vitamin A, pyridoxine and thiamine deficiencies are factors in the etiology of nephrolithiasis, it becomes obvious that a complete, balanced diet is particularly important.

The type of diet prescribed is determined by the acidity or alkalinity of urine, actual and desired, and by the variety of stones, but in all cases the intake of fluids (3000 to 4000 ml or more daily) is strongly encouraged to prevent the concentration of stone-forming minerals. Obviously the more the urine is diluted, the less are the chances of precipitation. Unfortunately, experience shows that a high water consumption is difficult to maintain over a long period in patients with chronic stone formation.

## ACID-ASH AND ALKALINE-ASH DIETS

The resultant acidity or alkalinity of a food burned completely outside the body indicates its potential acidity when burned inside the body. Most fruits and vegetables contain organic acids, but these acids are completely burned in the body. The resulting ash is alkaline, due to the high potassium, calcium and magnesium content; the organic acid oxidizes to carbon dioxide and water or forms bicorbonate. By contrast, a diet containing large amounts of protein will yield sulfuric and phosphoric acid and acidify the urine. Thus foods that, unlike fruits, do not taste acid, such as meat, fish, eggs, milk and cereals, will lower the pH of the urine.

The high-acid diet sometimes is prescribed for the patients in whom stones form more readily in an alkaline medium, with the hope that existing stones will not enlarge and new stones will not form. Such stones usually are made of calcium salts of phosphate, carbonate and oxalate. The objective is to keep the pH of the urine at 5 to 6. Products containing baking powder or soda are prohibited. The diet is high in eggs, meat, fish, poultry and cereals, with restricted intake of fruits, vegetables and milk.

The high-alkaline diet sometimes is used in treating patients with uric acid and cystine stones. It consists of vegetables and fruits (except plums, prunes, cranberries and corn) and restricted intake of meat, fish, poultry, eggs, milk and cereals.

## CALCIUM-CONTAINING CALCULI

Urine high in calcium favors the formation of calcium-phosphate and calcium-oxalate stones. Hypercalciuria may result from (1) a diet excessively high in calcium such as one based on milk, cream and ice cream, which was and too often still is used in treating peptic ulcers, in spite of the risk of atherogenesis, (2) excessive intake of proprietary antacids that are high in calcium salts, (3) excessive intake of vitamin D, which mobilizes calcium and thus increases urinary excretion, (4) immobilization after fractures and extended bed rest, and (5) osteoporosis. Dietary measures include a low-calcium and low-vitamin D diet, with the addition sometimes of sodium phytate. The sodium phytate forms an unabsorbable complex with calcium. Milk, cheese, and other milk products are limited to the equivalent of a maximum of two cups of milk daily; foods fortified with vitamin D are excluded. The Mayo Clinic Diet Manual* lists high-calcium foods that should not be over-consumed, including milk products, beet greens, collards, dandelion greens, kale, spinach, turnip greens,

---

*W. B. Saunders Company, Philadelphia.

salmon and sardines.

To compensate in part for the low calcium content of the diet, the protein intake should be reasonably high, since protein is believed to promote calcium deposition in the bones. Acid-ash foods, which lower the pH of the urine, may be a factor in keeping the calcium salts in solution. In fractures, when the plaster cast is removed, allowing some body mobilization, a normal calcium intake should be resumed.

## CALCIUM-OXALATE STONES

A universally accepted regimen has not been established for patients with recurrent oxalate stones. Large quantities of food high in calcium and oxalates should be avoided. Among the latter foods are asparagus, beet greens, spinach, sorrel, dandelion greens, cranberries, figs, gooseberries, plums, rhubarb, raspberries, black tea, chocolate cocoa, coffee, gelatin and pepper. Oranges, pineapples, strawberries, beans, brussel sprouts, potatoes, tomatoes and beets should not be eaten more than once daily.

Even a strict diet often does not prevent recurrence of oxalate stones, because endogenous production continues even with controlled exogenous sources. Gershoff and Prien (2) investigated the effects of daily oral administration of magnesium and vitamin $B_6$ on patients with recurring calcium-oxalate stones. Thirty-six patients were maintained for five years on 200 mg of magnesuim oxide and 10 mg of pyridoxine given daily. In 30 of these patients, stone formation either did not recur or was strikingly decreased. This may be partly explained by the combined effect of ash increase in the magnesium and citric acid ions on the urine's solvency. Whatever the explanation, the results are encouraging, although the authors indicate the difficulty of mainaining the interest and cooperation of the patients who have been calculi-free for a year.

## CALCIUM-PHOSPHATE STONES

For calcium-phosphate stones, a low-calcium, low-phosphate diet is usually recommended. Foods high in phosphate are milk,

milk products, eggs, organ meats (liver, kidneys, etc.), sardines, fish, roe, whole wheat bread and cereals, wheat germ, brown or wild rice, oatmeal and bran. Reasonable amounts of beans, nuts and meat in general are permissible. An excessive reduction in phosphates may cause a corresponding increase in citrate, with precipitation of citrate stones.

## URIC ACID STONES

An attempt is usually made to keep the urine alkaline so that the uric acid will remain in solution. Although the use of acidifying and alkalizing agents if more effective than diet alone, the diet should obviously support the medication that is used. If urinary alkalization alone is inadequate, overall protein intake must be restricted to 1 gm per kilogram of body weight, with restriction of purine intake.

## CYSTINE STONES

Low-protein diets have not been very effective in treating patients with cystine stones. An amino acid diet that is low in methionine and cystine, combined with a high fluid intake and alkalizing agents and a high-alkaline diet (to keep the pH of the urine above 7), has yielded encouraging results.

## REFERENCES

1. Smith, L. H. Jr.: Symposium on stones. Introduction. Books in the running brooks, sermons in stone. Amer. J. Med., 45:649, 1968.
2. Gershoff, S. N. and Prien, E. L.: Effect of daily MgO and vitamin $B_6$ administration to patients with recurring calcium oxlate kidney stones. Amer. J. Clin. Nutri., 20:393, 1967.

*Chapter 55*

# DIET AND RENAL DISEASE

T RANSPLANTATION, dialysis and diet are the
three basic methods for treating renal disease. The most desirable
of these methods is a successful transplant, since it is the only one
that allows the patient a normal existence. However, transplantation is limited by certain restrictions, the most obvious of
which is a lack of suitable donor kidneys.

Peritoneal dialysis and hemodialysis may effect remission and
stabilization of the disease but do not cure, and they require
permanent adjustment to an abnormal style of living. The best
adjustment to an artificial kidney seems to be in patients between
ages 21 and 41, who have achieve full growth but have not yet
acquired the problems of aging.

Dialysis therapy has several other disadvantages: (1) The patient
either must live with an indwelling cannula in his arm and the
attendant dangers of clotting or local infection or must have
repeated abdominal punctures to reinsert the cannula, (2) only a
few centers have professional and, especially, technical personnel
to perform long-term dialysis, and (3) the cost for in-hospital
dialysis is between $10,000 and $30,000 per patient per year. In
addition, the patient's condition may be aggravated by hypertension, anemia, heart disease, diabetes, neuropathies, or metastatic calcifications.

The increased availability of home dialysis units is taking some
pressure off the in-hospital facilities, but the home units also pose
problems. They must be installed in a stable home and operated
by reliable persons. The expense of maintenance and of chemicals
is estimated at $3,000 to $5,000 per year, after an initial
investment of $10,000 to purchase the machine and to learn its
operation.

Reprinted from *Postgraduate Medicine, 49* (No. 4), April, 1971.© McGraw-Hill, Inc.

Although more money is becoming available to establish dialysis centers and to train personnel, it will be some years before this therapy can be given to all who can benefit from it, and even longer before transplantation can be performed for all who need it. Thus, diet, the third method of treating chronic, progressive renal disease, should be carefully considered for each patient.

## DIETARY TREATMENT ALONE

Diet alone cannot cure renal disease or effect a remission for an unlimited period, but it can slow the progress of the disease, give the patient a new lease on near-normal life, and prolong the time between onset of disease and dialysis, transplantation or death. When diet alone becomes insufficient to maintain the patient, it may be used in conjunction with peritoneal dialysis or hemo-dialysis to lessen the number of hours each month the patient must use the machine.

Obviously, dietary regulation must be tailored to the often complex requirements of the individual, but the basic aims are simple: to conserve the remaining renal function, to prevent tissue breakdown and promote tissue repair, and to stabilize intake so that the impaired kidney can handle urinary excretion. Deviation from the prescribed diet, sometimes by adding only one hamburger, can cause symptoms to recur. Usually, the dietary intake of sodium, potassium, fluid and protein is restricted.

As kidney disease progresses, urine volume diminishes, con-centration and filtration rates decrease, and metabolites normally excreted in the urine build up to toxic levels in the body tissues. Common symptoms are anorexia, nausea, vomiting, edema, diarrhea and dyspepsia. Of the three basic dietary constituents, fats and carbohydrates present no problem in excretion. The end products of these two food types are carbon dioxide, expired through the lungs, and a small amount of water, lost through the skin, lungs and intestines.

Protein, however, presents a problem. Exogenous protein is ultimately broken down to urea, and endogenous or tissue protein is catabolized to creatine, which is also excreted in the urine. As urine volume diminishes, blood urea nitrogen levels rise. The theory that a high-protein diet adversely affects renal disease was accepted empirically for almost 100 years before it was confirmed by the discovery that the end product of protein metabolism is urea. For many years, protein-free or low-protein diets have been the standard prescription in renal disease.

In the first low-protein diets, the quality of protein and the number of calories were not considered. As a result, the unpalatable diet soon aggravated the initial anorexia and anemia. In the mid-1940's, Borst, of Amsterdam, was one of the first to insist on a high caloric intake with a low-protein diet to provide energy for physical activity and maintenance. His diet and other variations were highly successful in effecting short-term remissions. However, since the protein was of low biologic quality, the tissue protein gradually broke down trying to compensate for the missing essential amino acids.

In 1963, Giordano, followed by Giovanetti and other investigators, developed and tested similar low-protein diets in which the protein was of high biologic value and contained, by extrapolation from Rose's data, the minimal daily requirements of all essentail amino acids. Giordano believed that uremic patients with more than normal supplies of amino acids in tissue could use these acids endogenously to form the nonessential amino acids, provided the diet had adequate calories and enough essential amino acids.

The G-G diet aims at supplying 2000 to 3000 calories and about 20 gm of protein of high biologic value. Typically, the daily allowance inclueds one egg and three-fourths cup of milk. The 0.5 gm of methionine added for a time to complement the daily intake of amino acids has been dropped. To keep total nitrogen content low, only proteins of the highest biologic value are used, and appreciable amounts of grain and vegetable proteins are assiduously avoided. The rest of the diet consists of wheat-starch products from deglutinized wheat. Commercially available bread for phenylketonuric patients (PKU Bread) also may be used. In addition, the patient receives generous amounts of low-protein, low-potassium fruits and vegetables; ad libitum quantities of sugars and fats (in addition to the daily caloric allowance); a multivitamin preparation; iron tablets; and fluid intake limited to the level of fluid loss through lungs, skin and stools.

The G-G diet is satisfactory when some residual renal function (above a glomerular filtration rate of 2.5 to 3 ml per minute) is present or can be restored. The blood urea level decreases, gastrointestinal and neurologic symptoms improve or are entirely relieved, and appetite improves. The hemoglobin and hematocrit values decreased more slowly or stabilize in some patients and increase in others, and the nitrogen balance becomes neutral or slightly positive.

Adapted to national tastes, the G-G diet has been used with equal success in England and the United States. Berlyne and associates have found that patients on the diet are able to resume normal living during remissions. They also have found that a choice of caloric sources improves the outpatients' adherance to the diet. Heavy cream, sweet carbohydrates, ice cream, and even alcohol make up a substantial portion of calories for the British patients. In the United States, Franklin and associates have added a daily supplement of 5 gm of calcium carbonate to prevent severe metabolic acidosis and hypocalcemia.

Rubini and Kopple have tested an electrodialyzed whey containing lactalbumin and lactose as the source of high-quality protein, and after blending it with maltose, corn oil, sugar and flavors, have combined it with a diet low in proteins and electrolytes, high in fats and carbohydrates, and complemented with a vitamin supplement. Obviously, the success of the diet depends on careful adherence, which is partically a function of palatability.

As low-protein, low-sodium and low-potassium foods with various flavors and textures are developed, it will become easier to prescribe adequate diets and to persuade patients to remain within the protein limit even when cessation of symptoms tempt them toward indiscretion. Berlyne found that symptoms were renewed by even a 5 gm deviation from the diet. However, Rubini and Kopple found no critical advantage between a 10 gm and a 20 gm protein diet. They believe that adherence to the diet is greater when a 40 gm protein diet is allowed under very careful medical supervision. Other investigators have suggested increasing the use of endogenous urea by substituting alpha amino analogues of the essential amino acids for part or all of the dietary protein.

Obviously, the success of the diet also depends on maintenance of residual renal function, which decreases as the underlying disease progresses. Thus, dietary effectiveness will be greater in some patients than in others. Patients with polycystic disease may do well on the diet for as long as a year, whereas patients with pyelonephritis or chronic glomerulonephritis deteriorate more quickly.

In each case, symptoms recur when the filtration rate drops to 1.5 to 1 ml per minute. Serum creatinine and potassium rise, and pH falls below 7.15. Edema and neurologic symptoms return. Even in terminal patients, however, distressing symptoms appear to be fewer than in patients receiving one of the older low-protein diets. Gastrointestinal symptoms are absent and appetite remains good, often up to coma. However, bleeding from the skin, nose and muscle is common, and some patients feel increasingly agitated and doomed. At this stage, the physician should consider the practicality of a transplant or of dialysis.

## DIET AND DIALYSIS

When diet and dialysis are combined, the diet must be adjusted to compensate for the new conditions. The first consideration should be maintenance of caloric intake and restoration of salt and fluid balance. Since many, if not the majority, of patients accepted for long-term dialysis are usually hypertensive and in heart failure due to retention of sodium and water during the terminal illness, maintaining a sodium-restricted diet between periods of dialysis and effectively limiting fluid intake become major problems. Acute weight changes are often used to monitor changes in hydration. Patients in dialysis usually lose most, if not all, renal function after treatment begins; thus, the fluid intake must be limited to the amount of fluid that can be disposed of by residual renal function and insensible body functions and in the feces. In severe hypertension, the sodium intake should be limited to 10 to 12 mEq per day, as it cna contribute to the hypertension.

Although dialysis quickly (but temporarily lowers the blood

levels of urea, uric acid, and creatinine, dietary protein still should be carefully regulated. Blood levels of more than 200 mg per 100 ml before dialysis are associated with the sometimes fatal "disequilibrium" syndrome and disturbed cerebral function during and after dialysis. Another factor seems to be the speed of dialyzation.

Strategy on protein intake depends on the patient's state. If he is severly undernourished, with protein depletion, protein intake must be increased until a positive balance is established. However, if he is adequately nourished, all that is required is sufficient protein to maintain equilibrium. In theory, this is 0.5 to 0.6 gm per kilogram of ideal body weight for a normal person, but 1 gm is safer. In practice, 10 to 15 gm of first-class protein (milk, egg or meat protein), with a total intake of between 0.5 and 1.0 gm per kilogram of body weight, is adequate to maintain a normal, nonpregnant, nonlactating adult.

In dialyzed patients, additional variables are introduced. Large amounts of protein are lost during peritoneal dialysis. Significant amounts of amino acids are lost during hemodialysis, particularly in well-nourished patients, and the loss is related to the duration of dialysis. Thus, the protein intake for these patients should be based on 1 gm per kilogram of ideal body weight, plus an allowance to replace amino acid loss in the dialysate. Obviously, such a rule is far from inflexible. A lower protein intake may be required until uremia symptoms are relieved. Protein intake is correlated with sodium intake; if sodium intake exceeds 12 mEq and blood pressure rises, protein intake should be decreased until blood pressure is under control.

Adequate caloric intake is important not only because it is indispensable to the patient's welfare but also because it has a protein-sparing effect.

When dialysis has restored serum calcium to normal levels, phosphorus, an end product of protein metabolism, can combine with calcium to precipitate insoluble calcium phosphate salts and produce metastatic calcification in tissues. The serum level of phosphorus should not exceed 7 mg per 100 ml.

Postassium is present in most foods and is particularly abundant in high-quality protein fruits and vegetables. Because myocardial toxicity from hyperkalemia is prevalent in dialyzed patients, the serum potassium should be maintained below 6 mEq per liter. As before dialysis, the intake of potassium usually can be controlled in the diet by carefully choosing the allowed fruits and vegetables and by preparing them in water to remove the potassium. Phosphate and potassium can be partially controlled by binding them insolubly in the intestine. Berlyne and collegues have recommended binding with calcium cycle ion exchange resins, because serum calcium is easy to measure accurately and the dosage can be controlled by monitoring blood levels.

Aluminum also can be ingested, but its toxic level is unknown.

Because there is some evidence that folic acid and possibly other water-soluble vitamins may be lost during dialysis, oral supplements of B complex vitamins and ascorbic acid are recommended. Iron levels may be considerably lowered due to blood loss during dialysis and from testing. Bone marrow stores may be a more reliable guide to the iron status than are the serum iron levels. In iron deficiency, supplemental iron should be given orally, or parenterally if it is not absorbed by the oral route.

## REFERENCES

1. Rubini, M. E. and Kopple, J. D.: Dietary management of end-stage uremia. Bull. N.Y. Acad. Med., 46:850-868, Oct. 1970.
2. Lotspeich, W. D.: Metabolic Aspects of Renal Function. Springfield, Ill, Charles C Thomas, 1959.
3. Merrill, J. P. and Hampers, C. L.: Uremia: Progress in Pathophysiology and Treatment. New York, Grune & Stratton, 1971.
4. Berlyne, G. M. (Ed.): Nutrition in Renal Disease. Baltimore, Williams and Wilkins, 1968.

*Chapter 56*

# DIET AND PERIODONTAL DISEASE

PERIODONTAL disease, one of the most wide-spread diseases of mankind, is not always spectacular or even obvious but can, over the long term, be highly injurious to the patient's health and well-being. The etiology of peridontal disease is complex and not yet fully understood. Its presence and course are known to depend both on external environmental factors and on the host's ability to resist and respond to challenges.

Periodontal disease has been with us for some time; the skull of Rhodesian man (circa 300,000 B.C.) shows evidence of a periodontal abscess. In modern times, a great increase has occurred in the incidence of conditions which can be classified, for our purpose, as periodontal disease. Wade (1), director of the department of periodontology, Royal Dental Hospital of London School of Dental Surgery, has stated that periodontal disease is so common among civilized races that few adults fail to show either the active disease or evidence of healed lesions. Incidence and severity increase with age. In persons from 25 to 35 years of age, tooth loss is attributed equally to tooth diseases and periodontal diseases. After 35, periodontal disease is the more common cause.

The physician's involvement in the treatment of periodontal disease is clear, if anatomic considerations are kept in mind. Periodontal diseases relate, not to the enamel and dentine of the tooth, but to the four-part aggregation of tissues called the periodontium, which binds the teeth to the jawbone structure of the cranium.

When teeth begin to form in the fetus, often as early as the sixth week of life, they metabolize nutrients. When the enamel covering forms and is calcified, however, metabolism is confined to the surrounding tissues. The cementum, periodontal ligaments,

Reprinted from *Postgraduate Medicine, 49* (No. 5), May, 1971.© McGraw-Hill, Inc.

bone of the alveolar process, and the outer covering or gingiva are constantly breaking down and renewing themselves throughout the lifespan. Their metabolic processes are the same as those of bone and soft tissue elsewhere in the body. Like other tissues, they react to body changes, aging, nutrient deficiencies, infection or disease. Wade (1) has listed 56 conditions which affect the health of periodontal tissue, including infections, endocrine imbalances, avitaminoses, blood dyscrasias, osteodystrophies and dermatoses. This does not take into account allergies, metal intoxications, irradiation, some poisons, and psychosomatic disorders. Conversely, bacterial infections in disease gingival tissue and periodontal abscesses will influence health or disease in the rest of the body. Also, discomfort involved in eating can alter the patient's eating habits and make it more difficult to maintain an adequate normal or therapeutic diet.

Clinical symptoms differ among the periodonatal disease, but in general they are: formation of plaque or calculus (composes of calcium carbonate, calcium flouride, and magnesium phosphate), which accumulates on the teeth and under the lossened gingival margin; inflammation and infection of the periodontal tissues; loosening and destruction of periodontal fibers; and resorption of alveolar bone, with consequent tooth mobility and loss.

## DIETARY FACTORS

Among many other contributing environmental factors, periodontists have identified a number of nutrients which, if absent from the diet or present in excess, can affect the onset and course of the disease. Perhaps the two most important and basic nutrients to be considered in the therapeutic diet are carbohydrate and protein.

### Carbohydrate

It is well known that simple sugars and soft carbohydrate foods that cling to tooth surfaces promote dental caries. The effect of ingested carbohydrates, particularly the simple sugars, is not so obvious. In a recent survey of dental literature on nutrition and periodontal disease, Clark, Chearaskin and Ringsdorf (2) cited studies showing that dietary sucrose enhances plaque formation and demonstrating that subjects given diets containing sucrose and glucose exhibited impaired gingival health and increased sulcus depth and tooth mobility. These authors suggested that excessive carbohydrate intake may contribute to the development of the disease by increasing the requirements for vitamins and essential minerals and by replacing some protein in the diet.

*Protein*

Protein deficiency has been implicated in periodontosis (resorption of alveolar bone and degeneration of periodontal fibers), which is especially common in persons living in economically deprived nations and in vegetarians. Protein-calorie deficiency can cause an increase in cornified cells among the buccal mucosal cells, a change that also occurs as a result of infection and aging. Protein deficiency may reduce resistance to toxins, antibody production, leukicyte activity, and adrenocortical function. Adequate protein is essential to horomonal function of endocrine systems, whose malfunction can seriously alter periodontal tissues, and to prevention of iron-deficiency anemia, which adversely affects health of gingival tissues, especially in female patients. In short-term studies, even healthy subjects seem to show improved gingival state, sulcus depth, and tooth mobility when dietary protein supplements are given.

Protein and vitamin D determine the effective metabolism of calcium, phosphorus and magnesium. In studies quoted by Clark, Cheraskin and Ringsdorf (2), subjects on a low-protein diet (0.67 to 0.97 gm per kilogram of boyy weight per day) absorbed an average of 5 per cent of dietary calcium and 32 per cent of dietary magnesium. When the same subjects received 2.1 to 2.6 gm per kilogram, 15 and 41 per cent of calcium and magnesium, respectively, were absorbed.

*Calcium, Phosphorus and Magnesium*

Calcium deficiency due to a deficiency in vitamin D will cause severe osteoporosis of the alveolar bone and resorption of formed cementum. Osteoid tissue forms to excess but does not calcify, causing a deformed pattern of bone growth and compression of periodontal ligaments. Since phosphorus is present in most foods containing calcium, patients rarely exhibit phosphorus deficiency alone. In experimental animals, induced phosphorus deficiency has caused defective bone growth and dental malocclusion. Experimental deficiency in magnesium has caused fibrous replacement of the marrow of the alveolar bone, widening of the periodontal membrane, lossening of the teeth, gingival enlargement, heavy calculus formation, and retarded tooth eruption.

## Fluoride

Studies seem to indicated a positive relationship between increased consumption of dietary fluoride and periodontal status in adults. The effect in adults may be related to retardation of osteoporosis by fluoride, which recent evidence suggests. Wade (1) has stated that high levels of experimentally injected fluorine cause extensive periosteal deposition at the muscle sites where osteoporosis in the bone has already formed, and that fluorine acts as an enzyme inhibitor.

## Vitamin A

Vitamin A deficiency causes replacement of epithelium with squamous cells, resulting in diminished saliva secretion, resorption of cementum, hypercementoses, and disturbed bone growth. Hypervitaminosis A may cause bone resorption and osteoporosis.

## Vitamin B Complex

Investigators have attributed herpeslike vesicles to lack of thiamine, and ulcerative gingivitis to lack of nicotinic acid. A deficiency of riboflavin can produce loss of crest in the alveolar bone, with consequent tooth loosening. Lack of pantothenic and folic acids has been cited as causing ulcerations of the gingiva.

*Vitamin C*

The clinical oral signs of scurvy as well known but rare today. However, suboptimal levels of ascorbic acid may be fairly common. Periodontal tissues constantly require new bone and cementum matrix. The effect of vitamin C is on mesenchymal cells, and studies have shown a positive response to supplements of ascorbic acid in patients with borderline intake.

*Vitamin D*

The effect of vitamin D deficiency on calcium absorption has already been mentioned. Hypervitaminosis D, a rare condition, causes osteosclerosis, calcification of the periodontal ligament, hypercementoses, ankyloses, and calculus formation.

*Vitamins E and K*

A definite relationship between vitamins E and K and periodontal disease has not been established. Vitamin E may influence gonadal function, which inturn may influence periodontal health. The intestinal synthesis of vitamin K can be inhibited in treating periodontal disease.

*Allergic Reactions*

Periodontal pathosis is thought to be, in part, an allergic response. Investigators cite deficiencies of vitamins C and B complex and essential amino acids as precipitating factors. Volunteers who were made deficient in pyridoxine and panthothenic acid showed impaired antibody formation. Some authors feel that high doses of vitamins A, C and $B_{12}$ may be antiallergenic in certain persons.

## DIETARY THERAPY

As can be seen from the preceding discussion, proper diet for periodontal patients is much the same as the recommended nutrient intake for normal good health. Of course, the emphases are different and in some patients the best diet for periodontal purposes may conflict with that recommended for other ailments, such as gastrointestinal diseases, heart conditions requiring a low-cholesterol diet, or bland diets for ulcer or hypertensive patients. Periodontist and physician should cooperated closely in their recommendations, so that the final diet will be the most beneficial possible.

From the viewpoint of the periodontologist, the optimal diet should maintain an acid-alkali balance at a pH of 7.4, which permits the most efficient cell metabolism. Diabetes or lengthy fasting may cause acidosis and result in dissolution of bone salts. Alkalosis, conversely, may reduce normal bone resorption.

Oral cleansing and gum exercise are important criteria in choosing specific foods. Firm, fibrous foods such as raw carrots, celery and apples or fresh vegetable salads promote natural cleaning.

A good prenatal diet is important not only for the usual reasons but also for the dental health of the fetus and mother, since this is the time when fetal dental tissues are forming and differentiating. Iron supplements are especially important.

Dividing the diet into three general categories is a valuable teaching device for the periodontal patient:

1. The "resistance" foods, which are rich in high-quality proteins (lean meat, fish, eggs, milk and cheese), vitamins and minerals. Fruits and vegetables should be served raw as well as cooked to increase masticatory exercise and in a variety to insure optimal nutrition. Citrus fruit should be included daily.

2. Foods which are necessary to complete dietary calorie requirements but should be used sparingly. These include breads and cereals, with whole grains preferred, ans saturated fats such as butter and most oleomargarines.

3. The "susceptibility" foods, which contain the simple sugars, particularly sucrose and glucose. These foods have few nutrients other than calories and increase requirements of vitamins and minerals for their metabolism, which may precipitate a deficiency of certain water-soluble vitamins when the patient is on a diet of borderline adequacy. A high sugar intake may trigger clinical

symptoms of diabetes mellitus, which has a strong link with increased susceptibility to periodontal disease.

## REFERENCES

1. Wade, A. B.: Basic Periodonotology. Ed 2. Bristol, England, John Wright & Sons Ltd., 1965.
2. Clark, J. W., Chearaskin, E., Ringsdorf, W. M. Jr: Diet and the Periodontal Patient. Springfield, Ill., Charles C Thomas, Publisher, 1970.

*Chapter 57*

# FOOD ALLERGIES

$F$OOD or gastrointestinal allergies reveal themselves in many ways: nausea, vomiting (which can go into actual paroxysms), colic, diarrhea, mucous colitis, spastic constipation, allergic rhinitis, labyrinthitis, conjunctivitis, angioneurotic edema, eczematoid detmatitis, perianal eczema and pruritus, urticaria, fatigue, irritability, and headaches (with migraines that may be delayed for hours after ingestion of the offending allergens). In a few, fortunately rare, cases generalized systemic reactions with circulatory collapse, shock or even death occur. "Food asthma" is seen occasionally in children and is usually associated with consumption of egg, wheat or milk.

The incidence of food allergy seems to decrease with age. An estimated 10 per cent of the population carries a genetic predisposition to allergic sensitization. In patients under two years old, most allergies (85 per cent) are associated with foods. There is evidence that the gastrointestinal tract of the newborn is relatively permeable to small amounts of undigested protein and may remain so until the age of six months. By the age of four years, ingestants and inhalants are of equal importance. After age eight, inhalants are more preponderant, and eventually no more than 15 per cent of new allergies are associated with foods. Often, allergies that were very prominent in small children show gradual improvement or spontaneous amelioration after the age of six. Nevertheless, many allergologist think that the prevalence of food allergies is greater among adults than among children even though allergies are more difficult to diagnose in older patients.

Allergens are usually proteins. Major alterations of the protein structure, as in digestion by proteolytic enzymes or in cooking, usually eliminate the allergenic property of the molecule. For

Reprinted from *Postgraduate Medicine, 47* (No. 6), June, 1970.© McGraw-Hill, Inc.

example, some persons are allergic to raw or pasteurized milk, but not to boiled or evaporated milk.

In rare cases, the original sensitizer may have traveled through the placental barrier. More commonly, the allergen sensitizes the patient after ingestion and travels in small undigested quantities through the intestinal barrier.

Theoretically, the number of foods that cause allergies is almost as great as the total number of foods. The most common allergenic foods are wheat, milk, eggs, seafood, chocolate, chicken, pork, corn, nuts and strawberries. Oatmeal, rye, oranges, cottonseed, legumes, tomatoes, potatoes, beef, mustard, cucumbers and garlic also are implicated. Rice, lamb, geletin, peaches, peas, carrots, lettuce, artichokes, sesame oil, and apples are rarely allergenic, but occasionally may cause severe symptoms.

There are two types of allergic responses to food. In one type signs and symptoms appear within minutes. Seafood, berries and nuts are most often associated with this rapid response. In the other type, characteristic of cereals, milk, eggs, chocolate, pork, chicken, beef, potatoes, legumes and oranges, the response may be delayed for hours. The allergen in some cases may be a breakdown product of protein digestion and diagnosis is obviously much more difficult, particularly if the allergy is multiple.

For infants, the most common allergenic foods are milk, eggs, cereal grains (particularly wheat), and sometimes orange juice. Repetition and the proportionally large amounts consumed may be factors in this high frequency.

Besides the fact that raw foods are more likely to be allergenic than cooked foods, the allergenic response is also conditioned by the patient's physiologic state. Eczema increases the patient's physiologic state. Eczema increases the hypersensitivity of infants. Immediately after an allergic crisis, a refractory period may follow during which the ingestion of allergens causes no further reaction. Certain drugs may increase or decrease the severity of symptoms. Seasons and emotional states also influence the severity of allergic reactions.

## DIAGNOSIS

The principal tools in establishing a diagnosis of food allergy are a family history of food allergies, a detailed diet history (supplemented if possible by a food diary), trial diets, elimination diets, provocative diets, and skin tests. The dietary methods are more important than skin tests; the latter are more useful in diagnosing allergies to inhalants or contractants. At best, only 40 per cent of foods showing positive results in skin tests are related to the signs and symptoms caused by the ingestion of these foods. Specificity of target tissue may be involved, or the extract may have been inactivated during preparation for the skin test. Scratch and patch tests may reveal skin sensitivity to so many different substances that interpretation of the results is almost impossible. Thus, skin tests are just one of the confirmatory elements in the diagnosis.

Since allergies appear to be strongly conditioned by heredity, a thorough family history of allergic reactions to foods is useful. A detailed diet history, as quantitative as possible and verified by cross-checks as to nature and amount of foods, is essential. The mother should be questioned at length on the diet given to the infant. Afterward, she should again report symptoms as well as specific foods she suspects. Although most mothers report positive reactions well and their judgment is usually sound for foods that cause immediate reactions, a negative food history is not conclusive when one is dealing with foods that cause reactions hours (sometimes a day) after ingestion. This phenomenon may also induce the mother to incriminate the wrong food. A food diary kept by the mother is highly useful and should include intake of medicines, vitamins and tonics.

The older patient should be questioned on the effects of the foods he thinks are involved in his allergies and on the periodicity of both specific food ingestion and lalergic reactions. It is important to examine the patient's food dislikes because these are often unconscious protective devices based on repeated unpleasant experiences. In infants an intense dislike for cow's milk coupled with allergic sympatomatology should alert physicians to the possibility of hypersensitivity to milk. In older patients the symptoms may have been forgotten but the dislike remains, and the symptoms may follow ingestion of milk-containing foods, while milk itself is avoided.

Because food consumed as components of snacks or larger dishes tends to be forgotten, food allergies are often difficult to characterize until the patient keeps a detailed food diary. The patient should list all foods, all condiments, and all side dishes and sauces and note the time he eats and the time symptoms occur. This may establish a correlation between repeated allergic reactions and repeated ingestion of suspect foods. These foods are then excluded from the diet, and their allergenicity is tested by a dietary "on-or-off"method. Sometimes omission of the suspect foods eliminates all sympoms for a long experimental period. Often, symptomatic experimentation with more rigid elimiantion diets is necessary.

Elimination diets are used when symptoms are so frequent that allergens in a commonly eaten food or allergens contained in a variety of foods are suspected. The trial diet included only foods known to be hypoallergenic. All foods not specified must be regidly excluded. If no reactions occur after the patient has been on this diet for 15 days, the physician adds other foods at the rate of one every four or five days until the offending substance is clearly identified. When this substance is removed, other additions are resumed.

For infants, the basic diet is soybean milk, rice cereal, and a multivitamin preparation. For adults, the basic diet is cooked rice, pure rice cereal, and rice biscuits (with no other admixed cereal); canned peaches or pears; lamb (cooked without other fat); carrots; gelatin desserts made with the permitted fruits; water; salt; sugar; and jams and jellies made from the permitted fruits. A multivitamin supplement should be given, possibly as the first supplement, because the diet is otherwise deficient. For infants, the foods first added should be those of low allergenicity.

Stage 1 of the diet can be cereals other than wheat, lamb gelatin, carrots, squash, bananas and applesauce; stage 2, other cereals (still no wheat), other vegetables and fruits and pork or bacon; stage 3, wheat products;stage 4, beef, evaporated milk, raw vegetables and fruits, hard-boiled egg yolk; stage 5, soft egg yolk, well-cooked egg white, and bottled milk; stage 6, other foods. A similar sequence is followed for adults, although the basic diet is much more inclusive. Once the offending food is found, it must be clearly identified and the form of the food to which the patient is sensitive must be characterized.

The only effective long-term treatment is usually permanent exclusion of the allergen. In children, hypersensitivity to an allergen may decrease past the sixth year or past adolescence, so cautious reintroduction of the food may be attempted from time to time. In acute cases antihistamines are sometimes useful. If epinephrine relieves abdominal pain, allergy probably causes the pain.

## MANAGING THE FOOD-ALLERGIC INFANT

The nutritional state of infants with food allergies is often poor for a variety of reasons. Before diagnosis the infants may reject a variety of foods; during diagnosis whole classes of food may have to be excluded.

Certain consequences of the allergy, such as recurrent allergic rhinitis with nasal obstruction, edema of the intestinal mucosa, or recurrent diarrhea, may interfere with ingestion or with the absorption of a number of nutrients. If the allergenic food contains essential nutrients usually provided by it alone, the nutritional problem is serious and, unless it is well managed, growth and development will be compromised. Wheat can be replaced by rice, later oats and barley; egg by chicken and other baby meats; and citrus juice by other vitamin C-fortified fruit juices or by ascorbic acid.

Milk is not so easily replaced by other foods. Allergy to breast milk is very rare. Allergy to raw and pasteurized cow's milk is much more frequent, with an incidence reported from 0.3 to 2 per cent or more. Casein does not seem to be involved. In evaporated milk, lactoglobulin (most potent sensitizer) and lactalbumin (most potent) are heat-denatured and therefore safe for many infants. In other infants, goat's milk (which contains different lactoglobulins and lactalbumins) is well tolerated. If neither evaporated milk nor goat's milk is tolerated, soybean milk formulas are indicated (Mull-Soy®, Neo-Mull-Soy®, Similac®, Isomil$^{TM}$, Sobee, Prosobee®, Soyalac®). Meat-base formulas and protein hydrolysate mixtures, like the soybean milk, fortified with calcium lactate can also be used.

Even the soybean milk or meat-base formulas can contain allergens. Some pediatricians have successfully used casein hydrolysates, but the amounts compatible with absence of diarrhea may not permit optimal growth. For infants with multiple allergies, however, this may be the best solution. When milk is replaced by such mixtures, the vitamin and mineral adequacy of the diet must be checked.

Careful management of the allergic pregnant woman's diet prevents or at least decreases the chances of sensitization in the infant. She should avoid foods to which she is sensitive and limit daily milk intake to two glasses of evaporated, calcium-fortified milk. She should continue this regimen during lactation and breast-feed the baby as long as possible.

## FOOD SOURCES FOR THE ALLERGIC PATIENT

Proper labeling and knowledge of food sources are often indispensable if the sensitive patient is to avoid allergies (1, 2). Unfortunately, neither is widespread. For example, if corn is the allergen, it must be remembered that baking powders may contain cornstarch; monosodium glutamate may be derived from corn (or beets, soybean or wheat); or corn oil, which contains some protein, may be found in mustard, mayonnaise or catsup.

Similarly, products containing milk are white bread, cakes, custards, candies, ice cream, cream soups, sauces, noodles, macaroni, infant foods, whipped cream and cream substitutes, butter, and most margarines. Wheat flour is found in breads, crackers, cakes, macaroni, spaghetti, gravies, cream sauces, soups, breakfast cereals, certain sausages, and various infant foods. Eggs are found in custards, certain puddings, ice cream, certain candies, cakes, muffins, mayonnaise, and glazed breads, rolls and pretzels (3).

Obviously, an allergic child's mother will need extensive help to know what foods the child should avoid, as well as what foods can be used as substitutes not only for main dishes but as ingredients in recipes used to cook safe foods. The help of a competent dietitian or dietetic outpatient service is indispensable.

## REFERENCES

1. Sheldon, J. M., Lovell, R. B. and Mathews, K. P.: A Manual of Clinical Allergy. Ed. 2. Philadelphia, W. B. Saunders Company, 1967.
2. Gelfand, M.: Important allergens easily overlooked. In Prigal, S. J. (Editor): Fundamentals of Modern Allergy. New York, McGraw-Hill Book Company, 1960.
3. Feeny, M. C.: Nutritional and dietary management of food allergy in children. Amer. J. Clin. Nutr., 22:103-111, 1969.

*Chapter 58*

# DIETARY CONTROL OF DIABETES

## TRIAL AND ERROR

INSULIN was discovered in 1921. Within a year, its use had altered the clinical course of diabetes from that of a fairly short-term, fatal disease to that of a long-term, chronic illness that predisposes to death from other causes.

The increased incidence of diabetes is due to several factors: Diabetics no longer die early from lack of insulin or from acute infection, diabetic women can produce babies, the prevalence of diabetic genes in the national genetic pool is increasing, and the present mode of life and nutrition may predispose to diabetes. The American Diabetes Association has estimated the minimal number of diagnosed and undiagnosed cases of diabetes in the United States at about 10 million. Of the known diabetics reported by the Bureau of the Census survey in 1964 to 1965, 70 per cent were 45 years of age or older when the disease was diagnosed (50% were 45 to 64 years old; 20% were 65 or older). In far less than 1 per cent, the diagnosis was made before age 25.

These statistics would lead one to believe that various diets have been tried systematically on large groups of patients for long periods. However, this is hardly the case. In regard to insulin and other antihyperglycemic agents, we know a great deal about certain effects of various diets on blood glucose. For example, reducing excessive weight considerably improves the prognosis in respect to control of hyperglycemia, and large amounts of sucrose in meals cause wide swings in blood glucose levels that are difficult, if not impossible, to prevent even when insulin dosage and meals are synchronized. However, we know too little about other aspects of diabetes control, such as the long-term effects of

Reprinted from *Postgraduate Medicine, 50* (No. 2 and 3), Aug. and Sept., 1971.

diet on the complications of diabetes: atherosclerosis — particularly atherosclerotic disease of the heart and small vessels — retinopathy, nephropathy and neuropathy.

It would be unduly pessimistic, however, to think that we have not learned a great deal about the relation of diabetes and dietotherapy in the past 50 years.

## History of Diabetic Treatment

Diabetes was known in the three main cradles of medicine as early as the sixteenth century. The "Ebers Papyrus," which dates back to 1552 B.C., described a disease characterized by polyuria, emaciating but painless. Susruta, the Hindu writer, described a "honey-urine" disease. Ancient Chinese texts spoke of a disease characterized by polyphagia, polydipsia and polyuria.

Empirical treatment based on drugs and diets was practiced. Archigenes of Apamea used opium and diet; the Galenic school prescribed emetics, narcotics and diet, and Avicenna, an Arabian physician and the first to suggest a nervous origin for diabetes, used a combination of fenugreek, lupine and wormseed — an early form of the starvation diet. Willis, a seventeenth-century English physician, established diet as the primary treatment and fed his patients milk and barley water, using limewater to replace the "salt" lost in the urine. He began the practice of tasting urine as a means of diagnosis, but believed the "wonderfully sweet" taste came from the "salt," which had been isolated by Paracelsus.

By the beginning of the eighteenth century, carbohydrate restriction was solidly established in most prescribed diabetic diets and continued, often in extreme form, until insulin became available. Some diets were highly unpleasant and presumably short-lived.

By the second half of the nineteenth century, Bouchardat and other French physicians were prescribing more palatable foods, but maintained the principle of eating as little as possible, especially restricting carbohydrates. With daily urine tests for excess sugar, Bouchardat demonstrated the efficacy of moderate exercise in increasing carbohydrate tolerance. He saw his dietary principles confirmed by the effect on his patients of the privations of the siege of Paris in 1870 to 1871.

In the early 1900's, Naunyn and Allen were the foremost exponents of undernutrition and carbohydrate restriction. Naunyn taught that all foods directly or indirectly contributed to the amount of sugar in the blood; thus, the most important aspect of a diabetic's diet was total caloric intake. Allen carried undernutrition to the extreme of reducing carbohydrates to less than 30 gm per day and of decreasing the daily caloric allowance of his young patients to the extent that they were often confined to bed. Their life expectancy was doubled, however, from 1.3 to 2.9 years, and the advent of insulin therapy returned some of the survivors to a near-normal life.

Joslin, an associate of Naunyn, reported that from 1897 to 1914, Naunyn's treatment resulted in an average survival time of 4.9 years after diagnosis of diabetes; from 1914 to 1922, with Allen's more drastic methods, the average rose to 6.1 years. When insulin became available, the average rose steadily from 7.5 years in the period from 1922 to 1925 to 14.5 years from 1945 to 1955. An increasingly larger number of Joslin's patients continue to be physically sound after 25 years of control with diet, insulin and exercise.

These advances are striking, but diabetes still ranks high (fifth) as a cause of death in the United States, and hundreds of thousands of persons are victims of its complications. The fact that insulin therapy has liberalized the starvation diet has reopened the issue on the type of diet that will allow the diabetic the longest life free of complications.

The finding that all foods in various proportions give rise to glucose has been superseded by the findings that glucose can be used to a certain extent through administration of insulin and that all dietary carbohydrates are not metabolized in the same way. Disaccharides, sucrose in particular, are hydrolyzed in the cells of the intestinal wall, and starches are hydrolized in the lumen. Sucrose increases triglycerides, whereas a greater proportion of starch in the diet often reduces triglycerides and cholesterol. Thus, the nature and rates of absorption of carbohydrates must be considered when discussing the role of carbohydrates in the diabetic diet.

Another grave question arose as the role of saturated fats in hypercholesterolemia and atherosclerosis became more manifest and as the prolongation of the diabetic's life made cardiovascular disease an increasingly greater risk. Data from the Joslin Clinic show a mortality rate from cardiovascular diseases of 46.8 per cent from 1922 to 1929 and of 76.6 per cent from 1956 to 1962.

In 1970, Pell and D'Alonzo reported that during a 10-year study, death was caused by heart disease in 45 of 370 diabetics but in only 16 of 370 matched controls. Even when such factors as hypertension, overweight, kidney disease, or preexisting heart disease were excluded, the diabetics had two to three times the normal rate of morbidity from heart disease. Such data question the desirability of a low-carbohydrate diet, which is automatically a high-fat diet.

### Epidemiologic Studies Raise Questions

Recent epidemiologic studies have raised more questions than they have solved. At the very least, they do not confirm the desirability of a low-carbohydrate diet for all types of diabetes. For example, a 1968 survey in Japan showed a prevalence of diabetes comparable to that in the United States; yet, in Japan, diabetes is not a major cause of death, juvenile diabetes and ketosis are rare, and atherosclerotic complications are relatively infrequent.

The Japanese diet is traditionally low in total fat, cholesterol, animal protein, and simple sugars, and it is high in total carbohydrate (national average is 381.6 gm per day), of which 337.4 gm are polysaccharides. A Japanese male with diabetes mellitus is usually allowed about 350 gm of carbohydrate (starch) and 30 gm of fat per day. Chinese medical customs are reported to be similar.

In 1969, a report was published on the treatment of 123 diabetic members of the Armed Forces of India. The men received tolbutamide, phenformin, hydrochloride, or insulin, or a combination of two or all of these agents, and were given a diet containing 520 to 570 gm of carbohydrates, 120 to 140 gm of protein, and 70 to 75 gm of fat, with a total of 3,010 to 3,515 calories per day. The results showed no unusual problem of control or of complications in spite of the high carbohydrate content.

In a recently published survey of 10 countries of Asia and Central and South America, caloric intake and overweight were the most consistently associated factors in diabetics of all ethnic groups. Sucrose consumption and diabetes seemed to be correlated in some areas, but the correlation between total carbohydrate consumption and diabetes tended to be negative.

## Three Types of Diet Control

The apparent diversity of study results has led internists in Western countries to investigate three very different types of diets for diabetic control. The traditional diet, still in common use and generally recommended in recent medical textbooks, closely regulates carbohydrate intake to a maximum of 40 per cent of total calories, more generally from 125 to 200 gm per day, with an average of 150 gm. Protein is restricted to 1 gm per kilogram of body weight per day (1.5 gm in certain complications). The fat content makes up the remaining calories needed to maintain the ideal (lean) body weight. Increasingly, the fat component is manipulated to increase the polyunsaturated and decrease the saturated triglycerides and to reduce cholesterol.

Impressed by the Japanese results and mindful of the increased risk of atherosclerosis in diabetics, other investigators have tried a high-carbohydrate, low-fat diet, containing 250 to 500 gm of starch and 50 gm or less of highly polyunsaturated fat. Some reports show that the diet has lowered cholesterol and triglyceride levels and that good control has been maintained without added insulin and undue difficulty in managing blood glucose levels.

The third diet seems much more hazardous. The patient may eat normally as long as he is without symptoms, including acetone in the urine. With this diet, hyperglycemia and glucosuria are common, ketosis occurs frequently, and triglycerides and cholesterol are often elevated. Early enthusiasm regarding dietary freedom for the patient – and the physician – has faded as long-term follow-up has revealed the frequency of complications.

## Comment

Diet appears to be an essential part of diabetic treatment. There is general agreement on the need for a nutritionally adequate diet, containing sufficient protein, vitamins and minerals; water and electrolyte balance; strict weight control; a regular pattern of intake, balanced with insulin therapy and exercise; extremely moderate use of alcoholic beverages; and avoidance of loads of sucrose and other rapidly absorbed carbohydrates.

Debate continues, however, on the ideal balance between carbohydrates and fats (which may vary with the patient) and on the degree that the lipid component of the diet must be manipulated to avoid atherosclerotic complications.

## PRESENT NUTRITIONAL BASIS

In the United States, a large proportion of patients with maturity-onset diabetes are obese. The most important dietary measure for these patients is restriction of caloric intake to reduce their weight to that of normal young adults of the same sex and body build. Weight reduction should be gradual — usually not more than 2 lb per week, which corresponds to a deficit of 1000 calories per day. Achievement of the desirable weight is almost always associated with better control of blood glucose and serum lipid levels. Sometimes, weight control through dietary restriction improves glucose tolerance sufficiently to obviate drug or even insulin therapy. (In one large series, one-third of the patients were controlled by weight reduction alone.)

Undernutrition is undesirable and should be avoided, especially in patients with growth-on-set diabetes. Since insulin became available, there has been no rationale for underfeeding the diabetic. The growth pattern of the diabetic youngster need not deviate appreciably from the normal growth pattern.

There are a number of reasons why regular exercise is particularly important in maintaining diabetics. Some years ago, Jean Christophe and I showed through systematic studies of glucose utilization what had been known empirically for decades: namely, that in diabetics receiving a baseline dosage of insulin, exercise acts as an additional dose. My associates and I also have shown that exercise is effective in controlling weight and can be instrumental in reducing blood cholesterol.

Food intake must be spaced in such a way as to balance administered insulin and physical activity, thereby averting hypoglycemia and excessive hyperglycemia.

## Protein

The classic daily allowance of 1 gm of protein (half of high biologic value or animal origin) per kilogram of body weight gives healthy adults a margin of safety to compensate for variation in protein quality, maintain adequate reserves, and allow for possible increases in requirements resulting from the normal stresses of an active life.

If the diabetes is not under perfect control, and particularly if infection or some other complicating factor is present, additional protein may be required to offset losses from excessive gluconeogenesis and ketogenesis due to impaired glucose utilization. Patients with nephropathy or malabsorption lose additional protein in the urine and feces and thus may require more protein. Psychologic stress makes control of diabetes more difficult and may cause additional nitrogen losses.

Thus it seems reasonable for certain diabetics to take up to 1.5 gm of protein per kilogram per day if this is not contraindicated by hepatic and renal conditions. Several clinics routinely order 75 gm of protein for diets of less than 1500 calories and a minimum of 100 gm for diets of more than 1500 calories.

## Carbohydrate

Minimizing wide swings in blood glucose levels reduces the chance of taxing the already inadequate mechanisms of glucose utilization and disposal. Therefore, large individual loads of carbohydrate should be eliminated, especially when they include concentrated and refined carbohydrates, sucrose in particular. Many diabetics have been reported to be under good control on diets containing a large proportion of starch, but there is universal agreement that sucrose should be avoided as much as possible. (Recent studies even suggest that sucrose plays an etiologic role in persons genetically susceptible to diabetes.)

Other factors such as total caloric intake and exercise must be considered, but carbohydrate intake must be timed so that it roughly synchronizes the peak of insulin action with that of carbohydrate availability.

As stated earlier, opinions vary on the optimal percentage of caloric intake represented by starches, but most clinicians tend to limit carbohydrate intake to about 40 per cent of the calories. Reducing carbohydrate below that value means prescribing a diet very high in fat, with all the dangers attendant in an athero-sclerosis-prone population. In any event, carbohydrate intake should not be less than 125 gm per day. Lower intake tends to be associated with excessive ketogenesis and gluconeogenesis.

## Fat and Blood Lipids

Two countervailing considerations are applicable in determining the amount of fat in the diet: (1) Many clinicians consider that diabetes may be easier to control in a patient on a diet low in carbohydrate and therefore high in fat, and (2) the association of diabetes with a very high risk of atherosclerotic disease precludes use of fat, particularly saturated fat.

Levels of cholesterol and triglycerides tend to be higher in diabetics (especially in cases of maturity onset) than in non-diabetics of the same age. Lipids, particularly triglycerides, increase in acidosis and decline when acidosis is controlled. Atherosclerosis also is much more common in diabetics, with triglycerides, in particular, associated with coronary artery and atherosclerotic diseases. Neither cholesterol nor triglycerides seem implicated in small vessel diseases (retinopathy, glomerulosclerosis, neuropathy), which do not appear to be atherosclerotic. Athero-mata of the medium and large arteries generally are associated with elevated serum lipid levels.

Eruptive lesions on the extensor surfaces of arms, legs, trunk and buttocks (xanthoma diabeticorum) may occur with high elevation of serum triglycerides, usually as a result of long-term, poorly controlled diabetes; the lesions usually disappear with control of the diabetes. Intractable hyperlipemia occurs in rare lipo-atrophic diabetes and to a lesser degree in the Kimmelstiel-Wilson syndrome, a form of diabetes associated with a nephrotic syndrome.

It is obvious from the foregoing that at least some forms of hyperlipidemia respond to adequate control of diabetes. The relationship of hyperlipidemia to impaired carbohydrate metabolism is still obscure and at present we can only recommend a piecemeal approach. Three important aspects have already been mentioned: careful control of the diabetes, weight reduction, and avoidance of sucrose. The first may or may not be effective; the second may still be the most effective method of controlling lipid elevation.

Besides making control of diabetes more difficult, sucrose may be specifically associated with a rise in triglycerides. It appears prudent to modify the lipid component of the diet to attain the lowest feasible serum levels of cholesterol and triglycerides. The cholesterol level is best lowered by reducing the cholesterol content of the diet to less than 300 mg per day, reducing the total fat content to less than 40 per cent of the calories (unless the patient has carbohydrate-induced hypertriglyceridemia), and selecting a higher proportion of fats composed of polyunsaturated fatty acids. Triglycerides may be lowered through weight reduction, and in lipid-induced hypertriglyceridemia, through restriction of lipids. (If the condition is carbohydrate-induced, fat must be increased as carbohydrate is reduced and the composition of the diet watched carefully.)

The proportion of fat may be manipulated by limiting eggs to no more than two per week; by replacing, as much as possible, whole milk, cheese (other than low-fat cottage cheese), beef, pork and mutton with fish and poultry; and by replacing butter and saturated shortenings with polyunsaturated oils (safflower, cottonseed, corn) and margarines.

A capable and imaginative dietitian, always important in managing diabetes, may also be able to achieve at least partial control of atherosclerosis by dietary means.

## Vitamins and Minerals

The dietary requirements of vitamins and minerals in a diabetic patient under adequate control are similar to those of a normal person and should conform to the recommended dietary allowances of the Food and Nutrition Board. The recommmended amounts of fruits and leafy green vegetables; fresh meat, poultry or fish; and enriched cereal products should insure adequate intake. A daily maintenance multivitamin tablet is added insurance but the patient should remember that only a varied diet will provide the minerals required. (Such trace minerals as zinc and chromium have generated interest lately because of a possible role in carbohydrate metabolism; impaired glucose tolerance in some elderly persons seems to improve with supplementary dietary chromium.)

Abnormal utilization of nutrients, particularly vitamins, may occur in patients with poorly controlled diabetes, infection, or other complication. Vitamin supplements up to three times the recommended dietary allowances may then be desirable.

## Water and Electrolytes

In the absence of complications, the diabetic's intake of water, sodium and potassium need not differ from that of normal persons, although a large intake of water and avoidance of excessive sodium are useful prophylactic measures. Poorly controlled diabetes is likely to be associated with deficits of water, sodium, potassium, and possibly other cations. These deficits obviously must be corrected immediately. The quantity of water consumed should be at least 1 ml per calorie of food ingested per day. In any instance of anorexia, nausea or vomiting (whether associated with poor diabetic control or other illness) fluid and electrolyte balance should be maintained by oral liquid supplements or, secondarily, by parenteral preparations. Concommitant hypertension or renal, hepatic or vascular disorders may complicate electrolyte balance.

## Alcohol

Many diabetics tolerate a small amount of alcohol but it goes without saying that allowing it depends as much on the patient's self-control as on his general condition. Diabetics are particularly prone to having fatty livers; even the slightest sign of impaired liver function is a strict contraindication of alcohol.

## General Aspects

As in all lifelong regimens, the physician and dietitian must take into account the patient's age and sex, food preferences, economic status, and the way in which his food is acquired, prepared and consumed. The dietary rationale should be discussed with the patient in a two-way exchange. He must understand why the total amount of food is limited, why specific foods are limited or proscribed, and why distribution in intake during the course of a day is important. The simplest terms should be used in the dietary explanation.

From the great variety of foods and of meal (or snack) patterns compatible with adequate control of diabetes, only those most compatible with the patient's taste and life-style should be selected. Above all, any patient who expends large amounts of energy should not be subjected to unnecessary (and dangerous) periods of hunger; meal patterns should be tailored to his needs. A high-protein meal may be needed in the late evening to prevent midnight and early morning reactions. In this case, the rest of the daily rations should be adjusted accordingly.

The dietitian may have to spend considerable time with the patient and his family; home visits are invaluable.

## REFERENCES

1. West, K. M. and Kalbfleisch, J. M.: Influence of nutritional factors on prevalence of diabetes. Diabetes, 20:99-108, Feb. 1971.
2. Pell, S. and D'Alonzo, C. A.: Chronic disease morbidity and income level in an employed population. Am. J. Publ. Health, 60:116-129, Jan. 1970.
3. Marble, A. et al., Eds. Diabetes Mellitus, 11th ed. Philadelphia, Lea & Febiger, 1971.
4. Malins, J.: Clinical Diabetes Mellitus. London, Eyre & Spottiswoode, 1968.
5. Innami, S. and Mickelsen, O.: Nutritional status — Japan. Nutr. Rev., 28:275-278, Oct. 1969.

*Chapter 59*

# LOW-SODIUM DIETS

## MILD RESTRICTION

IN our studies of the nutritional knowledge of professional and lay groups, Dr. Johanna Dwyer and I found, as expected, that physicians knew much more about the physiology and biochemistry of nutrition than did educated laymen. However, in regard to foods, the physicians were not much more knowledgeable than many laymen and were much less knowledgeable than dietitians. Thus, it would appear that patients who must be placed on special diets would benefit a great deal from a dietitian's instruction.

Because the physician is the authority behind the patient's advised dietary changes, which may be drastic, it is imperative that he give the patient, and spouse, general instructions about the diet before they see the dietitian. The advice "Just cut down on sodium intake" is almost useless in most cases, for patients tend to equate sodium with visible salt — that in the saltshaker — and will ignore the sodium that is already present in foods.

It is hoped that this chapter will be useful in defining the broad lines of instruction to the patient who must follow a mildly restricted low-sodium diet.

The patient must understand that while salt contains sodium, sodium is not necessarily equivalent to salt. Sodium chloride is about one-half sodium; monosodium glutamate contains only about one-third as much sodium. Soy sauce contains large amounts of sodium. Sodium is also present in drinking water 1 to 1500 mg or more per quart); medicines such as alkalizers, antibiotics, cough remedies, laxatives, pain relievers, and sedatives; and some compounds taken as medicine, such as bicarbonate of soda.

Reprinted from *Postgraduate Medicine, 19, 50* (Nos. 6 and 1), June and July, 1971. © McGraw-Hill, Inc.

Sodium is naturally present in all foods, but the amount varies. Some foods such as avacados and unsalted nuts contain very small amounts of sodium; others such as milk and meat contain much larger amounts. A 10-oz can of commercially prepared stew may contain as much as 9000 mg of sodium.

The patient also must be told how to measure sodium content. Milligrams mean little to most Americans, many of whom do not even recognize the gram as a unit of weight. With a diet mildly restricted in sodium, the patient is not required to measure his intake in milligrams, but to give him an idea of the quantities he must deal with, the dietitian should translate grams into more familiar weights and measures. It is usually a revelation to the patient that 1 gm equals only about one-thirtieth of 1 oz and that 1 mg is one-thousandth of 1 gm.

Since the average American diet contains about 6000 mg of sodium per day, the unrestricted intake of sodium equals only one-fifth of 1 oz per day. Normal cooking measurements can give a further idea of the amount of sodium in various compounds. For example, the sodium content per teaspoon of soy sauce is 365 mg, monosodium glutamate 765 mg, baking soda 1000 mg, and table salt 2300 mg.

Even before the patient consumes any food, he can reduce his sodium intake by checking his medicine chest and water supply and making any necessary adjustments, such as rinsing his mouth well after using tooth cleansers and mouthwashes, some of which contain large amounts of sodium. With regard to the diet itself, the patient should remember the following general rules. It must be emphasized, however, that these rules pertain only to a mildly restricted low-sodium diet.

1. Halve the usual amount of salt, monosodium glutamate, and soy sauce used in cooking and at the table.

2. Use baking soda only for baking and not in boiling vegetables or as an alkalizer.

3. Avoid food cured with salt, preserved in brine, or very high in salt.

4. Avoid commercially prepared foods with unlabeled salt content (canned stews, frozen dinners, and soft drinks, except low-sodium dietetic preparations), for the water and syrup in

## SODIUM CONTENT OF FOODS IN A MILDLY RESTRICTED LOW-SODIUM DIET

**Foods that may be eaten (fresh, frozen, canned)**

**Low in sodium**

Fruits: all fruits and fruit juices

Fats
  Avocado
  Butter, margarine
  Cooking oils or fats
    (except bacon fats)
  Cream, sweet or sour
  Mayonnaise
  Unsalted nuts

**Moderately high in sodium**

Vegetables: all kinds, except those listed
  under "Foods to avoid"

Breads and cereals
  Barley          Oatmeal
  Bread: white and Rice
    whole wheat   Tapioca
  Biscuits        Farina
  Muffins         Dry cereals
  Matzo           Crackers
  Grits           Griddle cakes
  Cornbread         and waffles
  Cornmeal        Macaroni
  Cornstarch      Noodles
  Wheat meal      Spaghetti
  Rolled wheat

**High in sodium**

Milks          Meats
  Whole          Beef        Liver
  Skim           Pork        Tongue
  Buttermilk     Lamb        Chicken
  Powdered       Veal        Duck
  Evaporated     Rabbit      Quail
                 Brain       Turkey
                 Kidney

Fish: all kinds, except those listed under
  "Foods to avoid"

Cheeses (lightly salted
  Swiss
  American cheddar
  Cottage

Eggs: in moderation
Other foods
  Alcoholic beverages   Honey
  Fountain beverages    Molasses
  Baking chocolate      Leavening agents
  Cocoa                   Baking powder
  Candy                   Baking soda, for
  Coffee or coffee          baking only
    substitute          Potassium
  Gelatin                 bicarbonate
  Pudding mixes         Yeast
  Syrups

which they are packed may contain large amounts of sodium.
Read the labels of canned vegetables and do not add salt to those
already salted.

5. Do not use a salt substitute or meat tenderizer unless
prescribed by a physician. Some of these products have ingredients
that can be harmful in certain diseases.

6. Dietetic foods are made for various purposes and are not
necessary in a mildly restricted low-sodium diet. However, if used,

SODIUM CONTENT OF FOODS IN A MILDLY RESTRICTED LOW-SODIUM DIET (continued)

**Foods to avoid (very high in sodium)**

Meats  
(salted or smoked)  
  Bacon  
  Bologna  
  Corned beef  
  Ham  
  Luncheon meats  
  Sausage  
  Salt pork  

Fish  
(salted or smoked)  
  Anchovies  
  Sardines  
  Caviar  
  Dried cod  
  Herring  

Cheeses  
  Processed cheese  
  Cheese spreads  
  Roquefort<sup>TM</sup>  
  Camembert  
  Other strong cheeses  

Peanut butter,  
  unless low-sodium  
  dietetic  

Vegetables (salted or packed in brine)  
  Pickles, sauerkraut, etc.  

Flavorings  
  Commercial bouillon  
  Catsup  
  Celery, onion or garlic salts  
  Chili sauce  
  Meat extracts, sauces or tenderizes,  
    unless low-sodium dietetic  
  Prepared mustard  
  Relishes  
  Salt substitutes  
  Cooking wine  

Miscellaneous  
  Breads with  
    salt topping  
  Potato chips  
  Pretzels  
  Popcorn  

  Other salted snacks  
  Salted nuts  
  Olives  
  Bacon and bacon fat  

**General reminders**

Milks, meats, fish, cheese and eggs are quite high in sodium.

Vegetables, breads and cereals have moderate amounts of sodium, which vary greatly among the different vegetables.

Fruits and fats are low in sodium or have only trace amounts.

Highly salted snack foods should be avoided.

Halve the amount of salt, soy sauce, and monosodium glutamate used in cooking and at the table.

Do not add salt to foods already salted in freezing and canning.

Try different flavorings except those listed under "Foods to avoid."

Do not use a salt substitute unless the physician has recommended it.

When eating out or buying prepared canned or frozen foods, try to avoid those with an unlisted salt content.

they should carry the label "low-sodium dietetic."

7. Experiment with flavorings. The selection is large and the combinations are varied. The French, who are among the world's best cooks, undersalt rather than oversalt food, depending rather on herbs and spices to vary and emphasize flavor.

8. Remember that in spite of restrictions on certain foods, a healthy body still needs a balanced diet. The local public health service and dietetic and heart associations can give help in planning meals and often sponsor cooking classes in sodium-

restricted foods.

Foods that may be eaten or should be avoided in a diet mildly restricted in sodium are listed in convenient tabular form above. Neither this list nor this discussion should supplant the advice and guidance of the dietitian in individual cases; hopefully, this material will orient the patient before he consults with the dietitian.

Several points regarding the food list should be noted. Milk is the food with the highest sodium content (about 120 mg per 8-oz cup). Two cups of milk daily are usually sufficient for adults, except lactating mothers. Meats, fish, cheese and eggs are next highest in sodium content, containing about 25 mg per ounce. Vegetables vary considerably in sodium content, but this is not important in mildly restricted low-sodium diets, unless like sauerkraut, the foods have been packed with salt. Fruits are very low in sodium (about 2 mg per serving) and fats, unless deliberately salted (butter, margarine, nuts, etc.), have almost no sodium.

The diet list takes into account only the sodium content of foods. If the patient is also on a reducing diet or one of the other specialized diets, the dietitian will need to make modifications in the list.

## SEVERE RESTRICTION

Many foods are forbidden to the patient on the mildly restricted low-sodium diet described above, but the range of choices is wide compared with that for the patient whose sodium level is limited to 1000 mg per day or less. This patient must become aware not only of the average sodium content of all foods he might consume but also of many less obvious ways in which sodium may enter his diet.

The patient on the severely restricted low-sodium diet must accept the fact that many foods are forbidden. He must also become aware of the variability in sodium content in different water systems. A patient restricted to 1000 or 500 mg of sodium per day cannot afford to drink or cook with water containing more than 120 mg sodium per quart; 2 qt of water containing 120 mg sodium will acount for 240 mg of his total daily allowance. Therefore, the patient, dietitian or physician must check with the local health department or have the water supply analyzed for sodium content. If the sodium content is too high, distilled (not spring) water should be used. The patient should not drink water treated by home water softeners, as they contain sodium.

Low-calorie soft drinks can be made with high-sodium water and must be avoided unless the composition is ascertained and found to be satisfactory. Low-calorie drinks may also contain sugar substitutes made with sodium. The patient should check the labels to be sure they specify "calcium" cyclamate or "calcium" saccharin, since compounds with sodium may be labeled simply as saccharin or soluble saccharin. Artificially sweetened products other than diet drinks should be avoided unless their labels clearly state their ingredients. So-called low-sodium dietetic foods should still be avoided if the food is on the disallowed list. For example, carrots, even if prepared without salt, are not low-sodium vegetables. The same may be true of beans or salmon.

The patient should be prepared to read all labels carefully. He must avoid not only salt, artificial sweeteners with sodium, monosodium glutamate, and baking soda, but also brine, baking powder, sodium propionate, disodium phosphate, sodium benzoate, sodium sulfite, and sodium hydroxide. The words "soda" and "sodium" and the symbol "Na" are clues that foods should be avoided however, these are not always easy to find on labels.

Sodium compounds are used in commercially prepared foods to inhibit mold, retard spoilage, and give smooth texture and quick-cooking qualities. Even headache remedies may be high in sodium; the patient should not take any medication without specific permission from his physician. Baking powder and soda must not be used in home baking, but yeast, sodium-free baking soda, and potassium can be substituted. The last two items can be found in stores where dietetic foods are sold.

Eating in a restaurant can present a problem. It is better for the patient to go hungry than to risk ingesting a large amount of sodium by taking chances on unknown foods. In restaurants it is wisest to order broiled meats, inside slices of roasts, an egg poached or boiled in unsalted water (only one egg a day is

## SODIUM CONTENT OF FOODS IN A
## SEVERELY RESTRICTED LOW-SODIUM DIET

**Foods that may be eaten**

**Low in sodium or negligible sodium**

Fruits (about 2 mg per serving, e.g. one apple)
  Fresh, frozen, canned or dried and juices
  All kinds except tomatoes, provided no
    sodium compound has been added in
    processing

Fats
  Unsalted spreads
  Unsalted salad and cooking oils
  Unsalted nuts
  Cream, if used like a fat, should be
    confined to about 2 tbsp per day

Other (used in normal quantities)
  Honey
  Brown sugar
  White sugar
  Maple sugar
  Jams
  Jellies
  Homemade sodium-free candy
  Chocolate (baking, semisweet, bittersweet)
  Plain gelatin
  Coffee, tea, and coffee substitutes

**Moderately high in sodium**

Cream (about 11 mg per ounce)

Vegetables (fresh, frozen, or dietetic canned)
  About 9 mg per ½ cup serving:

| | |
|---|---|
| Asparagus | Okra |
| Broccoli | Onions |
| Brussels sprouts | Summer squash |
| Cabbage | Winter squash |
| Cauliflower | Tomato juice |
| Chicory |   (low-sodium dietetic) |
| Cucumber | Green peas |
| Eggplant | Green or red peppers |
| Endive | Pumpkin |
| Escarole | Radishes |
| Green beans | Rutabagas |
| Lettuce | Turnip greens |
| Mushrooms | Wax beans |

About 5 mg per ½ cup (starchy vegetables):

| | |
|---|---|
| Beans | Parsnips |
| Lentils | Sweet potatoes |
| Dried peas | White potatoes |
| Corn | |

Breads (about 5 mg per serving)
  Low-sodium breads, rolls, crackers
  Unsalted matzo
  Melba toast
  Unsalted popcorn, pasta, rice, barley, flour
  Cooked cereals: farina, grits, oatmeal,
    wheat meal
  Dry cereals: puffed rice, puffed wheat,
    shredded wheat, and other cereals with
    less than 6 mg sodium per 100 gm

**Relatively high in sodium**

Milks (about 120 mg per 8 oz cup,
2 cups per day)
  Whole and skim
  Reconstituted powdered and evaporated
  Unsalted buttermilk
  Plain yogurt (6 oz) may be substituted for
    1 cup milk

Meats and poultry (fresh, frozen, or
dietetic canned; about 25 mg per ounce,
5 oz per day)

| | |
|---|---|
| Beef | Liver (beef or calf only |
| Lamb |   once every two weeks) |
| Pork | Rabbit |
| Veal | Chicken |
| Fresh tongue | Duck |

Fish
  All kinds except those prescribed on
    moderately restricted diet; fresh only;
    must be well rinsed

Meat substitutes
  One egg per day
  Unsalted cottage cheese
  Low-sodium cheese
  Low-sodium peanut butter

## SODIUM CONTENT OF FOODS IN A
## SEVERELY RESTRICTED LOW-SODIUM DIET (continued)

**Foods either too high in sodium to be
allowed or which should be avoided
because sodium content is unknown**

Milks
  Salted buttermilk
  Commercial milk foods, e.g. ice cream,
    sherbert, malted milk, milkshakes,
    instant cocoa mixes

Protein foods
  Meats              Fish
    Brains             Canned
    Kidneys            Salted or smoked
    Canned, salted     Shellfish
      or smoked        Frozen
  Cheeses
    All kinds except low-sodium or
      unsalted cottage cheese
  Peanut butter (except low-sodium variety)

Vegetables
  Regular canned vegetables or juices
  Frozen vegetables that contain salt
  Artichokes
  Beets and beet greens
  Carrots
  Celery, celery leaves, and celery seeds
  Chard
  Dandelion greens
  Hominy
  Kale
  Mustard greens
  Sauerkraut
  Spinach
  White turnips

Fruits
  Dried or frozen with sodium sulfite or
    salt added
  Olives
  Canned tomatoes, tomato juice, or
    tomato puree

Breads
  Regular commercial breads, crackers,
    and bread mixes
  Cooked cereals with sodium
  Dry cereals with more than 6 mg per 100 gm
  Self-rising meals or flours

Fats
  Salted butter and margarine
  Regular salad dressings
  Bacon and bacon fat

Beverages
  Beverage mixes
  Soft drinks
  Fountain beverages
  Commercial bouillon
  Tomato juice
  Cocoa and chocolate-flavored beverage
    powders

Sweets
  Commercial candies and gelatin desserts
  Rennet tablets
  Pudding mixes
  Molasses

Seasonings
  Flavored salts
  Catsup
  Chili sauce
  Prepared mustard
  Salted horseradish
  Meat and vegetable extracts
  Meat sauces and tenderizers
  Soy sauce
  Worcestershire sauce
  Olives
  Pickles
  Relishes

allowed), or a raw vegetable or fruit salad without dressing (cooked vegetables are often seasoned with salt or monosodium glutamate). Planes, trains and hotels sometimes can provide special foods if notified in advance, but the safest method is to carry a supply of low-sodium dietetic foods on trips and to pack lunches to take to work.

All products on the list of foods to be avoided on the mildly restricted diet described earlier must be avoided on the severely restricted diet. Additional foods, particularly meats and milk products, are now forbidden. Some may surprise and even puzzle the patient. For example, a few vegetables (of many, fortunately) have too much sodium to be allowable foods, except very occasionally as a bit of flavoring or a garnish. One hundred grams (about 3 oz) of raw carrots contains about 47 mg of sodium; even in the dietetic pack, carrots have 39 mg of sodium per 100 mg. Beets, celery and spinach are other vegetables relatively high in sodium; 100 gm of raw spinach contains 71 mg of sodium. Raw fresh tomatoes have only about 3 mg per 100 gm, but canned tomato juice contains 200 mg per 100 gm.

Milk and meats, needed as sources of protein but highest in sodium of allowable foods, are restricted to two 8-oz cups and 5 oz per day, respectively. Vegetables high in sodium are removed from the list; only vegetables listed as having moderately high, low or negligible sodium content can be used. Sodium compounds in foods are forbidden. The only change for a regimen lower than 500 mg per day would be to use low-sodium milk rather than ordinary milk. Since low-sodium milk is expensive and difficult to obtain, it is the last food to be added to the list. Caloric content can be increased by adding servings of any permitted food except milk, meat and eggs.

The diet may be planned as follows. If the diet should be limited to 1000 mg of sodium per day, the prescribed component of the ration should provide only 500 mg; the patient may they choose according to his taste from among ordinary forbidden sodium compounds or foods to make up the extra 500 mg. The supplementary component is usually small. For example, whether the diet allows 500 mg or 1000 mg of sodium, it is usually made up of a fixed amount of basic (protein) foods and a set amount of vegetables moderately high in sodium; calories are adjusted by varying low-sodium foods. Specifically, 500 mg of sodium equals a scant 1/4 teaspoon of salt or 3/4 teaspoon of monosodium glutamate, one-half of a commercial bouillon cube. 1 cup canned tomato juice, one serving of cooked cereal or pasta made with salt, or 1/2 cup of drained sauerkraut. Each of the following contains 200 mg of sodium: 1 oz of canned tuna; 2/3 cup salted buttermilk; 1/2 cup seasoned carrots, spinach, or other forbidden vegetable; five salted nuts, or two slices of drained bacon; 50 mg of sodium is found in each of the following: 3 oz of shrimp, 1 oz of natural cheddar cheese, 1 tablespoon of catsup, one slice of regular bread, 1 teaspoon of salted butter, 1/2 cup of raw carrots or celery, or 1 1/2 teaspoons of regular mayonnaise.

At a level of 500 mg of sodium per day or below, no additions can be permitted.

The more restrictions are tightened, the more necessary it becomes to emphasize the positive aspects of the diet to some patients. Good health is certainly one such aspect, but it sometimes is difficult for the patient to keep it in mind. The advice of a dietitian may help the patient adhere to his diet. Dietitians are trained to think of food in terms of cooking a finished product, and a few are even gourmet cooks themselves.

If the patient has not already discovered the pleasures of experimenting with foods, the many possibilities of flavoring with herbs, spices and wines, and the special taste of fresh as opposed to canned or frozen foods, this is a very good time to start. A few suggestions: sweet butter and lemon juice on asparagus; green peppers, tomatoes, and chili powder with corn; dill, thyme, marjoram, nutmeg, or unsalted French dressing with green beans; onion, mushrooms, mint, or lettuce with fresh peas; mace, onion, parsley, chives or scallions with potatoes; ginger, cloves or nutmeg with winter squash; onions and green pepers with summer squash; basil, chervil or tarragon with tomatoes; sweet butter and dill with salmon or other fish; mushrooms and tarragon with eggs; bay leaf, cumin or oregano with veal; rosemary with lamb; garlic and sage with pork; bay leaf, thyme, marjoram, onion, dry mustard, or nutmeg with beef; paprika or sage with chicken; fruits with almost any meat or poultry as an accompaniment or glaze. Drinking wines (with the physician's permission) with most meats, poultry, fish, fruits and desserts will usually improve the morale of patients on a low-sodium diet. An imaginative cook can produce what is still a palatable diet, in spite of the severe handicap presented by salt restriction.

The low-sodium diet will be with the patient for a long time, and he will generally adhere to it in the measure that it can be made to seem an endurable challenge rather than an impossible, confusing and tasteless burden.

## REFERENCES

1. Food and Nutrition Board: Sodium-restricted diets: The rationale, complications, and practical aspects of their use. Washington, D.C., National Academy of Sciences — National Research Council, 1954.
2. American Heart Association: Your 500 mg. Sodium Diet — Strict Sodium Restriction; Your 1000 mg. Sodium Diet — Moderate Sodium Restriction; Your Mild Sodium-Restricted Diet. American Heart Association, 44 East 23rd Street, New York, N.Y. 10010.

*Chapter 60*

# NUTRITION AND CANCER

## NUTRITIONAL PROBLEMS CAUSED DIRECTLY BY TUMORS AND BY DISEASES ASSOCIATED WITH THE PRESENCE AND GROWTH OF TUMORS

L ET us at the onset limit the scope of this chapter. We shall not deal with possible nutritional etiologies of various types of cancer. There are a number of theories, some of them bolstered by cogent facts, which suggest that certain types of tumors may originate in the continual presence of certain foods or factors in the diet. However, none of these theories has reached the stage which calls for an urgent readjustment in our dietary habits similar, for example, to that associated with attempts to prevent atherosclerosis by dietary means. The present chapter will instead be concerned with the nutritional disturbances caused by cancer and cancer-related diseases and with those brought about by drugs, radiation and surgery used in the treatment of cancer and with the dietary measures which can be taken to minimize these disturbances.

Neoplastic diseases are commonly (though not universally) accompanied by three systemic effects: a negative nitrogen balance, a speeded up basal metabolic rate, and anorexia.

A severe anorexia can appear well before any obvious contributing cause, such as intestinal obstruction, endocrine disorder, anatomic lesion, or sepsis. The anorexia is often accompanied by mental depression (with fear or guild feelings frequently obvious) which complicates treatment further. And it occurs during a period of active progression of the disease when the drain caused by tumor growth makes excellent nutrition particularly urgent for the patient's welfare. There are few reports of lowered basal

Reprinted from *Postgraduate Medicine, 50* (No. 4 and 5), Oct. and Nov. 1971.

metabolic rate in the face of active malingancies; some patients have a rate within the normal range, but the rule, first noted by Pettenkofer and Voit in a leukemic patient almost 100 years ago, is that basal energy production is considerably increased. Thus both the anorexia and the increased basal metabolism contribute to the body wasting that is seen so often. The caloric expenditure is usually decreased during periods of remission.

While a negative nitrogen balance is most often observed in metabolic studies of patients with actively growing tumors, nitrogen equilibrium and even a positive balance have been observed in some such patients, suggesting that the growing tumor retains nitrogen even while the host tissues are losing it. Cases where the tumor n t only appeared to feed upon the nitrogen in the diet, but also on the nitrogen of healthy tissues have been reported. As in the case of the basal metabolic rate, the situation seems to be reversed with tumor regression. After effective therapy, the normal tissues again retain nitrogen, and also appear to incorporate some nitrogen from the inactive tumor.

More extensive studies in experimental animals using radioactive amino acids confirm these suggestions. In fact, investigators have considered the active tumor a "nitrogen trap," comparing it to a dead end street from metabolic pool to tumor. More recent studies indicate that there may be some exchange of nitrogen between tumor and host, but it is clear that, once incorporated in the protein material of the growing tumor, the amino acids tend to remain there rather than take part in the turnover process seen in normal tissues. In rats, rapidly growing tumors have been shown to draw nitrogen from host tissue so as to maintain their growth rate even when the host is on a very low-protein diet. Other studies have shown that, even when the diet contains what appear to be adequate amounts of protein and calories, and even, finally, under forced feeding, the host could not indefinitely maintain a favorable weight and nitrogen balance. Even on an adequate diet, as the tumor continued to grow it eventually depleted surrounding tissues.

A neoplasm thus ultimately has a unique effect on its host. Granted, it has been demonstrated that organ regeneration is possible in starved animals, or that pregnant rats on a protein-free diet can produce viable young; growth at the expense of the host is not unknown. But growth which eventually destroys the host, even with every attempt to meet nutrient requirements, is characteristic of the cancerous cell. Pregnant mice and mice with transplanted tumors were studied over the same period. They increased their dietary intake by the same amount as compared with normal controls. The pregnant mice were able to create fetal tissue at a rate double that of the tumor growth and still gain body weight. The mice with tumors lost 25 per cent of their body weight in the same three weeks. We are still unable to explain this phenomenon.

This lack of understanding of the basic mechanisms involved in the nutrition of tumor cells and in the nutritional interrelationship between tumor and host is one of the factors which cast doubt on the extent of the benefit, if any, to be derived from hyper-alimentation of human patients during an active phase of cancer growth. A number of clinical studies suggest the possibility that the beneficial effect of a high dietary intake of calories and protein may be temporary. For example, Pareira (1) found that it was possible to reverse the rapid weight loss of terminal cancer with tube feeding, but only temporarily. Patients force-fed by Terepka and Waterhouse (2) gained in body weight, but much of the gain was merely intracellular fluid, and in some, there was a suggestion that tumor growth was accelerated during the feeding period. Levenson and Watkn (3) also noted the increase in tumor activity with introvenous high-calories feeding and found that the cancer patients stayed in negative nitrogen balance in spite of the treatment. Instead, their basal metabolic rate increased, and on discontinuance of the feeding they lost weight rapidly. It may be noted that most such tests were conducted using artificial feeding; against the usual background of anorexia and depression, and considering the many reasons for discomfort associated with eating in the normal way, the problem of getting most patients to consume merely an adequate number of nutrients is paramount in ambulatory or outpatient situations. A letter to the Editor of *Lancet* published November 8, 1969, provides an interesting footnote. It cited the case of cancer outpatient, who, on hearing that many cancer victims die of starvation, literally force-fed himself at every opportunity. According to the correspondent, the patient not only succeeded in feeding himself adequately, but there was a subsequent remission in the disease, which the correspondent suggests may have had some connection with the eating regimen.

Besides these nutritional problems usually encountered in any type of neoplastic disease, other nutritional disturbances are the result of more specific tumors. The most obvious of these are the consequence of lesions or obstructions in some part of the alimentary or gastrointestinal tracts. The simplest is an interference with food intake by partial or complete obstruction which must be removed surgically, substituting artificial feeding for oral intake until food can again be taken normally. When such an operation has to be performed in the stomach or the intestinal tract, it ususally also results in digestive disturbances and/or malabsorption if any condition has been created which produces an insufficient or ineffective intestinal absorptive surface.

Malabsorption can also result from involvement of the pancreas, pancreatic duct, and common bile duct, all of which will interfere with formation or secretion of digestive enzymes and ancillary substances, or of bile salts. Biliary obstruction can also lead to prothrombin deficiency. Digestion of fats and the fat-soluble vitamins is affected, and can cause vitamin D deficiency with consequent osteomalacia. Protein and electrolyte absorption may be impaired. Leukemia, lymphoma, and solid tumors which infiltrate the small bowel or mesenteric lymphnodes significantly impair absorption of a number of nutrients, copper among them. Folic acid depletion is frequently seen in leukemias, lymphomas, and tumors of the head and neck.

In patients with abdominal tumors, gastrocolic or jejunocolic fistulas may result in bypass of the small bowel, causing not only significant malabsorption, but also electrolyte and fluid disturbances. Diarrhea and steatorrhea are seen in the Zollinger-Ellison syndrome in many cases where the pacreatic islet cell adenoma is malignant, in bronchogenic carcinoma, and in intestinal cardinoid tumors.

In addition to the nitrogen imbalance common to most cancer conditions, protein can be lost through malabsorption and through enteropathies associated with gastric carcinoma or lymphomas (4).

Fluid and electrolytes are lost primarily through vomiting and diarrhea. Water-soluble vitamins poorly absorbed from the gastro-intestinal tract may be lost concurrently. Fluid and electrolyte imbalances are also seen in patients with active, widespread liver and cardiac metastases and hepatic or heart failure, with ascites caused by hepatic and ovarian carcinomas, with renal failure due to obstruction of the urinary tract by tumor, urates or paren-chymal neoplasms, and in patients with extensive edema caused by obstruction of venous or lymphatic drainage. Diarrhea in patients with villous adenoma and adenocarcinoma of the colon as also been observed to cause severe electrolyte imbalance.

Tumors which influence hormone production and secretion also alter electrolyte metabolism. Malignant tumors or the lung have been reported to cause increased sodium losses and hyponatremia; this complication has been attributed to an uncontrolled secretion of antidiuretic hormone. Hyperadrenocorticism is seen in non-adrenal malignant tumors of the thoracic cavity. The patients show increased steroid production and pronounced hyperplasia of the adrenals. Extracts of some tumors have produced material with activity like that of adrenocorticotropic hormone. Amino acid analyses of extracts from Zollinger-Ellison tumors, have shown that they contain material virtually identical in com-position to one or both of the gastrin peptides found in normal mucosa. It appears probable that the gastric hyperacidity seen seen in this syndrome results from release of this material from the tumors.

Hypokalemia, characteristically seen in patients with hyper-adrenocorticism, is also observed in malignancies of the intestinal tract. Hypoanatremia, often an accompaniment of lung tumors, has also been seen in medullary corcinoma of the thyroid associated with excess secretion of calcitonin and an increase of urinary sodium and phosphorus.

Hypercalcemia is a feature of breast cancer, particularly when metastases of the bone are readily demonstrable, and of osseous ,cancer. Patients with breast cancer also have been seen to exhibit an abnormally high rate of iron clearance, which has slowed somewhat massive doses of androgens.

Anemia is often seen in cancer patients; sometimes it is a direct result of nutritional factors, such as the anorexia, but more commonly it is related to other causes: malabsorption of vitamins and protein, hormonal imbalances, suppression of prothrombin synthesis, an increase in hemolysis or bleeding of ulcerated lesions such as in the peptic ulcer of the Zollinger-Ellison syndrome, or in gastrointestinal fistulas.

From a nutritional as well as from a general medical viewpoint, cancer is not the only disease process to be considered in patients with active neoplasms. Concomitant illnesses, renal, metabolic, cardiovascular — all of which have nutritional implications — must also be considered. Cancer in its turn initiates other disease processes, which in their turn cause other nutritional problems. For instance, bronchial adenoma and other argentaffinoma can cause the carcinoid syndrome or serotonin excess, which in turn produces symptoms of nicotinic acid deficiency; renal carcinoma causes polycythemia; various carcinomas alter systemic thrombosis and cause bleeding; thymoma causes myasthenia gravis and depresses erythropoiesis. Malignant lymphocytoid plasma cells cause macroglobulinemia, and multiple myeloma can produce amyloidosis. It is possible that uterine fundus cancer can cause diabetes mellitus. All of these secondary or tertiary phenomena have nutritional implications.

It is obvious that there can be no nutritional cure for any of these nutritional problems; there is probably no long-term nutritional therapy which can adequately make up the nutrients lost in the malabsorption syndrome or appropriated by the growing tumor. The only effective therapy once the diagnosis of cancer is established is excision or destruction of the neoplasm by surgery or other methods. What nutrient therapy can accomplish is to give the patient strength during the treatment period, prepare him to better withstand the traumas of treatment, and make his life a little easier if the disease is incurable.

## PROBLEMS CAUSED BY TREATMENT OF CANCER WITH DRUGS, RADIATION AND SURGERY

### Chemotherapy

It is now widely recognized that hormones used in therapy can produce a number of metabolic aberrations which, in turn, can be mitigated by appropriate nutritional measures. The adreno-corticosteroids, depending on the type, dose, and length of treatment, may cause significant losses of protein, calcium and postassium. Estrogens may cause nausea and vomiting unless the dose is increased gradually; when they are withdrawn, fluid retention and internal bleeding can occur. Estrogen therapy in metastatic breast cancer has also been reported to have caused rapid and acute, finally fatal hypercalcemia in some patients. It has been suggested that prednisone may effect a reversal if serum calcium levels do not rise with cessation of estrogen therapy. In other cases, cortisone has been used.

Androgens such as testosterone have an anabolic effect and can be used beneficially to improve nitrogen retention. However, they also bring about retention of fluids and sodium; hepatitis is also occasionally seen in androgen therapy. Synthetic drugs, (unfortunately, still very costly) have been developed which mimic the anabolic effect of androgens while producing less side-effects. Insulin, at one time used as an appetite stimulant can cause acute hypoglycemia, and is not recommended by comparison with other alternatives, including alcoholic stimulants.

Folic acid antagonists, the amcthoptcrins, cause damage to areas of rapid cellular proliferation other than the neoplastic tissues, especially the bone marrow and the gastrointestinal mucosa. Functionally, the intestinal alterations are much like those seen in sprue: in particular, a decrease in absorptive capacity for the test substance xylose and for nutrients. It has been demonstrated by electromicroscopic examination that intestinal cells show alterations after a patient has received a single intravenous injection of methotrexate at doses of 2 to 5 mg per kg body weight. Such changes are prevented by giving the metabolite, citrovorum factor, by simultaneous infusion with the antimetabolite at a rate of 6 mg every 6 hours. The infusion can also be used to correct any electrolyte imbalance.

The fluoridated pyrimidines, such as 5-fluorouracil, injected intravenously against solid tumors, affect the gastrointestinal mucosa, producing stomatitis and diarrhea. Morphologic changes, much like those seen in pernicious anemia, are seen in epitheliala as well as cancer cells, with megaloblastic bone marrow a not infrequent concurrent change.

Actinomycin D, used in a number of different types of cancer, and often in conjunction with radiation therapy, causes gastro-intestinal changes with fluid loss and diarrhea, as well as marked hematologic alterations.

Monoamine oxidase inhibitors, used in palliative therapy and before other forms of treatment to relieve the mental and emotional depression seen in many cancer patients, have well-known toxic effects when taken in conjunction with foods containing pressor amines, such as cheese. They can also be directly toxic to a few patients, with strong adverse effects on the central nervous system (5).

### Radiation Therapy

Radiotherapy can unfortunately also cause serious nutritional problems, some of which may not be noticeable for some months and even years after the treatment is over.

Effective radiation therapy used against cancers of the oro-pharyngeal region can destroy the sense of taste, a seemingly minor and benign effect compared with the cancer itself. But it is one which can make a major difference to a patient who may be suffering as well from loneliness, depression, anorexia, and perhaps nausea and diarrhea as well. Such a patient often feels that there remains little reason to eat; when the incentive of taste is also removed, special attention must be given to making food appealing in other ways, such as appearance and aroma.

The intestinal damage caused by radiation can be more serious. The small bowel is especially susceptible to ionizing ratiation which can cause edema and congestion as well as paristalsis, inducing either over-or under-activity. Intestinal radiation may also produce endarteritis in the small vessels; the intestinal wall may show fibrosis, stenosis, necrosis, and ulceration. These, in turn, may result, over an extended period, in hemorrhages, obstruction fistulas, diarrhea and malabsorption. Necrosis may become generalized, so that the indurated bowel is surrounded by fibrous tissue.

Radiation therapy in small children at doses considered safe for healthy liver tissue (which is supposedly quite radioresistant) was observed to result in gross liver damage, with decreased uptake of radionuclides and subsequent atrophy in both hepatic and reticuloendothelial cells. Apparently, the liver in children is quite susceptible to radiation damage (5).

## Surgery

Many of the surgical procedures used in cancer are also used in other diseases, but resections of the oropharyngeal area, total esophagectomy, and total gastrectomy are most often used in cancer patients. There are a number of advantages to resection, especially in the upper alimentary tract and the small bowel, such as relieve of obstruction and control of blood loss and electrolyte disturbance. The disadvantages are mechanical difficulties in food ingestion or the necessity for long-term dependence on tube feeding in radical resection of the oropharnygeal area, and gastric stasis, malabsorption, and fistula or stenosis caused by tube feeding in esophagectomy and esophageal reconstruction. Malabsorption of fat is espically noticeable, and may be related to the bilateral vagotomy which is a part of the surgery. The gastric stasis and diarrhea seen in some of these patients make pyloroplasty or gastroenterostomy necessary. The same effects have been seen in patients undergoing surgery of duodenal ulcers. Decreased intake is apt to result from the feeling of gastric fullness after an inadequately small meal. The number of feedings must be increased to compensate for the small meals (6).

Gastrectomy can be followed by a number of serious nutritional distrubances. The severe dumping syndrome which appears in some patients is related to rapid intestinal absorption of dextrose. Nausea, cramps, epigastric fullness, sweating and flushing, faintness, as well as tachycardia, tachypnea, and pallor are frequently observed. The symptoms diminish with time, but can easily lead to a strong aversion to eating. It is possible that the gastrointestinal and vasomotor disturbances are related to serotonin release, or to release into the bloodstream of a material like the polypeptide bradykinin.

Steatorrhea is common after gastrectomy, although it varies in intensity in different patients. In a series of patients subjected to total gastrectomy the absorption range was found to be 41 to 97 per cent, but only a very small proportion of the patients were in that part of the range above 92 per cent (the "normal" range). Losses of nitrogen in the feces are usually no greater than 1-2 grams per day above average.

The dumping syndrome, bile regurgitaition, and similar unpleasant or painful complications increase the risk of malnutrition in free-living patients, unless careful attention is given to meal planning. A regimen of "nibbling" rather than large meals separated by long intervals and a choice of foods high in protein, moderate in fat, and restricted in carbohydrate are often found helpful. Sometimes liquid is restricted at meals, and in grave steatorrhea, fat intake must be lowered further.

Phytobezoar can be a problem in gastrectomized subjects, for bulky, fibrous, or inadequately chewed foods can be impossible to digest, and obstruction can result. The patient must be instructed to chew all foods well, and to avoid those which the stomach, with its impaired function, cannot cope with adequately. Another cause of steatorrhea in gastrecomy can be bacterial overgrowth in the afferent loop. Malabsorption may also result, and antibiotic therapy or even another operation may be needed.

Total or near-total gastrectomy also means removal of cells which secrete intrinsic factor. Vitamin $B_{12}$ is therefore no longer absorbed and, after a period of time, macrocytosis and pernicious anemia will result unless $B_{12}$ therapy is undertaken. Even with partial gastrectomy there is apt to be a deficiency of the fat-soluble vitamins, iron, and vitamin $B_{12}$. Calcium metabolism appears to be affected in 30 to 40 per cent of gastrectomized patients studied, and may be related to the deficiency of the fat-soluble vitamins, vitamin D in particular. Bone pain and osteomalcia may be the result.

Ablation of the small intestine affects absorption to a greater or lesser degree depending on the site and extent of the operation. Physiological studies have shown that most nutrients are absorbed in the proximal part of the small bowel. Therefore, localized resection of the ileum will probably be associated only with loss of vitamin $B_{12}$. Resection of the jejunum still leaves the ileum to absorb significant amounts of the other nutrients. Extensive resection of the distal part of the small intestine will cause steatorrhea and creatorrhea, as well as malabsorption of $B_{12}$. If the remaining duodenum and jejunum are sufficient to absorb glucose and the rest of the vitamins and minerals, the pateints can be put on a low-fat, high-protein diet with injections of $B_{12}$.

Massive resection, which takes all but a few feet of the proximal jejunum, will cause malabsorption of all nutrients. A low-fat diet, many small "nibbles" of solid foods, and parenteral administration of $B_{12}$ and other vitamins and minerals will be needed.

Sodium and fluid losses are usually seen immediately following ileostomy. They usually become less and are stabilized by the tenth day. After this, the patients lose from 300 to 600 ml water, 40 to 100 mEq of sodium and 2.5 to 10 mEq of potassium. Greater losses are seen in some patients with gastroenteritis, intestinal obstruction, and sweating.

The "blind loop syndrome" of gastrectomized patients has long been known. It is associated with the appearance of a blood condition very like that of pernicious anemia. The immediate causes of the syndrome vary; improperly draining loop in Billroth II gastrectomy, multiple jejunal diverticuli, or enterostomies are some of them. In all cases, an area of stasis appears in the intestine. Malabsorption, particularly of vitamin $B_{12}$ but also of the fats and fat soluble vitamins, proteins, and minerals follows. Carbohydrate absorption may also be impaired. There is an apparent local growth of abnormal intestinal flora, and the stasis must finally be eliminated by surgery. Tetracyclines can be used temporarily to combat abnormal bacterial proliferation.

Pancreatectomy (which also inevitably implies partial gastrectomy) means loss of digestive enzymes, and so leads to losses of proteins, fats, minerals, and vitamins in the stools, as well as to the disorders associated with gastrectomy. The diabetes mellitus seen in these patients is hard to control precisely, despite the fact that the insulin requirement is small.

Ileal bladder construction can control, to some extent, the disturbances in acid-base balance and hyperchloremic acidosis seen after ureterosigmoidostomy, when the bladder is removed and the ureters implanted into the sigmoid colon.

It may not be necessary to state that should therapy be successful and result in prolonged survival, should all acute short-term nutritional disturbances resulting from the presence of the neoplasm and from its successful excision, irradiation and chemotherapy be surmounted, there is still need for the long-term monitoring of all nutritional indices. Only if this is done at regular intervals can preventable secondary deficiencies be avoided.

## REFERENCES

1. Pareira, M. D., Conrad, E. J., Hicks, W. and Elman, R.: Clinical response and changes in nitrogen balance, body weight, plasma proteins, and hemoglobin following tube feeding in cancer cachexia. Cancer, 8:803-808, 1955.
2. Terepka, A. R. and Waterhouse, C.: Metabolic observations during the forced feeding of patients with cancer. Am. J. Med., 20:225-238, 1956.
3. Levenson, S. M. and Watkin, D. M.: Protein requirements in injury and certain acute and chronic diseases. Fed. Proc., 18:1155-1190, 1959.
4. Watkin, D. M.: Nitrogen balance as affected by neoplastic disease and its therapy. Am. J. Clin. Nutrition, 9:446-460, 1961.
5. Shils, M. E.: Nutrition in neoplastic diseases, in Wohl, M. G. and Goodhart, R. S.: Modern Nutrition in Health and Disease, 4th ed. Philadelphia, Lea & Febiger, 1968. (5th ed. in press, 1971.)
6. The First National Conference on Cancer of the Colon and Rectum. Cancer, 28(1), July 1971.

*Chapter 61*

# IATROGENIC MALNUTRITION

$A$NYONE who has practiced medicine or worked with nutritional problems among medically unsophisticated families is depressingly familiar with the malnutrition induced in sick children by well-meaning parents. A child with diarrhea is adjudged incompetent to digest anything but sugared water, a fever is "starved," and at best, illness is thought to necessitate "very light" meals, grossly inadequate calorically and often deficient in nutrients. In Africa, Asia and Latin America, the "experienced" grandmother's advice not to feed a sick child is often the decisive factor that pushes a young patient into protein-calorie malnutrition. In the Southwest, marasmus and kwashiorkor seen recently among children of migrant workers were due to a combination of patients taking the pyridoxine antagonist desoxypyridoxine, perhaps because it increases the rate of excretion of pyridoxine. The neuritis that often accompanies isoniazid

Less recognized, but infinitely more frquent in the United States, is the malnutrition resulting from long-term administration of drugs in chronic disease. Because of the seriousness of the disease under treatment, the need for continuous control, and the worry that side-effects of the drugs may complicate the course of therapy, all too often the tendency is to concentrate on specific aspects of the condition and forget the possibility or likelihood of long-term nutritional impairment.

Some deleterious effects of drugs on nutrition are well known and are anticipated during treatment. Isoniazid causes signs resembling those seen in patients taking the pyridoxine. The neuritis that often accompanies isoniazid therapy can be prevented by giving large dosages of pyridoxine (over 150 mg per day) from

---

Reprinted from *Postgraduate Medicine*, 49 (No. 3), March, 1971. © McGraw-Hill, Inc.

the beginning of treatment. Another tuberculostatic, para-aminosalicylic acid, causes malabsorption of vitamin $B_{12}$ and lowers serum folic acid values, probably through interference (by competitive inhibition of folic acid?) with the absorption process.

Neomycin causes lesser-known changes resembling those seen in idiopathic steatorrhea: excessive fecal losses of fat, electrolytes (especially potassium), nitrogen, and free fatty acids, as well as malabsorption of carotene, vitamin $B_{12}$, glucose, iron, lactose and D-xylose. The loss of fat and fat-soluble nutrients seems to be proportional to the dose of neomycin; 6 gm causes twice the loss that occurs with 3 gm, and 12 gm four times the loss. Elimination of gluten or oral glucocorticoids does not affect the steatorrhea; only cessation of the neomycin therapy reverses the condition.

The physician must carefully watch and compensate for other well-known nutritional side-effects of therapeutic agents. Anorexia, nausea, vomiting and diarrhea (side-effects of hypotensive drugs) often follow administration of large dosages of guanoxan. Diuretics cause potassium depletion, usually moderate unless the patient is already depleted by hyperaldosteronism, cirrhosis with ascites, or the nephrotic syndrome; such reactions occur particularly with the benzothiadiazine derivatives. Glucosteroids cause excessive loss of calcium and phosphorus that results in osteoporosis. Cholesterol-lowering agents bind bile salts and cause a loss of fat-soluble vitamins, such as the loss of vitamin K which occurs during cholestyramine therapy.

Often misunderstood and thus not monitored is the undramatic, slowly developing malnutrition resulting from long-term, apparently innocuous drug therapy. Because there are no side-effects initially, the physician and the patient may not be aware of the chronic impairment the agent is causing. The term "iatrogenic malnutrition" seems appropriate to characterize this situation, which can be exemplified by two instances: the apparently rare finding of megaloblastic anemia consequent to a course of oral contraceptives and the much more frequent incidence of folate deficiency, osteomalacia and rickets accompanying therapy with anticonvulsant drugs.

Necheles and Snyder (1) recently described two patients on oral contraceptives who had severe megalobastic anemia, characterized by a hemoglobin value less than 5 mg per 100 ml, hematocrit less than 13 per cent, serum folate less than 3 ng, and vitamin $B_{12}$ less than 200 pg per milliliter. Of various treatments, only folic acid therapy gave a positive response. In testing the role of progesteronal agents, these investigators measured the peak rise in serum folate concentration in volunteers to determine absorption with and without such agents. When given alone, crystalline folic acid and folate polyglutamate caused peak increases in serum folate of 10 to 23 ng per milliliter in all subjects. After two cycles of oral contraceptive therapy, serum response to free folic acid was in the same range, but orally administered polyglutamyl folate did not increase serum folate more than 8 ng per milliliter in any subject.

Oral contraceptives may increase the rate of renal clearance or tissue utilization of conjugate folate, but they more likely limit absorption. Whatever the explanation, obviously we must add an important nutritional deficiency syndrome to the growing list of the possible side-effects of oral contraceptive agents.

Epileptic patients taking anticonvulsants tend to have a folate deficiency. In studying a large group of epileptic children on anticonvulsant drugs, Miller (2) observed a substantial number with low serum folate. The anticonvulsants did not significantly affect the values for hemoglobin, hematocrit, erthrocytes, mean corpuscular volume, and mean corpuscular hemoglobin, but in several children who had "slight" macrocytosis, the serum folate level was below 5 ng per milliliter.

Of the drugs studied, diphenylhydatoin sodium (Dilantin®) appeared to be the most critical in this regard. Two-thirds of children taking this preparation had serum folate levels below 5 ng per milliliter, compared with only one-third of patients taking other drugs. Diet apparently was not a variable.

Some investigators have reported anemia and macrocytosis in patients taking anticonvulsants. In addition, at least one study has shown that in patients receiving polyglutamyl folate, administration of phenytoin prevented a rise in serum folate, even though these patients had shown a marked response before phenytoin was given. Free folate caused an increase in serum folate whether or not phenytoin was given.

These examples indicate the need to monitor serum folate, and if necessary, to supplement the diet with free folic acid.

Even more serious risks of anticonvulsant therapy are osteo-malacia and rickets. We have known for some time that an appreciable number of young epileptics show roentgenographic and biochemical evidence of osteomalacia, the severity depending on the duration and dosage of drug therapy. Richens and Rowe (3) recently reported a study of 160 treated epileptics 16 to 70 years old; 22.5 per cent (36 patients) had serum calcium levels below 9 mg per 100 ml, but none of 80 controls had levels below this value. They ruled out the possibility of differences in serum albumin concentration as a cause of the different levels and seamingly eliminated serum phosphorus and vitamin D intake as factors. Serum calcium definitely tended to vary inversely with the number and dosage of drugs given. Pheneturide appeared to have the most unfavorable effect on the serum calcium level, followed by primidone and phenytoin. Phenobarbitone had the least effect on serum calcium.

These authors detailed case studies of a 16-year-old boy and a 61-year-old woman. The boy had been on anticonvulsants since five months of age, most recently phenytoin and primidone. At 13 years of age he had a slightly low serum calcium level. At age 15 a folate deficiency was seen, and folic acid was added to the regimen. Skeletal x-rays showed no pathologic change, but a biopsy specimen of the iliac crest showed osteomalacia. The patient was given whole-body irradiation with ultraviolet rays; he also received vitamin $D_2$ in a dosage of 50 ng daily for two and one-half weeks and then three injections of 350 ng at weekly intervals. After two months, a biopsy specimen of the iliac crest showed a normal histologic pattern.

The woman had taken phenytoin and primidone for many years, and symptoms developed slowly over five years. She had irregular vertebral collapse, serum chemical changes typical of osteomalacia, and amino-aciduria. She also responded to treatment with vitamin $D_2$ and ultraviolet irradiation.

In addition to these two patients, two others (one with a history of megaloblastic anemia) responded to vitamin D therapy. The authors suggested that even with an adequate intake of vitamin D, hepatic enzyme induction by the anticonvulsant drugs leads to increased turnover of vitamin D and hence to tissue deficiency. Another possibility in anticonvulsant therapy and must be watched for and corrected.

Such instances of drug-related malnutrition will probably increase over the years. It appears more and more obvious that any long-term therapeutic course demands detailed periodic examination of the patient's state of nutrition to prevent development of iatrogenic malnutrition.

## REFERENCES

1. Necheles, T. F., Snyder, L. M.: Malabsorption of folate polyglutamates associated with oral contraceptive therapy. New Eng. J. Med., 282:858-859, 1970.
2. Miller, D. R.: Serum folate deficiency in children receiving anticonvulsant therapy. Pediatrics, 41:630-635, 1968.
3. Richens, A., Rowe, D. J.: Disturbance of calcium metabolism by anticonvulsant drugs. Brit. Med. J., 4:73-76, 1970.

*Chapter 62*

# TASTE TESTS AS DIAGNOSTIC TOOLS

$A$BNORMALITIES in hearing and vision have been used as diagnostic tools for many years, not only in the therapy of diseases of the corresponding sense organs but also in the study of more general diseases which affect the function of the ear and the eye early or characteristically. Recently (largely through the efforts of one patient and enthusiastic investigator, Robert I. Henkin, of the National Heart Institute, Bethesda, Maryland) abnormalities in taste have begun to loom as an additional group of symptoms which can be used as diagnostic aids in a number of pathologic situations (1).

## ANATOMY AND PHYSIOLOGY OF TASTE

The anterior two-thirds of the tongue is innervated by a branch of the facial nerve (chorda tympani), and the posterior part by a branch of the glossopharyngeal nerve; a V-shaped groove (sulcus terminalis linguae) separates the two areas. The fungiform papillae are in the anterior two-thirds and contain one to eight taste buds. The posterior third contains larger, circumvallate papillae with many taste buds. Both types of papillae also contain unmyelinated free nerve endings. Papillae, taste buds, and free nerve endings are also found on the surfaces of the hard and soft palates, pharynx and larynx.

The tongue receptors record all four "tastes" (salt, sweet, sour, bitter) but seem particularly sensitive to salt and sweet. The palate also records all four modalities of taste but appears most sensitive to sour and bitter. The pharyngeal and laryngeal receptors are sensitive to all four varieties of taste, but less so than the tongue

Reprinted from *Postgraduate Medicine*, *43* (No. 5), May, 1968.© McGraw-Hill, Inc.

and palate. Physiologically the various methods of measurement of taste acuity which have been devised (1) determine two types of thresholds, the detection threshold and the recognition threshold. The detection threshold is the lowest concentration of a substance which the patient can detect as being different from water. The recognition threshold is the lowest concentration of a substance which the patient can identify as being salty, sweet, bitter or sour.

## TASTE ABNORMALITIES DUE TO ANATOMIC ABNORMALITIES

A common taste abnormality is that caused by artificial dentures covering and fitted closely to the palate. In line with the preceding review on the physiology of taste, it is hardly surprising that patients wearing such dentures show increased detection and recognition thresholds for sour and bitter (2). As could also be expected, thresholds for sweet and salty are not affected.

Patients with the high arched palates characteristic of Turner's syndrome show increased detection and recognition thresholds for sour and bitter, while their thresholds for salt and sweet are normal (3). Henkin has shown that patients with submucous clefts of the dorsal hard palate, hypoplasia of the basicranium, hyposmia, and skeletal growth retardation show a characteristic abnormality called "recognition hypogeusia," in which the recognition threshold for each of the four tastes is elevated while the detection thresholds are normal (1). The patients are unaware of any taste abnormalities; these can be detected only through determination of the thresholds.

Anatomic abnormalities of the surface of the tongue are also, predictably, associated with taste abnormalities. In lichen planus, as in situations where the surface of the tongue is infiltrated by a tumor, taste acuity is lost, as it is following processes which affect the innervation of the lingual surface, such as postdiphtheritic neuritis, glossopharyngeal neuralgia, Bell's palsy, or sarcoidosis (1). Various surgical lesions, certain head injuries, or irradiation of the mouth as part of treatment of malignancies may also affect taste.

Henkin and Kopin (4) have shown that patients with familial

dysautonomia cannot detect any difference between water and saturated solutions of sodium chloride, sucrose or urea, or between water and 0.3 N hydrochloric acid, and cannot recognize these solutions as being salty, sweet bitter or sour. This situation obviously is related to the absence of fungiform and circumvallate papillae. The sulcus terminalis linguae is also absent (1). Methacholine, an acetylcholinelike substance, produces spontaneous crying with tears (missing in this syndrome), as well as a return of detection and recognition thresholds to normal, a phenomenon which suggests that the anatomic abnormality is not alone responsible for the taste abnormality (4).

## TASTE ABNORMALITIES DUE TO DRUGS

Gymnemic acid decreases the taste of sweet and bitter without altering that of salt or sour. The hallucinogen psilocybin increases taste sensitivity in all its modalities (5). Many other rarely used drugs have similarly been reported to have differential effects on the various taste thresholds.

The significant decrease in taste acuity occurring in about 30 per cent of a large group of patients receiving D-pennicillamine has been systematically investigated (6). When the decrease in taste acuity occurred, it was seen in each of the four modalities of taste. The patients were aware of it. They complained of a "metallic taste" and had to add more salt or sugar to their food to have it taste salty or sweet. They felt that foods were without flavor. When use of D-penicillamine was stopped, taste acuity did not return to normal for four to eight weeks.

Henkin suggested that copper depletion is an essential element in development of this condition. D-Penicillamine is a metal chelator. When it is given to patients with Wilson's disease to lower the serum level of copper (elevated because of deficiency of the copper-carrying protein ceruloplasmin), a decrease in taste acuity correlates with the decrease in serum copper. Henkin hypothesized that copper may participate in an enzymatic reaction which either initiates or maintains the taste response, that it might be a component of a "protein complex" necessary for maintaining the normal taste-bud integrity (biopsy specimens of fungiform papillae of patients with decreased acuity following D-penicillamine administration fail to show taste buds), or that it may participate in the electrochemical mechanism of taste reception. Whether copper deficiency operates through taste abnormalities, as Henkin has surmised, and causes the geophagia observed in copper-deficient infants, in individuals with nutritional dwarfism, and in copper-deficient cattle seems to this reviewer more speculative.

## TASTE ABNORMALITIES IN DISEASE

Patients with untreated adrenocortical insufficiency show enormously decreased detection thresholds, with many of them able to detect concentrations less than one-hundredth of those perceived by normal subjects (7). Cessation of therapy, similarly, is accompanied within a few days by a considerable drop in the detection thresholds. Treatment with desoxycorticosterone or other sodium-potassium-active sterols does not alter the heightened taste sensitivity, which responds only to sufficient dosage of carbohydrate-active steroids.

Patients with panhypopituitarism also have a massive drop in each of the four detection thresholds, which return to normal only in response to treatment with carbohydrate-active steroids. Patients with nonsalt-losing congenital adrenal hyperplasia show an analogous increase in taste detection acuity and a decrease after suppressive therapy with carbohydrate-active steroids (6).

Other endocrine disturbances have been accompanied by changes in sensitivity to glucose, both in experimental animals and in patients with diabetes (5). For that matter, various phases of the menstrual cycle and of pregnancy have been reported to be characterized by variations in taste sensitivity (8). Patients with pseudohypoparathyroidism show an increased detection and recognition thresholds of sour and bitter, although thresholds for salt and sweet are within the normal range (6). Treatment which lowers serum phosphorus and raises serum calcium does not alter the taste thresholds. The decreased taste acuity, like pseudo-hypoparathyroidism itself, seems to be inherited as an X-linked dominant characteristic.

Some otherwise normal individuals show an increased sensitivity to the bitter taste of substances such as para-ethoxyphenylthiourea or phenylthiocarbamide (PTC), while others show congenital taste blindness for one or another of the four modalities of taste. Interest in such abnormalities is heightened by the possible association with the carrying of genes for certain diseases. For example, increased sensitivity for all taste modalities has been reported among patients with cystic fibrosis (9) and among their mothers (4).

## CONCLUSION

It will be some time before taste (and olfaction, which has been even more neglected) joins vision and hearing among the senses which are routinely tested, but evidence accumulated recently is intriguing. As is reflected in the medical work reviewed here, there is a renewal of interest in both the normal physiology and the psychology of taste, and the exploration of possible fields of practical application of this knowledge is expanding. It appears that measurements of taste acuity are already a tool reliable enough to give valuable indications on the course of treatment with an agent such as D-penicillamine or carbohydrate-active steroid. They are also already of importance in diagnosing various pathologic conditions in the oral region and in diagnosing and perhaps following the genetics of various admittedly rare conditions. Further advances in this field will be followed with interest.

## REFERENCES

1. Henkin, R. I.: Abnormalities of taste and olfaction in various disease states. In Kare, M. R. and Maller, O. (Editors): The Chemical Senses and Nutrition. Baltimore, Johns Hopkins Press, 1967, pp.95-113.
2. Strain, J. C.: The influence of complete dentures upon taste perception. J. Prosth. Dent., 2:60, 1952.
3. Henkin, R. I.: Hypogonadism associated with familial hyposmia. Clin. Res., 13:244, 1965.
4. Henkin, R. I. and Kopin, I. J.: Abnormalities of taste and smell thresholds in familial dysautonomia: Improvement with methacholine. Life Sci., 3:1319, 1964.
5. Fischer, R. Griffin, F. and Rockey, M. A.: Gustatory chemoreception in

man: Multidisciplinary aspects and perspectives. Perspect. Biol. Med., 9:549, 1966.

6. Henkin, R. I.: The role of taste in disease and nutrition. Borden. Rev. Nutr. Res., 28:71, 1967.

7. Henkin, R. I. and Solomon, D. H.: Salt-taste threshold in adrenal insufficiency in man. J. Clin. Endocr., 22:856, 1962.

8. Glanville, E. V. and Kaplan, A. R.: The menstrual cycle and sensitivity of taste perception. Amer. J. Obstet. Gynec., 92:189, 1965.

9. Henkin, R. I. and Powell, G. F.: Increased sensitivity of taste and smell in cystic fibrosis. Science, 138:1107, 1962.

## Chapter 63

# VITAMINS AND MENTAL DISORDERS

$I$N the course of my travels across the country, I have encountered mounting interest in the possibility that enormous doses of certain vitamins may be beneficial to schizophrenics and other mentally ill patients. Linus Pauling's (1) famous (or notorious) publication in *Science* has given the older claims of proponents of massive vitamin therapy some scientific respectability. On the basis of distant extrapolations (e.g. the cure of the psychologic signs of pellagra and of vitamin $B_{12}$ deficiency by appropriate vitamins, and consideration of growth rates of *Neurospora* mutants), Pauling, the greatest living chemist, suggested the likelihood that certain psychiatric patients have general or brain tissue requirements many, many times greater than normal. Only massive vitamin supplementation can satisfy these requirements and permit normal brain function.

In 1952 two Canadians, Hoffer and Osmond (2), using very large doses of niacin and ascorbic acid on adult schizophrenics, initiated the "megadose" vitamin treatment for mental illness. As early as 1939, Sydenstricker and his co-workers had reported the successful treatment of patients with severe psychiatric symptoms by the use of large doses of nicotinic acid (0.3 to 1.5 gm per day), but there was a presumption of pellagra even though physical signs were absent. Hoffer and Osmond have customarily used very large doses of nicotinic acid or nicotinamide (3 to 18 gm per day), together with 3 gm of ascorbic acid per day. The rationale for using nicotinc acid or its amide was essentially based on the favorable psychologic effect of these agents on pellagrous patients and on Sydenstricker's reports. The rationale for using ascorbic acid is not as clear.

The observation that guinea pigs have a twentyfold range of required intake of ascorbic acid has led some investigators to estimate that certain types of patients might require as much as 15

Reprinted from *Postgraduate Medicine*, 45 (No. 4), April, 1969.© McGraw-Hill, Inc.

gm of ascorbic acid a day, presumably on the supposition that the variability in man may be much greater than in the guinea pig. It should be noted that 15 gm is 200 times the allowance of 75 mg that the Food and Nutrition Board of the National Research Council at one time recommended for the American population (presumably already taking into account individual variations) and is considered by most to be extravagantly high.

However, 15 gm is not the highest value claimed to be therapeutically beneficial. Herjanic and Moss-Herjanic (3) have given a patient up to 110 gm of ascorbic acid per day. Such gigantic doses are predicated not just on "chemical individuality" but on the theory (as yet unproved) that schizophrenia is characterized by either a massive rate of destruction of ascorbic acid or a block to the passage of ascorbic acid through the bloodbrain barier.

(The argument that administering megadoses of water-soluble vitamins is both cheap and safe compared with other treatments – a statement that I readily concede – could be invalidated by the emotional cost of disappointed expectations on the part of the patient's family) This is even more probable since children recently have been given vitamin therapy as often as adults.

Children have been treated daily with niacin (30 mg to 6 gm), ascorbic acid (100 mg to 6 gm), pyridoxine (5 mg to 400 mg), and pathothenic acid (25 mg to 900 mg). These studies have not been systematic, as even Rimland (4), one of the enthusiasts of vitamin therapy, recognizes. In a recent review he conceded that "findings must be presented in anecdotal form." The reports of physicians he quotes appraise results of vitamin therapy as being from "most encouraging" to "absolutely fantastic." Results reported by parents show a similar range. Rimland discounts the placebo effect in exploring favorable results for the following reasons: (1) Many of the cases represent "single clinical experiments" conducted on a "trial and error" basis independent of each other; yet, they show surprising consistency in converging toward nicotinamide and vitamins $B_6$ and C (and sometimes pantothenic acid). (2) Improvement shown is enormous. (3) Other drugs tried almost always have had no effect, so that the very existence of a placebo effect is doubtful. (4) Discontinuing or reducing dosage caused deterioration of the state of the patient. (5) Error in filling prescriptions resulted in observed changes in the state of the patient.

I am a nutritionist, not a psychiatrist. In spite of this, I venture to take issue with Rimland and his fellow enthusiasts on the basis of the vagaries of the course of schizophrenia. While clinical observations collected by careful and interested observers should never be discounted and are profitably used as the foundation of a working hypothesis, it seems to me impossible to test the value of a treatment for schizophrenia (short of total, permanent cure, which is not the case here) except through the most meticulous double-blind procedure. Then neither the attitude of the therapist nor the description of the effects of the therapy can be biased in any way, and the analysis of results can be completely objective. Failure to observe these precautions led to the announcement a decade ago that alcoholism could be cured by large doses of vitamins — also a theory predicated on the fact of individual chemical variation extrapolated to a theory of "partial genetotropic block" and badly tested experimentally.

The evidence presently available does not appear to support the claims that megadose vitamin therapy is a successful treatment for schizophrenia. On the other hand, it can be taken as sufficient to justify systematic experimentation on well-fed patients, using an appropriate sample of the sick population; controlling intake, activity and the effects of hospitalization and other environmental factors; and using tight diagnostic criteria and well-defined methodologic precautions such as a double-blind technics. Even though I am doubtful of results at this point, the cost of mental disease is such, in suffering and in resources, that such an investigation, however expensive, can be justified. On the other hand, results to date do not suffice to raise the hopes of parents of schizophrenics. If this is exaggerated skepticism, so be it. All I ask to be proved wrong is solid evidence. No one will be more pleased if it is forthcoming.

## REFERENCES

1. Pauling, L.: Orthomolecular psychiatry. Science, 160:265-271, 1968.
2. Hoffer, A. and Osmond, H.: How to Live With Schizophrenia. New Hyde Park, New York, University Books, Inc., 1966.
3. Herjanic, M. and Moss-Herjanic, B. L.: Ascorbic acid test in psychiatric patients. J. Schizophrenia, 1:257-260, 1967.
4. Rimland, B.: High Dosage Levels of Certain Vitamins in the Treatment of Children With Severe Mental Disorders. San Diego, California, Institute for Child Behavior Research, 1968.

# PART VII

## The Safety of Foods

*Chapter 64*

# FOOD ADDITIVES AND NUTRITION:
# A PRIMER

T HE emotional response to the government ban on cyclamates and the voluntary industry ban on monosodium glutamate has acquired, in some persons, an almost hysterical character. The widespread fear that our food supply is poisoned, the belief that all sorts of vague symptoms experienced by aging individuals and specific syndromes such as various types of brain damage can be explained on the basis of some mysterious toxic agents introduced into our daily food by a supposedly callous and greedy medical-industrial complex may well drive tens of thousands of American families into food fads and secondary deficiencies.

Under such conditions of uncertainty, persons should turn to their physicians. Unfortunately, even when physicians have had some instruction in nutrtition it almost never entails consideration of food, let alone food additives. This situation should be remedied. A few observations on each category of additives may be useful, this chapter describes the various types of food additives and comments on the situation that produced the recent flurry of attention and action in this field.

## COLORING MATTERS

None of the dyes used in both natural and manufactured foods has any nutritional value. They originally were used because many food products lost their natural color when processed, and pale tints tend to discourage consumption. As "synthetic" foods replaced the original products, artificial colors were introduced to "reinforce" taste. Banana ice cream made with artificial banana

Reprinted from *Postgraduate Medicine, 46* (No. 6), 195, 1969 (revised 1971). McGraw-Hill, Inc.

flavor will not be accepted unless it has the color as well as the flavor of banana. Obviously, while the restoration of the original color of a product can be justified nutritionally, the second use described cannot. Nor can the introduction of completely arbitrary colors in new products be justified, except on purely esthetic grounds.

## PRESERVATIVES

Unlike many other kinds of additives, preservatives as a class have an obvious nutritional usefulness in that they help make possible the greater abundance and variety of foods that characterize industrial societies. They are used to prevent spoilage caused by bacteria, fungi and molds and may be used to prolong the "keeping quality" of foods. Some of them, such as benzoic acid, sulfur dioxide and sulfites, have been used for many decades, and are on the "generally recognized as safe" (GRAS) list (with some reservations). (This, incidentally, does not necessarily guarantee complete safety; various countries are reevaluating some of these compounds.)

Hydrogen perioxide is allowed for treating milk at temperatures around 120° to 125° F as an alternative to pasteurization in making certain types of cheese. (Before coagulation the residual peroxide is destroyed with catalase, however). Boric acid and borax are permitted in certain countries. Some antibiotics also have been used to retard spoilage of fish, meat, poultry, etc. Small doses used in processing these foods, or in ice-cooling them, can increase the conservation time considerably, a factor important in transporting meat over great distances or preserving fish caught out at sea. Because a prolonged intake of antibiotics can increase susceptibility to various infectious agents and can cause changes in the intestinal flora resulting in secondary bacterial or fungal infection, candidomycoses, and invasion of the organism by resistant microbial strains, various countries have applied greater or lesser degrees of restriction on their use. In the United States, the earlier authorization of tetracycline-type antibiotics as a preservative was rescinded by the FDA. Tolerances for antibiotics in foods in this country range from 0 to fractions of a part per million. None can be added to foods. The tolerances, when set, recognize the amounts that may come through from feeding growth promoting substances to the animals. The tolerance in milk is zero in all cases. In certain other countries, notably in the Soviet Union, antibiotics are still in use to preserve fish and meat. In general, to be authorized for use in foods in these countries, antibiotics should be free from toxicity, should not affect the quality of food, should have a wide spectrum of anti-bacterial activity, and should be readily inactivated when the food is heated, processed or stored for a given period. (Chlortetracycline is an example of one such antibiotic.) The use of antibiotics is usually accompanied by chilling or freezing.

## ANTIOXIDANTS

Antioxidants, which inhibit oxidation of foods during storage, are used essentially to prevent the spoilage of fat. As such they protect the taste of fat and prevent the formation of objectionable (and dangerous) peroxides. They preserve the content of the fat in polyunsaturated fatty acids and fat-soluble vitamins.

## ACIDS AND BASES

Acids and bases are used to give tartness or acidity to certain foods and beverages or to alter the acid-base balance of the medium. For example, the pH of the medium is lowered in a number of canned products, and the pH of jams and jellies is altered to prevent crystallization. Organic acids such as tartaric, citric and lactic acids are used to acidify fruits or fruit juice preparations; acetic acid is used in pickling various foods and in salads and relishes. Carbonic acid is used to make beverages effervescent. Organic acids are used in a number of confectioneries and orthophosphoric acid in soft drinks. The main bases used in baking powders in bakery products are sodium carbonate, potassium carbonate, and sodium bicarbonate. Some bases also are used to produce effervescent beverages.

## FLAVORING AGENTS

Food flavors are often complex mixtures with 10 or 15 different ingredients, both synthetic aromatic substances and natural essential oils, fruit juices and extracts. These flavors are used in preparing confectionery products, both alcoholic and nonalcoholic beverages, syrup, dessert powders, and ice cream. Some synthetic aromatic substances such as vanillin and diacetyl are used directly in foods (for example, vanillin in ice cream, diacetyl in margarine to give it a milky odor). The number of synthetic aromatics is increasing rapidly. Many are similar to the aromatic substances found in essential oils, but a number have their own distinctive scent and do not structually resemble aromatic oils. This is one of the areas of greatest toxicologic uncertainty at present.

## ARTIFICIAL SWEETENERS

Artificial sweeteners have been the focus of much attention as a result of the ban on cyclamates. Cyclamates were under suspicion for about a year after experiments indicated that they were mutagenic to the chick embryo when injected into the egg. While this evidence was still under investigation by a special committee appointed by the National Academy of Sciences (and while the appropriateness of action was under debate), the report by scientists at Abbott Laboratories that at high concentration, cyclamates caused bladder tumors to develop in rats brought about the automatic enforcement of the Delaney Amendment and the immediate ban on manufacturing, with bans on sales to follow. It must be noted that the decision was thus taken on grounds independent of the prolonged discussion on the significance of the chick embryo data and that the relevance of chromosomal changes in one set of experiments to carcinogenicity in the other remains, to my knowledge, unknown.

Saccharin, which is the main surviving sweetening agent, has been used since before the beginning of this century and is presumed safe; it acts at concentrations much smaller than those used for cyclamates. It has been recently reevaluated by a National

Academy committee and its safety has been reaffirmed, at least for the present.

## TASTE ENHANCERS

The main taste enhancer is monosodium glutamate. It, too, has been in the news as a result of Dr. John W. Olney's work at Washington University, St. Louis. He demonstrated that injected and stomach-fed doses greater than, but still of the same general order as those found in baby foods caused hypothalamic lesions in groups of infant mice, rats and rabbits and in a rhesus monkey (1, 2, 3). These lesions in turn led to disorders of regulation of food intake and of endocrine regulation. The work corroborates the extreme sensitivity of infant nervous tissue to this compound which was indicated by earlier work on the retina done by other researchers in the late 1950's, and has recently been confirmed in this writer's laboratory (4). This type of sensitivity to monosodium glutamate appears to be limited to infant mammalians; the ability to detoxify glutamic acid by producing glutamine develops progressively as the infant animal ages. Beech-Nut, Gerber and Heinz, the three major infant food manufacturers, have discontinued the use of monosodium glutamate in preparing baby foods. Some adults are sensitive to large doses (5).

## GELLING AGENTS, STABILIZERS AND EMULSIFIERS

Gelling agents, stabilizers, and emulsifiers (including "modified" starches that serve the same purpose as gelling agents) are used for technological reasons. For example, pectin, sodium alginate (processed from algae), agar, vegetable gums, and cross-linked starches are used to keep jellies, baby foods, and other preparations in a set state and to prevent various ingredients from settling. Stabilizing agents such as agar, vegetable agaroid, sodium alginate, methylcellulose, and sodium caseinate are used in various areas to keep ice cream creamy. Calcium lactate, calcium chloride, disodium pyrophosphate, and sodium triphosphate are used to improve a variety of products (fish cakes, sausage products, potato flakes, etc.)

Emulsifiers are used primarily in producing margarine, bread, and bakery products. Closely related to emulsifiers are plasticizers and anti-splattering agents (such as combinations of monoglycerides and diglycerides of $C_{16}$ or $C_{18}$ fatty acids). Inorganic salts such as potassium and magnesium carbonates and complex organic substances such as phosphatides are also used.

## IMPROVING AGENTS

This catchall group, sometimes taken as a more general classification embracing the two preceding groups, includes compounds used for glazing confectionery and improving the shine of bakery products, and compounds and enzymes that improve the taste and consistency of certain foods. Improving and "polishing" agents comprise a number of compounds which may come under suspicion, including organic substances such as lecithin and phosphatides. Inorganic compounds, particularly nitrates and nitrites which are used in the meat industry, are also under suspicion. As a result of the activity of denitrifying bacteria, nitrates are gradually metabolized into nitrites. In young animals, nitrites cause methemoglobinemia. Lowering the nitrate content of suasage products and other processed meats seems desirable. Bleaching agents (such as hydrogen peroxide) may be added to this "catchall" category.

Finally, enzyme preparations can also be included in the group of improving agents, both in the baking industry and in tenderizing meat. No adverse effect has been reported.

## CONCLUSION

It is essential to remind alarmed patients that our food supply is actually much safer than it used to be when spoilage and microbial infestation meant a constant risk of gastroenteritis and other food-borne diseases for both infants and older individuals. Obviously the screening of new compounds by regulatory agencies, the U.S. Food and Drug Administration in particular, should be thorough. The substances on the GRAS list certainly should be submitted to the same searching review. This, incidentally, means that additional means should be given to the FDA.

A unified code for all states also would help. For that matter, I strongly think that additional criteria for accepting new compounds, such as clear usefulness to the consumer, should be introduced; these by themselves would reduce the number of new additives and would increase the safety of our food supply. Still, even now we can eat with far more safety than our grandparents did.

Finally, it may be useful to point out to the patient that absolute safety is not of this world. Cancer existed millions of years before chemical additives were invented. Natural foods probably contain carcinogenic, mutagenic and other toxic substances that we have not yet identified. And, of course, no one who smokes is on good grounds to worry about food safety!

## REFERENCES

1. Olney, J. W.: Brain lesions, obesity and other disturbances in mice treated with monosodium glutamate. Science, 164:719, 1969.
2. Olney, J. W.: Glutamate-induced retinal degeneration in neonatal mice. Electron microscopy of the acutely evolving lesion. J. Neuropath. and Exp. Neurol. 28:455, 1969.
3. Olney, J. W.: Brain lesions in an infant rhesus monkey treated with monosodium glutamate. Science, 166:386, 1969.
4. Arees, E. A. and Mayer, J.: Monosodium glutamate-induced brain lesions: Electron microscope examination. Science, 170:549, 1970.
5. Morselli, P. L.: Monosodium glutamate and the Chinese restaurant syndrome. Nature, 227:611, 1970.

*Chapter 65*

# FOOD-BORNE DISEASES AND CONSUMER PROTECTION

$P$ROTECTING the consumer against unwholesome food traditionally has been the role of three organizations: the Meat and Poultry Insepction Division of the United States Department of Agriculture; the Food and Drug Administration of the United States Department of Health, Education, and Welfare, an agency of the United States Public Health Service; and state and local food and drug organizations and inspection departments. Large commercial organizations (e.g. Campbell Soup Company) have their own monitoring organizations, which often detect contamination before public authorities can. In spite of the fact that this network of organizations has not completely eliminated outbreaks of food poisoning, our food supply is much safer than it was one or two generations ago.

## MEAT AND POULTRY INSPECTION

Following Upton Sinclair's description of a Chicago packing-house in his novel "The Jungle," meat inspection as we know it today began with passage of the Meat Inspection Act of 1906, which was supplemented by the Poultry and Poultry Products Inspection Act of 1957. The USDA Consumer and Marketing Services administers both of these acts. Today federal agents inspect about 85 per cent of commercially slaughtered livestock and 86 per cent of poultry sold off farms. In addition, each year federal agencies regulate the processing of more than 20 billion pounds of meat and 2 billion pounds of poultry.

Unfortunately, federal inspection regulations do not apply to farmers who slaughter their own livestock on their own farm, or to

Reprinted from *Postgraduate Medicine, 48* (No. 2), August, 1970.© McGraw-Hill, Inc.

meat and poultry plants that sell all their products within the same state in which they are produced to nonfederally inspected establishments or nongovernmental agencies. While the administrative and legal reasons for such exemptions are clear, from the viewpoint of the consumer — and therefore of the medical and public health worker — there is no possible justification for such exemptions.

## THE FOOD AND DRUG ADMINISTRATION

The FDA administers several federal acts that deal in whole or in part with food regulation. These include the Tea Importation Act of 1897, the Filled Milk Act of 1923, the Import Milk Act of 1927, and the Food, Drug and Cosmetic Act of 1938. The latter prohibits interstate commerce in adulterated and misbranded foods, establishes safe tolerance standards for food additives, color additives and pesticide residues, and grants authority for pre-clearance review.

In the case of substances that are considered to be carcinogenic in any amount in any animal species, the tolerance rating is zero under the Delaney Amendment, a stricture hotly debated by industry and some academic scientists. The report of the White House Conference on Food, Nutrition and Health (1) includes a reasonable discussion of the Delaney clause. The Filled Milk Act pertains to standards of identity rather than to safety as such and the Import Milk Act to requirements for permits to import dairy products.

The FDA is primarily a law-enforcing agency and as such is in constant contact and collaboration with federal, state and local agencies that perform similar or related activities. Several hundred field inspectors periodically inspect food plants and warehouses, but they are too few in number to do the thorough job that the agency would like to do; the number of inspections and successful prosecutions is also very small. The moral authority of the FDA and the possibility of adverse publicity ultimately are its main assets in enforcing the laws.

## PUBLIC HEALTH PROGRAMS

The USPHS has guarded the public against health hazards in

food since 1906, when its predecessor, the Marine Hospital Service, investigated typhoid fever cases in the District of Columbia and identified milk as one of the vehicles. Ever since, the USPHS has set sanitation standards for milk. As a result of the 1925 typhoid fever outbreak, in which consumption of contaminated oysters caused 1500 cases and 150 deaths, the program was broadened to include criteria for sanitary breeding, harvesting and processing the shellfish. Later, the agency set sanitation standards for control of food service in public eating places, frozen desserts, food and beverage vending machines, poultry processing, and ice manufacturing. Many state and local agencies have adopted these standards as the basis for their sanitation laws and regulations. It must be admitted, however, that state and local codes and enforcement are usually the weakest link in protecting the consumer against food-borne disease.

## SURVEILLANCE OF FOOD-BORNE DISEASE

In 1966, the National Communicable Disease Center instituted a national program of voluntary surveillance for food-borne diseases. They were prompted to do so by the realization that in spite of existing controls, food-borne disease is still a major public health problem. Analyses of the results of the first two years of operation (1966 and 1967) (2, 3) were published only this year, but the main conclusion is still valid.

Data on food-borne outbreaks were derived from a variety of sources: reports by state and local health departments to the NCDC; investigation by Epidemic Intelligence Service officers in collaboration with state and local authorities; and reports received from the FDA, from HEW's Division of Food, Milk, and Interstate Travel Sanitation, and in a few cases from the news media. Improved reporting undoubtedly accounted for the rise from 181 outbreaks with 8000 cases in 1966 to 273 outbreaks with over 22,000 cases in 1967.

The city of New York and California lead in reporting, not because of unusually hazardous conditions in those places, but because they have made special efforts to investigate and report outbreaks of food-borne illness. Of the 50 states, the District of

Columbia, and Puerto Rico, 37 reported in 1966 and 42 reported in 1967. Those not reporting in 1967 included Arizona, Delaware, Iowa, Montana, New Hampshire, North Carolina, Puerto Rico, South Dakota, Utah and Wyoming.

For the purpose of surveillance, food-borne diseases have been classified as bacterial, parasitic, viral, chemical, "other" and "unknown." Bacterial causes accounted for 60 per cent of the outbreaks. Illness due to *Salmonella* other than typhoid bacilli occurred in 12,000 people in 27 outbreaks, making this organism by far the most common cause of food poisoning in 1967. *S. typhimurium* was the predominant serotype.

*Clostridium perfringens* caused illness in 2500 persons in 19 outbreaks in 1967. In 1966 it had ranked with *Salmonella* as the foremost infecting agent. The third most common cause of bacterial food poisoning was *Staphylococcus* (32 outbreaks with 1,339 cases in 1967), followed by *Shigella* (six outbreaks with 547 cases). Only five confirmed and two suspected cases of botulism occurred in 1967, a record low since 1899, when the disease was first recognized in the United States. There were two deaths. Other bacterial food poisonings in 1967 were the result of *S. typhosa* (51 cases), enteropathogenic *Escherichia coli* (70 cases), and *Brucella* (six cases in Alaskan Eskimos who had eaten raw caribou bone marrow).

Viral gastroenteritides were limited to nine outbreaks of food-borne or water-borne viral hepatitis that involved 196 persons. Trichinosis affected 47 individuals (39 isolated incidents and three outbreaks involving eight individuals). Water-borne amebiasis was reported in one family of five persons.

In spite of recent emphasis on the possibility of food-borne chemical poisoning, only six episodes involving 32 people were reported in 1967. There were three outbreaks of so-called Oriental food poisoning or Chinese restaurant syndrome that affected 18 persons. This syndrome is characterized by sudden onset of numbness, paresthetic ache, and dizziness occurring within half an hour after the subject has eaten soup in an Oriental restaurant. The course of the syndrome lasts less than two hours but the symptoms are extremely distressing. At present the evidence indicates that susceptible individuals manifest this syndrome after consuming an excessive amount of monosodium glutamate.

In terms of size, outbreaks of food poisoning from *Staphylococcus* tended to be smaller than those caused by *Salmonella* or *C. perfringens*. In terms of vehicles, salmonellosis was caused most often by contaminated turkey, beef, eggs or milk; *C. perfringens* infections primarily by beef; staphylococcal illness by beef, pork and vegetables; viral hepatitis most often by contaminated water; and botulism by home-canned foods. Those who have an aversion to banquets will be confirmed in their bias by the fact that more than 50 per cent of all infections were contracted at banquets. Restaurants and homes were second as locales of infection.

Obviously such reports, important though they are, represent only "the tip of the iceberg," in the words of Woodward and colleagues (4). The 1700 outbreaks causing illness in 115,000 people are probably but a fraction of the unreported cases, although they may comprise many of the larger outbreaks. While most large-scale food-borne and water-borne infections are usually controlled, reports such as those of the NCDC emphasize the ubiquitousness of pathogenic organisms and the need for constant surveillance and vigilance to prevent outbreaks.

## CONCLUSION

The panel on safety of the White House Conference on Food, Nutrition and Health (1) rightly emphasized the need for better reporting of food-borne disease outbreaks to the NCDC; improvement of laboratory testing for microbiologic safety of foods through a joint effort of industrial, governmental, academic and private laboratories; a more effective system for food plant inspection; passage of a stronger National Food Sanitation Act; greater publicity on food safety, including information on naturally occurring toxic substances in foods, microbiologic hazards of foods, and methods by which these risks can be lessened; stronger controls on the quality of restaurant foods; and review of regulations on trade secrets. Certainly, in terms of public education, to give but one example, people should be warned that refrigeration does not necessarily insure the safety of food for an indefinite length of time.

# REFERENCES

1. Mayer, J. (Editor): White House Conference on Food, Nutrition and Health; Final Report. Washington, D.C., U.S. Government Printing Office, 1970.
2. Foodborne Outbreaks: Status Report for 1966. National Communicable Disease Center. Washington, D.C., U.S. Government Printing Office, 1970.
3. Foodborne Outbreaks: Status Report for 1967. National Communicable Disease Center. Washington, D.C., U.S. Government Printing Office, 1970.
4. Woodward, W. E., Gangarosa, E. J., Brachman, P. S. and Curlin, G. T.: Foodborne disease surveillance in the United States, 1966 and 1967. Amer. J. Public Health, 60:130-137, 1970.

# ADDITIONAL REFERENCE

1. Hayes, J. (Editor): Protecting Our Food. The Yearbook of Agriculture. United States Department of Agriculture. Washington, D.C., U.S. Government Printing Office, 1966.

# PART VIII
## Dietetics

*Chapter 66*

# DIETETICS LOOKS TO THE FUTURE

## DEVELOPMENT OF THE DIETETIC PROFESSION

$\text{D}$IETETICS, soon to mark 50 years as an organized profession, is being subjected to much the same identity searching as must have preoccupied the 98 charter members. The gist of the problem seems to be, How can one person be a generalist and at the same time be recognized as a specialist with a unique knowledge and a special service to render? This question is not unlike the one the medical profession solved by making medicine a field of graduate (postcollege) study and creating specialty boards.

Dietetics as a separate organized profession dates back to the founding of the American Dietetic Association (ADA) during World War I. From the beginning, at the Cleveland conference in 1917, it appeared that the profession had diverse activities: dietetics in hospitals involving outpatients as well as inpatients, food administration, community nutrition, teaching nutrition, dietetics in military and various government services, research science, managing quantity food services, etc. As could be expected, the immediate interest of the convention in 1917 was military hospital dietetics, infant feeding, and the National Food Administration program of the late President Hoover. The convention was also preoccupied (as the ADA still is) with defining standards of excellence and professional goals and educating future dietitians.

The Association grew steadily, and in 1932 the *Journal of the American Dietetic Association* was started. During the depression, the Association assisted with relief feeding, local and national projects, and a massive effort in counseling low-income groups in budgeting and menu planning. During World War II, it actively

Reprinted from *Postgraduate Medicine, 40* (No. 2), August, 1966.

assisted with problems of hospital dietetics under a variety of field conditions. Seventy-two per cent of the ADA members were engaged in the activities of the armed forces or the American Red Cross. Because these activities were successful, the number and responsibilities of dietitians were expanded, not only in hospitals and the armed forces but also in schools, colleges, health departments at the various levels, and community services.

## SPECIALIZATION IN DIETETICS

The largest percentage of ADA members work in hospitals, an area with a wide range of dietetic activities.

The therapeutic dietitian is concerned with corrective diets rather than food preparation. She gives preliminary guidance and instruction in the rationale of special diets that will be continued after the patient leaves the hospital. She is also responsible for special instruction to student nurses, dietetic interns and, in a number of hospitals, medical students.

Obviously, a therapeutic dietitian must have a good scientific background in the biochemistry of nutrition, physiology of digestion and metabolism, function of nutrients in enzyme systems, maintenance of acid-base balance, role of minerals in enzymatic functions and in the operation of the heart and central nervous system, and the pathology of nutrition, including the increasing number of inborn metabolic errors with nutritional overtones; some therapeutic dietitians have learned to operate a metabolic service. The dietitian's knowledge of food composition should be of inestimable value for the physician.

The outpatient-clinic dietitian, also concerned with diet therapy, works with patients in planning menus and budgeting and preparing food. She deals with dietary problems of obesity, infant feeding and various infirmities (e.g. lack of teeth) and with the nutritional aspects of specific medical problems. She also assists the inpatient dietitian with patients whose dietary regimens will continue after they leave the hospital.

The teaching dietitian is concerned primarily with education. She may conduct hospital classes for pregnant women, obese patients, etc., or she may teach adult education classes, hospital and public health nurses and social workers, or be concerned with international programs, community or state rehabilitation services, or civil defense projects, or she may perform a combination of these activities.

The food administrator is expert in quantity food planning and preparation, kitchen services, bakery production, etc., and is responsible for the food standards and general nutritional policies of the hospital for which she works. Because she selects and purchases food and cooking, serving and storage equipment, she must be proficient in accounting, buying procedures, equipment and facility designing, and quality control. She is also a personnel manager, hiring food and service personnel and training dietary employees.

Dietitians specializing in dietotherapy and food management serve in the armed forces and U.S. Public Health Service hospitals as commissioned officers and in Veterans Administration hospitals as civil service workers. Dietitians are employed as food administrators in private schools; public schools, some of which have government-supported lunch programs with positions at city, county and state levels; social service and welfare agencies, such as children's homes and convalescent hospitals; industrial organizations, and universities. Public health agencies employ dietitians in appreciable numbers as instructors for community groups, public health nurses, social workers, etc.

## TRAINING IN DIETETICS

The American Dietetic Association supervises the training of dietitians. After four years of undergraduate education, usually with a major in foods and nutrition, the graduate trains as an intern in an approved hospital or food administration service for at least one year.* Three years of experience under ADA supervision may be substituted for the internship; this must be in one or no more than two of the following fields:

1. A responsible position in a dietetic department in a hospital or in the food service of a school, college or commercial or

*A list of approved dietetic internships for each state is available from the American Dietetic Association, 620 North Michigan Avenue, Chicago, Illinois 60611.

industrial organization having at least two full-time dietary staff members. In hospital positions this is interpreted to mean one year in administration and one year in therapeutics. The third year may be in either area.

2. A position in public health nutrition or a clinic with a nutrition program.

3. A responsible position in the area of foods, nutrition or equipment with a publication, a business organization, or a radio or television network.

4. Faculty status at an accredited college or university, including extension service, with the responsibility for teaching such subjects as foods, nutrition or food service management.

The candidate for ADA membership must be endorsed by three persons of whom at least two are ADA members (one a former supervisor) and one a former teacher in a major field. Membership is contingent on satisfactory scholastic and work performance. A much smaller number of ADA candidates become members by obtaining a master's degree in public health nutrition, food, nutrition, food service management, or related fields and sufficient qualifying experience.

The ADA provides opportunities for continuing education: study programs, workshops, the annual national convention, the Journal, and, for some of the younger members, fellowships for graduate work.

Although the dietetics profession is firmly established (membership in the ADA is now 18,000), there is room for improvement. The following suggestions may be useful to physicians and dietitians. These comments are concerned more with therapeutic dietitians and others engaged in nutrition work than with food administrators.

## DIETITIAN AND PATIENT:
## A CLOSER RAPPORT?

The dietitian influences the lives of many patients in the measure that she becomes involved with them. Sometimes dietitians appear reluctant to act as though the patient is "their" patient or client. To those who would protest that the nurse and physician have, perforce, more intimate rapport with the patient as a person because they are in actual physical contact with him, I would answer that the psychiatrist and social worker often achieve an even closer patient rapport without such contact. Too often education, professional training and custom fail to stress the necessity or desirability of close rapport, and the dietitian's attitude is more that of a technician or, at best, a substitute teacher who feels that the regular teacher may resent her becoming too closely involved with the students.

Yet, if the dietitian is to change habits as basic, ingrained and bound with emotional, cultural and economic factors as are food habits, wisdom (and common courtesy) command that she know a great deal about her patient and that she be accepted by him as an understanding and well-meaning friend. Unless she supplements the patient's dietary history with considerable information about his intellectual, cultural, socioeconomic and familial backgrounds and has a sound perception of him as a person, she cannot communicate more than a few prescriptions and recipes, and these, at best, will be but of transient value.

In some ways, a dietitian is in a better position than the physician to know the patient, because she and the questions she asks do not represent a threat, particularly to the patient's economic status, interpersonal family relations, and attitude toward health and health fads. It is relatively easier, especially in dealing with a woman, to get a more accurate picture of the family's economic status by discussing food prices and the portion of income budgeted to food than by knowing the total income, even if this information is available. Similarly, a discussion on how meals are taken during the day — which members of the family eat together, which eat outside the home and where, and the pattern of food intake during weekends and holidays — clearly reveals the family structure in a way that, again, can hardly be regarded as prying or threatening.

Finally, whereas the physician's questions on understanding the disease or on possible lapses into dietary faddism will immediately put the patient or his family on the defensive, a quiet conversation about the role of food in maintaining health or curing a particular disease will easily reveal any susceptibility to quackery. At the end of an hour's session (and a good dietary interview followed by an understandable prescription and advice of lasting value cannot take less time), the dietitian should have information that will be useful both as a basis for her own therapeutic procedures and to the physician. It is regrettable that only the experienced and most successful dietitians are thoroughly informed about their patients and that they rarely pass on this information to the physician in charge.

When dealing with long-term problems, such as arthritic conditions, in which known nutritional factors are not entailed in the etiology of the disease but often present numerous difficulties in its treatment, a close rapport among dietitian, patient and the patient's family is particularly important. The dietitian can foresee many of the complications that may occur − obesity and increased immobility, loss of appetite and malnutrition, awkwardness and difficulty in caring for the family − and act quickly to alleviate them. This often means seeing the patient in his home environment, another dimension for rapport which is too often neglected.

## THE DIETITIAN'S EDUCATION: A BROADER BASE?

I contend that a dietitian's general background and training do not adequately prepare her for the interpersonal aspects of her work. At a time when all medical schools accept students with varied academic backgrounds, even if it means the scientific knowledge of a number of their students will be minimal, the American Dietetic Association continues to insist on admission requirements I believe are too rigid and exclusive. Students can be admitted to medical school on the basis of college training with a major in almost any academic discipline from art to zoology, provided they have an acceptable scholarship and have absolved some requirements in the sciences, such as organic chemistry. However, the student entering the school of dietetics must have a major in foods and nutrition. She usually has a weak background in the humanities and social sciences even though her work will be concerned mainly with patients and teaching. In effect, her college background, emphasizing the chemistry of foods and the bio-chemical aspects of nutrition, is more similar to that of medical technicians than of teachers, including science teachers, or of physicians.

It would appear more reasonable for the dietetics profession to seek girls of varied college interests and majors who have had sufficient basic chemistry (general and organic) and biology (some anatomy and physiology) to take courses in food chemistry, biochemistry, diet therapy, etc., at the graduate level. Girls with such broad backgrounds should be able to cope more rapidly and adequately with the interpersonal aspects of dietetics. This would open a larger area for recruiting a good selection of potential students. Although in theory students who are not food majors may enter the school of dietetics at the graduate level, in fact it is rarely done.

It should be possible for very good students to quickly acquire at the graduate level the knowledge that students today are slowly acquiring at the undergraduate level, to feel more at ease when working with other professionals who have been trained at the postcollege level, and to be taught disciplines to which present-day nutritionists are not exposed. One such discipline is physical anthropology. The dietitian could relieve the physician of measuring and weighing the child having feeding problems and the obese patient. If she were taught to use calipers to measure subcutaneous fat, she could follow the variation in the patient's composition (particularly that of the obese child or adolescent). Training in somatotyping would enable her to better appraise problems of growth, weight reduction and malnutrition. Studying the patient's physique, including determination of skinfolds (the arm skinfold is the easiest to determine and the best indicator of fat content), will increase the dietitian's involvement and rapport with him.

## THE DIETITIAN AND THE PHYSICIAN: BETTER COMMUNICATIONS?

I have suggested that future dietitians could receive broader training and more systematically develop a closer relationship with their patients. I would like to emphasize that although I believe these are desirable targets, many of our present dietitians, particularly among the more experienced, are distinguished women who have acquired through self-application a broad cultural basis and an impressive knowledge of human beings. Their training, of course, gives them considerable competence in foods and nutrition and they are well informed about therapeutic nutrition.

Most good dietitians are not utilized to their fullest potential. They should be encouraged to contribute to the information recorded in the patient's history and chart. Furthermore, they should stop passively translating nutritional prescriptions (often impossible to put into practice because no known mixture of natural foods corresponds to the combination of grams of protein, fat, etc., requested) and volunteer their knowledge and experience to the physician. The dietitian should also be encouraged to take responsibility for reeducating, for example, obese patients, not only in food habits but also in organizing a schedule, including exercise habits, substitute interests, etc., to maintain a more hygienic weight and mode of life. Usually, the physician does not have the time or, in some aspects, the skills to adequately study the patient's food habits or to effectively teach caloric content, desirable food portions, and low-calorie, low-fat or low-salt cooking, yet he will often make a quick (and misunderstood) attempt to do so rather than spend a fraction of that time explaining the medical problem and the desirable nutritional objectives to a good dietitian and rely on her to do a thorough job.

A good therapeutic dietitian should be taken on doctors' rounds and asked, whenever appropriate, to comment on the dietary aspects of a patient's problem and treatment. She should be given a chance to acquaint young house officers with her field of competence so that they can understand what information she requires to function well and in what area she is an expert deserving of their attention. Before a patient is discharged from the hospital or admitted to the outpatient clinic, the dietitian should be given sufficient information about his problem and ample time to effectively instruct him. The information she obtains should be made available to other therapists.

Recently, physicians in group practices have added dietitians to their staffs to instruct mothers who have children with pediatric problems and patients who are obese or pregnant or have some disorder, such as heart disease. Dietitians who are associated in such groups and paid on the basis of services rendered to each patient develop a closer relationship with "their" patient, the desirable goal I mentioned previously.

## THE DIETITIAN IN THE FUTURE
## HEALTH ORGANIZATION

Undoubtedly, we are entering a period which will tax the nation's medical resources. Our population is proportionately increasing more rapidly than is the number of physicians. The growth is particularly rapid within the groups at the two extremes of age, the very young and the old, who have the greatest medical needs. Passage of the Medicare Act entitles a number of aged poor to treatment that formerly was beyond their reach. The anti-poverty campaign will also increase the demand on our medical services. To maintain a high quality of medical care under these conditions, we will need to better utilize our professional personnel, broaden their roles, and give them suitable assistance.

The dietitian can play an important role in this process by relieving the physician of numerous tasks that are in her field or immediately related to it. I have discussed a number of these tasks. Conversely, if she is to be an effective therapist and teacher, she must be freed from a number of tasks that nonprofessionals can perform. The development of good catering services for patients without special nutritional problems may decrease the administrative requirements for food preparation services, particularly in small and medium-sized hospitals, and permit more emphasis on dietotherapy. The availability of instant "special" diets, for example, for phenylketonuric or galactosemic patients, may also simplify the dietitian's tasks. Although I do not advocate preventing all dietetic executives from becoming food administrators, the long-term solution, in many cases, may be to employ food managers (with training similar to that at the School of Hotel Administration, Cornell University) who have been exposed to sufficient nutrition to realize that they must follow the advice of a competent therapeutic dietitian concerning special diets and dietary problems.

The dietitian's time also can be freed for more professional tasks if she (or the outpatient dietetic department) is given adequate secretarial and nontechnical help, and if she is able to use the hospital data-processing system. Relieved of nonprofessional tasks, the dietitian can be a much more effective assistant to the physician.

*Chapter 67*

# ON-THE-JOB NUTRITION TEACHING
# IN THE HOSPITAL

Written in collaboration with Johanna T. Dwyer

THE winds of change that blow into our universities are motivating present-day medical students to take new interest in preventive medicine, including nutrition. Both the federal government and medical schools are responding to these new interests, and we believe that federal money will soon be available for teaching nutrition in all our medical schools.

Meanwhile, what Dr. Robert H. Barnes, Jr., of Seattle, has called the "doctors' dietary antics" continues in our hospitals. Hospital staffs give more special diets to patients than could conceivably be necessary. Many physicians seem uncertain about what they want their patients to eat, and confuse (or exasperate) the dietitian by asking for diets so impossibly high in protein and low in everything else that, in the words of the old tale, "There ain't no such animal."

The situation obviously must be remedied. The attitudes of house officers and student nurses training in hospitals suggest that they are aware of the weakness of our nutrition practices and are eager to improve their knowledge. Furthermore, the ways in which they express their dissatisfactions and their aspirations indicate that much of the needed education should take place in the hospital.

## NUTRITION AND THE YOUNG PHYSICIAN

We surveyed the attitudes of interns and residents in two

Reprinted from *Postgraduate Medicine, 46* (No. 4,), October, 1969.© McGraw-Hill, Inc.

Harvard-affiliated hospitals through a detailed questionnaire. Most of these young physicians (71%) felt that nutrition had not received sufficient attention in their medical curriculum. Only 29 per cent felt that their training had been adequate in this regard. When they were asked how important knowledge of nutrition and diet therapy is to the doctor on duty in the wards, 14 per cent answered, "extremely important"; 57 per cent, "very important"; 24 per cent, "fairly important"; and only 5 per cent, "unimportant." Sixty-two per cent of the house officers felt that other doctors did not have adequate knowledge of nutrition and diet therapy. Only 28 per cent felt that older doctors (including attending physicians) knew enough about nutrition. Thus, it is obvious that bright, otherwise well-trained young physicians feel that knowledge of nutrition and diet therapy is highly significant in treating hospital patients.

The house officers felt that nurses should be properly trained in nutrition and that many nurses had insufficient training. They were impressed with the dietitians' knowledge. An overwhelming majority of the young physicians (80%) felt that nurses and dietitians worked well together; 10 per cent did not know, and 10 per cent felt that they did not work well together, primarily because the nurses did not know enough about nutrition.

We found that none of the physicians interviewed had had a formal nutrition course during medical training. The information they had accumulated came mostly from occasional lectures on subjects related to nutrition or from working up patients with diseases that required diet therapy. They felt that additional lectures on clinical topics of interest to them, ward experience with specific patients with dietary problems, and informal chats with dietitians about therapeutic diets were the most useful in learning clinical nutrition.

It seems obvious to us that hospitals that have a staff member with specific interest in and information on nutrition or a therapeutic dietitian capable of clear exposition should use such a resource by organizing frequent presentations on specific cases, illustrating various aspects of nutrition. In hospitals that do not have a therapeutic dietitian or a potential clinical lecturer, dietitians should participate in patient care with house officers.

Discussing the prescription of therapeutic diets with the dietitian and seeing a meal prepared and even consumed may be the most important teaching aids.

Young physicians should realize that the average dietitian has had four years of home economics training with a major in nutrition, some graduate courses in the subject, a dietary internship, and a varying amount of practical experience. Furthermore, precisely because her approach to the patient is noncharismatic, low key and nonthreatening, she can obtain invaluable information on the interpersonal relationships in the patient's family, on the family's true economic picture, and on the attitudes of the patient and his family about medicine, quackery or faddism. Encouraging the dietitian to add her significant findings to the notes kept at the foot of the patient's bed may provide additional learning experiences for the young physician.

## NUTRITION AND THE STUDENT NURSE

In one of the Harvard-affiliated hospitals, we also asked student nurses whether nutrition and diet therapy received proper emphasis in the curriculum. The great majority (77%) expressed satisfaction, 18 per cent felt that these subjects were not emphasized enough, and only 5 per cent felt that they received too much emphasis. Similarly, when the students were asked how important knowledge of nutrition and diet therapy is to the nurse on duty, 26 per cent answered, "extremely important"; 59 per cent answered, "very important"; and 12 per cent "fairly important." Three per cent did not feel that it was important.

Student nurses felt that most registered nurses with whom they had come in contact did not know enough about nutrition and diet therapy to optimally care for patients. They were even harsher in their opinion of physicians' knowledge in these areas. Eighty-five per cent of the student nurses felt that the physicians with whom they had contact did not know enough about nutrition and diet therapy. Only 2 per cent were positively impressed with the physicians' knowledge of nutrition.

With regard to their own training, the student nurses disliked the "nutrition" course, while they enjoyed the "diet therapy" course. These answers clearly indicated that the student nurses preferred a disease-oriented, action-directed approach to the one emphasizing the intellectual aspects of nutrition. This impression was reinforced by the student nurses' evident interest in their three-week rotation as student nurse-dietitians on the hospital wards. Again the picture that emerged from the students' behavior and expressed preferences was the desirability of frequent, direct involvement with dietitians.

## CONCLUSION

Hospitals tend to consider the dietitian as a technician involved with "things" rather than one involved in patient care. This tendency is often reinforced by the fact that the dietitian has had relatively little experience in professional interpersonal relationships besides her own relationship to the patient. Yet it seems obvious that young people being trained in the health professions in the hospital are conscious of the importance of nutrition, unimpressed with the erudition of older members of the health professions in this regard, and eager to benefit from the dietitian's knowledge. A wise chief of staff or medical director of a hospital will see that his dietitians work daily with house officers and student nurses, teaching by example what they are doing.

*Chapter 68*

# THE SCHOOL LUNCH PROGRAM:
# A FACTOR IN CHILDREN'S HEALTH

THE school lunch program, one of the largest Federal efforts in the field of public health, is important in the nutrition of more than 70 per cent of the nation's children. Besides supporting the school day nutritionally with a satisfactory meal and insuring a minimum nutrient intake which, if other meals are calorically adequate, would prevent at least the more severe deficiencies, the school lunch program has served as a powerful tool of nutrition education. In the past this educational effort has been directed at teaching about new foods, the structure of a balanced meal, and the virtues of a varied diet. With so much of our adult mortality due to atherosclerosis, obesity and diabetes — conditions whose causes have nutritional components — the school lunch program can and should be an important agent in preventive medicine.

For these reasons the pediatrician, school doctor and general practitioner should be familiar with the organization, practice and limitations of the school lunch program. The fact that areas which most need school lunches are still deprived of them shows a serious deficiency in our national health organization, and physicians mindful of what the school lunch program has done for the well-being of the nation's children should be particularly interested in correcting this unfortunate situation.

## HISTORY

The extraordinary Benjamin Thompson, Count Rumford, the American-born physicist, inventor and statesman who married Lavoisier's widow, is credited with originating the school feeding

---

Reprinted from *Postgraduate Medicine, 39* (No. 1), January, 1966.

program in 1790 in Munich, Germany, as part of a campaign against vagrancy among children. Aside from this isolated instance, however, the responsibility of providing noon meals for schoolchildren remained with the home until the ravages of the industrial revolution on the health of the proletariat made obvious the need for special feeding programs.

While workers and schoolchildren were not necessarily in a worse state of nutrition than housewives and preschool children, they were more accessible; thus school lunches and industrial feeding facilities were the early consequences of the widespread character of malnutrition.

France was the first country to have a network of school *cantines.* In 1867 the city of Angers began serving a noon meal, prepared by the "people's kitchens," for two cents to children who could afford to pay and free to others who could not pay. The provision of inexpensive and free school lunches was incorporated in the 1882 law which made elementary education compulsory.

England, facing the crisis of the Boer War, found that three-fifths of the men called to colors were unfit — essentially, medical authorities believed, because of malnutrition. This situation created such an uproar, both among the public and finally in Parliament, that the Provision of Meals Act of 1906 transferred school feeding from charitable to educational institutions and considerably extended the scope of the program. Local schools were authorized and encouraged to organize the necessary facilities and buy the equipment which would provide warm lunches for both paying (twopence) and nonpaying children.

By 1910 most other European countries (with the exception of Russia and Spain) had developed similar lunch programs and breakfast programs in certain cities, such as Oslo. Local authorities realized that such programs were necessary in the discharge of their responsibility for the health of the children as well as their incentives for education. An examination of the menus served to British children of that period shows that the meals were high in starch, usually satisfactory in proteins, and almost always very low in minerals and vitamins. Typical menus would be pea soup, baked jam roll and bread; Irish stew, suet pudding and bread; and meat in batter and bread.

It was not until 1894 that school lunches were started in the United States with the pioneering efforts of Ellen H. Richards, one of the founders of the home economics movement in this country. To be sure, a number of philanthropic agencies had observed that the provision of inexpensive noon meals for schoolchildren was beneficial to them, especially those in the poorer sections of large cities where large families, working mothers and low incomes resulted in great concentrations of indigent and undernourished school children.

In 1853 the Children's Aid Society of New York City founded an industrial school and, in the belief that a free noon meal would prevent or delay students from leaving school to earn their living expenses before they had acquired a basic education and knowledge of a trade, the school provided lunch for its pupils. National support, however, was lacking for such a venture, and the home-packed school lunch — often nutritionally poor, sometimes absent — continued to be the almost universal solution to the problem of feeding children at school.

By 1890, following the work of Magendie, Voit, Rubner and others in Europe and at the time Atwater was pursuing his epoch-making studies (including development of a table of food composition and model menus) at the Connecticut Agricultural Station, the time had become ripe for such efforts as those of Mrs. Richards. Nutrition was again recognized to be an essential component of health. Well-fed children made better pupils. Concerned parents, educators and social organizations were realizing that inexpensive meals should be provided within the local school systems, at least for the indigent.

Mrs. Richards convinced the Boston School Committee that only approved foods should be sold in the schools, that meals should be centrally prepared, and that facilities should be provided in the various schools to reheat the prepared food. The city of Boston provided funds to maintain the lunchroom, serving equipment and fuel; private contributions enabled Mrs. Richards to start the New England Kitchen, where the food was prepared for the schools.

In 1907 the Women's Educational and Industrial Union replaced Mrs. Richards and the New England Kitchen, providing lunches at the cost of a penny for Boston children who could afford it and free for those who could not. These women were motivated not only by their concern for the health of the children, but also by a desire to demonstrate that women could organize and direct a large-scale social program. As the program expanded, the staff added a superintendent of lunchrooms and a director of school lunches, who were entrusted with the administration of food preparation, delivery and finances. The Committee On Hygiene of the Homes and Schools Association (the forerunner of the Parent-Teachers' Association) advised the program, particularly with respect to the numerous anemic children, in an effort to prevent tuberculosis. Crackers, dates, milk and applesauce were served to those children who returned home for their noon meal. The overall system functioned well, at least until the 1920's.

Other cities began to emulate Boston. In Philadelphia the sale of penny lunches, started in elementary schools by the Star Center Association, a private philanthropy, was taken over and extended by the board of education. In 1909 the board granted funds to the William Penn High School for hiring a trained dietitian, installing and maintaining suitable cooking equipment, and paying utilities charges. The cost of food was covered by the price charged for the lunches. This division of cost became standard budgeting procedure for school cafeterias throughout the United States.

New York City Public School 51 began serving lunches in 1908, and the program soon spread to other schools. The organizers considered that one-third of the child's daily nutritional requirements should be provided which, in practice, meant one-third of the calories. Attention was paid to the food habits of the nationalities inhabiting each section. For example, on a Friday in an Irish section, the children would get cheese sandwiches and cocoa while in an Italian section the would be served macaroni and two slices of Italian bread. A special three-cent meal was provided at 10 a.m. for anemic and crippled children. Unfortunately, no provision seems to have been made for completely indigent children.

In 1914 New York became the center of two movements to improve the school lunch service. One group, concerned with the spread of communicable diseases, fought to require medical examinations, tests for typhoid, and vaccinations for smallpox for school lunch employees. The second group, concerned with the continuing widespread malnutrition among children of various national origins, fought for standardization of all recipes used in the New York City schools in order to provide satisfactory food of uniform content and value. Cleveland, Cincinnati, Rochester, Chicago and Louisville, among other cities, developed similar school lunch programs before World War I, with private charities generally pioneering at the beginning and the school system taking over and extending the programs.

The advent of World War I accelerated the growth of the school lunch movement. As enlistees and draftees pressed into the examination rooms, the effects of malnutrition were visible in a large number. As in Britain during the Boer War, the resulting public outcry was seen as pressure on local authorities to feed schoolchildren.

## MODERN DEVELOPMENTS

The present structure of the school lunch program dates essentially from the Depression years. With undernourishment, and even famine, a serious visible threat to the nation due to unrelieved unemployment affecting millions, it was urgent that the Federal government step in. An early measure was the allotment of government surplus food to school cafeterias. To make this available where cafeterias did not exist or where local authorities could no longer support them, the government in 1933 started Federal aid through the Reconstruction Finance Corporation. By 1934, 40 states had gained Federal assistance under provisions of the Civil Works Administration and the Federal Emergency Relief Administration. The preparation of school lunches was incorporated into projects of the Works Progress Administration and the National Youth Administration. A 1935 Federal law formalized the channeling of surplus food commodities into school lunchrooms. There is little doubt that this measure was responsible for saving millions of American children from malnutrition and, in some cases, starvation.

The dramatic increase in employment brought about by World War II decreased the need for emergency relief operations. At the same time, the need for long-term supporting operations was clearly established.

From 1944 to 1946 the school milk and lunch programs were operated under the Secretary of Agriculture. Since June 1946 these programs have operated under authority established in the National School Lunch Act (Public Law 396). This act provided a permanent method of Federal grants to local schools, required that the state match these funds in a 3 to 1 ratio, and made surplus commodities available for direct distribution to nonprofit lunch programs in elementary and high schools, nonprofit summer camps, child care centers, and other welfare agencies. The law also specified that, in order to qualify, recipients must make sure that the meals served "meet minimum nutritional requirements prescribed by the Secretary on the basis of tested nutritional research."

The purpose of the National School Lunch Act was stated as twofold: "The improvement of the health and well-being of the nation's youth and the assurance, both immediately and in the period of postwar reconversion, of a substantial market of agricultural production." The act was then supplemented by milk program legislation initiated in September 1954 pursuant to Public Law 690, which authorizes partial or total reimbursement for milk served with lunches.

## NUTRITIONAL STANDARDS

The established pattern of the "A" lunch acceptable to the Department of Agriculture is planned to meet one-third of the child's daily nutritional requirements. Amounts vary somewhat with age according to physiologic standards, with children in the early grades receiving somewhat less than the amounts listed below and children in older groups, particularly boys, receiving more. An average is as follows:

1. Two ounces (edible portion) lean meat, poultry or fish; or 2 oz cheese; or one egg; or 1/2 cup cooked dry beans or dry peas; or 4 tablespoons peanut butter; or an equivalent quantity of any combination of these. To be counted in meeting this requirement, these foods must be served in a main dish alone or in more than

one other menu item.

2. A 3/4 cup serving of two or more vegetables or fruits, or both. Full-strength vegetable or fruit juice may be counted to meet not more than 1/4 cup of this requirement.

3. One slice of whole-grain or enriched bread, or a serving of corn bread, biscuits, rolls, muffins, etc., made with whole-grain or enriched meal or flour.

4. Two teaspoons of butter or fortified margarine.

5. One-half pint of unflavored fluid whole milk as a beverage.

## NUTRITION EDUCATION AND THE FUTURE OF THE PROGRAM

Besides furnishing nutrients, the school lunch program is designed to improve food habits. Many states and school systems accomplish health education by supplementing the child's exposure to the variety of foods served in the lunchroom with lectures in science and health classes on the value of good nutrition and the role of various nutrients, as well as information in posters, leaflets, films, etc.

It has been found over and over again that the conjunction of the laboratory or clinical experience – in this case the daily consumption of a varied meal – and formal instruction was vastly more effective than either alone. The Department of Agriculture and private organizations such as the National Dairy Council, The American Dietetic Association, schools of home economics, etc., have developed useful material illustrating the chemical concepts of nutrition.

Emphasis on increased consumption of dairy products, meat, eggs and fruit in the school lunch program, together with the rise in national income, has been instrumental in changing for the better the consumption of many important nutrients, in particular vitamin A, riboflavin, ascorbic acid, iron and calcium.

This is not to say that we should rest on our laurels. First, many children from poor and uneducated social groups in rural areas and city slums are still not receiving a school lunch, a matter of concern to pediatricians, general practitioners and nutritionists in these areas. I am ashamed to admit that, in spite of my efforts, my home base of Boston with its many poor Negro and white children still lacks a lunch program in its elementary schools (while the suburbs enjoy the benefits of the Federal-and-state-subsidized program). This situation remains despite surveys showing the miserable food habits of many of these children and the fact that a number come to school without any food or money and are fed at the teacher's expense.

Second, the varying nutritional requirements of different children still receive insufficient attention. In several school systems, including some excellent ones, the small obese girl and the star athlete are offered the same dessert. A heavy pudding, perfect for an active boy, is a deplorable dish for the girl with a weight problem. Skim milk is often unobtainable because its widespread distribution would not fulfill another official aim of the school lunch program — to open a market for surplus agricultural commodities, of which butter is one. Substituting skim milk for part of the whole milk in the program would further increase butter surpluses and make the probem of their disposal more difficult.

Finally, although heart disease is the leading cause of death in the United States and obesity is widespread among children (up to 20% of the children examined in the suburbs of Boston) and even more widespread among adults (perhaps as much as one-half of all middle-aged men), very little attention has been given so far to the possibility of using the school lunch program as a long-term tool in preventive medicine. Youngsters could be taught to control sensibly their caloric intake as a function of their requirements and to limit their intake of saturated fats and sugar.

With the health problems associated with overconsumption of saturated fats and calories becoming more acute each day, the school physician may wish to consult with the school dietitian or the director of lunch programs to integrate the school lunch programs into the armamentarium of preventive medicine.

## ADDENDUM

A good general summary of the school lunch program in the United States can be found in the following:

Cronan, M. L.: The School Lunch. Peoria, Illinois, Chas A. Bennett Co., Inc., 1962.

The following pamphlets may be obtained free of charge from the United States Department of Agriculture, Washington, D.C.:

Food Donation Programs. Pamphlet No. 667, June 1965.

Food Service in Public Schools. Marketing Research Report No. 681, November 1964.

National School Lunch Program. Pamphlet No. 19, March 1964.

Planning Type A School Lunches. Pamphlet No. 264, April 1955.

The Why and How. Pamphlet No. 372, July 1958.

Dietitians and administrators who desire guidance in buying may find helpful the following pamphlets from the United States Department of Agriculture, Washington, D.C.:

Food Buying Guide for Type A School Lunches. Pamphlet No. 270, June 1955.

USDA's Consumer and Marketing Service. Pamphlet No. 661, June 1965.

*Chapter 69*

# FOOD HABITS AND NUTRITIONAL
# STATUS OF AMERICAN NEGROES

 $T$ HE publicity given to the problem of securing
equal civil rights for our Negro citizens has tended to obscure
many of the other problems American Negroes face. Indeed in
recent years the collection of information on medical, nutritional
and social characteristics of the Negro population seems to have
ceased. Since the publication of Gunnar Myrdal's famous pre-
World War II book, "An American Dilemma," no comprehensive
study of the life of the American Negro has appeared.

This may be a fruitful time to review briefly what we know of
"Negro" food habits in the United States. Oddly enough, what
makes such a review important is the very fact that these food
habits mirror, with some distortion, the food habits of the white
citizens of the same region and and of the same (generally very
low) income level (1). In the past 15 years, large numbers of
American Negroes have migrated from the rural South and on to the
urban South and on to the urban North. The Northern physician,
used to thinking of Negro food habits as being essentially those of
poor Northerners, often does not realize that Southern-born
Negroes have a very different nutritional background and are
extremely vulnerable to malnutrition. Not only are their food
habits extraordinarily poor to start with, but in the process of
adjusting to their new environment they may relinquish whatever
protective foods they consumed in their native habitat.

I shall examine in succession how food is obtained by the
poorer Negroes (the great majority) in the South and in the North,
those food habits that are somewhat more characteristic of
Negroes, and the nutritional consequences thereof. Negro migrant
workers will be discussed briefly because this population group is,

Reprinted from *Postgraduate Medicine, 37* (No. 1), January, 1965.

medically speaking, the most "vulnerable." The food habits and nutritional status of Negroes in the higher socioeconomic classes will not be considered, as they appear to be essentially indistinguishable from those of their white counterparts.

## HOW FOOD IS SECURED IN THE SOUTH

Negro sharecroppers in the rural South purchase much of their food, often on credit in advance of the harvest. Usually, the shopping is done once a week by the head of the household. When food is grown for their own consumption, the women are usually deeply involved in its production. Children, especially girls, are also put to help. The children also collect wild greens and berries. Fishing is extensively done, mostly by men and boys. Catfish and other fish are caught in the rivers, and crabs, shrimp, clams and crayfish are collected along the seaboard. Squirrels and rabbits are hunted.

In the "urban" South, much of the food consumed by Negroes is still home-grown in backyard vegetable gardens and chicken coops. The majority, however, is purchased, generally at large supermarkets. There are few stores owned and operated by Negroes, and these tend to be small neighborhood stores where prices are higher than in chain stores. Among lower-income Negro families in Southern urban centers, leftovers brought home by the woman domestic worker are considered an integral part of her wages and may constitute an appreciable fraction of the family food supply.

## HOW FOOD IS SECURED IN THE NORTH

Negroes in the North are essentially urban dwellers, so home-grown food is of relatively little importance except in some small towns of the Middle West and West. Large markets as well as small stores in Negro areas often stock foods familiar to the Southern Negroes: turnips, mustard greens, kale, okra, plantain (favored by West Indians), and such parts of pork as chitterlings, hog jowl and salt side. Because many of the women work and cash is short, much of the shopping is done in small amounts by children who are told what to buy and have neither the knowledge nor the opportunity to take advantage of bargains. Lack of storage facilities also precludes more economical quantity buying. Industrial and school feeding programs make a proportionately greater contribution to the nutrition of Northern than of Southern Negroes.

## FOOD HABITS IN THE SOUTH

In the South as in the North, Negroes who have not migrated consume foods similar to those consumed by white persons of the same income level, although the proportions may be different. Breakfast usually consists of biscuits without a spread, a beverage (water, tea or Kool-Aid®), an animal protein food two or three times a week, and cereal or a fat "meat" (fat back) the other mornings. The cereals used are cooked oatmeal, rice and grits, served with margarine. Rural Negro families rarely eat cold cereal with milk and sugar. Among protein foods used are eggs (relatively rare), brains, canned mackerel, salt herring, sausage and fried chicken. The servings of these foods are usually very small. A serving of sausage may be less than an ounce, and a small chicken may be cooked for a family of 8 or 10 persons, the father receiving the meatier portion. Fruits, fruit juice and milk are seldom consumed. Yellow cheese, considered a treat, may be consumed on Sunday mornings.

The noon and evening meals tend to be similar except that an animal protein food, if served at all, is served at only one of the meals. The evening meal often consists of leftovers from the noon meal. An animal protein food (lard, fat meat, fish or eggs) may be served at one of these two meals two to three times a week, usually with a cooked vegetable (generally potatoes or cabbage). Corn bread, almost always served with greens, or light bread and a beverage make up the rest of the meal. In addition a large panful of biscuits is usually made at breakfast time, and these are available for the children to eat throughout the day. When sweet potatoes are plentiful, a large panful of these may be baked in the morning and left for the children to eat. Tomatoes, cucumbers and melons are eaten directly from the garden during the summer in the rural areas; in the same way, during the winter, some children eat turnips. When a dessert is prepared, it is usually a sweet potato pie or molasses pudding.

The Negro city dwellers in the South tend to have similar food habits except that fewer green vegetables are available. They are heavy consumers of flour, baking powder, fats (fat back and, only recently, some margarine), rice, grits, corn meal and sweet potatoes. They consume small amounts of fish, meat (preferentially salt pork, bacon and fresh pork) and poultry (2). Consumption of fresh vegetables is low; consumption of citrus fruits is negligible. Milk consumption is substantially lower among Negro than among white families; in many Negro families water is the only or main beverage consumed with meals. This lower milk consumption is largely a reflection of lower income (3), but even in Negro families whose income is comparable to that of white families the milk consumption may be lower (4).

## FOOD HABITS IN THE NORTH

The food habits of Northern-born Negroes appear to be similar to those of other Northerners when income, type of employment and housing are taken into account. Southern-born Negroes living in the North tend to retain Southern food habits, often at great inconvenience and cost. The food habits of Negroes living in large Northern cities are often profoundly affected by their crowded living conditions. It is not uncommon for several families to share an apartment designed for one family. Many lodgers must pay a separate charge for kitchen privileges, and this may lead them to dispense with cooking altogether. When several families share a kitchen, they are likely to wait their turns rather than to plan for cooperative meals. Cooking is accelerated, and the frying pan is the utensil used most often. The meat tends to be fat (salt pork, bacon), and the grease is used to cook vegetables.

Among Negroes in Northern cities, the majority of whom are poor, a large proportion of the mothers work, and feeding the children is often a difficult problem. Typically the mother gives them breakfast and, if they are under school age, leaves them in the care of another woman. If they are of school age and the school does not have a lunch program (as the Boston grade schools do not), they are given money and allowed to fend for themselves at lunchtime. Elaborate but often unreliable arrangements are made to have small children fed by 6 o'clock if the mother has not returned by then.

The food habits of Southern-born Negroes living in the North appear to be particularly erratic. They spend a substantial amount of money for Southern foods of very limited nutritional value such as fat back and grits. Little use is made of the increased variety of available foods.

## NUTRITIONAL STATUS OF AMERICAN NEGROES

In the absence of a large-scale survey covering the various habitats and economic classes of American Negroes, it is difficult to make a general statement concerning their nutritional status. It can be fairly stated that in general their nutritional status is inferior to that of white persons in the same geographical areas; in some cases it is vastly inferior. The reasons appear to be multiple. Chief among them are the lower earning power of the Negroes and their lower economic level. (In Georgia, for example, which is by no means the poorest Southern state, three-fourths of the Negroes have an annual income of less than $600 per person.) Various recent surveys indicate that the diets of more than 60 per cent of Negro families in both rural and urban areas of the South are "obviously inadequate," compared with less than 25 per cent of white families. Only 10 per cent of the Negroes consume diets that are "obviously adequate," and the diets of 15 per cent are "probably adequate"; respective figures for white families are 45 and 20 per cent (3). The Negro diets are characterized by monotony, a restricted choice of foods, and a low intake of "protective elements." While the caloric requirements are generally covered for all members of the family, the protein intake of the children tends to be only borderline. At least 25 per cent and perhaps as many as 35 per cent of Southern Negroes have a low calcium intake. Likewise the iron intake of perhaps one-third or more is low. The intakes of thiamine, riboflavin and nicotinic acid are low in 12 to 15 per cent of the population, vitamin A requirements are not adequately covered by the diets of perhaps as many as 50 per cent, and vitamin C intake is inadequate for much of the population, particularly in urban areas, for several months each year.

It is impossible to describe the nutritional status of the Negro population in the North even in approximate terms, because hospital records are not analyzed according to race and because surveys covering Negro areas do not seem to have been conducted in recent years. Careful perusal of the records available in large cities as well as the collection of impressions of experienced physicians, dietitians and health administrators leave little doubt that our Negro slums represent the greatest concentration of anemias, growth failures, dermatitides of doubtful origin, accidents of pregnancy, and other signs associated with malnutrition. A number of cases of acute malnutrition are seen each year among the Negro patients including, occasionally, such full-blown syndromes as kwashiorkor (5).

## NUTRITIONAL PROBLEMS OF NEGRO MIGRANTS

There are a number of "migrant streams" or migratory farm forces in the United States, several of them numbering tens of thousands of laborers and their families. One of the largest of these moves "on the season" from Florida to upstate New York. This "Atlantic Coast migrant stream" has been studied fairly intensively by such agencies as the Florida State Board of Health and the Children's Bureau of the United States Department of Health, Education, and Welfare (6).

Although an increasing number of Puerto Ricans and other "whites" are entering this stream, it is estimated that Negro workers still constitute 90 to 95 per cent of its labor force, with more than 50 per cent coming from Georgia. This is a poorly educated group, the median grade completed by adult workers being of the order of six; perhaps as many as one-fourth of the adult men have never had formal education. Many households are quite large (7% consisting of more than 10 persons) but many others are made up of a single person (13.3%) (6). "Serial monogamy" appears to be the rule, with no solid data available on the distribution of marital status in the legal sense. The enormous majority of migrants appear to have been driven to this life through economic necessity rather than by choice. It is not unusual for migrants to follow the stream for 10 or even 20 years.

As would be expected, the poverty, ignorance and nomadic life are attended by nutritional problems incomparably more serious than those of Southern or Northern urban Negroes. For example, the public health study conducted in 1961 among Negro migrant agricultural workers in Palm Beach County, Florida, under the auspices of the Florida State Board of Health, disclosed cases of scurvy, rickets, nutritional edema and marasmus. One case of kwashiorkor in a three-year-old girl was found; it responded to treatment over a period of several months. A high percentage of the children examined fell in the lower percentiles of the Stuart grid. Dental health was extraordinarily poor both in children and in adults. Food habits were deplorable due to lack of money, space and cooking equipment which limited both the availability of protective foods and their preparation. Flour, grits and breads constituted the bulk of the calories, with supplements of beans, the tails and ears of pigs, pigs' feet, neck bones, chicken, fish and some cheese, but practically no milk except for infants (who were fed milk exclusively, well beyond the age at which solid foods should have been given). Our migrant Negro population appears to have the highest proportion of malnourished individuals.

## CONCLUSION

Good nutrition should never be taken for granted in a patient, whatever his age or economic status. This article obviously constitutes the plea of a nutritionist to physicians to be particularly on guard when dealing with Negro patients. So much has been said about the United States being the best-fed country on earth, about our main nutritional problem being overnutrition, and so on, that it is easily forgotten that millions of our fellow citizens are poor, ignorant and ill-fed. In the 1960's a very large proportion of these are Negroes, and their nutritional problems are compounded by the fact that many of them are living in alien or at least non-native environments. Considerable time may have to be spent to elucidate the food habits of such patients, analyze them, determine their inadequacies and correct them through reeducation and perhaps with the aid of foods available through governmental and private agencies. The difficulties of dealing with nutritional problems associated with growth failure, pregnancy, diabetes, heart disease or obesity are compounded in such patients. In many instances the services of a dietitian experienced in the social, psychologic and economic aspects of dietary prescription among such groups is almost a necessity if the physician is not going to spend too much time on nutritional education. Whether the physician will tackle this task himself or will delegate it to a dietitian, the realization by the doctor that it must be tackled is a prerequisite to successful treatment.

## REFERENCES

1. Joffe, N. F. and Walker, T. T.: Some food patterns of Negroes in the United States of America and their relationship to war time problems of food and nutrition. Report prepared for the Committee on Food Habits, National Research Council, 1944.
2. Meat choices for family meals in selected cities, Alabama-Georgia. Agricultural Stations of Alabama, Georgia, Kentucky, Mississippi, South Carolina, Tennessee, Texas and Virginia cooperating. Southern Cooperative Series Bulletin No. 77, 1961.
3. Anderson, E. L.: Dietary practices of Negro and white families with crippled children in five counties in eastern North Carolina. Reproduced by the Children's Bureau, United States Department of Health, Education, and Welfare, with permission of the Department of Public Health Nutrition, Schools of Public Health, University of North Carolina, 1963.
4. Consumption and demand of fluid milk and fluid milk substitutes in the urban South. The Agricultural Experimental Stations of Alabama, Arkansas, Georgia, Louisiana, Mississippi, North Carolina, South Carolina, Tennessee, Texas and the U.S. Department of Agriculture cooperating. Southern Cooperative Series Bulletin No. 53, October 1957; also Dickens, D.: Use, knowledge and attitudes concerning milk products by home-makers. Mississippi State University Agricultural Experiment Station Bulletin 643, April 1962.
5. Mayer, J.: Kwashiorkor. Postgrad. Med., 26:98, 1959.
6. Browning, R. H. and Northcutt, T. J., Jr.: On the season. Florida Board of Health Monograph No. 2, 1961.

## Chapter 70

# NUTRITIONAL QUACKERY

N O one knows just how much money nutritional quackery costs Americans each year; the American Medical Association estimates that it is between $500,000,000 and $1,000,000,000. But nutritional quackery does not just cost money: it also systematically undermines the confidence of American people in their food supply, in their physicians, and in their universities. When garlic pills are sold to treat high blood pressure and when raisins are sold as a cancer remedy, the cost may be high indeed!

## HOW NUTRITIONAL QUACKERY WORKS

Nutritional quackery operates by undermining the public's confidence in reliable sources of information, and this undermining often goes unnoticed or unrecognized by those in a position to counter it. To enable you to recognize nutritional quackery in action, here is how it works: The quack depends for his profits on convincing people that the foods they buy through regular retail outlets are poisoned by preservatives and insecticides, and that they are "devitalized" by the use of "chemical" rather than "natural" fertilizers. The medical profession and the universities are alleged to be in league with the food manufacturers in their exploitation of the public.

What should people do about this exploitation? The quacks tell them that the only remedy is to consume foods that have not been exposed to such nefarious influences. This is why even such apparently innocuous institutions as "nature food" or "health food" stores are dangerous. These stores drain off a lot of money

Reprinted from *Consultant* February, 1963.

that should go for normal, wholesome, nourishing foods and for needed medical care. Elderly people, especially those who are not well educated, are especially vulnerable to this exploitation.

In some cases "nature" foods are outright frauds. The Food and Drug Administration recently found a little "factory" in Boston where labels of well-known food cans were ripped off and new labels substituted. The new labels assured the public that the food had been grown without insecticides and without chemical fertilizers. This "special care" supposedly justified hiking up the price!

## BUSINESS BASED ON DISTRUST OF MEDICINE

Aside from the fact that people are being exploited, physicians should realize that the very existence of the "health foods" business is based on distrust of medicine. This leads the consumer to the ultimate step — medical quackery.

Many "nutritional" supplements are sold door-to-door as part of daily "family programs." Printed matter that advertises these supplements is worded very carefully to avoid federal penalties. But door-to-door salesmen — and one organization alone employs thousands  are under no such restraint. Salesmen will promise that their supplements will prevent or cure dandruff, heart disease, cancer, gout, and arthritis. They make great capital out of what they claim their products will do to retard senility or to rejuvenate sexual functions. And what do these miraculous preparations actually contain? Usually haphazard amounts of vitamins plus such "natural" compounds as powdered alfalfa, water cress, soy beans, or kelp! And what do the salesmen say if they are investigated? Usually they will deny that they ever made such claims, or will say that what they said was misunderstood. They point to the innocuous labels and printed advertising to support their innocence.

## SELLING SEAWATER INSTEAD OF
## THE BROOKLYN BRIDGE

Seawater recently became a nutritional fad. Seawater, someone discovered, is a source of minerals. It obviously is . . . of the same minerals that are found in foods. The fact that seawater is a good source of iodine and fluorine, usually proclaimed as deadly poisons by the very proponents of food fads, does not seem to hinder the quackery entrepreneurs. The presence of fluoride is apparently outweighed in their evaluation by the delightful cheapness and abundance of their raw material. Another great advantage, shared by few manufacturers: the raw material is also the finished product! Who would bother to sell the Brooklyn Bridge when he can sell the Atlantic and the Pacific?

Another aspect of nutritional quackery, and one that could be corrected by administrative action and education, is the nutritional quackery that goes with athletics. There isn't a fad diet or a quack preparation (including royal jelly) known to man that is not advocated somewhere by a coach or athletic director to boys or girls under his care. School and college physicians should ascertain what advice, diets, and prescriptions are given under the sponsorship of the department of physical education.

The nutritional quackery that exists in the field of obesity therapy is so obvious and so prevalent as to be a national scandal. Less well recognized is quackery in treating arthritis. Whenever people lose hope of being cured by medical treatment – because there is no known cure – they listen to quacks. A study of a large population of arthritic patients revealed that half of them have gone to quacks and have followed faddist dietary treatments at various times.

## MEANS OF MISINFORMATION

The means by which the public is misinformed about nutrition are many. I have already mentioned the "health food" and "nature food" shops, which are often centers for distributing quack literature as well as antifluoridation propaganda, and the door-to-door salesmen who give the most dangerous misinformation. "Health" lecturers are an important source of misinformation, too, whether they operate through speeches to live audiences or through radio, a medium licensed by the federal government and therefore a public responsibility. The Food and

Drug Administration has tried recently to get some of the better-known quack nutritional lecturers off the air, but so far has had only indifferent success. Magazines and newspapers have difficulty in resisting the lure of advertising profits, so they, too, have become media for disseminating nutritional misinformation.

What can we do about all this? First, we need to resolve not to stand idly by while this fad information is given to the public. Our professional organizations ought to be enrolled in an effort to provide sound information that will counteract faddist propaganda. The American Medical Association recently created machinery that will permit it to exercise some restraint over literary nutritional quackery perpetrated by some of its members.

## DOCTORS SHOULD SPEAK UP

The medical profession must speak up against nutritional quackery even though it may result in our being subjected to personal abuse and an occasional law suit. We must explore avenues through which we can inform the public. The schools are one place this can be done, not by adding a few more assemblies to an already confused curriculum, but by insisting that all high school students complete at least one good course in human biology and physiology so that they will know how to recognize fraudulent claims. Coaches and athletic directors, if properly educated, would be natural allies in health campaigns.

We need to give more support to the Food and Drug Administration and, in many states, to local food and drug administrations so these agencies will be given the personnel and authority they need. Finally, we must learn to use the mass media. We must cultivate our relationship with newspapers, radio, and television and stand ready to help them as consultants so as to enable us, in turn, to apply pressure to eliminate quackery and bring sound information before the public. There is a reluctance among medical and academic people to enter the public arena, but it is essential that they do. Somebody is going to advise the public on its diet and it should be the people who know what they are talking about.

# PART IX

## The White House Conference, Hunger and Nutrition Policy

*Chapter 71*


# OPENING STATEMENT AT THE FIRST SESSION OF THE SENATE COMMITTEE ON NUTRITION AND HUMAN NEEDS, 1968

I FEEL honored to be asked to appear before this body, and to be the first witness to be so asked. I am sure that I speak for all U.S. nutritionists when I say how pleased we are that the United States Senate, and the members of this Committee in particular, recognize the importance of sound nutrition for the welfare of our people and are interested in the improvement of the national diet. Because I do have the privilege of being the first witness to testify, I see myself as responsible for giving this Committee a broad picture of our nutritional problems rather than a detailed analysis of any single aspect.

We have too long been content to repeat that "we are the best fed country on earth." While we have good reasons to be proud of our agricultural production records and of the work of our public health and extension nutritionists, three major considerations militate against excessive complacency on our part:

First, a considerable number of published studies document the fact that a large number of our people, situated economically in the lowest fifth of the nation, are too poor to feed themselves properly under the conditions in which they live. The existence of this type of malnutrition has been dramatized lately by various reports and television programs. Government surveys (HEW) are bringing in controlled facts on statistically valid stratified samples which are confirming and reinforcing many of the pictures produced by these hearings and reportings. I understand that this evidence will be presented to you soon. It appears that present corrective governmental measures are inadequate in many areas and under various conditions to deal effectively with malnutrition due to poverty.

Second, a great many of our people are uninformed about nutrition, put themselves on inadequate diets, and are frequently the prey of food faddists and quacks. This is true, in particular, of adolescents, old people, and sufferers of chronic conditions such as arthritis or overweight.

Third, the national diet is extremely high in saturated fats. Together with the physical inactivity characteristic for our adult males (and unfortunately, of a growing number of our young people) and the obesity so prevalent in our population (and again, as our studies have shown, so directly related to physical inactivity), this high-fat diet is probably largely responsible for the pandemic of coronaries and other cardiovascular diseases which are afflicting our land and nullifying the effect of medical advances at least as regards our national life expectancy.

Let us look at these three areas in more detail.

## 1. MALNUTRITION AND POVERTY

Government and university studies have shown repeatedly that a great many of our people have highly inadequate intakes of a number of nutrients. Anemia and growth retardation are frequent among the poor as are accidents of pregnancy. In general, it appears that we have five main areas of malnutrition:

(a) Unemployed or partly employed poor: Many of these are in the Deep South — in particular, ex-cotton workers displaced by changes in crops from cotton to corn and by the use of new machinery. It has perhaps not been pointed out enough that many are in other areas, such as Appalachia.

(b) Migrant workers: The eastern "stream" is mostly made up of Negroes and Puerto-Ricans, the western "stream" is mostly Mexican. Both contain many ill-fed children and adults.

(c) Indians in the Southwest and elsewhere: There appear to be great differences between tribes and between reservations, but a substantial proportion of our Indian citizens appear to be in a poor state of nutrition and of health.

(d) The very poor in big cities: Many very poor individuals and families are not receiving welfare payments; many are not in areas or groups included in nutrition programs. Some cities have no school lunches or have school lunches only for certain grades. Some poor people who have migrated from other areas (e.g. Puerto Rico, the rural South or border states) try to reconstitute in northern cities, at very high cost, the often inadequate diet to which they were used.

(e) The nutritional situation of certain Indians and Eskimos in Alaska appears to be bad or at least precarious. Data available to me are inadequate for judgment.

How can we cope with these problems?

I believe that an expanded program of free food stamps, commodities and supplementary nutritional programs, such as day-care and school meals, could if conducted on a large enough scale, have a considerable impact on malnutrition due to poverty. In advocating the removal of payments on food stamps and commodities, at least for the very poor, I am not blind to the need for responsible accounting. At the same time I want to point out that reluctance on the part of the Secretary of Agriculture to use his full authority and remove price tags for the very poor and indifference of many officials at the local level have been greater problems in the past than difficulties of control. Social welfare agents should be less involved in control, more in welfare (the reverse may be true for law enforcement agencies). I would suggest that the licensing, by federal standards, of voluntary associations and groups, could be a way to create responsible bodies which could undertake to distribute free food stamps and commodities, conceivably with some financial help. Possible abuses could be checked by the Internal Revenue Service; the Department of Agriculture would retain responsibility at the federal and state level for the programs.

Greater incentives may have to be given cities so that they will expand their school lunch programs (and day-care feeding programs) to all children. At present these are fragmentary. For example, I am ashamed to have to report that in my own city of Boston (where school lunches were invented), the enormous majority of our elementary schools do not have a school lunch program. Children in the wealthy suburbs are subsidized and have such a program, while children in the urban core, whose parents or only parent work all day, are often reduced to buying soft drink and a doughnut, do without such a program (or are subsidized by their teacher).

*All these programs ought to be monitored in terms of actual intake of food by people, and nutritional status of recipient groups, not just in terms of money spent.*

Finally, I want to emphasize that *we cannot continue to have our surpluses (and indirectly our subsidies policy) dictate our nutrition programs.* We have inherited from the thirties (when economists believed that the Depression — and its attendant miseries — derived from agricultural "overproduction", when a quarter of the population were farmers, and when the farmers were the poor) a system of subsidies which though they have been frequently altered since, are by no means directed at producing the type of "surpluses" which would be most useful for feeding programs. As a result, our children and our poor are often fed whatever tends to accumulate as a result of these economic policies, rather than the types of food they really need. (Some of our surpluses, e.g. butter, are often equally unusable for foreign relief as well). It is high time that we reverse this policy; we should determine on nutritional grounds, not on economic grounds the foods required by our feeding programs and then go ahead and produce them. If we have surpluses, at least let us have the right surpluses.

## 2. NUTRITION EDUCATION

The ignorance of our people as regards the caloric value and the nutrient content of foods as well as the nutritional requirements, is appalling. This ignorance is responsible for some of the malnutrition we see in this country. It also makes the fortune of quacks who prey on our people and, in spite of the efforts of federal authorities, make fortunes selling useless "dietary supplements", quack "reducing" diets and faddist books, etc. Hundreds of millions of dollars thus become unavailable for sound nutrition and legitimate health expenditures.

In the long run, I am convinced that we shall not be able to avoid the increasing flood of nutritional (and health) quackery which threatens the nutritional status of many of our fellow citizens until states adopt a requirement for a course in human physiology (including nutrition) before graduation from high school (similar to the requirement for an American history course which many states have set). Meanwhile, I believe that we are failing to make use of a great national asset by not utilizing the competence of the Agricultural Extension Service more fully for nutrition and home economics education among the rural poor. There is no fundamental reason why the service could not be extended to work in urban areas as well. (Or it could serve as a nucleus for the creation of a similar service – with a different sociological orientation – under the aegis of the Department of Housing and Urban Development.)

We can also hope that the Public Health Service, through appropriate measures, will encourage the development of better nutrition teaching in the medical, dental, and nursing schools, and that fluoridation of the water supply will be universally accepted.

### 3. NUTRITION AND DEGENERATIVE DISEASES

In the course of the past 20 years we have as a nation quadrupled our health expenditures (tripled per capita). Health is now the third largest user of manpower. Yet during that period, our life expectancy at 20 has not increased and our position has tumbled, particularly for men (we are now, I believe, 37th). The main reason for our poor showing is our growing mortality from cardiovascular diseases. This is in turn related to our diet – extremely high in saturated fats; to our lack of physical activity – adult males are now almost immobile in urban areas, children do less and less; to the prevalence of obesity – itself probably largely due to the fact that as shown in our laboratory, the "minimum" appetite of inactive subjects is higher than their energy expenditure so that people who exercise very little are more likely to get fat. We need to do much more for the nation's fitness. Children need a daily program of exercise rather than the bi-weekly exposure they now get. Greater effort must be put into those children who need it most, instead of concentrating exclusively on athletes; sports and games which can be practiced through life must be taught rather than simply team games played in schools. And we must increase enormously the facilities available to adults for exercise (presumably, in part by having facilities which can be used both by the schools and the community). Exercise improves weight control, maintains vessels elastic, can create collateral circulation to replace partly occluded arteries, and may lower cholesterol and blood pressure. When it is realized that exercise facilities are not simply "recreation", but fill an urgent health need relating to our main cause of death, we may hope that federal support for the construction of such facilities will be forthcoming. (Certainly, the achievements to date of the various presidential fitness committees have been meager.)

We can and we should facilitate changes in the national diet which will lower the total fat content of the diet and shift as much as possible of the dietary fat from "saturated" fats to "polyunsaturated" fats. Such changes have been shown to lower blood cholesterol and the risk of coronaries. In particular, we should encourage the precise labeling of the content of the various fatty acids in various oils and fats. Together with proper nutrition education this should reward manufacturers who have, in fact, produced more healthful fats. We should encourage the development of leaner meat and enormously increase our catch and our consumption of fish. Finally, last but not least we should put more emphasis on preventive cardiovascular medicine which can save (and keep healthy) millions of Americans (even if we continue to admire feats of surgical virtuosity which prolong the life of a few).

Whether we are dealing with the problems of the poor or the problems of the rich, we have to readjust our priorities before effective action can be taken.

*Chapter 72*

# A SOCIAL PHARMACOPEIA FOR NUTRITION

THE American public — including the medical profession — has been shocked by the extent of malnutrition due to poverty in the United States, as revealed by the "Hunger, U.S.A." report of the Citizens' Board of Inquiry into Hunger and Malnutrition in the United States, the CBS reports on hunger and malnutrition, and a number of magazine and newspaper articles. The hearing of the Senate's Select Committee on Nutrition and Human Needs and the preliminary reports of the Department of Health, Education, and Welfare confirm the substance of the less official and more sensational reports. As many as 10 per cent of our fellow citizens are ill-fed because they are too poor. Certainly we can take little pride in the long ignorance of this fact, for basically we have had the information all along in statistics on child mortality, anemia, growth rates, prematurity and the accidents of pregnancy.

As chairman of the new National Council on Hunger and Malnutrition in the U.S.A., I know very well that no nationwide program to eradicate malnutrition can succeed without the help of the nation's physicians. Conversely, physicians practicing in poverty areas can help their patients immeasurably by helping to monitor and correct governmental programs.

## SOME MYTHS

First let us dispel some widespread misconceptions about the nutrition programs.

Myth — The really poor have access to adequate surplus commodities and food stamps if they are in danger of starving.

Reprinted from *Postgraduate Medicine*, 45 (No. 3), March, 1969.© McGraw-Hill, Inc.

Fact — Only 5.4 million of the more than 29 million poor participate in government food programs, and the majority are not the poorest.

Myth — Poor children are fed at least one good meal a day through the National School Lunch Program.

Fact — At most, one-third of poverty-stricken children attending public schools participate in school lunch programs. Many of the poorest areas in big cities have no program for elementary schools. Despite express provision in the National School Lunch Program Act that children from poor families shall "be served without cost or a reduced cost," a majority of poor children must pay the full price for the school lunch or go without.

Myth — Progress is being made as a result of massive federal efforts in which multimillion dollar food programs take care of more people now than ever before.

Fact — Participation in government food programs has dropped 1.4 million in the last six years. Malnutrition among the poor has risen sharply over the last decade.

In 1967 there were 8,876,700 poverty-stricken families (including one person households), tabulated by the government on a sliding scale which relates income to household size. These families comprise 29,900,000 persons, only 18 per cent of whom are covered by either of the two main food programs, commodities and stamps. Of the six million children of school age in these families, only two million received free lunches.

## AVAILABLE PROGRAMS

In theory we should be able to insure each poor American a decent diet, either through Social Security and welfare programs or the food assistance programs.

1. Commodity distribution program for needy families — The federal government distributes to needy families some of the food it buys to bolster the farmers' income (Section 416 of the Agricultural Act of 1949). These foods, called basic commodities, are provided in the form of cornmeal, corn grits, flour, nonfat dry milk, peanut butter, rice and rolled wheat. The so-called Section

32 money (Section 32, PL 320), which comes directly to the Secretary of Agriculture without appropriation by Congress, is intended to keep farmers' prices high and to provide for those in need, but usually only a small part is used. Of the $700 million received in 1967, some $500 million was returned to the Treasury or carried forward. Less than $150 million was used in connection with commodity or food distribution programs.

2. Food stamp program – This program was designed to correct the deficiencies of the commodity program by letting the poor choose their own foods. The bonus coupons they buy multiply their food-purchasing power at local stores. The law requires that the Secretary of Agriculture set prices at a rate equivalent to the "normal expenditure" for food, which he does by determining average expenditures for families of different sizes and income.

3. School lunch program – This program has the potential for directly alleviating hunger and malnutrition among poor children of school age.

## DEFICIENCIES AND WEAKNESSES OF THE PROGRAMS

One basic deficiency is that over 300 of the poorest counties have no programs because local authorities have not requested them. The USDA has the power to start programs where the need is evident but has been reluctant to override county authority. Some counties discontinue programs during harvest time to assure an abundant labor supply at subsistence wages. In counties where commodities are distributed, they seldom reach a majority of the poor. Some persons are arbitrarily barred; others are unable to go to distribution centers and transport the commodities. "Surpluses" may be unfamiliar or unusable, and the commodities do not furnish the basis for a nutritionally adequate diet.

Food stamps are too expensive for the very poor. When commodity distribution is replaced by food stamps, participation drops drastically. As income rises, a larger proportion must go to pay for food stamps. Most counties are unwilling to adjust prices for seasonal income. The poor have to pay for stamps in a lump sum and buy a minimum amount – at the same level each month – or they are dropped. Single persons cannot participate. In addition, food stamp offices are often inconveniently located and have short, sporadic hours. By the USDA's own standard, the money value of stamps falls consistently and deliberately below the amount necessary to secure a minimally adequate diet. This inadequacy is increased by the practice of many local stores of raising prices on food stamp distribution days.

We have already seen how fractional the contribution of school lunch programs is to the problem of nutrition of the poor. "Consumer education programs," often mentioned as aids to these programs, are in practice nonexistent, and the contribution of the public assistance programs in feeding the poor is limited. Most states administering federal welfare monies do not pay the minimal amount necessary for subsistence as estimated by their own or federal standards – and incidentally pay less than the amount to which families are entitled by law.

## WHAT THE DOCTOR CAN DO

A firm stand by organized medicine supporting to the limit federal, state and local efforts to wipe out hunger and malnutrition in the United States would be of immeasurable help. More directly, the doctor can help in his own area by pressing for commoditiy and food stamp participation by his county; for sufficient publicity of such programs, with clear indication of the location of offices; for ease of access and help with transporting commodities; for financing of stamps, as well as for requests by local authorities to the USDA to have food stamps made free when necessary (the Secretary of Agriculture has the authority to do so under Section 32, PL 320); and for organization of school lunch programs in all schools, particularly in poverty areas, with meals for children who need them, under conditions that safeguard the dignity and self-respect of our very young fellow citizens who live under difficult circumstances.

*Chapter 73*

# WHITE HOUSE CONFERENCE ON FOOD, NUTRITION AND HEALTH, 1969

 $T$ HE hunger and malnutrition John Steinbeck described so vividly in "The Grapes of Wrath" did not disappear after the Depression. Agricultural abundance and prosperity benefit most of us, yet the poor remain in a condition similar to that of the Joad family in Steinbeck's book.

The publication of "Hunger, U.S.A.," the CBS documentary, "Report on Hunger," the hearings of the Senate's Select Committee on Nutrition and Human Needs, and the National Nutrition Survey have shown that a large number of our poor live in a deplorable state of malnutrition and many of them are hungry. The American population is alarmed by these findings. They know now that distributing food baskets to the poor will not solve this enormous problem. The time has come to develop a national nutrition and food distribution policy, a policy based on human need and not predicated by agricultural subsidies.

The White House Conference on Food, Nutrition and Health, December 2, 3 and 4, 1969, will meet to lay the foundation for such a national nutrition policy, to advise President Nixon on the best methods to eliminate hunger and malnutrition in the United States, and to create an awakened public opinion that will seek action on the recommendations made.

The Conference will consider methods through which the nutritional status and dietary intake of the American people can be continually monitored and evaluated. Three panels will study nutritional status. The first panel, chaired by Dr. James P. Carter, assistant professor of nutrition, Vanderbilt University School of Medicine, will discuss actual methods for collecting clinical, biochemical and dietary data needed to determine nutritional

Reprinted from *Postgraduate Medicine, 46* (No. 3), September, 1969.© McGraw-Hill, Inc.

health. Currently available methods are cumbersome, time-consuming and expensive. We need to develop new ways to monitor the nutritional status of our entire population to detect any existing malnutrition.

The second panel, chaired by Dr. D. Mark Hegsted, professor of nutrition, Harvard University School of Public Health, will develop standards to evaluate nutritional status. This is a difficult problem. For example, not all children will fall above the fiftieth percentile on a growth curve. We need to know, however, what point below this percentile is unacceptable and perhaps indicative of nutritional inadequacies. Dietary needs differ; not everyone will eat the recommended dietary allowances every day. What is the range of tolerance? When is a diet inadequate for a particular individual?

A design for continually evaluating the nutritional status of a population is meaningless without methods for carrying it out. The third panel, chaired by Mr. William Carey, former assistant director of the Bureau of the Budget, will discuss the administration of a national nutrition policy.

The health of several groups in our population may be impaired if they are improperly fed. In a national nutrition policy, vunerable groups such as pregnant women must receive special consideration to insure their having an adequate diet. Dr. Charles U. Lowe, scientific director, National Institute of Child Health and Human Development of the Department of Health, Education, and Welfare, assisted by Dr. Howard Jacobson, the noted San Francisco obstetrician, will chair the panel examining special nutritional problems of the pregnant woman and her infant.

During childhood and adolescence, food patterns become habits and the foundation of nutritional status is laid. These early years are also the period of rapid growth, and the demand for several nutrients is higher than at any other time of life. A panel chaired by Dr. Samuel J. Fomon, professor of pediatrics, University of Iowa, will discuss nutrition policy for children and adolescents in relation to their needs and existing programs and consider nutrition education for adolescents and methods for improving the health and fitness status of children.

Improperly balanced diets are known to cause or aggravate

several degenerative diseases. A panel chaired by Dr. Ancel Keys, director of the Laboratory of Physiological Hygiene, University of Minnesota, assisted by Dr. Irvine Page, Cleveland Clinic cardiologist, will recommend changes in diet to prevent such conditions as cardiovascular diseases, dental caries, and obesity.

In our culture, the aging, especially the poor, are often isolated and forgotten. These people may have a limited education and be immobilized by their poverty and physical disabilities. The problems of the aged, while primarily social, have many health and nutritional manifestations. Dr. Edward L. Bortz, chief of medical services, Lankenau Hospital, Philadelphia, and former president of the American Medical Association, will chair the panel on aging, which will discuss methods to make attractive and palatable foods available and methods whereby meals and food can serve to alleviate social isolation and loneliness in the elderly.

Another panel, chaired by Dr. W. H. Sebrell, R. R. Williams Professor of Nutrition, Columbia University, will look at nutritional personnel in the health systems. The panel will discuss methods for increasing their effectiveness in caring for the sick in hospitals and clinics and possible ways of extending their expertise into the community.

The unique nutritional problems of the wards of the federal government — Indians, Eskimo, the people of Guam, Samoa and Micronesia, migratory workers, and the residents of the District of Columbia — will be examined by a panel chaired by Dr. William J. Darby, professor and chairman, department of biochemistry, Vanderbilt University School of Medicine. A special study of Puerto Rico may be included in this panel's discussion.

The principal component of an effective nutrition policy is food. Once the nutritional status and nutrient demands of the population are clearly defined, the necessary foods to meet these requirements must be made available. Hunger and malnutrition will be eliminated only if our agricultural policies are sensitively geared to respond to the needs of the poor. A panel chaired by Mr. William B. Murphy, president, Campbell Soup Company, will examine current levels of food production and projected changes in the food supply in relation to nutritional needs. The recommendations made will clearly specify what changes in the supply of traditional staples are needed, what trends in food production should be encouraged, and what agricultural policies need to be eliminated.

In the last 10 years, scientists have made tremendous advances in food technology. We now have the technical capability to produce in our laboratories food that is nearly an exact facsimile of traditional foods. The area of new foods is exciting and promises some solutions to malnutrition. However, we must develop standards so that simulated food offers at least comparable quantity and quality of nutrients available in its traditional counterpart. Dr. Richard S. Gordon, vice-persident, Monsanto Company, will be responsible for the panel on new food.

The next panel, chaired by Mr. Donald M. Kendall, president, Pepsi Cola, Inc., will deal with the overall problems of safety evaluation of foods. Safety of food processing, components of convenience foods, and the vast, complicated area of food additives will be examined. Finally, Dr. Emil M. Mrak, chancellor emeritus, University of California at Davis, will head a panel to review the procedures used to grade quality of food.

Nutrition education is of paramount importance in a national nutrition scheme. Previous efforts have been largely ineffective, and most Americans are abysmally ignorant about the most elementary principles of applied nutrition. A national nutrition policy will become a working reality only if we find new effective ways to educate the population in the basics of food and nutrition.

Nutrition is often presented in the primary and secondary schools as an afterthought to biology or hidden in the curriculum in home economics courses. A panel chaired by Dr. George M. Briggs, professor and chairman of nutrition sciences, University of California, will tackle the problem of making nutrition education a key part of the curriculum in primary and secondary schools.

Ignorance about nutrition is not confined to laymen. Most physicians graduate from medical school with only a cursory understanding of nutrition. Consequently, when the practicing physician is confronted with a nutrition problem, he is forced to rely on pharmaceutical supplements for treatment. A panel chaired by Dr. Grace A. Goldsmith, professor of medicine and dean, Tulane University School of Public Health and Tropical Medicine, will discuss methods for improving nutrition education in medical, dental and other professional schools.

Fully aware of the difficulty of changing food habits, a panel chaired by Dr. Cecile H. Edwards, chairman, department of home economics, Agricultural and Technical College of North Carolina, will discuss improving the general nutrition education of the public. This panel will also look at the problems of training nutrition aides and volunteers working in poverty areas and the potential role an expanded extension program may play in urban community education.

Food faddists have used the media for years to misinform the American public, yet reliable nutrition educators have sadly neglected this persuasive and effective educational tool. A panel chaired by Dr. Philip L. White, secretary, Council on Foods and Nutrition, American Medical Association, will consider using the media for nutrition education and other methods for reaching and educating disadvantaged groups. Included in this assignment will be methods for offsetting misinformation and food quackery.

Many inequities remain in our food distribution system. Our middle-class suburbs have an abundance of supermarkets, but few are in the urban ghettos, forcing the poor to shop in expensive small markets. Supermarkets that do serve the ghettos often have lower-quality food and higher prices than those in the suburbs. A panel chaired by Dr. David L. Call, H. E. Babcock Professor of Food Economics, Cornell University, will look at our food distribution system, with special attention to the components of food prices and food distribution in poor areas.

The traditional family structure has undergone radical change. Women, especially poor women, are forced to work outside their homes to support their families. The food industry has responded to this change by producing convenience foods and thus has almost eliminated the traditional role of the mother as the preparer of food. Inadvertently, these changes have acted to further weaken the family structure. It seems useful to examine these trends to see if anything can be done through nutrition to reinforce the family structure. This difficult assignment will be the responsibility of a panel with the noted scholar Dr. Kenneth Clark, president of the American Psychological Association, as chairman.

The delivery of food and money for food to the poor has come under sharp attack — and justly so. For the last several years, we have spent more and more money to feed the poor but have fed fewer and fewer people. We need to devise a workable system that is integrated with our welfare assistance programs and solidly based on the needs of the people these programs serve — the poor. Dr. Stanley Gershoff, associate professor of nutrition, Harvard University School of Public Health, will chair this panel.

Food-catering institutions have streamlined and centralized food service. The lessons learned and the technics used may well help solve some of the federal government's institutional feeding problems. Mr. Harvey T. Stephens, executive vice-president, Automatic Retailers of America, Inc., will chair the panel that will discuss new ways to provide meals for federal installations.

All the panels described have been concerned with the federal government's role in feeding the poor and improving the nutritional status of the entire population. However, the effectiveness of voluntary support may be the critical element in a successful nutrition policy.

The food industry has within its structure tremendous untapped resources. Food chains, on their own initiative, might develop a far-reaching and effective consumer education program in food purchasing and budgeting. Five panels will discuss what the food industry can do to help feed the poor properly. The first will be on agricultural production. Mr. C. W. W. Cook, chairman, General Foods Corporation, will lead the panel on food manufacturing and processing. The next panel, headed by Mr. Augustine Marusi, chairman, Borden, Inc., will discuss food packaging and labeling. A panel on food distribution and retailing will be chaired by Mr. Donald S. Perkins, president, Jewel Companies, Inc., and the last panel, headed by Mr. James P. McFarland, chairman, General Mills, Inc., will deal with food promotion and advertising.

Last, but certainly important, are panels that deal with voluntary citizens' groups. Women's organizations, community action groups, churches, men's organizations, university faculties and the students, and consumer organizations will be called on to use their resources to bring the needs of the people they serve to the Conference and then to implement Conference recommendations in their communities and to explore ways of implementing them on a national scale.

At the White House Conference, we will have segments of the entire population on panels. We hope to involve the entire population with the purposes and issues of the Conference. Many physicians will participate on the panels, and the entire medical community will be called on to implement the recommendations stemming from the Conference.

This will not be a scientific meeting. We will bring together persons who, although conversant in nutrition, will be asked to use their creative energies to invent socially feasible solutions to the problem of hunger and malnutrition. The real limits and challenges at the White House Conference will be economic, social and political.

## Chapter 74

# LETTER OF TRANSMITTAL TO THE PRESIDENT

The following is the letter of transmittal accompanying the report of the first White House Conference on Food, Nutrition and Health, from Dr. Jean Mayer to President Nixon.

December 24, 1969

Dear Mr. President:

I have the honor to transmit to you the report of your first White House Conference on Food, Nutrition and Health. You announced on May 6, 1969, that you would call such a Conference to advise you, the Congress, and the American people on the development of national policy aimed at eliminating hunger and malnutrition due to poverty and at improving the nutritional health of all Americans. On June 11, 1969, you appointed me to organize the Conference.

A great deal of preliminary work was done during the summer and the fall of 1969 by twenty-six panels and by eight task forces. The panels were made up of academic, medical, industry, and agriculture experts, as well as citizens chosen because of their particular concern rather than expertise. The task forces represented vast segments of our population such as social action groups, women's organizations, industrial and consumer interests, professional organizations and religious denominations. All 800 or so participants in the preparatory work were highly conscious of their responsibility and spent considerable time in work and travel to insure that the 2200 additional members of the Conference be

Reprinted from *Postgraduate Medicine, 47* (No. 2), February, 1970.© McGraw-Hill, Inc.

provided with thoughtful and detailed provisional recommendations and background material.

Panel and task force members met for the whole week starting Sunday, November 30. The full Conference started on December 2, when you addressed nearly 5,000 persons at the opening plenary session. The Conference lasted three days, during which groups were meeting in 30 different rooms with intense and constructive discussions taking place. Following your instructions, the membership of the Conference — and of each discussion group — was as broad as possible. University professors and students, physicians, old and young, industry leaders and technicians, representatives of consumer organizations, members of all main religious denominations and of minority organizations, members of women's organizations with membership totaling over 60 million women, labor leaders, representatives of health organizations, agricultural and trade organizations, social action groups from all economic levels ranging from the National Association of Manufacturers to various organizations dealing with the very poor — and last but not least, over 400 of the very poor themselves: black, Mexican-Americans, Puerto Ricans, white, Indians, Alaskan natives, inhabitants of the Pacific trusts and territories, and of our Caribbean dependencies and migrant laborers were brought together to discuss the recommendations submitted to them by the panels and the task forces.

The recommendations which this volume contains were the final outcome of the deliberations of the Conference. As such, their sponsorship is much broader than that of the original groups which prepared the preliminary recommendations.

Because the identification of undernourished and malnourished groups is basic to any corrective program, three panels dealt with various aspects of the surveillance of the state of nutrition of the American people. The surveillance system they designed can also be used for the monitoring of the effectiveness of federal and state and local corrective programs. They recommend that prime responsibility for such a surveillance system be placed in the Department of Health, Education, and Welfare. Detailed recommendations concerning administration, methods, standards and personnel are given in the first section of the Report.

Section II deals with the specialized problems of certain specific groups: pregnant and nursing women, children and adolescents, adults prone to degenerative diseases, the sick, the aging, as well as groups for which the Federal Government has statutory responsibility — inhabitants of Guam, American Samoa, the U.S. trust territories, the citizens of Puerto Rico and the Virgin Islands, the American Indians and Alaskan natives, the migrant workers, inhabitants of the District of Columbia, and the military. All panels of this section emphasized that special programs could only be considered on the basis of adequate provision of food stamps in adequate amounts — including the provision of free food stamps for the very poor, a realistic family allowance, or a combination of the two programs. All panels also emphasized the desirability of better health services with a strong nutrition component. Nutrition education was considered an essential part of all special programs (though it could not replace food or money for food). The panels dealing with children, adolescents and adults emphasized the need for better facilities for exercise as well as nutrition programs. The requirements for services as well as food or money are particularly apparent for the aging. The fact that a thorough overhaul of the administrative machinery dealing with special geographic groups is long overdue, that greater emphasis must be placed on health and human values will be apparent to you as you read the recommendations dealing with these categories of Americans.

The four panels dealing with various aspects of our food policies all directed their recommendations at simplifying legislation, permitting greater innovation by industry in the development of new and better foods while, at the same time, insuring better protection of the consumer than is available now as regards safety, grading of quality, and meaningful disclosure of content and nutritional value. The recommendations of these panels should lend themselves particularly well to the rapid development of legislative proposals.

Four panels dealt with education at preschool and school, university, and community levels as well as with the use of the various media. The recommendations of panels concerned with school and academic interests should greatly improve the quality of nutrition teaching from Head Start to medical school. Community programs suggested better uses of community aides and of feeding programs in popular nutrition education. The group dealing with the media was particularly innovative in their suggestions concerning the use of radio, television, reading material, symbols and slogans, and suggested constructive ways by which media could cooperate with educators. Again, all four panels predicated their recommendations on the availability of vastly improved food programs, including free food stamps and free school lunches, or adequate cash assistance. A subpanel headed by a well-known judge made important recommendations pertaining to misinformation and deception through the media.

Four panels dealt with problems of food distribution. Commercial distribution of food of good quality at the lowest possible price will be greatly facilitated if the type of Government and managerial assistance recommended is made available to food distributors in poor rural and city areas.

The family is and should continue to be the basic unit for delivery of food. A number of recommendations pertaining to family recipiency of food, and of services rendered to the family by the Government and the community, and to the continued role of philanthropic foundations were evolved by a far-seeing panel. Recommendations dealing with Government food programs and family assistance were very thoughtfully designed by a cooperative and hard-working panel. They recommend basic improvements in certification, administration, and level of support of the various food programs. In particular, they analyzed the need for self-certification for food stamps, suggested novel and more uniform methods of distribution, and recommended cheaper schedules and free food stamps for the very poor. They described desirable improvements of commodity distribution programs while these still exist. The relevant panel recognized, as did other concerned panels, that food programs should be eventually replaced by income maintenance at an adequate level and discussed various estimates of long-term goals. The panel also discussed specific changes in the financing and administration of school lunch programs.

The panel dealing with mass-feeding programs, which had a high level of competence in this specialized field addressed itself to schools, hospitals, Veterans Administration, military and penal feeding systems, and suggested measures which would insure large possible economies as well as detailed improvements in existing methods of feeding communities.

Panels entrusted with advising Government emphasized the need for more concentrated and centralized authority concerning nutrition: They recommended that an officer at subcabinet level head nutrition activities of the Department of Health, Education, and Welfare and that coordinating nutrition activity be continued in the Executive Office of the President.

The panel dealing with agriculture made far-reaching recommendations concerning, among others, vocational technical training of workers in agriculture, modernization of land use, tenant contracts, farm credit, agricultural extension, aid in establishment of cooperatives to meet the needs of deprived small farmers in America, and suggested other measures to bring net income for producers and farm laborers to the level of others in the U.S. economy.

Industry leaders were most cooperative and forward-looking in their consideration, in four panels, of problems of food manufacturing and processing (including the preparation of enriched and more nutritious foods), of retailing and distribution (with particular emphasis on those measures which would help poor consumers), of packaging and labeling (including the meaningful description of significant nutritional information), and of promotion and advertising (including the launching of large-scale effective nutrition education programs).

The panels dealing with voluntary action by farmers and industry as well as the primarily professional panels emphasized the need for urgent measures to combat the more acute problems of hunger and malnutrition due to poverty, to improve the outreach and quality of existing food programs and to insure an increased buying power for our poorest citizens.

Very much the same type of concern was expressed, in somewhat more detailed and forceful language, by task forces representing citizens' groups. A joint resolution was presented by the community action task force, the women's organization task force, the students' task force, the consumers' task force, the religious action task force, and the health organizations' task force. This joint statement was presented for a vote to the Conference as a whole at the closing plenary session, not for specific approval of all points but for a general expression of the groups on order of priorities. The health task force and many professional persons were strongly in favor of free school lunches as soon as possible for needy children but not for all other children who could afford to pay. A very large part of the audience, while enthusiastically in favor of the concept of family assistance and desirous of seeing support at a realistic level permitting good nutrition as well as the acquisition of other necessities, was not willing to be committed to a single target figure, unrelated to geography, work incentives, and minimum wages, and unaccompanied by any order of magnitude of time of achievement. The final vote had, therefore, a symbolic significance only, representing essentially an endorsement of principles. In some ways, this may well increase its significance. The first priority — need for urgent action — was the one which received universal support from panels, from the task forces and from the Conference. You were gracious enough to converse at length on this point with some of the delegates from the Conference. I know that they and their colleagues deeply appreciate the fact that their President shares their concern.

While the recommendations of the Conference are arousing active interest within your Executive Office, in the executive departments, at state level and in both Houses in the Congress of the United States and while I know that under your leadership tremendous strides will be made in the implementation of many or most of them, I believe that the greatest contribution of the Conference may well be of a different order.

The demonstration that at a time when divisions and confrontations are common in our land, forceful and sometimes militant Americans of all walks of life and persuasion can be brought together and, after spirited discussion, agree on common priorities in the service of the Country and of one's fellow man is deeply reassuring. The fact that conservatives could be shown to display compassion and a desire for reform, that liberals could be shown to display restraint and responsibility, that the young could work with the middle-aged, that academics could speak in intelligible fashion to the poor, that minorities could see the common interest, that the majority could demonstrate a new concern for the minorities — all this made the meeting, in the words of an eminent bishop, a member of the Conference, "as close to a mass religious experience as any event in [his] lifetime." Scores of letters from participants received since the end of the Conference confirm that this was a very general feeling.

Let me conclude this letter of transmittal by thanking you for the honor you bestowed upon all nutritionists in the Nation, and upon me personally, in asking me to organize the Conference. I want also to express my gratitude for the complete freedom you gave me in selecting the detailed topics and the membership of the Conference, for your continued counsel and support, and for your trust in the soundness of the results. I can think of no historical example of a Presidential Conference as completely divorced from any partisan influence, as broad in its membership, and as free in its expression as this, the first White House Conference of your Administration. All of us who had the privilege to participate in this unique venture hope that you will find its long-term achievements worthy of your confidence.

Sincerely,

(Signed) Jean Mayer
Special Consultant to the
President

## Chapter 75

# OPENING SPEECH AT THE WHITE HOUSE FOLLOW-UP CONFERENCE ON FOOD, NUTRITION AND HEALTH, 1971

THERE are two extreme opinions, unfortunately both of them widely held, which are equally destructive of our values and our chances for progress: one view, often found among those who have benefited handsomely from our economic development in the past thirty years such as many in organized labor and in the management of large business, which holds that we can do no wrong and that any criticism of our system is based on exaggerations if not on downright inventions. Such people have tended not to believe that there were widespread malnutrition and illness due to poverty in the United States and have considered almost as subversives those who described these conditions. According to their view, there are no consumer problems in our country, and consumerism is just the work of a small minority eager for cheap publicity. The contrary opinion is popular among the young, the intellectuals and the poor: the country can do nothing right, successive administrations, the present one in particular, conspiring with vested interests have deliberately kept millions of our fellow citizens in abject poverty and peonage. As for the food industry, they hold that it is plotting night and day to poison the American people, with the overt complicity of the regulatory agencies. Neither group will find comfort in our proceedings. But the great majority of our people will. For I believe that the picture that we are examining today is one of important progress but also one of large remaining tasks. Under the leadership of a President who was the first to make "the elimination of hunger in America for all time" a national goal, with the help of a Congress inspired and prodded by the debates of the members of the bipartisan Senate Committee on Nutrition and Human Needs, and through the handwork of two devoted and hardworking Secretaries at Agriculture and HEW, the country has made more progress in the fight against hunger in the year since the White House Conference than it had in the twenty-five years since the end of World War II. Since the White House Conference, the number of food stamp recipients has gone from 2 to nearly 10 millions; the monthly family allotment has been increased by 50 per cent and the price has been decreased to nothing for the very poor. The number of children receiving free school lunches has essentially doubled, to about 6 million. And several accessory programs have shown similarly great leaps forward. Every state of the Union has had its own Conference on Hunger and Nutrition and is developing local programs in addition to the Federal effort. These are great achievements for which we can thank not only the Administration and the Congress but also great national organizations, in particular the women's organizations so ably orchestrated by our women leaders at the Conference. And yet at the same time, facts keep on reminding us that the millenium has not arrived and that there is still a lot to do to help people who somehow fall between the cracks of existing programs.

Let me illustrate this statement by a striking example. In January, I spent a little time in Denver, Colorado, and had an opportunity to look at the health and nutrition picture of migrant workers. I can describe it in a few figures. Since the period of the White House Conference, the University of Colorado Medical Center has admitted seven children with kwashiorkor, and literally dozens with more or less advanced cases of marasmus. These diseases, as you know, are acute forms of the protein-calorie malnutrition syndrome. Pediatricians there have demonstrated unequivocally that many of these children who superficially appeared to have recovered from the acute malnutrition syndrome never recovered normal growth and remained permanently retarded mentally. The perinatal figures also reflect the poor state of health and nutrition of the migrant families in Colorado: a fetal wastage of over 70 per 1000 and an infant mortality of 63 per 1000, well over three times the national average. Besides their poor housing, a family mean actual income of $1,885, and the need for infants to travel with their parents, migrant families are not, in practice, included in the Medicare-Medicaid hospitalization programs, are refused admission in the private hospitals of Denver (unless they have, for example, $300 in cash at the time of delivery) and are not eligible for food stamps while travelling (or for that matter in Texas in their home counties during the winter months). They are not eligible for unemployment compensation. These people, may I remind you, are not people who are waiting for the Government to support them. They are men who are killing their wives and their children trying to get work — and subsidizing both the food industry and the consumers out of their misery. They are fools, honorable fools, but fools. Their wives and their children could receive better care, better housing and better education if they moved North and went on welfare. I believe that we have in this room the people who can be instrumental in stopping this national scandal — through pressing for the Family Assistance Program, eligibility for unemployment compensation for the migrant, permanent certification for food stamps, permanent eligibility for Medicare-Medicaid, nurses, nutrition Aides and teachers in the migrant stream, and a more humane attitude among farmers, the food industry, physicians and hospital administrators and many of us Sunday Christians that we are.

Let me add, in case you think that I believe that all such dereliction occurs far from my home town, that while I see steady progress in the development of food programs in Massachusetts, Boston is as good a city as any to see their shortcomings. The progress of the school lunch program has been agonizingly slow with thousands of very poor elementary school children still not able to avail themselves of this national resource. Food stamps are by and large not available. As for the commodity program, I can only tell you of what goes on in the Center nearest my laboratory, 1280 Tremont Street in the heart of Roxbury. Of the twenty-plus commodities theoretically available, only 15 have ever been listed, and seven were in fact being distributed as of the beginning of this week. Butter, evaporated milk (a very unpopular item, although you can cook with it, you can't use it as a plain milk beverage), chicken, lentils for soup (a very unfamiliar item to all but a small minority), sweet potatoes, shortening and corn syrup (another difficult item to use). This constitutes obviously the most preposterously unbalanced diet: there has been no cheese for 3 months, no peanut butter, no macaroni, no potatoes, no fruits, no vegetables, (applejuice, a pleasant but nutritionally not very useful juice is "on order") as well as no instant dry milk (which is popular as a plain milk beverage and can also be used for cooking), no other meat or fish for many weeks. It is impossible to obtain even halfway decent nutrition for healthy people with this combination of foods. (For example, there is no source of vitamin C, hardly any of B vitamins, etc.) As for those who have any health problem at all, dietitians of the Peter Bent Brigham Hospital who man the nutrition outpatient departments in the health centers are at their wit's end. I understand the problems of a program which is being phased out and whose personnel may well be demoralized. But in that case, let us stop the program now and transfer immediately the 2 million Americans still on it to food stamps. Let me say that I am convinced that in the cases I have just cited, the failure is not a purely federal one. State and local authorities and the citizenry at large do bear much of the responsibility. The older I get, the more I am convinced that, in the long run, the most difficult, the most intractable problems are the local problems. The Federal Government has done much more, in the enlargement of the scope and the better administration of its programs, than have the states, and municipalities. It still has to develop better feedback from local communities. It also must develop a greater measure of leadership and inspiration which will make local functionaries and local elected officials feel that when programs do not function as they should, blaming Washington is not enough: they — and all of us — fail until the programs succeed.

Finally, a word about consumer problems. There again, the achievements are important. The Food and Drug Administration, the Federal Trade Commission, the Office of the Assistant to the President for Consumer Affairs are to be congratulated for elaborating new regulations which will go a long way towards informing the public and increasing its protection against the hazards of pollutants and of insufficiently tested additives. The food industry has, in the past twelve months, considerably increased the scope of its enrichment programs which now embrace thousands of items hitherto unfortified and developed a number of attractive and informative presentations of nutrition education material, usually based on the food group concept. On the third of February, one large food chain inaugurated its nutrient labeling program; it will be followed in short order by several others.

This is excellent. But I am not sure that all of us understand yet the full scope of the needs. The percentage of processed foods in our diet has jumped from perhaps 10 per cent in 1941 when both our present enrichment policy and the food group approach (seven food groups in those days, actually a vastly more informative method) were designed, to about 50 per cent nowadays. One-third of the meals (and 40% of the money spent on foods) are now taken outside of the home. In addition, I believe that the following factors are highly important: like all our industries, the food industry desires to be a "growth" industry. Because the population of the United States is growing slowly, and individual intakes are declining as a result of decreased physical labor and decreased walking, the overall picture is not, inherently, a growth picture. To make it a growth picture, industry is incorporating more and more services into the food: the housewife does not buy potatoes or flour any more, but frozen french fried potatoes or ready-made frozen cake. This decreases the women's work, but it does largely eliminate the savings in price due to our increasingly efficient agriculture. It also makes food subject to the same inexorable increases in labor costs which afflict all industrial goods and services. The much greater resistance of the public to increases in food prices than to other increases is driving industry to look constantly for cheaper material, such as replacement of expensive meat by inexpensive textured vegetable protein for example. This alone need not be accompanied by a decrease in nutritional value (we can replace one type of protein by another of sufficient biological value) provided we do not further eliminate at the same time, the vitamins and trace minerals which are *not* included in our 30-year-old enrichment program. What I am afraid will develop unless we are careful is a "horsepower" race with more and more of a few vitamins and minerals being added to all foods while twenty equally important nutrients, which happened not to have been limiting in 1941, (and some of which may not be known now) are left out of a more and more processed diet. As the population pressure and manpower costs increase, this may pose real problems to our population. Some of these problems may be with us already. Now that our "urgent" hunger problems are beginning to be under control, we must attack vigorously our "important" consumer problems. We need a vigorous research effort into trace minerals and "secondary" vitamins requirements and we need a more rapid procedure than we have to establish at least tentative recommended allowances for those secondary vitamins and trace minerals, otherwise our quickly evolving food supply will no longer be adequate. The trend toward highly processed foods can probably no longer be reversed. Let us make sure that we make them as nutritious as we know how.

I would suggest that we ought to devote one-tenth of one per cent of the Nation's food bill to nutrition research. We also need to educate our public to the continued value of the primary foods — fruits, vegetables, meat, fish, eggs, milk, whole grain cereals — particularly until we have a truly comprehensive nutrition policy. At present let us recognize that the bulk of advertising is directed at promoting highly processed snack foods and such things as candy, soft drinks, and alcoholic beverages, which can only be consumed at the expense of the primary foods. I would also suggest that the nation ought to spend one-tenth of the food advertising bill (or another one-tenth of one per cent of the food bill) on nutrition education programs aimed at promoting not only increased knowledge of the significance of nutrients (food groups obviously are inapplicable for the highly processed foods — what food group is a pizza?) and at understanding of nutrient labeling but also at promoting actual change in attitudes as well.

Finally, we are making constantly more demands of our Food and Drug Administration as regards safety from involuntary additives such as pollutants, retesting of voluntary additives, better labeling, clearer and more understandable standards. But we are not giving the FDA the additional resources which it needs to do the job. There again, I would suggest that one-tenth of one per cent of the Nation's food bill is not too much to spend to monitor its safety and nutritional value. These three components totalling three-tenths of one per cent — 3 cents for every ten dollars — would enormously improve our knowledge of nutrition, the wholesomeness of our food supply and our food habits.

If we do this, we may at the same time be on the road to solving some of our important general medical problems as well as our nutrition problems. Whether we consider our number one killer, cardiovascular diseases (which has prevented our men from improving their life expectancy in the past twenty years in spite of a more than quintupling of expenditures for health — over 70 billion last year!) or the most widespread of all diseases, dental caries, we shall not solve these as long as our people consume over 100 pounds of sugar per person per year and almost as much by weight (much more by calories) of saturated fat. The combination of food technology and nutrition education gives us a chance to do what medicine alone cannot do, and would save a great deal of money, as well as suffering in the long run. It will be a difficult road but we should start right now.

I think that what has been done in the past year is impressive enough to give us the confidence we need to solve our problems. We have made a great start. Let us not relax our effort.

*Chapter 76*

# SUMMARY OF FOLLOW-UP CONFERENCE
# ON FOOD, NUTRITION AND HEALTH, 1971*

THE consensus of the Follow-up Conference was that the Administration ought to be commended on the many important steps already taken; in particular, the wide expansion of the Food Stamp Program and of the School Lunch Program. These achievements have already been presented in the preliminary booklet distributed to all members of the Conference as well as in the presentation of Secretary Hardin. The Conference also wants to congratulate the Administration on some of the measures it has introduced before Congress. The principle of welfare reform, exemplified in the concept of a Family Assistance Program, is excellent and the enactment of such a measure at a level of support adequate to support the health, nutrition and human dignity of the recipients is an indispensable step in fulfilling basic national goals. The Conference also welcomes the fact that the Administration has introduced a number of measures such as unemployment compensation for migrant workers, which it hopes it will again push forward vigorously in the coming session of Congress.

The Conference also takes cognizance of the fact that a considerable voluntary effort had been made by a number of citizens' groups and by the food industry. The change in climate in many sections of the food industry with its new emphasis on the nutritional aspects of food and its enrichment and fortification programs is an important step in making our overall food supply more nutritious.

*This summary report was prepared by a drafting committee composed of the following: Professor David Call, Dr. Stanley Gershoff, John Holloman, M.D., Professor Michael Latham, Professor Jean Mayer (Chairman) and Patricia (Mrs. Joseph H.) Young.

While a great deal has been done, a great deal remains to be done.

1. We are concerned over the fact that full extension of national programs, the Food Stamp Program and, in particular, the School Lunch Program will require substantial increases in funding, if all eligible poor people are to be covered, which is the President's announced policy. Currently there are 4 to 5 million eligible children denied the benefits of the Free and Reduced Price Lunch Program. If this gap is to be removed in the near future, more money will be required. Also it is reasonable to assume in the year ahead 3 million or more eligible people will be added to the Food Stamp Program. These necessary increases in participation will be impossible if the 1972 budget allocations remain unaltered. We are distressed that the level of funding for food programs in the 1972 budget allows for no real growth in participation. We are also concerned that this whole topic of funding was not presented at the Follow-up meeting.

2. Another area of concern is that many programs are mutilated at the interface of federal and state or local governments. Three factors appear of importance to minimize this difficulty. First, more money must be made available to local governments to support the costs of implementing and maintaining food programs. Relatively small amounts made available for outreach and certification should reap large returns. Such increased resources at the local level should allow for a greater flexibility in the use of these funds to fit the special needs of each area or locality. Second, it is essential that federal directives be couched in more clear, curt terms so that local authorities understand without any possible doubt the federal intent to reach every poor child or every poor person who is eligible for food programs. At present too many directives are couched in such language as to create loopholes for those local authorities who are unwilling to fulfill legal requirements. National eligibility standards for child nutrition programs similar to those enacted for food stamps must be defined without any possible ambiguity. The combination of clear, enforced, federal standards and greater local flexibility and resources ought to permit a broader reach of federal programs than exists presently. Third, it is the consensus of the Conference that poor

use has been made of voluntary organizations in the fight against hunger. Often the tremendous talent, energy and even money of volunteers is spent fighting the various levels of government rather than in extending and multiplying the outreach and services of official bodies. The fight against hunger could serve as an exciting pilot project in demonstrating the potential of the partnership between the government and its private citizens. It would seem that a mechanism within government to facilitate this must be created. We urge that much more serious consideration be given to this matter. In general, the articulation between federal goals and the enormous resources in manpower and goodwill represented by voluntary organizations has never been satisfactorily bridged. We urge that much more serious consideration be given to this matter especially in an attempt to involve volunteer groups at the local level. The use of citizens' advisory committees at various levels of government, as regards both poverty and consumer programs, still needs to be developed.

3. As regards the administration of nutrition programs, the overwhelming consensus of the Conference is that the need for coordination of nutrition programs emphasized at the White House Conference still remains unfulfilled. The establishment of the Food and Nutrition service in the USDA was a welcome step in the right direction. The Conference notes with satisfaction the program of Government reorganization including the creation of a Department of Human Resources and emphasizes the necessity of including all food and nutrition activities under the leadership of an officer of sufficient rank within that new Department. At the same time, the Conference recognizes that this reorganization of the Executive Branch will take time to be effected and urges that the coordination between existing agencies responsible for nutrition programs be improved with a clear designation to professionals and to the public as to whom, in the Federal Government, is responsible for what area.

As regards the content of these programs, we feel that it ought to be made clear to professionals as well as to the public that we need a rational balance between action and knowledge. We do not know all we need to know about nutrition or food quality and safety, yet we must make decisions about new foods, old foods, additives, pesticides and environmental contaminants. At any moment, our decisions should be balanced and sophisticated, recognizing that our knowledge is incomplete and that we must, therefore, choose among risks that cannot fully be known. (For example, shall we choose at the moment persistent pesticides or current supplies of food and fiber?) We should recognize the relation between decisions on food and nutrition and other elements of our social fabric and should be reluctant to make extreme decisions of acceptance or abandonment without full and informed consideration of the consequences of such decisions.

This general statement has very specific implications from the point of view of the setting up of nutritional standards and of safety standards by regulatory agencies. There is a general agreement that the existing machinery to provide scientific advice from the nutrition community to regulatory agencies and to industry  needs overhauling and speeding up. Recognizing that knowledge is approximate, the agencies need the best possible scientific advice at any one time in order to function, and this advice must be forthcoming when they need it. This also poses an obligation for the regulatory agencies to look ahead for emerging problems and to seek solutions before those problems reach "crisis" proportions. In line with this we are greatly encouraged by the FDA's acquisition of the Pine Bluff Facility and their movement into a broader-based, long-term research effort. Proper coordination with other scientific groups should provide a stronger effort in the future.

Finally, it is the consensus of this Conference that while nutrition education is as important as ever, there is greater and greater recognition that the scope and the techniques of nutrition education need drastic review. The inception of new methods of labeling foods requires the development of new methods of nutrition education. Nutrition education must also accept responsibility for instructing the public as to the principles on which both requirements and standards of safety are based so as to free the continued atmosphere of crises which discussions of our food supply seems to have engendered in the past year or two. The willingness of the food industry to become actively involved through the efforts of the Food Council of America and the

Advertising Council is a large step forward and further efforts should be encouraged and supported. Voluntary regulation of media advertising, particularly with regards to children, and a greater participation of media in providing information are desirable.

Specific comments on the response of the Government to the recommendations of the White House Conference on Food, Nutrition and Health and comments on the Follow-up Conference would be summarized as follows:

In general, members of the Conference felt that there is a continuing need for nongovernmental review of progress in domestic food and nutrition programs. They were pleased with the fact that the Government had held a Follow-up Conference and sent material throughout the year to the participants of the 1969 Conference. They appreciated the fact that a summary report had been prepared and that the various departments concerned had been asked to comment on the 1969 Conference recommendations. On the other hand, they were generally disappointed with some aspects of the Follow-up Conference. Holding the meeting in Williamsburg, Virginia, not only made it inconvenient for people to attend, it also, inappropriately, gave the appearance that the Administration had something to hide. The conferees were disappointed that they were given little advance knowledge about the meeting and no opportunity to seek out from Government sources and from members of the original panels and task forces detailed information concerning the action taken during the past 14 months on their recommendations. The comprehensive report prepared by Government departments and agencies, which was delivered about a week before the Conference did not in many cases provide adequate information on the disposition of the recommendations of the White House Conference. In fact, many of the recommendations were missed and even more importantly, the comments were so incompletely and carelessly prepared that the interests of the Government were poorly served. The following are but a few examples taken from the groups of Panel V:

1. The recommendation that the family commodity distribution program be transferred to HEW was rejected in the following way:" . . . But we maintain that commodity programs are of a

different nature. Their primary thrust is to help balance the agricultural economy rather than to provide income substitutes. They serve a different constituency than that concerned with health and nutrition." This is absolutely contrary to what the Department of Agriculture has publicly stated. It is the first time that the Government has agreed with the charge that the family commodity programs are to help the producers, not the consumers. Is this an official position?

2. The recommendation that until free school lunches are universal, Congress authorize by law the use of food stamps to pay for school lunches was rejected with the comment that food stamps should not be diverted for school lunches when a program specifically for that purpose already exists. It appears that the respondent did not read the recommendation. The recommendation was to cover the period during which the program was not fully functioning. At this time there are still 4 to 5 million school children without the means to acquire the school lunch offered in their schools.

3. The recommendation that the large-scale mass feeding expertise of the Armed Forces and the Veterans Administration be used in the national commitment to combat hunger and malnutrition was rejected on the ground that the recommendation was not appropriate to the missions of the two agencies. This is an astounding answer! Has our bureaucracy become so compartmentalized and inflexible that even on issues of major social importance one agency of Government can not expect help even in the sharing of expertise from another?

4. The recommendation that a National Council for Food and Nutrition be established in the Executive Office of the President was rejected in the following way: "The Council feels strongly that placing a unit in the Executive Office at a level immediately under the President may well raise its effectiveness by investing it with a claim on the President's time and attention. But that positioning must be at the expense of his attention to other activities thus may result in a net loss of overall effectiveness." An answer written this way certainly could be interpreted as meaning that the problems of hunger in the U.S. are not important enough to distract the President. Whoever wrote it did him no service.

One could go on and on with other examples but these surely illustrate why some conferees found the Comprehensive Report prepared for the Follow-up Conference so disappointing. It is fortunate that in some important food and nutrition areas, the Government's actions speak louder than these words. We want to again emphasize in conclusion, that the task remaining is still very large. We urgently seek the continuing commitment of all governmental bodies so that those gains achieved to date will not be viewed as success in the fight against hunger, but only as an encouraging start toward solving a most critical social problem.

# PART X
## Nutrition and the World

Chapter 77

# NUTRITION:
# FIRST PRIORITY IN WEST AFRICA

IN the course of the past few years we have been repeatedly exposed to a series of tempting syllogisms concerning malnutrition in Africa. The argument runs something like this: Africa is the emerging continent; we should do something for the Africans; they are malnourished; we have food surpluses; ergo, by donating our surpluses to Africa we can remedy their nutritional problems, get them started on their economic development, reduce or eliminate our vexing problem of agricultural surpluses, make friends at very little or no cost, and feel virtuous at the same time.

Unfortunately, the fact that this course of action can be stated in such simple and almost self-evident terms does not necessarily make it right or wise. While the problem of malnutrition in Africa is both acute and solvable, the solution cannot rest on such an oversimplification.

First and foremost, we have the wrong surpluses: while there are occasional famines in very limited areas, the major nutritional deficiency is of good quality protein, and our surpluses are essentially cereals and butter. Skim milk and soy beans are no longer surpluses. Available supplies of these are already fully used, particularly by international organizations. Meat and fish have never been surpluses.

Second, these countries are essentially agricultural countries: 95 per cent of the population is engaged in agriculture or in the occupations ancillary to agriculture. The tragedy is that in spite of this they are not self-sufficient as regards foods, largely because the main incentive to farmers so far has been the high price of cash (rather than food) crops. The dumping of free agricultural

Reprinted from *Harvard Alumni Bulletin*, 63:594-598 May, 1961.

commodities on their markets is the last thing that could help African countries achieve harmonious economic growth. It would make it even more difficult for the farmers to be assured of prices high and stable enough to provide the incentive necessary to make the national economy independent of costly food imports. As we shall see, what they need is not more (and free) lower grade food, but the education, the means, and the incentive to produce better food.

It is as dangerous to generalize about Africa as it is to generalize about Latin America. Even if we limit ourselves to West Africa, the area with which I have had the most contact (and the area with most of the new countries), we are dealing with a region which shows considerable diversity in wealth and degree of cultural development. By and large, the countries of West Africa are the former various territories of the French and British colonial empires. Exceptions are Portuguese Guinea, which is still a colony in the most depressing nineteenth century meaning of the term; and Liberia, which, while politically independent, has been economically dominated by a few American companies, is particularly devoid of any professional personnel, and has not the best reputation currently for good government.

Senegal, Ghana, and the Ivory Coast are the richest states and those which have the greatest concentration of education administrators and technical personnel, including physicians and engineers. The degree of development is exemplified by the proud claim of an official booklet distributed by the Republic of the Ivory Coast to the effect that the country has more cars and trucks per one hundred people than Spain and Portugal. Nigeria, first in size, comes next in wealth and education, probably followed by Guinea and Sierra Leone, while such states as Togo, Mali, the Republic of Niger, the Chad, and the Centrafrican Republic are at the other end of the spectrum as regards income and availability of technical personnel.

Political regimes show an equal diversity. While by and large all these countries are devoted to a one-party system, a number, such as Senegal, Nigeria, and the Ivory Coast, show a certain degree of democracy (that this is, after all, compatible to a point with a one-party system is exemplified by Vermont and some of our

Southern states). By contrast other countries, such as Mali, Ghana, and Guinea, tend towards much more absolute authoritarianism.

The soils of the region are predominantly the end products of progressive surface disintegration of eruptive rocks, in particular laterite, a porous clay-like brown, red, or yellow rock, high in ferrous oxide and aluminum hydroxide. Such soils are highly leached and potentially very productive if sufficient standards of management, including sufficient fertilizer application, are used. At present, however, methods of soil management are primitive and fertilizers rarely used.

From a nutritional viewpoint, it is useful to view West Africa as divided into four areas or population groups: (1) the coastal area, (2) the forest zone, (3) the northern savannah, and (4) the large cities. These are in part determined by the mean annual rainfall which varies between 60 and 100 inches in the forest zone, 30 and 60 inches in the southern part of the savannah, and usually even less in the northern end of the savannah which eventually emerges into the Sahara desert. In some areas the forest zone goes practically to the sea, with the coastal area reduced to a very thin band.

It is important to realize that West Africa is one area of the globe where population pressure has almost nothing to do with the nutritional situation. With the exception of the large cities, such as Dakar, Accra, Abidjan, Monrovia, and Freetown, which are crowded and rapidly increasing in population, the whole of the area is sparsely populated. One of the most populated countries, Ghana, with an area as large as that of England, only has 6 to 7 million people. The Ivory Coast, almost as large as France, has 4 or 5 millions. With its vast surface and its primitive agriculture West Africa would present essentially the same food problems were its population half what it is.

The coastal area is better fed than the interior when and where fish is available. Harbors, however, are few, craft are inadequate, and the ocean fish supply is highly seasonal. The paradoxical result is that more centrally located populations, living near the Volta River and its tributaries, often have more fish than coastal populations, and that fish often travel from inland toward the coast.

The coastal area usually exists on cassava (manioc), a starchy root of negligible protein content, and on corn. Plantains (non-sweet large bananas), yams, eggplants, onions, and palm nuts are relatively rare components of the diet. Meat is expensive, and eggs are only occasionally eaten and then not by the most vulnerable groups, e.g. children, or pregnant or lactating women. The foods consumed in the large cities (which are predominantly coastal) reflect production in the surrounding territories except that imported wheat, flour, corn, and sugar play a large role and accentuate further the dominance of carbohydrates in the diet.

The agricultural population of the forest zone is often predominantly occupied in the growing of cash crops (such as cocoa, bananas, fruits for canning, coffee, and rubber) and largely relies on imported food supplies. The main food crops are plantains and cocoa yams, with cassava tending to replace these because it is even easier to cultivate. Corn, green leaves, and palm oil are consumed in appreciable quantities. Rice consumption is limited to some areas. Fish and legumes are consumed in very small amounts.

The tribes of the northern region and the northern countries generally have very distinctive crops. Their staple foods are bullrush millet and sorghum, cereals with higher protein content than the coastal and forest staples. A variety of oil seeds and fermented locust beans and baobab seeds are frequent dietary items. Shea butter (from the seeds of *Butyrospermum parkii)* is an important item of export as well as of domestic consumption. Green leaves eaten either fresh or powdered, are also important. Fish powder and guinea fowl are eaten not infrequently but in very small amounts. Cattle, goats, and sheep are used for religious sacrifices and as a source of cash rather than as a source of meat. This area, which is by and large the most sparsely populated, is the region which is periodically subjected to acute — and often dramatic — food shortages. Stores of foods are practically nonexistent; if the rains fail, the only foods available may be wild leaves and other "bush foods." Sometimes even these fail. The lack of roads, of efficient administrative methods, and of communication usually prevents supplies from moving into the areas before the famine comes to an end. This is the one zone, incidentally, in which limited amounts of our cereal surpluses could be profitably used in small "food banks."

Important infectious and parasitic diseases throughout West Africa are malaria, tuberculosis, yaws, leprosy, trypanosomiasis (some forms of which are popularly known as "sleeping sickness"), onchocerciasis (the ocular localization of this filarial infestation causes "river blindness"), schistosomiasis (the fact that the agents, cercarial larvae, go through a stage where a snail is the obligatory host complicates irrigation developments), and guinea worms. Investigations and control of these diseases have been vigorously pursued in formerly British and French territories and it is to be hoped that the impetus will not be lost.

In West Africa, as elsewhere in Africa, food habits and agricultural practices are bad and tend to keep protein out of the diet. In most parts of Africa meat is rarely consumed, even where cattle and goats are numerous. Owners consider the beasts to be their capital. As a result, cattle are eaten exceptionally; they are consumed only during religious festivals or when they die of old age or disease. Chicken and eggs are reserved for gifts and game is becoming scarce. Milk is expensive and sold to the towns; prevalent hygienic conditions often make it a poisonous fluid anyway. Ignorance of nutrition, ease of cultivation, and high yield combine to make high-calorie low-protein starchy staples more popular.

The fact that the cultivation of the crops usually falls to the women, already burdened with other work, tends to preclude the raising of low-yielding crops such as vegetables and legumes. When cash crops such as cocoa, cotton, or peanuts displace the traditional food crops of an area, or when a family moves to a city and takes up wage employment, the tendency is to buy prestige foods such as white bread and sugar rather than add needed proteins to the diet. The money earned by the rural farmer is often earmarked for luxuries, and is spent on more useless cattle, additional wives, or clothes and ornaments for the home.

The nature and frequency of prevalent nutritional diseases are not surprising in view of the dietary pattern described above. Malnutrition is widespread throughout the country. An indirect measure of malnutrition is the very high ratio of mortality of small children to infant mortality. Even in relatively developed Ghana, more children die between the ages of one to five than during the first year, a ratio which has been shown to be a sure index of malnutrition. (Infants of less than one are also the prey of infectious diseases, but they are fed breast milk and thus are not deficient in protein).

While the sporadic and patchy famines in the northern savannah areas have attracted more attention, chronic protein deficiency throughout the region is the outstanding type of malnutrition. Throughout West Africa it results in blood disorders which are so widespread that anemia is characterized as such in hospitals only if hemoglobin levels are below 50 per cent of normal. The most widespread form, sometimes improperly characterized as "iron deficiency anemia," appears to be far less due to parasitosis (including malaria) than is usually taught. It responds well to protein supplements (which may be devoid of iron, such as dry skim milk). It is also likely that malnutrition makes the organism more vulnerable to a number of parasitic diseases.

Incidence and prevalence of tropical ulcers is another indication of the extent of protein deficiency. Tropical ulcers are characterized by the rapid development of exploding blebs on a previously sound skin surface followed by a quickly destructive gangrenous process affecting muscles, tendons, nerves, vessels, and even the periosteum of bones. They may develop as the result of traumas or minor skin infections in a malnourished individual, and do not heal until the patient receives a sufficient amount of good quality protein. In a little town in northern Ghana which I visited two years ago, one-third of the boys in the secondary school (though members of the upper social stratum in the area) were hospitalized for tropical ulcers.

The form and manner in which protein malnutrition expresses itself in young children in West Africa is characteristically related to the availability of calories. Along the coast and in the forest zone calories are abundant and kwashiorkor is the prevalent form of protein malnutrition in small children. This extremely widespread disease, which in many areas is observed in practically all recently weaned infants and of which no area in West Africa is exempt, is characterized by cessation of growth, edema, discoloration of the hair, intensely fatty liver, fibrosis of the pancreas, swelling of the parotid and other salivary glands, cracking, peeling, and discoloration of the skin, and (unless treated in time with enough good quality proteins) early death. Kwashiorkor is particularly full-blown in the cassava-consuming areas of the forest region. This is not surprising in view of the extraordinarily low-protein content of that root which forms the basis of the gruel fed recently weaned infants. Kwashiorkor, incidentally, is a Ghanan name meaning "displaced infant" and refers to the fact that it attacks children when they are weaned, often because a young sibling is on the way.

In the northern savannah where caloric intakes are lower and may fall to starvation levels if the rain fails, "marasmus," rather than kwashiorkor, is seen in younger children. Marasmus is really a state of undernutrition rather than malnutrition, and while it may be more impressive to the uninitiated, it is actually much more reversible than kwashiorkor in that it responds quickly to good food and recovery appears complete. Kwashiorkor, which can be considered really a case of carbohydrate intoxication, appears to leave the liver and perhaps other organs permanently damaged. Cancer of the liver is highly prevalent in adults in those areas where children have kwashiorkor.

Compared to the protein shortage, other features of malnutrition in West Africa are far less important. Vitamin A, riboflavin, and calcium are low in patchy areas, and there are areas of simple goiter in regions where the iodine content of the waters and soil is low and no sea salt is consumed. There are also occasional cases of bleeding gums, neuritis, edema, and unusual anemia which are probably related to other vitamin and mineral deficiencies.

The economic consequences of the state of malnutrition are appalling. Not only is it a threat to health and vigor and thus to productivity, but in addition these agricultural countries spend an enormous proportion of their relatively scarce resources in importing high-protein foods for their upper classes. For example, the Ivory Coast, which exports for a low price substantial amounts of good quality protein in the form of pressed peanut cakes and dried fish, imports for eleven times their cost the same amount of protein in the form of canned meat, milk, and fish products.

Incidentally, this particular bill is greater than the amount spent by the country on trucks and industrial equipment.

These facts should make it clear why many nutritionists and economists believe that West Africa's first priority is the development of its agriculture in the direction of food crops. To be sure, the public health needs of Africans are very obvious, but to increase the survival and hence the size of a population without increasing its food production and its nutritional status is hardly a desirable program.

Similarly, the spread of popular education is a fine and necessary thing, but it must be realized that the enormous majority of the children to be educated live in small and miserable farming communities; they not only need better food while they learn, but they also need better opportunities when they leave school. For most of them again this means better farming opportunities.

Finally, industrial projects are very tempting, and to new countries the larger the more tempting. But history has shown over and over that to develop a heavy industry and thus a concentrated large urban proletariat without first making sure that the workers and their families have readily available cheap and adequate food is a sure road to disaster. All of these other goals are desirable, but they must be based on cheap and adequate crops of wholesome food.

Given this premise, there are many ways we can help. First, we can help agricultural and nutritional education programs. The first educational need concerns the governments of these new countries; they are groping to find their way and can easily be influenced by outsiders, for better or for worse; they must be educated to recognize the importance of their food problems and to coordinate their efforts to meet them.

A U.N. mission in Ghana (consisting of Professor B. S. Platt of London and myself) was successful in convincing Mr. Nkrumah to create two years ago a Food and Nutrition Committee at the ministerial level to coordinate food policy and nutrition education. This committee, in turn, has already initiated action to teach physicians, teachers, agricultural extension workers, and community development officials to recognize, treat, and prevent the more widespread nutritional diseases; it has found ways to popularize the value of certain cheap foods such as dried fish and of new foods such as recently introduced types of beans and peas. (These, which contain over 20% of good protein, seem to offer the best hope of quickly improving the amount and the quality of the diet.) Adult education groups and schools have been enrolled to change food habits. (Incidentally, in spite of much that has been written on the fixity of food habits, these can be changed fairly readily. The best proof of this is that most of the malnutrition problem in Africa is associated with the culture of corn and cassava, neither of which is indigenous to the region, or with the imports of flour and sugar in the cities.)

Similarly, the interministerial program of school feeding, school gardening, and nutrition education programs sponsored by UNICEF which I was associated with in the Ivory Coast seems to have already a decided impact on attitudes toward nutrition in that country. The United States can furnish physicians, adult education personnel, and extension workers to help in these developments.

West Africa needs a great deal of help as regards research and education in agriculture. This area also needs the means to put recent teachings into effect. There are no first-class schools of agriculture in West Africa; there are some small schools at the college level and some at the secondary school level; they need to be fortified with outside faculty, expanded in their research and in their teaching facilities, given mechanical equipment and laboratories, and inspired to acquire the necessary research attitudes.

Similarly, the agricultural experimental stations established by the colonial powers have in the past dealt with cash crops; very few have dealt with food crops and with animal husbandry. In order for West Africa to know what it needs to know about the potentialities of indigenous and imported varieties of domestic animals and food plants, these all-important centers of research and extension should be developed.

The United States has done the most thorough work in agricultural research and agricultural extension of any country and has much to teach in this field. West Africa needs tractors; in vast, tribe-owned areas they can readily be used and they cause man to work, and to work in agriculture. We can help to finance their imports; returns should be more than adequate for repayments.

More than anything, West Africa needs fertilizers, particularly phosphate; these can completely transform the character of the local soil and miltiply yields by an enormous factor. Cheap fertilizer is more helpful than free food, and we can help Africans to finance their imports, especially as our production potential in this field is considerably in excess of our needs. Later we can help West Africa to find local sources of phosphate and other necessary minerals.

We can also help them set up the small or medium-sized industries which are most necessary for the development of food crops. Fertilizer plants for the maintenance and repair of agriculture equipment, mills, plants for the canning and preparation of foods, capital equipment for the fishing industry including the establishment of small harbors, the provision of cheap but serviceable fishing craft and that of canning and drying facilities need to be obtained with our help. I believe that it is essential that we convince our new African friends that their most urgent need is the development of the subsistence agriculture; that only when they meet their nutritional requirements will they be able to preserve the capital they can acquire through their cash crops and their mines and use it for the development of their countries. We should concentrate our economic assistance on this aspect (and its corollary, cheap power probably from oil also in surplus) for rural areas. We should not at this stage encourage the more spectacular but premature large-scale industrial projects such as steel and aluminum combines, even for the sake of political propaganda.

*Chapter 78*

# CROP DESTRUCTION IN VIETNAM

I AM addressing myself in this chapter to the practical and the ethical implications of our destruction of rice crops and grain stores, by chemicals and by fire, in South Vietnam. I am not addressing myself to the problem of the morality of using chemical agents in wartime, as did our colleagues in their letter in the issue of 21 January, page 309. Nor am I addressing myself to the problem of the general morality of the Vietnam operations, except to say that I think we can all agree that obviously for many Americans the emotions are not as simple as those aroused in previous wars by the unprovoked attack on Pearl Harbor, the gas-ovens of Auschwitz, or the clear-cut violation of the United Nations Korean mandate. With the ends thus debatable — or at least debated — the means become particularly important in their practical consequences as well as in their morality.

In wartime, the ethics of means always pose difficult problems. Having spent five years of war as a forward artillery observer and as commander of artillery units, I know all too well that my contribution to the demise of the Wehrmacht was accompanied by the demolition of houses, churches, and works of art and by the killing and wounding of children, women, and civilian men in Africa, Italy, France, and Germany. Still, while knowledge that this was so forced me — and all Allied officers in similar positions — to extreme care so as to minimize such casualties, some such casualties were in the last analysis unavoidable if we were to conduct successful operations and eliminate the Nazi nightmare.

The situation seems to me entirely different when we consider the crop and stores destruction program in South Vietnam. The aim of the program is to starve the Viet Cong by destroying those

Reprinted from *Science, 152*, April, 1966.

fields that provide the rice for their rest — and field — rations. This
aim is, in essence, similar to that which every food blockade (such
as the one imposed against the Central Powers in World War I) has
attempted. As a nutritionist who has seen famines on three
continents, one of them Asia, and as a historian of public health
with an interest in famines, I can say flatly that there has never
been a famine or a food shortage — whether created by lack of
water (droughts, often followed by dust storms and loss of seeds,
being the most frequent), by plant disease (such as fungous
blights), by large-scale natural disturbances affecting both crops
and farmers (such as floods and earthquakes), by disruption of
farming operations due to wars and civil disorders, or by blockade
or other war measures directly aimed at the food supply — which
has not first and overwhelmingly affected the small children.

In fact, it is very clear that death from starvation occurs first of
all in young children and in the elderly, with adults and
adolescents surviving better (pregnant women often abort; lactating mothers cease to have milk and the babies die). Children
under five, who in many parts of the world — including Vietnam —
are often on the verge of kwashiorkor (a protein-deficiency
syndrome which often hits children after weaning and until they
are old enough to eat "adult" food) and of marasmus (a
combination of deficiency of calories and of protein), are the most
vulnerable. In addition, a general consequence of famine is a state
of social disruption (including panic). People who are starving at
home tend to leave, if they can, and march toward the area where
it is rumored that food is available. This increases the prevailing
chaos. Families are separated and children are lost — and in all
likelihood die. Adolescents are particularly threatened by tuberculosis; however, finding themselves on their own, they often band
together in foraging gangs, which avoid starvation but create
additional disruption. The prolonged and successful practice of
banditry makes it difficult to rehabilitate members of these gangs.

I have already said that adults, and particularly adult men,
survive usually much better than the rest of the population. Bands
of armed men do not starve and — particularly if not indigenous to
the population and therefore unhampered by direct family ties
with their victims — find themselves entirely justified in seizing

what little food is available so as to be able to continue to fight. Destruction of food thus never seems to hamper enemy military operations but always victimizes large numbers of children. During World War I, the blockade had no effect on the nutrition and fighting performance of the German and Austrian armies, but — for the first time since the 18th century — starvation, vitamin-A deficiency, and protein deficiency destroyed the health, the sight, and even the lives of thousands of children in Western Europe.

We obviously do not want to take war measures that are primarily, if not exclusively, directed at children, the elderly, and pregnant and lactating women. To state it in other words, my point is not that innocent bystanders will be hurt by such measures, but that only bystanders will be hurt. Our primary aim — to disable the Viet Cong — will not be achieved, and our proclaimed secondary aim — to win over the civilian population — is made a hollow mockery.

## Chapter 79

# STARVATION AS A WEAPON:
# HERBICIDES IN VIETNAM

C ROP destroying agents are "good examples of strategic weapons." So said a 1960 report of the Senate Foreign Relations Committee, adding that the eventual result of their use "would be something of the same nature as a blockade cutting off vital foods and supplies" (1).

These strategic weapons are now being used on food crops in Vietnam. A U.S. Government spokesman explains that food is as important to the Viet Cong as weapons, and that herbicides are used "where significant denial of food supplies can be effected by such destruction" (2).

In the first nine months of 1966, the 12th Air Commando Squadron sprayed about 70,000 acres of crops, mostly rice. The acreage of croplands sprayed has by now risen to about 150,000 (3). These figures do not include accidental drifting of sprays onto agricultural land from the defoliation being carried out over a much larger portion of South Vietnam.

There is as yet little direct evidence from Vietnam of the effects of crop destruction on the Viet Cong: no data on starvation of persons who can be categorically defined as "Viet Cong;" no reports that Viet Cong prisoners have been found to be physically incapacitated by malnutrition; no clear evidence of a lessening of the Viet Cong will to fight. Yet it is clear that malnutrition is common among Vietnamese civilians, whether due to diet deficiencies unrelated to the war, to food problems resulting from other war conditions — military and economic, to the conscious efforts of denying food to the Viet Cong, or to a combination of all three.

Information justifying the program has never been released by

Reprinted from *Scientist and Citizen*, 9:15, August-September, 1967.

military or other U.S. Government sources. In the absence of such data, we must turn to other, less direct information and to historical inferences. In spite of the paucity of information from Vietnam, the effects of food denial as a weapon are no mystery. We can turn to well-documented sources for answers to the questions:

How does a food shortage affect a population?

Which elements of the population are most affected?

Is starvation an effective strategic weapon?

The answers to these questions can then be related to the situation in Vietnam.

The effects of starvation on the human body are well known and were described in detail in a number of publications immediately following World War II. Famine affects different elements of the population in different ways and to different degrees; this has been observed in famines occuring in peacetime as well as in war. The author has personally observed famines on three continents, one of them Asia.

Finally, although herbicides have not been used in previous wars, the creation of famine through blockade has been frequently used and there is historical evidence of its effects.

## EFFECTS OF STARVATION

The first and most obvious effect of starvation on the human body is the wasting of its fat deposits. A nutrition survey of South Vietnam in 1959 found that the average weight of civilian males was 105 pounds (4), suggesting that such body fat deposits would generally be meager in Vietnamese to start with.

The stomach and intestines, heart and lungs are affected next; the size of the liver is drastically diminished. The intestinal lining becomes thin and smooth, thereby losing some of its absorptive capacity, and diarrhea results. Thus starvation is a self-accelerating process, particularly in children; because of intestinal damage the food that is available is poorly absorbed and undernutrition increases correspondingly. The damaged lining of the stomach fails to secrete hydrochloric acid, which is important for digestion. Both blood pressure and pulse rate fall.

Early effects of starvation are cessation of menstruation in women and impotence and loss of libido in men. Hair is dull and bristling and in children abnormal hair grows on the forearms and back. The skin acquires the consistency of paper and not infrequently shows the irreversible dusty brown splotches which are permanent marks of starvation. In extreme cases, particularly among children, the lips and parts of the cheeks are destroyed.

The body becomes susceptible to infection and disease. The psychologic state deteriorates rapidly; the individual becomes obsessed with food, mentally restless, apathetic and self-centered.

A recent paper prepared by Physicians for Social Responsibility for Senate hearings on the refugee problem summarized the medical problems in South Vietnam (5). It pointed out that malnutrition is widespread among South Vietnamese civilians; beri-beri, night blindness and anemia are found frequently; kwashiorkor, a form of protein malnutrition, occurs and is a major component of the problems of wound healing and resistance to infections; infant and child mortality is high. Kwashiorkor is a deadly disease affecting children after weaning. It causes degeneration of the liver, pancreas and intestines, edema, and eventually death. Diseases associated with malnutrition, such as tuberculosis, are rampant. Although it is impossible to know to what extent these problems stem from the crop destruction program, there can be no doubt that if the program is continued these problems will grow.

In many parts of Southeast Asia, there are food shortages in the best of times, and any strain on the food supply, whether from political factors or natural disasters, may result in famine. In East Pakistan, for example, when food production is as little as ten per cent below normal, disastrous famine ensues (6).

Such a famine occurred in 1954 and 1955. For seven years prior to this time, beginning with the partition of India and Pakistan in 1947, large-scale migrations of Moslems had created a tremendous refugee problem and placed heavy additional demands on the food supply. In 1954 and 1955, the Brahmaputra River and tributaries flooded, destroying homes and crops and disorganizing transport. This writer was in India in 1954 and observed some of the aspects of the famine which followed the flood and reached serious proportions in spite of the efforts of the Pakistan and Indian governments and outside help from the U.S. and other nations.

A recent nutrition survey of East Pakistan found that even under "normal" conditions adult males are better fed than other groups (7), while twenty-six per cent of all liveborn children in that province die before their fifth birthday. This contrasts with 2.4 per cent of European children who die before age five.

This imbalance was aggravated in the Brahmaputra famine. As in all famines, small children were affected first and overwhelmingly. They were the first to die; older children and the elderly followed. Pregnant women not infrequently aborted, lactating mothers ceased to produce milk and the babies died. In addition to the food shortage itself, disruption and chaos typical of refugee populations were aggravated as people fled the flood areas and migrated in search of food. Thus social conditions also victimized the weaker elements of the population. The primary and secondary education systems which the Pakistan government had been struggling to develop were brought to the verge of collapse (8).

A general consequence of famine is the social disruption, including panic, which accompanies it. Starving people attempt to journey to other areas where they hope to find food and chaos increases. Weakened by lack of food, they are susceptible to disease, and these factors interact with one another, disease adding to social disorganization which in turn makes disease more difficult to combat.

In Vietnam, migration has already been set in motion by military attacks on villages, or fear of such attacks, and by the destruction of agricultural lands already referred to. At Senate hearings on refugee problems in South Vietnam and Laos, Frank H. Weitzel, Acting Comptroller General of the United States, gave the number of refugees in South Vietnam in fiscal year 1965 as 600,000, six times what had been expected (9). In November an additional statement from Mr. Weitzel gave a total of 719,000 but said 258,000 were classified as resettled. At the end of 1966, *The New York Times* put the figure at a million, growing at a rate of about 70,000 a month (10). A July 3, 1967 news item states that almost 2 million refugees are now in government resettlement camps — one in every seven South Vietnamese (11).* These recently uprooted people are a different population from the 1955 refugees from North Vietnam who, according to the South Vietnamese government, are now resettled.

In 1965, refugees were almost 100 per cent women, children and older men (12), and this remains true.

Twenty-six years of almost uninterrupted war have placed strains on the food supply, especially severe in the last two years. South Vietnam, which exported 49 million metric tons of rice in 1964 (13), must now import it. Figures for 1966 are not yet available, but 240,000 tons were imported in 1965 (14).

The medical-nutritional picture in South Vietnam is typical of an underdeveloped country ravaged by war. Infant mortality is estimated at twenty-five to thirty per cent, more than ten times that of the U.S. Maternal death rate is twenty-five times that of the U.S. Life expectancy at birth is about thirty-five years. In an environment where sanitation is primitive and medical facilities are in short supply, a great additional hazard is the risk of epidemics which can grow like wildfire in a weakened, starving and migrating population.

Bubonic plague is endemic, and although only eight cases were reported in 1961, the number is said to have risen to 4500 in 1965 (5). Malaria is also endemic, and the appearance of a form of the disease which does not respond to traditionally effective drugs is a matter of grave concern. Cholera and smallpox have been habitual fellow travelers of Asian famines, with influenza and relapsing fever also frequent.

In 1965 alone the number of cases of cholera in Vietnam increased by 25,000, according to the World Health Organization (15). In that same year Dr. Howard Rusk reported that among refugees "tuberculosis is highly prevalent, as are skin infections, intestinal parasites, trachoma and other diseases of the eyes, typhoid and leprosy" (16).

## STARVATION IN PREVIOUS WARS

What has been the effect of food denial as a weapon in previous

---

*Officials of the Agency for International Development were quoted in the *St. Louis Post-Dispatch,* October 12, to the effect that the total number of refugees in South Vietman in August, 1967, was 2,008,098.

wars? Has it reduced the effectiveness of the fighting men in the blockaded nations? Has it been decisive in bringing victory to the besiegers? What has been its effect on civilians? A study of three examples from wars fought within the past hundred years goes a long way toward answering these questions.

## The Siege of Paris

Paris was under siege by the Germans for 129 days in 1870-71, during the Franco-Prussian War. One of the reasons given by the government for surrender was the lack of food within the city. However there was a desperate military situation in the rest of the country. Prior to the siege, one of the main French forces was defeated at Sedan, during the siege, the other was defeated at Metz. Thirty-six new divisions were organized and equipped from Tours, but a number of them were driven into Switzerland, where they were disarmed and interned.

According to Baldick (17), the death rate in Paris rose from 3,680 in the first week to 4,465 in the third — and presumably still higher as the siege dragged on for eighteen weeks. The winter was severe so that people suffered from cold as well as hunger; epidemics swept the city, with smallpox the biggest killer.

Melvin Kranzberg describes the effect of the food shortage on the people of Paris:

> With the exception of the dent made in their pocketbooks the rich did not suffer from famine during the siege. . . . As for the poor, the men were not badly off, but the women and children suffered. The men could get enough to eat and perhaps too much to drink merely by enlisting in the National Guard (18).

## Blockade of the Central Powers

In the early days of World War I, the western Allies were optimistic that the hunger engendered by the blockade of the Central Powers — Germany, Austria-Hungary and the smaller countries allied with them — would help win the war quickly. After the war, the importance of the blockade may have been exaggerated by German historians in order to play down military defeats; it may have been underestimated by British, French and American historians. The fact remains that it took four years of the combination of blockade and military action to defeat the Central Powers.

Famine edema, a relative increase in the water content of the body, was observed in civilians in Hamburg in the winter of 1916-17, in Berlin in January, 1917, in Vienna and the Rhineland later the same year. In 1918, it became common throughout Central Europe. Tuberculosis, which is closely related to malnutrition had been decreasing, and reached its lowest point in 1913. It began to rise in 1914 and continued to rise throughout the war. In Vienna, the mortality rate from tuberculosis rose almost 100 per cent; in Germany, 44 per cent (19).

The excess of deaths in the civilian population during each of the war years, over the number of deaths for the year 1913 totaled 762,796.

These figures represent the number of deaths which under "normal circumstances" presumably would not have happened. They were probably due to a combination of the food shortage with other factors. Medical care of civilians suffered because of the army's drain on medical personnel and facilities. There was a shortage of fuel because importation of coal was reduced by the blockade and internal distribution was disrupted by the war. Although most of the war was fought on French and Russian soil, the Austro-Hungarian Empire was invaded, with some of its villages and countryside becoming a battleground.

If the figures above are compared with deaths in the army it can be seen that civilian deaths in excess of normal may have been about half as great as the army losses. However, it must also be said that the very war conditions which cause excess civilian deaths, make reliable statistics difficult to assemble.

George A. Schreiner, an Associated Press correspondent, spent the first three years of the war in Germany and the nations allied with it, including considerable time with the armies on both eastern and western fronts. He states that many men in the army received better food than they had as pre-war civilians. He says that the army "came first in all things" and that when it became necessary to reduce the bread ration, this was made good by

| | DEATHS IN THE ARMY | | DEATHS IN THE CIVIL POPULATION |
|---|---|---|---|
| | On the battle-field and through wounds | Through sickness | Due to the Blockade |
| 1st War Year | 451,506 | 24,394 | 88,235 |
| 2nd War Year | 330,332 | 30,329 | 121,174 |
| 3rd War Year | 294,743 | 30,190 | 259,627 |
| 4th War Year | 317,954 | 38,167 | 293,760* |
| Postwar due to the War | 62,417 | 10,902 | |
| Total | 1,456,952 | 133,982 | 762,796 |

*To end of 1918

These tables are taken from an article which appeared in the *Duetsche Medizinische Wochenschrift,* Berlin, April 10, 1919, *Vol. 45,* No. 15 entitled "Von der Blockade und Aehnlichem," by Dr. Ruth M. Rubner and are reprinted from "Blockade and Sea Power," by Maurice Parmalee, Thomas Y. Crowell Co., N.Y., 1924. (Minor errors in totals corrected by S/C.)

increasing the meat and fat ration (20). Schreiner quotes a "food dictator" as saying that thousands of the aged poor were going to a premature death.

## The Siege of Leningrad

The most recent, the most lethal and yet the most completely ineffective use of starvation as a strategic weapon of war was the siege of Leningrad by the Nazis in World War II. It closed around the 3 million people of the city on September 8, 1941. For four months only 45,000 tons of food were brought by water, air and finally by the road across the ice of Lake Ladoga, and this was expected to sustain the military as well as the civilian population. Late in January, 1942, a corridor was opened which permitted both the importation of food and the evacuation of large numbers of people, but the siege was not completely lifted until two years later. By this time almost a million people — about a third of the city's population — were dead from hunger, cold, and their attendant diseases, and from the bombing and shelling of the city.

As in the previous cases, the soldiers defending the city had better rations than the civilians, although their rations, too, had to be cut on November 20, 1941 when things were at the worst (21). Hospital records for the starvation period show some of the effects on infants and pregnant mothers: an increase in stillbirth and premature birth and a rise in neonatal mortality (22).

The early and worst parts of the siege were accompanied by German victories elsewhere in the nation; German armies came within a few miles of Leningrad homes and factories where people continued to live and work. Nevertheless, the troops besieged along with the city defended it successfully and eventually broke the blockade.

While historians differ in assigning significance to these blockades as effective military techniques it is clear from all three of these examples that food denial in war affects the fighting men least and last, if at all, and is therefore unsuccessful unless accompanied by military victories by the blockaders. It is hardest on civilians, particularly children and the elderly; where economic class divisions are sharp, it is particularly hard on the poor.

## DESTROYING FOOD IN VIETNAM

The increasing use of herbicides in Vietnam suggests that the U.S. military plans to enlarge the area where food crops will be destroyed.

News stories have reported other methods being used in the food denial campaign. In areas under the political control of the Viet Cong, U.S. and South Vietnamese troops may establish temporary military control long enough for a "harvest protection" operation. This is carried out by entering the area at harvest time, holding off Viet Cong rice collectors while peasants are required to sell their surpluses to the government or to the commercial market and then withdrawing (23).

The agricultural area in the demilitarized zone and just to the south of it has been rendered completely unproductive as have special areas in the immediate proximity of Saigon (Operations Junction City and Ceder Falls in the "iron triangle"). As many as 600,000 Vietnamese have been removed from agricultural productive labor and are now residing in camps (24).

Rice that has already been harvested may be destroyed. Sometimes it is dumped into large pits and covered with shark repellent or other obnoxious compounds; attempts have been made to burn or scatter it. Captured rice has been dumped into the Rachbenggo River by U.S. troops.

According to General William W. Berg, U.S. Air Force Deputy Assistant Secretary of Defense, "Our combat units are well aware of the food shortages in South Vietnam and are not wantonly destroying captured rice whenever it can be salvaged and put to local use. However, in a fluid combat situation, available time, manpower and transportation will not always permit removal of captured goods to a safe area" (25).

Charles Mohr has reported in *The New York Times* that the troops have found rice to be "one of the most maddeningly indestructible substances on earth. Even with thermite molten-metal grenades, it virtually will not burn. The scattering of rice does not prevent its collection by patient men" (23).

These practical difficulties suggest one reason for the use of chemical sprays. Another, and perhaps the most important reason, is that it entails a more efficient use of personnel.

"What's the difference between denying the Viet Cong rice by destroying it from the air or by sending in large numbers of ground forces to prevent the enemy from getting it?" a Pentagon spokesman asked. "The end result's the same; only the first method takes far less men" (26).

Whatever method is used, the examination of past wars and famines makes it clear that the food shortage will strike first and hardest at children, the elderly, and pregnant and lactating women; last and least at adult males and least of all to soldiers.

That these conclusions apply to Vietnam as well is suggested by the Vietnamese nutrition study carried out in 1959 by Americans and South Vietnamese under the latter's Committee on Nutrition for National Defense, in which an equal number of army and civilian Vietnamese were compared (27).

"In the general sense, the nutritional status of the military is superior to that of the civilian population, without appreciable differences between Army, Navy, and Air Force," says the study. While the average civilian male weighs 104.3 pounds, his counterpart in the military weighs 113.0 pounds. And, for those who might suppose the difference results from military selection procedures favoring bigger men from the general population, the study reports:

> Inductees (Quang Trung) weighed 107 pounds on the average, the lowest weight among any of the military. A group of similar men completing their basic training (Quang Trung) has an average weight of 114 pounds, suggesting that the change from a civilian to a military diet resulted in a prompt weight gain, in spite of the strenuous activity of basic training. Considering the combined military services, continuation of such weight gain during the first year of military life was further evidenced by the weight gain from an average of 107 pounds for those in the service less than three months to an average of 118 pounds for those with six months to one year of service.

South Vietnamese army medical care is also superior to that available to civilians, as Dr. John Reed of the U.S. Public Health Service testified on his return from working with Vietnam refugees: ". . . there are only about 800 qualified physicians in the Republic of South Vietnam. Of this 800, 500 are in the military service. Of the remaining 300, approximately half, or 150, are in private practice in Saigon, so this leaves only about 150 doctors for the entire rural population in South Vietnam" (28).

This refers to the South Vietnamese government side, but on the other side, Viet Cong soldiers may likewise be expected to get the fighter's share of whatever food there is. Whether extra rations are enforced by an organized government structure or confiscated by armed bands of guerrillas, the end result is the same. Unless direct evidence to the contrary from U.S. observations in Vietnam is forthcoming, this conclusion seems unavoidable: from a military viewpoint, the attempt to starve the Viet Cong can be expected to have little or no effect. What it can be expected to do is to add to a flow of refugees already far beyond the capacity of the program designed to care for them.

The history of modern war has been one of increasing involvement of civilians. Starvation as a weapon is an aspect of such involvement, one which has the peculiar property of inflicting suffering on civilians while doing little damage to the military. To destroy crops — with herbicides or in any other way — is therefore to employ a weapon whose target is the weakest element of the civilian population.

## REFERENCES

1. Senate Committee on Foreign Relations, Subcommittee on Disarmament, "CBR Warfare and its Disarmament Aspects," Washington, D.C., 1960.
2. Donnelley, Dixon, Assistant Secretary, Dept. of State. Letter to Arthur Galston and other plant physiologists, September 28, 1966. Published in full in *BioScience,* January, 1967, p. 10.
3. Langer, Elinor. "Chemical and Biological Warfare (II): The Weapons and the Policies," *Science, 155:* 303. These numbers were supplied to *Science* in January by the Pentagon.
4. "Republic of Vietnam, Nutrition Survey, October-December, 1959," A Report by the Interdepartmental Committee on Nutrition for National Defense, July, 1960.
5. Collins, J. L., Ervin, Frank, Levi, Vicki and Savitz, David. "Medical Problems of South Vietnam," Physicians for Social Responsibility, Boston, January, 1967.
6. United Nations Commission for Asia and the Far East. "Multi-Purpose River Basin Development, Part 2B Water Resources Development in Burma, India, and Pakistan," Bangkok, December, 1956.
7. Pakistan Ministry of Health (in collaboration with the University of Dacca and the U.S. Nutrition Section, Office of International Research, National Institutes of Health). "Nutrition Survey of East Pakistan, March, 1962 – January, 1964," U.S. Department of Health, Education and Welfare, May, 1966.
8. "Pakistan 1955-1956," Pakistan Publications, Karachi, 1956.
9. Weitzel, Frank H. Testimony before Hearings of the Subcommittee to Investigate Problems Connected with Refugees and Escapees of the Committee on the Judiciary, United States Senate, Eighty-Ninth Congress, July 13-September 30, 1965. U.S. Government Printing Office, 1965.
10. *The New York Times,* October 9, 1966.
11. Arnett, Peter and Faas, Horst. "American Claims of Progress in Vietnam Disputed," *St. Louis Post-Dispatch* (AP), July 3, 1967.
12. Rusk, Howard. "Refugee Crisis in Vietnam," *The New York Times,* September 12, 1965.
13. "Statistical Yearbook, 1966," U.N., 18th Issue, New York, 1967, p. 277.
14. Faltermayer, Edmund K. "South Vietnam's Economy," *Fortune,* March, 1966, p. 228.
15. "Refugee Problems in South Vietnam," op. cit., p. 137.
16. *Ibid.,* p. 366.
17. Baldick, Robert. "The Siege of Paris," B. T. Batsfor Ltd., London, 1964.

18. Kranzberg, Melvin. "The Siege of Paris, 1870-1, A Political and Social History," Cornell University Press, Ithaca, New York, 1962.
19. Keyes, Ancel, et al. "The Biology of Human Starvation," 2 Vols., University of Minnesota Press, Minneapolis, 1950.
20. Schreiner, George A. "The Iron Ration," Harper and Bros., N.Y., 1918.
21. Werth, Alexander. "Russia at War," E. P. Dutton and Co., N.Y., 1964.
22. Antonov, A. N. "Children Born During the Siege of Leningrad," *J. Pediatrics, 30:*250-59, 1947, quoted by Keyes.
23. Mohr, Charles. "U.S. Spray Planes Destroy Rice in Viet Cong Territory," *The New York Times,* December 21, 1965.
24. ABC Broadcast, July 2, 1967.
25. Berg, Gen. William W. Letter to Senator Jacob K. Javits, May 18, 1966.
26. Welles, Benjamin. "Pentagon Backs Use of Chemicals," *The New York Times,* Sept. 21, 1966.
27. "Republic of Vietnam Nutrition Study," pp. 1, 85, 62.
28. "Refugee Problems in South Vietnam and Laos," p. 134.

*Chapter 80*

# FAMINE IN BIAFRA

D URING February a technical group which I headed returned from a mission to Biafra. We traveled with a United States Senator and with the full knowledge and encouragement of the State Department. The report of our mission was made to the President and the Secretary of State. While we spent only a short time in Biafra, the composition of our group — a nutritionist, a pediatrician and epidemiologist, a professor of agriculture, and an expert on transportation and logistics — and the fact that we all were familiar with black African problems, several of us with the area itself, allowed us to use our time most efficaciously. In addition, the Biafran government officials, physicians and experts of all types were completely cooperative, trustworthy and open. We were able to traverse the entire country and thus saw a great deal for ourselves.

What I call Biafra here is the area now administered by the government of the Republic of Biafra. This area comprises about 7,250 square miles, approximately the area of Massachusetts. It is not the original Biafran area (about 29,000 square miles) that declared its independence on May 30, 1967. For the Nigerian government, of course, there is no Biafra, only a "rebel" government and "liberated" or "reconquered" territories.

After consulting with numerous statistical and medical departments of the Biafran government and observing the present population of villages (compared with their prewar population) and the number and size of refugee camps, we estimated the present population of Biafra at between 8 and 9 million inhabitants. These represent 4.5 million original inhabitants of the present area of Biafra, approximately 5 or 6 million refugees (about 2 million from Western and Northern Nigeria who fled the

Reprinted from *Postgraduate Medicine, 45* (No. 4), April, 1969.© McGraw-Hill, Inc.

1966 pogroms there, with the rest from the three-quarters of the original Biafran area which has been occupied by Nigerian troops), minus the 1 to 2 million people who have died in the famine. This range for the mortality due to famine seems the most accurate of the figures given us. The estimate of 2 million by the International Red Cross seemed high, while the government estimate of 1 million seemed decidedly low. The estimate of 1.5 million dead tallies well with the mortality data that we were able to obtain from parish priests and ministers.

It can be noted, parenthetically, that the figure of 8.5 million for the Biafran population bears little resemblance to the figure of 3 to 3.5 million given to me repeatedly at State Department briefings and at the U.S. embassy in Nigeria. The mortality figures believed by U.S. officials were equally wide of the mark. However, before our mission, no member of any U.S. government agency — let alone any professionally trained persons — had gone to Biafra to personally assess the situation.

On the Nigerian side of the fighting front, our officials do have more or less unencumbered access to any area and are not restricted by self-imposed diplomatic limitations. The USAID measles and smallpox inoculation teams operating on the Nigerian side have arrived at figures of 800,000 refugees in camps, 200,000 "floating" in and out of camps, and 1 million refugees not in camps in areas under federal control. Adding these figures to those for Biafra gives an idea of the magnitude of the displacement of people and of the relief problem posed by the Nigeria-Biafra conflict.

The extent of the caloric and protein malnutrition and the scope of outright famine have been so overwhelming as to make the Nigeria-Biafra conflict one of the great nutritional disasters of modern times. To fully understand the situation, we must remember that before the war, Biafra was a fertile producer of such food as yams, cocoyams, cassava and palm oil, but had to import nearly 80 per cent of her protein needs. This included all the milk, much of the meat, a considerable tonnage of fish, and large amounts of beans and groundnuts (peanuts). Because of the Biafrans' industriousness, their tendency to spend a somewhat higher proportion of their income on food than did neighboring populations, and the primary attention they paid to their children's nutrition, the prevalence of kwashiorkor was much less than the local agricultural pattern would have suggested.

Some data on the diet and the prevalence of nutritional diseases in Biafra before the war are an indispensable background to full understanding of the present catastrophe. Such information is available in a number of competent surveys conducted in Biafra and Eastern Nigeria before the war. In general, it can be said that the main source of fat in the diet was palm oil, providing a good source not only of polyunsaturated fatty acids but also of carotene (provitamin A) throughout the year. The main sources of calories were high-carbohydrate foods, mostly low-protein tubers, cassava, yams and cocoyams. Smaller quantities of cereals were also available, i.e. corn (maize) and rice. Yams, cocoyams and corn are seasonal plants, but cassava grows and is available throughout the year.

As indicated, the protein supply was largely imported. Beef came from Northern Nigeria and constituted the main source of meat. To lessen this dependence on imported meat, Biafra had made great efforts to develop a poultry industry. Unfortunately, this industry, like animal husbandry generally, depended on imported animal feed and, hence, was vulnerable to the blockade as well as to the elimination of stock and competition with human needs. The vegetable proteins, beans, groundnuts and soya, came from Northern Nigeria.

Vitamins and most minerals were usually adequate in the Biafran diet during the rainy season, when leafy vegetables were available. During the dry season, vegetables have always been in short supply and the supply of vitamins (other than vitamin A) and iron correspondingly low.

The nutritional disaster has gone through several phases. From the beginning of the blockade, which antedated the war by several months, until the spring of 1968, the general nutritional level steadily deteriorated. From that time on the situation, already serious, worsened precipitously. It was characterized by outright starvation among refugees, particularly those still on the move, and kwashiorkor (acute protein deficiency in a situation where calories are less deficient or adequate) among the regular inhabitants. It is difficult to give figures, but a minimum estimate, which we checked by several means, is 500,000 deaths from August through October and as many for the rest of 1968.

Since the end of October, the nutritional situation has improved in the refugee camps due to activities of the relief agencies. In particular, the prevalence of overt kwashiorkor has decreased among the children within the past three months. However, we did not see one single child in these camps whom we would describe as being in a satisfactory state of nutrition. Kwashiorkor and marasmus were still rampant. Kwashiorkor affected not only the one-to four-year-old age group, to which it is usually confined, but also many children up to age 12, many adolescents, and even a number of adults. Signs of caloric and protein deficiency were everywhere in evidence, and we saw many smooth tongues and much anemia. However, we saw no clear-cut examples of specific vitamin deficiency even though we heard the term mentioned and almost every physician and nurse we saw requested vitamin pills. Of course, it is possible that if the diet becomes more exclusively dependent on certain staples, overt vitamin deficiencies may appear.

The situation has improved much more slowly, if it has improved at all, in the villages. Relief distribution does not reach many of them, and their populations have grown tremendously as a result of returning relatives and other refugees. Those areas which are the beneficiaries of feeding stations and kwashiorkor stations fare somewhat better, but the aid given by these stations is limited. Supplies are so short that only small amounts of high-protein foods can be distributed (e.g. in one area, 3 to 5 oz of CMS formula, a corn-soybean-dry skim milk prepack; 1 oz of powdered milk; and 1 oz of stock fish — theoretically three times a week but in fact once every 10 days). The distribution also has to be made under conditions of extreme difficulty. Distribution centers and refugee camps are bombed and strafed if any concentration of people is manifest in the daytime; thus, all mass feeding activities have to be conducted in darkness.

The nutritional problems are aggravated by the difficulties in distributing foods. Movement of supplies and medical personnel is most difficult, particularly when they are clearly labeled with Red

Crosses. The Red Cross in general gives no protection in Biafra. As hospitals, kwashiorkor centers, and other health areas marked with the Red Cross were bombed and strafed, the emblems were removed or camouflaged on the ground. Displaying the Red Cross visibly increased risks. Assembling large numbers of people (up to 8000) — many of them sick, all of them weak, most of them children, women and elderly people — in long lines in utter darkness presents obvious difficulties. These difficulties are magnified in the areas near the front, where distribution by truck is often impossible.

On both sides of the line the civilian populations are starving. The estimate of a million dead in the area of Biafra occupied by the Nigerians (an estimate given by U.S. medical personnel who are members of USAID measles-smallpox vaccination teams on the Nigerian side) shows that the kwashiorkor and starvation band extends beyond Biafra in many directions. Relief expeditions into the front area under Biafran control and incursions to help Biafrans on the other side are dangerous forays and remain at best irregular.

In general, although the nutritional situation is better now than it was last fall, I must emphasize its precariousness. The improvement is almost entirely due to the airlift. Inasmuch as the airlift is funneled into an airport which is being bombed every night, its very existence is threatened, and the amount of food it can deliver depends on the length of the bombing. In addition, the proximity of a period when food supplies are normally short, the intensification of air attacks, and military operations designed to cut roads that carry an important part of the food supply mean that the life of every Biafran child is hanging by a slender thread.

As can be expected, serious medical problems are associated with the famine. These problems, which shall be reported in detail elsewhere (and are included in our public report to the President, now in press in the *Congressional Record),* include an enormously increased mortality from essentially all infectious diseases, particularly measles, whooping cough, chickenpox and tetanus; a surge of mortality and morbidity of disaster proportions from tuberculosis; increased mortality from malaria, and widespread diarrhea and dysentery. The dysentery obviously has infectious origins, but many cases of diarrhea are essentially sequelae to protein-calorie malnutrition, including adolescent and adult kwashiorkor. Severe anemias are common, especially among children and lactating and pregnant women; in hospital populations they are the rule rather than the exception.

The Biafrans' mental health is remarkably good. The people are determined despite reverses, and pursue their occupations in as normal a way as is possible under a near-famine situation and with daily bombing of civilian targets. All the physicians we talked with reported general sleeplessness, even among children, whose schooling has had to be discontinued because of the bombing and strafing of schools. (Lately a number of primary schools have been reopened. They are held in the forest, where it is hoped the children will not be seen because of the leaf cover.)

Our mission made a number of detailed recommendations to the President regarding the needed increase in shipments of food, drugs and other urgently needed relief material to Biafra. It is our hope — and our expectation — that these recommendations will be implemented. We also made some comments and recommendations concerning the work of private and international agencies in Biafra. Many such agencies, such as UNICEF, Caritas Internationalis, churches of the three major faiths, and increasingly the International Committee of the Red Cross, have performed outstanding service to mankind in Biafra. Physicians might be interested in what we had to say, by contrast, about the World Health Organization:

> WHO — There is very little that can be said in the defense of WHO's inaction in the face of one of the great medical disasters of modern times except that so far, more through luck than through foresight or the exercise of proper medical procedures, there has not yet been any large-scale infectious disease epidemic other than a deadly epidemic of measles. The personnel of WHO should remember that they are doctors and should not let political considerations stand between them and their patients. . . . We cannot emphasize too strongly that with a population weakened by famine, with millions of refugees, many of whom are on the march, only the closest epidemiologic surveillance and control and prompt medical action can prevent the spread of one or several large-scale epidemics. So far, the Biafran government has been able to exercise border control and territorial surveillance. They may be unable to act effectively in the absence of international medical help.

## Chapter 81

# STARVATION: MISSION FOR U.N.

To the Editor:

Although no one can predict when or where the next famine due to war or to a major national catastrophe will occur, we know that we can expect at least one such famine every year. We can also expect, unfortunately, that national and international response will be generally slow and inadequate.

Hundreds of thousands of civilians, particularly small children, died in Biafra during the Nigerian civil war because we did not have an international agreement outlawing famine as an instrument of war and because we did not have an international organization which can be automatically activated in times of disaster.

The UN organizations are slow to mobilize, their budgets entirely committed in advance to "regular" projects, and their competence lies elsewhere. The national Red Crosses are linked together by only the extremely weak League of Red Crosses which has no funds and no personnel to speak of. The International Red Cross is an exclusively Swiss organization, which functions best as an intermediary between warring nations to secure humane treatment for prisoners of war and is accustomed to diplomatic rather than to relief tasks.

The Pakistani catastrophe has emphasized once again the need for the creation of an international disaster relief organization that can train officials of all nations so that an agreed procedure can be followed into which international efforts can harmoniously blend, and then go into action the minute disaster strikes with "reserve" personnel and equipment.

The creation of such an organization in advance of any

Reprinted from *The New York Times,* Friday, November 27, 1970.

catastrophe is essential not only because it has to get to work immediately, but also because political problems always arise even in situations in which the disaster is not caused by war or civil war. Governments always tend to minimize the disaster and to claim that the situation is well in hand. The opposition always tends to maximize the disaster and to claim that the government is criminally negligent in its handling of relief operations. Problems of national prestige always arise with all governments reluctant to accept visible foreign help whatever the consequences for innocent victims.

At Stockholm last August a group of nutritionists of various nations, meeting under the auspices of the Swedish Nutrition Foundation and the Swedish Foreign Office, asked the Swedish Government to sponsor action in the United Nations to outlaw starvation as a legitimate means of war and to create an international relief organization.

The Swedish Government acceded to our request and is bringing these propositions before the United Nations. The pitiful spectacle of the fumbling national and international efforts at dealing with the East Pakistani disaster should be a signal for rapid and resolute action on both these areas.

JEAN MAYER

*Chapter 82*

# TOWARD A NON-MALTHUSIAN
# POPULATION POLICY

ONE theme of this essay is that food is only one of the elements in the population problem. Admittedly, at present, it is a major factor in some parts of the world; but there are large areas where the national food supply is a minor factor and others where it is not a factor at all. Furthermore, considering the world as a whole, there is no evidence that the food situation is worsening and there is at least a likelihood that food may at some time (20 or 30 years from now) be removed altogether as a limiting factor to population. Yet, to deny that the population problem is basically one of food for survival is not to deny that there is a population problem; it is in fact to remove the appearance of a safety valve and also to reveal the problem in its generality. For were we really to starve when the population reaches a certain magic number, this in turn would cause a drastic increase in child and infant mortality, decreased fertility, and a shortening of the average life span. In other words, it would cause the increase in population to be self-limiting. If the world can continue to feed — however badly — an ever-increasing number of people, this safety valve (however unpalatable, it would be a safety valve) is missing. And if lack of food is not a component of the definition of over-population, rich countries as well as poor ones become candidates for overpopulation — now.

Another theme is that there is a strong case to be made for a stringent population policy on exactly the reverse of the basis Malthus expounded. Malthus was concerned with the steadily more widespread poverty that indefinite population growth would inevitably create. I am concerned about the areas of the globe where people are rapidly becoming richer. For rich people occupy

Reprinted from *The Columbia Forum, XII* (2):5-13, Summer, 1969.

much more space, consume more of each natural resource, disturb the ecology more, and create more land, air, water, chemical, thermal, and radioactive pollution than poor people. So it can be argued that from many viewpoints it is even more urgent to control the numbers of the rich than it is to control the numbers of the poor.

The population problem is not new, although it has recently acquired new and dangerous dimensions. In all early treatments of the subject, considerations of population policy were not closely linked to economic concerns or the availability of food. Plato, who undertook nothing less than the projection of an ideal city-state in estimating the numbers needed for the various functions of citizenship, arrived at the figure of 5,040 citizens as the desirable size, adequate to "furnish numbers for war and peace, for all contracts and dealings, including taxes and divisions of the land." In *The Republic* he described his well-known eugenics proposal for public hymeneals of licensed breeders. His preoccupation was with the quality of man and of the state; not with the availability of food and other resources. Aristotle, who was concerned with certain of the economic consequences of overpopulation, though not specifically with food, warned in *Politics* that "a neglect of an effective birth control policy is a never-failing source of poverty, which is in turn the parent of revolution and crime," and advised couples with an excessive number of children to abort succeeding pregnancies "before sense and life have begun."

Plato and Aristotle did not go unchallenged. The Pythagoreans, in particular Hippocrates, opposed abortion. The Hippocratic oath contains the pledge: "I will not give a woman an abortive remedy." Of greater subsequent importance, the Romans, particularly Cicero, disapproved of the Greek views on population. They were not so much concerned with the quality of man as with the excellence of the Empire. Rome taxed celibacy and rewarded large families. Roman ideas, incidentally, were very similar to those of Confucius and his followers, also citizens of a large and expanding empire, and equally convinced that a numerous and expanding population should be promoted by wise rulers. The economic consequences of large populations were essentially ignored by the Romans; Confucius dealt with them by enunciating the rather intriguing formula: "Let the producers be many and the consumers few."

The Hebrews and the Fathers of the Church were similarly uninterested in the economic implications of population growth. Biblical and early Christian writers can, indeed, hardly be considered to have had a population policy, though their concepts of family life and of the dignity of man are as basic now as they were milleniums ago. Children were repeatedly designated as the gifts of God, with large families particularly blessed. The prescriptions of Saint Paul were somewhat more complex: while he stated that women could merit eternal salvation through bearing children if they continued to be faithful, holy, and modest, he praised virginity as more blessed than marriage, and dedicated widowhood as preferred above remarriage. Following Saint Paul, the position of Christians in sexual relations became variegated: from strict antinomianism, believers in all possible experiences, to fanatical ascetics who believed in self-castration to remove all possibility of temptation, with the center of gravity of Christian opinion somewhere between the traditional Roman double standard (strict virtue expected from the woman, somewhat more permissive rules for the man) and the more puritanical ideal of the Stoics.

In this ethical Babel, the absence of strict theological canons made it possible for intelligent citizens of a crowded and decaying empire to discuss the possible economic and political consequences of overpopulation. In *De Anima* Tertullian wrote: "The scourges of pestilence, famine, wars, and earthquakes have come to be regarded as a blessing to crowded nations, since they served to prune away the luxuriant growth of the human race." The position of the Church against abortion hardened in the third century, when Saint Hippolytus opposed Pope Calixtus I for showing too much leniency toward the abortionists, and reiterated the Christian position that the fetus is a person and not, as in Roman law, a part of the mother. Saint Augustine, rising from a Manichaean background and a personally unhappy sexual history, defined the purpose of Christian marriage as procreation, with abstinence permissible by mutual consent. This basis of the Christian marriage, unmodified by Thomas Aquinas or the medieval theologians, unmodified by Luther (an Augustinian, very much attached to the pattern of the order) was to survive far into the twentieth century.

In spite of theologians, Tertullian was echoed 1,300 years later in Botero, a sixteenth-century Italian writer, who held that man's productive powers are inferior to his reproductive powers, which do not diminish automatically when population increases. The population of the world, then, must be constantly checked by war and epidemics, the earth already holding as many people as it can feed. From Botero onward, concepts of optimum population size became indissolubly linked to economic considerations, but to economic considerations of the lowest order. Population limitation was advocated by writers, Malthus foremost among them, who felt they could demonstrate that population will inevitably rise to the very margin of food production capacity, with misery and vice the only consequences. The examples chosen were often unfortunate in the light of hindsight: Malthus based his prediction on an examination of the United States of the late eighteenth century. On the other side, mercantilist writers and rulers once again saw an increase in population as a guarantee of ample manpower for production and for war, and as a test of good government. Through the nineteenth century the debate continued. Malthusians saw the solution of economic problems due to overpopulation in continence and in more poverty — specifically, the repeal of the poor laws. The belief in the inevitability of starvation and the desirability of a *laissez faire* policy was in no small measure responsible for governmental inaction during the Irish famine. At the other end of the spectrum, Marx and Engels opposed Malthus as a peculiarly vicious and obsolete defender of capitalism. "Over-population" was a bourgeois invention designed to justify the poverty of the working classes. Improved production and distribution, not restriction of births, was the answer. A socialistic economy could thrive under all conditions of population growth, while an economy based on scarcity and high prices required birth control to mitigate its glaring deficiencies. Oddly enough, a number of modern Catholic philosophers have held a viewpoint not very different from that of Karl Marx.

The position of many Chinese leaders at present is a

combination of orthodox Marxist anti-Malthusianism and traditional Chinese predilection for large families. Others, echoing Francis Place and the liberal socialists, advocate the availability of the means of birth control so as to permit the liberation of women and their participation in the edification of socialism (being careful meanwhile to avoid any Malthusian implication).

Since the mid-nineteenth century, three profound revolutions have been taking place: a technological revolution, which promises to accelerate food production still faster; a demographic explosion, which is also accelerating and places the problem of population in an even more dramatic context; and changes in human attitudes, for which Harlan Cleveland has coined the felicitous expression, "the revolution of rising expectations." It is the contention of this writer that nothing is more dangerous for the cause of formulating a sound population policy than to approach the problem in nineteenth-century terms. By continuing to link the need for population control to the likelihood that food supply will be increasingly limited, the elaboration of birth control programs of sufficient magnitude will be held up for many years, perhaps many generations. In contemporary terms, it may well be that the controversy between Plato and Cicero makes more sense than that between the neo-Malthusians and the neo-Marxists.

That the magnitude of the population problem has increased dramatically in recent years is well publicized. Scholars have estimated that after hundreds of thousands of years of slow growth, the population of the world reached the quarter billion mark some time around the beginning of this era. It doubled to 500 million by 1650. Two centuries later it reached the billion mark. The next doubling took 80 years, with a population of 2 billion in 1930. It would appear that the world is on its way to the next doubling, to 4 billion in 45 years, by 1975; and a population of 8 billion may well be reached within the following 30 or 35 years unless rates of growth are drastically decreased. The present growth rate would lead to a population of 500 billion by the year 2200, and give the surface of all continents a population density equal to that of Washington, D.C. at present!

This increase has been due not to an increase in birth rates, but to a decrease in death rates. Around 1700, life expectancy at birth of European populations was about 33 years, and had increased little in the previous three to four hundred years. By 1950, life expectancy in Western and Central Europe and in the United States had increased to 66-69 years, an increase of over 100 per cent. This decrease in mortality rates is no longer confined to populations of European stocks. In 1946, the death rate of the Moslem population of Algeria was higher than that of Sweden in 1775. In 1954, in spite of generalized guerilla war on its territory, the death rate of this population was lower than that of Sweden in 1875. A similar telescoping of the drop in death rates is going on all over the world.

From a demographic point of view it must be noted that a drop in the death rate, with birth rate unchanged, not only results in an increase in the rate of population growth, but also produces an acceleration in the rate of growth itself: a decline in age-specific mortality rates in ages prior to the end of the childbearing age has the same demographic effect as an increase in the birth rate. In the United States, 97 out of every 100 newborn white females reach the age of 20; 91 reach the age of 50. In Guatemala, only 70 reach the age of 20; 49 that of 50. If the death rate in Guatemala fell within the next decade to somewhere near the 1950 United States level, a not unlikely development, this alone would increase the number of women reaching the beginning of the childbearing period by 85 per cent. Because of the high proportion of young people in underdeveloped countries generally — a country like Costa Rica has twice the proportion of people under 15 that Sweden has — this drop in the death rate in the pre-childbearing period has now and will have in the next few years a gigantic effect on the birth rate. Brazil had 52 million people in 1950, 71 million in 1960, and 83 million in 1966. If present rates prevail it should have 240 million by the year 2000, or 14 times the 1900 population. With a drop in mortality in the young age groups, the increase could be even more spectacular.

The significance of the demographic trends within this country is not generally appreciated. The United States, with a population of 200 million, has at present one-sixteenth of the earth's population on one-sixteenth of the land area. Though a number of underdeveloped areas are piling up population faster, we are accumulating about 2.2 million people per year, more than any increase before 1946. The rate of growth seems unimpressive, 1.1 per cent for the year 1967 (the highest rate reached was 1.8 per cent in 1946 to 1957). If the rate prevailing over the past five years persists, the population of the United States will reach 300 million by the year 1990. What most of us have tended to ignore is that the so-called baby boom of the postwar era followed a period of depression and very low birth rates: from 1920 to 1933 the birth rate had fallen steadily from 27.7 per 1,000 in 1920 to 18.4 in 1933. The absolute decline in births was less steep, because the numerical base of women of childbearing age was still growing. When the birth rate started rising in the early forties, the increase was applied to the still large number of women born between 1916 and 1924. Since 1945, the baby boom that has been so well publicized had actually been taking place on the basis of the shrinking group of women of childbearing age born since 1924. As of 1963, the last of the undersize groups had entered the reproducing age. From 1964 (when the first girls born in the big postwar years reached the age of 18), the number of women in the childbearing age has started increasing rapidly. While in 1940 there were 32 million women 15 to 44 years of age, in 1950 34 million, and in 1960 36 million (a very slow increase), there will be 43 million in 1970 and 54 million in 1980. While the birth rate is declining (and while a better index, the age-standardized general fertility rate based upon women of childbearing age only is also declining), the sheer existence of the number of women and girls alive now means that even in the unlikely event that the fertility rate fell to the historical lows of the depression years and never departed from it, the population of the United States would still more than double in the next century. The reader will, I trust, give me credit for not minimizing the problem of total population either at home or for the world at large.

With this picture of ever-increasing numbers of people, the first reaction among a portion of the public is that we are running out of space, that the "population density" is becoming dangerously high. This concept of "population density" — number of people per unit surface — has underlain the concept of "overpopulation" in the past. It is not very useful except where the primary resources are extractive (mining) and where the most primitive types of agriculture (independent of industry for fertilizers, machines, etc., and hence essentially dependent on area) and forestry prevail. It also presupposes that there is no industry to absorb surplus manpower. It is a concept of dubious value where non-extractive industries are dominant and where trade is possible. The high density band from Boston to Washington has an area of 14,000 square miles, an aggregate population of over 30 million (or over 2,000 persons per square mile), and very limited natural resources. The median family incomes is $1,000 more than for the United States as a whole. Can this area be said to be overpopulated from a material standpoint? To those who object that this area is part of a larger and less densely populated whole, one might point to prosperous Holland, or Belgium, or even Hong Kong, which, although trade with its hinterland is very meagre (imports from mainland China represent only 17% of total imports), not only houses 3.1 million people on 398 square miles (12,700 per square mile), but has shown an unexcelled increase in national product of 7 to 10 per cent per year — a doubling of real output within 10 years. Once one argues that a certain population density should be preserved, such as density with respect to capital for example, one is dealing with a much more complex concept. From it follows the idea that some sparsely settled countries need rapid increases in population, preferably through immigration, for optimal use of resources. The mental image of population density entertained by most people is, in any case, complicated by esthetic and social considerations, and "high density" is more likely to be ascribed to Calcutta than to Paris, to Costa Rica than to Denmark.

This leads us to the second and more popular concept, that overpopulation can best be appraised with respect to food resources and that the present rate of increase in the world's population is rapidly carrying us to the brink of or to actual starvation. It is my contention that this is not happening. Furthermore, I do not consider that my belief, which I shall now endeavor to justify, makes me an "optimist" as compared to the legions of conservationists, social scientists, etc., who have embraced a Malthusian "pessimism." If anything, this view makes me even more pessimistic about our chances of limiting the world's population at an early date: famine or the threat of famine is perhaps the worst method of limitation, but it would work.

World War II was not a Malthusian check. In spite of the horrendous numbers of soldiers and civilians killed, in spite of the massive genocide perpetrated by the Nazis, food production decreased much more than population. By 1945, intake per capita was 16 per cent lower than the 1934-38 average. The creation of the Food and Agriculture Organization, a specialized United Nations Agency that was endowed during its first years with particularly articulate spokesmen, dramatized the worldwide concern over the food siutation. The difficulties inherent in getting agriculture going while industry and the means of communication were not yet rebuilt, led to a generalized feeling of pessimism. Cereals, oils, meat, dairy herds were, in succession, the objects of great attention, the conclusion being in each case that prewar levels of production and consumption were not going to be reached for years. The chaotic state of international trade accentuated shortages, which UNRRA and various emergency agreements attempted to cope with on an *ad hoc* basis. And yet very quickly the situation improved. The oil shortage vanished first; while the gigantic ground nut scheme of the British government, which was supposed to mitigate it, was taking off to a very slow start, the reappearance in the channels of trade of adequate amounts of fats and oils eliminated the motivation for the scheme itself. United States production of cereals and animal products, which had grown during the war in spite of the lack of abundant manpower and the diversion of the chemical industry to military purposes, had to be slowed down as surpluses started accumulating, and, with their appearance, the threat of a collapse of agricultural prices loomed. By 1952-53, the worldwide rate of per capita production of food had overtaken prewar rates. Since then, the average rate of increase in the production of food for the world at large has been 3 per cent per year, while the population has increased on the average 1.7 per cent. In document No. 8148, the Department of State estimates that if individual consumption levels remained at the 1955-57 level, the world at large would show by 1975 an annual surplus of 40 million tons of wheat and 70 million tons of rice. (This estimate is based on the postulate that there will be no increase in rice production in Europe and North America, and no increase in wheat production in North America.) Actually, this slight but steady gain of food production over population is part of a secular trend. E. S. and W. S. Woytinski, in their monumental *World Population and Production,* estimate that since 1850 the increase in output has been more rapid than the increase in population.

As chairman of the National Council on Hunger and Malnutrition in the United States I have been talking of these evils at home for years. I have done extensive work in malnutrition in Asia and in Africa and have just returned from a trip to Nigeria and to Biafra, where I went to study the famine and the means to alleviate it. I am, therefore, as well aware of the widespread character of malnutrition as anyone in the world. Caloric undernutrition is still found in many parts of the world, and not always as a result of war or civil disorder, earthquakes or floods, invasions of insects and other parasites, or abnormally prolonged droughts. Protein deficiency — kwashiorkor where it occurs without accompanying caloric deprivation; marasmus when both caloric and protein intakes are inadequate — is encountered in varying degrees of prevalence among the young children of most countries of Asia and Africa and in many of Central and South America. Vitamin A deficiency is perhaps underestimated as a threat to the life, and the sight, of children of most of the same areas where protein deficiency is also seen. Riboflavin deficiency, thiamine deficiency (beri-beri in its various forms), and a number of other deficiencies are still very much with us. Still, there is no evidence that the situation is getting worse. The food balance sheets on which postwar pessimism was based are imperfect instruments. As an officer of FAO, I spent considerable time attempting to gauge such unknowns as figures for waste at the retail level and within families, and that portion of the food supply that does not move within the channels of trade (food grown by the farmer for his family is very inaccurately known, particularly as regards fruits and vegetables which tend to be underestimated). The nutritional standards against which available supplies are gauged are themselves being refined. As the results of additional experimental and clinical work become available, it is realized that a number of such standards — those for protein and calcium among others — were probably unnecessarily high. Even without such reevaluation, the evolution of food balance sheets, the only instruments we have to judge the race between food and population, make it apparent that most regions do show the same slow increase of per capita supplies exhibited by the world at large. It must be recognized, of course, that many of the worst nutritional scourges of mankind have been historically due as much to ignorance and to callousness as to lack of nutrients as such. Thousands of children die of protein deficiency in areas where the proteins which would save them do in fact exist and are often consumed in sufficient amounts in the very households where infants and toddlers die for lack of them. A faulty understanding of a child's needs may be the main reason he is denied some of the food consumed by his father and older siblings. As for man's inhumanity to man and its contribution to starvation, it could be illustrated by thousands of examples: cereals being shipped from Ireland under the protection of naval guns during the famine; stocks being withheld during the Congo famine to keep prices up; crop destruction policies in South Vietnam; the food blockade of Biafra.

Certainly as far as food is concerned ours is not one world. The United States government rents 20 million acres from our farmers so that they will not grow food on them. A study made at Iowa State University a few years ago suggests that 62.5 million acres ought to be similarly retired so that surpluses will not continue to be created in relation to the present market. Australia, Canada, New Zealand, Argentina, and France have been, or are at present, involved in similar efforts to restrict production.

Nor is this idling of food production restricted to highly developed countries. A recent study estimates that Ghanaian farmers work only an average of two hours a day in the cocoa area, the wealthiest agricultural area of the country.

It is fair to say that in most areas of the world the race between food and population would be more favorable to the development of adequate nutrition if the rate of population growth was decreased. But I believe that there are no grounds for saying in 1969 that the nutritional state of the world is getting worse. It is

not. And I believe that improvement in communication, availability of surpluses in certain countries, the existence of solid
international organizations, and the gradual improvement in
international morality make large-scale famines, such as the Irish
or the Bengali famine, less likely to occur in this era — except
perhaps in Red China because of its alienation from the two
richest blocs of countries. (It appears, moreover, that the food
situation in China has improved considerably in the past two
years, making the recurrence of famine there, as in India, more
remote.)

Bad as it is, the present is no worse than the past and probably
somewhat better. But what of the future? In absolute numbers,
the increase in population is likely to accelerate for some time.
Can the food supply be kept up? My contention is that for better
or for worse it can and will.

First, let us consider conventional agriculture. FAO's figures
indicate that 3.4 billion acres are at present under cultivation. This
represents less than 11 per cent of the total land area of the world.
Some experts — Prasolov, Shantz, Zimmermann — estimate the
area that can eventually be made arable at from 13 to 17 billion
acres. Colin Clark, director of the Agricultural Economics
Research Institute of Oxford, uses the figure of 19 billion acres,
but counts double-cropped tropical lands twice. (He considers,
incidentally, that if the land were farmed as well as the Dutch
farmers work their acres today, it would support 28 billion people
on a Dutch diet; if Japanese standards of farming and nutrition
were used, this area would support 95 billion people.)

The biggest potential increase of food production does not,
however, come from the extension of the area under cultivation,
but from the increase in the use of fertilizers. The phenomenal
increase in food production in this country has actually been
performed with a reduction in acreage farmed. By pre-World War I
standards of cultivation, it took one-and-one-half acres to support
an American. If such standards prevailed today, we would need to
add at least 40 million acres to our farm area every ten years, or
the equivalent of an additional Iowa every decade. In fact, we use
fertilizers instead. One ton of nitrogen is the equivalent of 14 acres
of good farmland. The use of between two and three hundred

thousand tons of nitrogen (and corresponding amounts of other necessary elements) per decade has obviated the need to discover another Iowa. And our use of fertilizer is less intensive than it is in Japan, where it is well over twice ours, or in Western Europe. (Incidentally, in spite of its already high standards of cultivation, Japan is still increasing its agricultural production at a rate of 3% per year.) India, Africa, and most of Latin America use only an infinitesimal fraction of Japanese or Western amounts of fertilizer, or none at all. Garst has estimated that an expenditure of ten dollars an acre per year for fertilizers would alone add 50 to 100 per cent to the low yields in underdeveloped countries. Applying this investment to an area of 1.5 billion acres would be the equivalent to adding at least 750 million acres to the crop areas of these countries, the equivalent of a continent bigger than North America. It is interesting to note that this primacy of fertilizers was recognized relatively late. In this country, the recognition dates back only to World War II, and has accelerated since the Korean conflict. In Japan, it dates back to 1950 or thereabout. And the leaders of the U.S.S.R. only recently realized that a large-scale increase in fertilizer output would be easier and more rewarding than the extension of cultivation to the "virgin lands."

There are many other advances in agriculture that have yet to be applied on a large scale. The identification of necessary trace elements and their incorporation into fertilizers and feeds have opened vast areas to cultivation and husbandry in Australia and elsewhere. Selective breeding of plants and animals has permitted the development of species with superior hardiness and increased yields. In the greater part of the world such work has hardly begun. Advances in animal health and nutrition have permitted the mass production of milk and eggs in indoor conditioners on a scale that was unimaginable a few years ago. The city of Los Angeles, for instance, is now an important and efficient dairy area. In some large installations, computers programmed to calculate the cheapest method of providing a diet of known energy and known content in 10 essential amino acids, total protein, and other nutrients, automatically set the controls that will mix basic staples providing the cheapest adequate poultry diet as they are informed of the latest commodity prices. Herbicides increase yields;

pesticides prevent losses from rodents, insects, and fungi. In many underdeveloped countries one quarter of the crop is lost before it reaches the consumer. Certain methods of preservation of foods by radiation have just been approved by the Food and Drug Administration. The control of weather by seeding clouds for rain; speeding cloud formation by heating lakes by atomic energy; the desalinization of brackish water by various methods, are entering the realm of practical feasibility.

Powerful though these methods of "classical" agriculture are, I believe that they will, within the lifetime of most present inhabitants of this planet, be left far behind as methods of food production. The general public is still unaware of some new developments, their promise, and the extent of the means likely to be expended in the next decade in bringing the results of research to practical application. Large-scale manufacture of food from petrochemicals started during World War II, when the Germans manufactured synthetic fats to feed forced labor groups. These fats did not conform to desirable standards of taste or safety (they contained a high proportion of branched-chain fatty acids not normally found in nature and probably not fully metabolized, and retained a petroleum-like odor). After the war, interest in "synthetic" fats persisted for a while during the years when it appeared that a shortage of natural fats was likely to be protracted. During the fifties, little or no work was done in this field, but recently some of the larger international oil companies have again become actively interested, and pilot plants are now in operation. Fatty acids, triglycerides (the constituents of our common oils and fats), and fully metabolizable simpler compounds, such as 1,3-butanediol, may soon be manufactured at very low cost for human food and animal feeds. While the promise of abundant and cheap atomic power, widely heralded for the morrow in the more immediate postwar period, has shown itself slow to be realized, it is coming, and it may well be that oil will be increasingly a raw material for food and plastics rather than a fuel.

As a potential source of food production, photosynthesis can be used much more efficiently in algae than in higher plants. With proper mineral fertilization and with the proper rate of removal of the finished products, one square meter may serve to support algae production sufficient to feed one man. And a large proportion of the calories produced — as much as one-half — are derived from protein; vitamins are also produced into the bargain. Several universities are working with a number of species, *Chlorella* in particular, and large industrial firms are yearly becoming more interested. The problems entailed in passing from the theoretically feasible to the economically feasible are formidable, but their solution is likely to be hastened for an unexpected reason. Interplanetary travel of long duration and the organization of distant stations require not only recycling of oxygen and waste water; they necessitate the fabrication of food and its integration into the recycling of oxygen, water, and excreta. Over the next two decades, an increasing fraction of the several billion dollars that the United States and the Soviet Union will spend every year for space travel is going to be channeled into life support systems. The money spent in the aggregate on new methods of food production will probably, during that period, dwarf the cost of the Manhattan Project. In many ways, we may have in space exploration what William James called "the moral equivalent of war." We will probably also have in it the technological equivalent of war, without the corresponding losses in men and in resources. The usable "fall-out" of such research is likely to be enormous. Certainly if economical harnessing of photosynthesis, through biological units or directly, can be realized under the hostile interplanetary, lunar, or martial conditions, it should become relatively easy to put it into effect on earth. All this is no longer science fiction. It is as much of a reality as the federal income tax. Obviously, a breakthrough in this field could for centuries altogether remove food as a limiting factor to population growth.

I hope I have said enough to show how dangerous it may turn out to be to link the population problem so closely to food, as so many writers have done. These have generally been conservationists and social scientists rather than agricultural or nutritional scientists, concerned — rightly — with the effects of crowding which they had observed. At the same time, not sure that the public and governments would agree with them that there was cause for concern, and action, based on these grounds, they have turned to the threat of a worldwide shortage of food as an easily understood, imperative reason for a large-scale limitation of births. Had they consulted nutritionists, agriculturists, and chemists, they might have chosen a more appropriate battleground. For if we can feed an ever-increasing number of people — even if we feed them as badly as many of our contemporaries are fed — their argument fails. And yet there is a need for the establishment as soon as possible of a sound population policy for the world at large.

There is, of course, another good reason for not tying population control to food: this tie eliminates from contention rich countries, and in particular surplus countries such as ours. Our population is increasing faster than it ever has; our major nutrition problem is overweight, our major agricultural problem is our ever-mounting excess production. Does anyone seriously believe this means that we have no population problem? Our housing problems; our traffic problem; the insufficiency of the number of our hospitals, of community recreation facilities; our pollution problems, are all facets of our population problem. I may add that in this country we compound the population problem by the migratory habits of our people: from rural farm areas to urban areas and especially to "metropolitan" areas (212 such areas now have 84% of our population); from low income areas to high income areas; from the East and Midwest to the South and Southwest; from all areas to the Pacific Coast; from the centers of cities to suburbs, which soon form gigantic conurbations, with circumstances everywhere pushing our Negroes into the deteriorating centers of large cities. All this has occurred without any master plan, and with public services continually lagging behind both growth and migrations.

Let us conclude with one specific example: 4 million students were enrolled in U.S. colleges and graduate schools in 1960, 6 million in 1965. The Bureau of the Census estimates that 8 million will seek admission or continued enrollment in 1970, 10 in 1975, 12 in 1980. No one questions our ability to feed these youngsters. But are we as a nation at all prepared for a near doubling of the size of our colleges and universities in 11 years?

Let us examine the other argument, that in certain ways the rich countries are more immediately threatened by over-population. A corollary of this is that the earth as an economic system has more to fear from the rich than from the poor, even if one forgets for a moment the threat of atomic or chemical warfare.

Consider some data from our own country. We have already said that "crowding" is certainly one of the pictures we have in mind when we think of overpopulation. The increased crowding of our cities and our conurbations has been referred to, but what of the great outdoors? In 1930 the number of visitor-days at our national parks was of the order of 3 million (for a population of 122 million); by 1950 it was 33 million (for a population of 151 million); by 1960 it was 79 million (for a population of 179 million); by 1967, 140 million (for a population of 200 million). State parks tell the same story: a rise in visitor-days from 114 million in 1950 to 179 million in 1960, an increase in attendance of over 125 per cent for a rise in population of less than 20 per cent! Clearly, the increase in disposable income (and hence in means of transportation and in leisure) becomes a much more important factor in crowding and lack of privacy than the rise in population.

Not only does the countryside become more rapidly crowded when its inhabitants are rich, it also becomes rapidly uglier. With increasing income, people stop drinking water as such: as a result we spread 48 billion (rust proof) cans and 26 billion (nondegradable) bottles over our landscape every year. We produce 800 million pounds of trash a day, a great deal of which ends up in our fields, our parks, and our forests. Only one-third of the billion pounds of paper we use every year is reclaimed. Nine million cars, trucks, and buses are abandoned every year, and while many of them are used as scrap, a large though undetermined number are left to disintegrate slowly in backyards, in fields and woods, and on the sides of highways. The 8 billion pounds of plastics we use every year are nondegradable materials. And many of our states are threatened with an even more pressing shortage of water, not because of an increased consumption of drinking fluid by the increasing population, but because people are getting richer and using more water for air-conditioning, swimming pools, and vastly expanded metal and chemical industries.

That the air is getting crowded much more rapidly than the

population is increasing is again an illustration that increase in the disposable income is perhaps more closely related to our own view of "overpopulation" than is the population itself. From 1940 to 1967 the number of miles flown has gone from 264 million to 3,334 billion (and the fuel consumed from 22 to 512 million gallons). The very air waves are crowded: the increase in citizen-licensees from 126 thousand to 848 thousand in the brief 1960-67 interval is again an excellent demonstration of the very secondary role of the population increase in the new overpopulation. I believe that as the disposable income rises throughout the world in general, the population pressure due to riches will become as apparent as that due to poverty.

I trust that I have demonstrated how dangerous it is to link constantly in the mind of the public the concept of overpopulation with that of undernutrition. I believe that it is dangerous to link it necessarily with poverty. It is absurd on the basis of any criterion of history, economics, or esthetics. Some countries are poor and densely populated. A few countries are poor and so sparsely populated that economic development (e.g. road building, creation of markets) becomes very difficult. It is easy to demonstrate that a couple with many children will be unable to save and invest. It is perhaps also true that, as the comparison to nineteenth-century France, England, and Germany suggests, at a certain stage of development, too low a birth rate (as in France then) decreases the ambition and labor of part of the population so that the savings expected from the decreased birth rate never materialize. (Losing wars because of a smaller population and having to pay a heavy tribute, as happened to the French at the conclusion of 1870-71 war, also nullified this advantage). The fact is that we are not yet in one world and that while in general it is true that population increases make improvement in nutrition and in delivery of social services more difficult, the relation of changes in wealth to changes in population has to be examined in each area on its own merits.

We have seen, furthermore, that there is more to the problem of population than the decrease in income consequent to overpopulation. We have seen that the increase in disposable income creates a population problem that is becoming every day more acute. The ecology of the earth — its streams, woods, animals — can accommodate itself better to a rising poor population than to a rising rich population. Indeed, to save the ecology the population will have to decrease as the disposable income increases. If we believe, like Plato and Aristotle, in trying for excellence rather than in rejoicing in numbers, we need a population policy now, for the rich as well as the poor. Excellent human beings will not be produced without abundance of cultural as well as material resources and, I believe, without sufficient space. We are likely to run out of certain metals before we run out of food; of paper before we run out of metals. And we are running out of clear streams, pure air, and the familiar sights of Nature while we still have the so-called "essentials" of life. Shall we continue to base the need for a population policy on a nutritional disaster to occur at some hypothetical date, when it is clear that the problem is here, now, for us as well as for others? Shall we continue to hide the fact that a rational policy may entail in many countries not only a plateauing of the population to permit an increase in disposable income, but a decrease of the population as the disposable income rises?